# TRADITIONAL AND ALTERNATIVE MEDICINE
## Research and Policy Perspectives

# TRADITIONAL AND ALTERNATIVE MEDICINE
## Research and Policy Perspectives

*— Editors —*
**Tuley De Silva**
**Theeshan Bahorun**
**Manoranjan Sahu**
**Le Mai Huong**

CENTRE FOR SCIENCE & TECHNOLOGY OF THE NON-ALIGNED AND OTHER DEVELOPING COUNTRIES (NAM S&T CENTRE)

2009
DAYA PUBLISHING HOUSE
Delhi - 110 035

ISBN 81-7035-614-8
ISBN 978-81-7035-614-1



**Centre for Science and Technology of the Non-Aligned and Other Developing Countries (NAM S&T Centre)**
Core-6A, 2nd Floor, India Habitat Centre, Lodhi Road,
New Delhi-110 003 (India)
Phone: +91-11-24644974, 24645134, Fax: +91-11-24644973
E-mail: namstct@gmail.com
Website: www.namstct.org

*Published by* : **Daya Publishing House**
1123/74, Deva Ram Park, Tri Nagar, Delhi - 110 035
Phone: 27383999, Fax: (011) 23260116
e-mail: dayabooks@vsnl.com
website: www.dayabooks.com
*Showroom* : 4760-61/23, Ansari Road, Darya Ganj
New Delhi - 110 002
Phone: 23245578, 23244987

*Laser Typesetting* : **Classic Computer Services**
Delhi - 110 035

*Printed at* : **Chawla Offset Printers**
Delhi - 110 052

Printed in India

# Foreword

This publication which contains the proceedings of the international workshop on Herbal Medicinal Plants and Traditional Herbal Remedies is a timely one because of the growing interest in herbal medicine. It has been thoughtful on the part of the NAM S&T Centre, New Delhi and the Institute of Natural Products Chemistry, Vietnam to have organized jointly this important workshop.

It is now clear that to achieve the goal of "Health for All" we have to promote a blend of tradition medicine and modern drugs. Unfortunately much of the knowledge on traditional medicine is getting lost and we can ill afford to remain silent spectators of genetic erosion among medicinal plants. Both dying wisdom and vanishing crops must be saved. This is why the World Health Organisation gave the slogan "save medicinal plants to save lives".

The Herbal Drug Industry is growing. Unfortunately in many cases, there is an expansion in the manufacture of drugs without concurrent efforts in improving the production of the needed medicinal plants. This leads to many of the important medicinal plants getting included in the Red Data books of conservation organizations. Immediate steps are needed to achieve a paradigm shift in raw material supply to drug companies, from collection to cultivation. This volume contains many useful papers written by leading authorities on the subject. I hope that this kind of interaction will foster greater south-south collaboration in the area of conservation, sustainable use and equitable sharing of benefits from the herbal wealth of developing nations. We owe a deep debt of gratitude to Dr. P. Pushpangadan, for this labour of love.

**Prof. (Dr.) M.S. Swaminathan**
*Member of Parliament and*
*Chairman, M.S. Swaminathan Research Foundation*
*(MSSRF), Chennai, India*

# Preface

Plant resources have provided the basic needs of life such as food, feed, fibre, fuel and shelter and will continue to provide these needs and much more on a renewable basis. Plants have also been a valuable source of flavours, fragrances, colourants, and phytochemicals for industries and pharmaceuticals. The rising incidence of health related problems in both developing and developed countries has prompted research in the development of drugs from leads identified from traditional medical uses as an alternative approach to manage new deadly diseases and those that have become resistant to available drugs. There is also a resurgence of interest on plant based medicines due to the undue side effects of modern therapeutic agents and their inability to cure diseases, many of them being for the treatment of symptoms. Herbal healthcare products could also help in uplifting the quality of life of the ageing populations.

On the policy perspective, the World Health Organisation has initiated global efforts to urge governments to take steps to upgrade the traditional medical systems and treatments of their respective countries through validation of their quality, safety and efficacy. Guidelines have been developed by the WHO on standardisation, quality control and analysis of herbal medicinal products. These initiatives have sparked considerable interest in the international health-related scientific community to re-evaluate traditional therapies based predominantly on the use of medicinal plants. Presently, research on the untapped plant resources and leads from traditional uses that would hopefully identify useful bioactive compounds/extracts with therapeutic relevance is being extensively carried out by scientists in developed and developing countries. Additionally the role of plant based products as dietary/health supplements, nutraceuticals, cosmecuticals and personal care products are being investigated and many countries have recognised the need for such products. It is clear from the high number of ongoing and completed studies in this research area that plant derived pharmaceuticals and healthcare products can meaningfully contribute towards the management of the biochemical and physiological functions of a wide range of disorders. However in many cases, the issue of mechanism of action and pharmacodynamics is a major concern and it is necessary to conduct research extensively focused on molecular level activities and clinical trials that will contribute to our understanding of the efficacy and safety of many extracts with therapeutic potential.

There are clear trends that the mainstream pharmaceutical research is moving away from single molecule or single target approach to combinations and multiple target approaches. Plant extracts containing several multiple pharmacological compounds have been reported to act on multiple molecular and cellular targets and such approach is gaining support in the development of drug combinations / extracts to fight diseases. There is growing evidence in support of the potential uses of medicinal plant derivatives and extracts as healthcare products that reduce the visits to physicians for minor ailments and as immunostimulants, anti-ageing products and rejuvenative agents that contribute to quality of life of the elderly.

The focus of this book "Traditional and Alternative Medicine: Research and Policy Perspectives" prominently encompasses the importance of traditional medicine in our modern health systems and discusses the potential applications of phytochemicals to assist biomolecular mechanisms and hence offer realistic and therapeutic possibilities. It includes review papers on production strategies, projection trends, regulatory status and IPR issues. Further reports are centred on the characterization and isolation of useful medicinal plant phytochemicals, clinical and bioactivity studies comprising antifungal, anticancer, antioxidant, enzyme inhibitory, hepato-protective and acetylcholinesterase assays amongst others. Finally, a series of comprehensive country reports provide an evaluation of the use of traditional heath care systems and related research output in Nigeria, Turkey, India, Laos, Vietnam, Mauritius, Myanmar, Nepal, South Africa, Indonesia, Brunei, Bhutan, Sri Lanka and Mongolia.

It was with this background that the NAM S&T Centre organised the International Workshop on Herbal Medicinal Plants and Traditional Herb Remedies in September 2007 in Hanoi, Vietnam. NAM S&T Centre continues to promote the fullest possible and mutually beneficial collaboration among scientists and technologists and scientific organizations from non-aligned and other developing countries. This book is reflective of the dedication of NAM S&T Centre to such a venture. We hope that this timely publication will contribute to an understanding of the status of research, policies and regulatory status of medicinal plants and their products in developing countries.

**Tuley De Silva**

**Theeshan Bahorun**

**Manoranjan Sahu**

**Le Mai Huong**

# Introduction

Herbs and traditional medicines are being extensively used for healthcare in almost all the countries since times immemorial. Ancient religious texts are replete with references on the use of natural products with medicinal properties. Because of local beliefs and practices and also from cost considerations herbal medicines remain a popular mode of treatment in the developing countries. Even in the industrialised society the rising cost of prescription drugs and ensuing side effects of the treatment make it highly attractive to use the traditional medicine particularly for minor ailments.

Modern system of medicine is based on sound experimental data, toxicity studies and human clinical studies, but in case of herbal medicine, on the contrary, the pharmacopoeia on herbal products is usually not available, standardization and quality control parameters for the raw material as well as finished products are virtually non-existent, and herbal industry lacks good manufacturing practices. Even the barest minimum standards of the medicinal plant products are not maintained or regulated and the quality of finished herbal products is often not monitored or is not up to the mark.

In addition, even though almost all the developing countries, specifically those sitting in the tropical belt, are a rich and abundant source of flora and phytopharmaceuticals, many medicinal plants are either getting scarce or are on the verge of extinction resulting into genetic erosion due to a huge public demand and also because a large number of modern drugs are extracted and developed from the plants. If this trend continues, the human race will lose some of the most important sources of future drugs, which will be lost by the mankind forever.

As such, there is an urgent need for the developing countries to take a fresh look at the status of medicinal plants, take up sustainable harvesting by balancing the commercial demand with the conservation of the valuable plants and their contribution to biodiversity and initiate extensive activity for the preservation of germplasm. In addition, they should develop their own technologies for processing of the crude drugs and export only finished products to the developed countries. Also to meet the increasing demand of raw materials for herbal medicines, the important medicinal plant species should be grown in fields based on advanced agricultural technologies instead of collecting the same from wild sources. The developing countries should strengthen their R&D efforts especially in the area of cultivation (which include agronomical techniques), use of modern tools of genetics and plant breeding, plant biotechnology, natural product chemistry, pharmacology and chemical engineering. If properly exploited with the modern tools of science, the developing countries can considerably increase their foreign exchange from export of products from medicinal plants and can also provide modern healthcare to the entire section of the vast rural population of their own countries. Finally, it is evident that if these herbal medicines have to reach a global market, adequate quality assurance is a dire necessity so that the consumers are assured that the herbal medicines do not contain toxic ingredients or such items that may have therapeutic action different from the claim made for the particular drug.

The Centre for Science and Technology of the Non-Aligned and Other Developing Countries (NAM S&T Centre) had organised an international workshop on 'Herbal Medicinal Plants and Traditional Herb Remedies' during 20-21 September 2007 at Hanoi in Vietnam jointly with the Institute of Natural Products Chemistry (INPC) of Vietnam and with the support of the Vietnamese Ministry of Science and Technology (MOST) and Academy of Science and Technology (VAST). I may also mention that considering the importance of medicinal plants, herbal and traditional medicines, natural products and related subjects for healthcare and economy in the developing countries, the NAM S&T Centre has identified this topic as a priority area for undertaking its scientific activities. In the past, the Centre had organized two international workshops, *viz.* 'Medicinal Plants: Strategies for Development of Herbal Drugs in the Third World Countries' at New Delhi, India in October 2002 and 'Herbal Medicine, Phytopharmaceuticals and Other Natural Products: Trends and Advances' at Colombo, Sri Lanka in June 2005 as well as an international training course on 'Natural Products–Drugs, Pharmaceuticals and Neutraceuticals for the Benefit of Mankind' at Karachi, Pakistan in February 2006. Consequently, the Hanoi workshop is the fourth activity of the Centre in the series. The Centre has also been executing a Fellowship scheme on Natural Products since the year 2006 in association with the International Centre for Chemical and Biological Sciences (ICCBS) at the HEJ Research Institute of Chemistry in Karachi, Pakistan through which the scientists from developing countries find opportunity to affiliate themselves with this Centre of Excellence and carry out their short term research work jointly/under the guidance of ICCBS experts.

Hanoi Workshop was spread over seven technical sessions beside the inaugural session. The overall technical programme of the workshop was coordinated by Dr. Le Mai Huong, Deputy Director, INPC and was attended by 34 senior foreign experts and specialists from 19 countries. Besides ten participants from India, the overseas participants included one each from Bangladesh, Bhutan, Egypt, Indonesia, Lao PDR, Mauritius, Myanmar, Nepal, Nigeria, Tanzania, Turkey; two from Brunei Darussalam, Germany, Italy, Republic of Korea, Sri Lanka, and three from Mongolia.

Moreover, 100 scientists from the host country Vietnam included the Heads and senior experts from the Institutes of Natural Products Chemistry, Chemistry, Ecology and Biological Resources, and Biotechnology and Department of Planning and Finance of VAST; Military Academy of Medicine; Academy of Traditional Medicine Pharmacy; National Institute of Malaginology, Parasitology and Entomology; Institute of Medicinal Materials; National University of Hanoi and Universities of Vinh and Tay Bac, and Animal Biotechnology Company.

The co-chairpersons of the respective sessions of the Workshop were Prof. Choudhury M. Hasan (Bangladesh) and Prof. Dr. Pham Quoc Long (Vietnam); Prof. Bounhong Southavong (Lao PDR) and Prof. Dr. Tran Van Sung (Vietnam); Prof. P. Pushpangadan (India) and Prof. Dr. Le Khanh Thuan (Vietnam); Dr. Mandsiakhan Zeveg (Mongolia) and Prof. Young Ho Kim (Republic of Korea); Prof. Dr. K. Husnu Can Baser (Turkey) + Dr. Le Mai Huong (Vietnam); Prof. Tuley De Silva (Sri Lanka) and Prof. Dr. Martin Hofrichter (Germany); and Prof. Manoranjan Sahu (India) and Prof. Dr. Nguyen Van Hung (Vietnam).

Plenary lectures in the Workshop were delivered by Dr. Le Mai Huong, Prof. Tuley De Silva, Dr. P. Pushpangadan, Prof. Choudhury M. Hasan, Dr. K. Husnu Can Baser, Prof. Dr. Martin Hofrichter, Dr. (Mrs.) S. N. Khan, and Dr. Emmanuel Orgah.The participants from Vietnam, who made scientific presentation during the workshop, were Prof. Dr. Phan Tong Son, Prof. Dr. Nguyen Van Hung, and Dr. Le Viet Dung. Among the overseas speakers presentations were given by Dr. P. Wangchuk, Dr. C. Regami, Dr. Mona H. Hetta, Dr. O.P. Singh, Prof. T. Bahorun, Dr. Soe Soe Win, Prof. M. H. A. Tissera, Dr. E. Innocent, Dr. Lancelot D'Cruz SJ, Prof. B. Southavong, Dr. C. Rajasekaran, Dr. Mridula Singh, Prof. Won Keun Oh, Dr. N. Pg Haji M. Kifli, Dr. B. D. Gupta, Dr. M. Sahu, Prof. Dr. M. Hofrichter, Dr. K. H. C. Baser, Dr. M. Sahu, Mr. Tariq Ahmad Butt and Dr. Ariyamuthu Sarswathy, Dr. Chua Kui Hong, Mrs. Adriana M. Lubis, Mr. Mandsiakhan Zeveg and Dr. Emmanuel Orgah presented the respective country reports on Herbs and Herbal Medicine in Brunei Darussalam, Indonesia, Mongolia and Nigeria.

The present publication comprises a compilation of 58 scientific articles and review papers. I would like to express gratitude to Prof. Dr. Chau Van Minh, Vice President of Vietnamese Academy of Science and Technology and Director of the Institute of Natural Products Chemistry; Prof. Phan Van Quy, Vice President of Vietnamese Academy of Science and Technology; Dr. Thai Van Tan, Deputy Director General (ICD), Ministry of Science and Technology of Vietnam and Dr. Le Mai Huong, Deputy Director, Institute of Natural Products Chemistry for support in their respective capacities that culminated in successful conclusion of the Hanoi workshop. I would also like to acknowledge the dynamic involvement and untiring efforts of Prof. Tuley De Silva, Prof. Theeshan Bahorun, Dr. Le Mai Huong and Dr. Manoranjan Sahu for technical editing of this publication, supplying the 'Preface' and for suggesting future course of action while reviewing the contents. I am indebted to Prof. M.S. Swaminathan, Member of the Indian Parliament and Chairman, M.S. Swaminathan Research Foundation (MSSRF), Chennai for sparing his valuable time in writing the 'Foreword'. My grateful thanks are also due to the Institute of Natural Products Chemistry (INPC) of Hanoi, Vietnam for providing generous financial support to bring out this publication. Last, but not the least, the valuable services provided by the entire team of the NAM S&T Centre, particularly by Mr. M. Bandyopadhyay, Dr. V.P. Kharbanda, Mr. Gaurav Gaur and Mr. Pankaj Buttan in compiling the presented papers and giving a shape to this volume are deeply appreciated.

I hope that this publication will serve as a valuable reference material for the entire community of the herbal medicine researchers, experts and practitioners and those particularly from the developing countries will find it useful in working out appropriate plans and programmes on increasing the importance of herbal medicine in healthcare.

**Arun P. Kulshreshtha**

*Director, NAM S&T Centre*

# Contents

## Part II: Phytochemistry

## Part III: Clinical and Bioactivity Studies

## Part IV: Country Reports

*Part I*

# Review Papers

# Part I

# Review Papers

# Chapter 1

# Herbal Medicines: From Research to the Production Line

***Emmanuel A. Orgah***

*Nigeria Natural Medicine Development Agency, Lagos, Nigeria*

*E-mail: emmaorgah@yahoo.com*

## ABSTRACT

In most developing countries, herbal medicines are produced using age-old methods, which affect their quality, stability and efficacy. The possibilities for value addition, processing and product improvement, and technical assistance for the industrial utilization of plant based medicines exists and remains a priority in the 21st century as over 80 per cent of people in these countries depend almost entirely on traditional medicines. This paper discusses the disadvantages of the traditional paradigm in the processing of herbal materials, the opportunities provided by natural product research for value addition and the need for qualitative industrial production of herbal medicines such that the efficacy and stability would be assured in order that herbal medicines may compete favourably in the global market.

***Keywords:*** *Herbal medicines, Quality management, Standardisation, Efficacy, Value addition.*

## 1.0 Introduction

Research in chemistry and bioactive components of indigenous flora of developing countries has been ongoing for many decades. Prior to the age of science, traditional medicine research was carried out at the level of traditional knowledge holders through precise observation and human experimentation by testing medicinal plant preparations on themselves after a process of identification, preparations and removal of toxins, modifications, correlation of dosages with specific types of illnesses, etc. As the following sequence will indicate, their research revealed which plants and what parts to eat as medicines, the optimal conditions for harvesting them and established a background for modern science to develop new drugs.

We have to go back in history to the time of the great Pharaoh herbalist Imhotep to find the real medicinal plants used at that time and to the surviving papyrus texts such as those of Edwin Smith and Eber, which documented nearly 1000 different substances and formulations (Cannell, 1998a,b). Egyptians have been found to document uses of various herbs in 1500 B.C. (Cragg 2001a, b; Holt 2002). Amazingly, they had no knowledge of the art of distillation, but relied on the techniques of enflourage, decoction, concoction, alcoholic extraction and cold expression. Many of the excellent extraction methods and brewing techniques found their origin in ancient Egypt and the wall paintings are full of the methods for purifying honey and fermenting grapes.

Theophrastus, a philosopher and natural scientist in approximately 300 B.C, wrote a *History of Plants* in which he addressed the medicinal qualities of herbs and the ability to cultivate them. The Greek botanist Pedanious Dioscorides, who was the physician to the Roman army, in approximately A.D. 100, produced a work entitled *De Materia Medica*, which today is still a very well known European document on the use of herbs in medicine. Galen, (A.D. 130–200), practiced and taught pharmacy and medicine in Rome and published over two-dozen books on his areas of interest. Galen is remembered in the term galenical and for his contribution to pharmaceutical science. Monks in the middle ages (fifth to the twelfth centuries) copied manuscripts about herbs and their uses (Cragg 2001a, b; Holt 2002). The 15th century herbalist Paracelsus (Theophrastus Bombastus von Hohenheim), seems to have been overlooked by the marketers and yet his theory on the Doctrine of Signatures is an ideal concept for the industry and over the centuries many of his theories have come to light and surprisingly have been found to work in many cases.

For Africa, a continent that is particularly dependent on herbal medicine, a collaboration of medicinal plant scientists from 14 countries established a pan-African pharmacopoeia–a database of plants with medicinal properties in 2006. The pan-African pharmacopoeia contains detailed profiles of 23 plants, including devil's claw, which is used to treat rheumatism; red stinkwood, whose bark provides an ingredient for prostate-cancer drugs; and African ginger, which is good for relieving headaches–The Economist Oct 5th (2006).

The pooling of knowledge has not only expanded our understanding of more plant species, but also revealed the way in which specific classes of plant molecule behave biochemically. However, despite the acknowledged importance of herbal medicines/medicinal plants to both the global economy and local household economies, their use is generally poorly organized and most are still processed using age-old techniques with little or no regard to quality control and Good Manufacturing Practices (GMP)

## 1.1 Research Evidence and Proof of Efficacy of TM

The pharmaceutical industry has its roots in the ancient art of herbalism. The first commercial pure natural product introduced for therapeutic use is generally considered to be the narcotic morphine, marketed by Merck in 1826, Newman (2000).

The first synthetic blockbuster drugs, Bayer's aspirin and heroin, introduced in 1899, were minor modifications of molecules extracted from, willow bark and poppy seed-pods respectively (The Economist 2006).

Herbal medicine has benefited tremendously from scientific research, as there are indications from literature that new drug development based on leads from traditional medicine has worked. This is not surprising because herbal medicine is guided by a long history of traditional clinical practice.

To give some examples:

- The anti-sickling agent NICOSAN™/HEMOXIN™ developed by the Nigerian National Institute of Pharmaceutical Research and Development (NIPRD) is a non–toxic, phytopharmaceutical product composed of extracts from four Nigerian plants, seeds, stems, fruits and leaves used in Nigerian traditional medicine as haematinics. Each plant is indispensable in the manufacturing of NICOSAN™/HEMOXIN™–a clear demonstration of synergy. Xechem Pharmaceuticals Nigeria Limited has developed refined and standardized small–scale formulations of NICOSAN™/HEMOXIN™ for consistent production in strict compliance with the recommended procedures and policies of the WHO.
- The bark of the African tree Pygeum (*Prunus africana*), harvested from wild trees growing in the mountain forests of Africa and Madagascar, is a very popular natural remedy for prostate disorders in some European countries such as Spain (*Prunus africana* factheet)
- Reserpine, extracted from the root of the Serpent-Root, *Rauvolfia serpentina*, a common plant in Nigeria is used for lowering blood pressure and as a tranquilliser.
- Rose periwinkle (*Catharanthus roseus)*, endemic to Madagascar, is widely cultivated for its alkaloids, vinblastine and vincristine, which are used for treating childhood leukaemia and Hodgkin's disease (Balick, 1996).
- The bark of the yohimbe, (*Pausinystalia johimbe)*, is used extensively in traditional health care systems in West Africa. It has become popular in Europe and the US for treating impotence, particularly before Viagra became widely available. Under US law, yohimbe is regulated as a dietary supplement, and yohimbine hydrochloride is an FDA-approved pharmaceutical drug for impotence. (Tyler, 1999).
- A local pharmaceutical firm in *South Africa* has standardised into tablets an herbal preparation, Sunderlandia® that is used as a tonic for diseases associated with significant loss of body mass. (AACHRD, 2002).
- NIPRD in *Nigeria* has reported two of the many herbal preparations that TMPs claim to be effective for the management of HIV/AIDS: Dopravil® and Conavil® on which phase II clinical trials are being conducted. (AACHRD, 2002).
- Research on evaluation of herbal preparations for the management of HIV/AIDS in some countries such as Burkina Faso, has reported a weight gain of up to 20 kilograms in some patients within four months of treatment.

Blood tests to monitor the level of immunity (CD4 and CD8 counts) of patients, has shown a marked increase in blood cell counts. (AACHRD, 2002).

- In *Tanzania, Warburgia* species are used effectively for the treatment of people living with HIV/AIDS (PLWA). (AACHRD, 2002).
- *Huperzia selago* (Fir Clubmoss) was traditionally used in traditional Chinese medicine. Huperzine A, an alkaloid isolated from leaves of the Chinese *Huperzia* species, is currently one of the most promising drugs for testing memory and learning loss in Alzheimer's patients and has been recently patented by the Chinese (Borman, 1993). Clinical trials in the US indicate that huperzine is considerably less toxic and more effective than tacrine, one of the few drugs currently approved by the FDA for Alzheimer's.
- Devil's Claw is an herbal therapy used commonly for rheumatism, arthritis, gout, muscle pain, and other degenerative disorders of the musculoskeletal system. They are produced in southern Africa and Namibia, the biggest exporter in the region. Just less than 200 tonnes were exported from Namibia between January and August 2000 (Cole, 2000).
- The root of a vine called *Radix pucrariae*, used for centuries in traditional Chinese medicine and consumed as food to treat alcohol abuse, was found to contain daidzin which suppresses the craving for alcohol in animals (Keung, 1995).
- Lee-Huang (1995) and her colleagues at New York School of Medicine isolated a protein, MAP 30, from another traditional Chinese medicine and a local Nigerian plant, bitter melon (*Momordica charantia* L), and found that it had multiple anti-HIV effects. The MAP protein is able to inhibit HIV-l integrase, one of the enzymes responsible for the virus's gene expression. This sort of activity is unique among anti-HIV agents and the development of integrase inhibitors is being vigorously pursued.

In some of these examples, although researchers sought and found single active substances, the source material was traditionally consumed as a food or nutraceutical, and all these agents were identified through ethno-botanical searching.

In industrialized countries, plants have contributed to more than 7,000 compounds produced by the pharmaceutical industry, including ingredients in heart drugs, laxatives, anti-cancer agents, hormones, contraceptives, diuretics, antibiotics, decongestants, analgesics, anaesthetics, ulcer treatments and anti-parasitic compounds. Around one in four of all prescription drugs dispensed by western pharmacists are likely to contain ingredients derived from plants (BGCI fact sheet). Of about 120 main prescription drugs currently in use, an estimated 75 per cent were located through ethno-botanical knowledge or folklore claims around 90 plant species.

Therefore, much of the population of the world still relies on herbs for its medicines. Used correctly, they can be extremely effective. However, the twin problems of herbal medicines are inadequate evidence bases for efficacy (what truly works and what does not), and quality control of a product that is not the result of standard production methods. *The Economist* 2006.

# 2.0 Traditional Paradigm of Herbal Medicines Production

## 2.1 The Old Production Paradigm

Many medicinal and aromatic plants are wild-crafted, usually without regard to Good Agricultural and Collection Practices (GACPs). In West Africa, for example, the vast majority of drug plants grow only in the wild, rather than being cultivated and in 1991, 80 per cent of the more than 700,000 tonnes of plant materials that were used for the preparation of decoction in traditional medicine and as ingredients in *officinal* medicine in China, were collected from the wild–BGCI Fact Sheet. This unregulated exploitation/usage of traditional medicine resources pose enormous challenges for the herbal medicine industry since development of quality herbal products based on established industry standards is hinged on adequate monitoring of raw materials.

The traditional paradigm of processing herbal raw materials into medicines involves such activities as pulverization, slicing, bleaching, soaking, dry frying, roasting, steaming, fermentation and sun-drying. Processed medicinal plants are subsequently sold directly to herbal dispensaries or practitioners that combine and administer herbs to patients or manufacturers who combine the herbs into therapies and sell to practitioners. This paradigm incorporates three concepts, which influences the way herbs are produced, marketed, and used.

- A nutritive approach in which foods are considered medicinal and some medicinal herbs are considered appropriate for everyday consumption
- An understanding that processing techniques used to prepare medicinal plant fractions for consumption affect the energetic, chemistry, and efficacy of the product, and
- A reliance on traditional formulations to achieve the desired therapeutic result. For traditional medical practitioners, no firm distinction between food and medicine exists (Yang, 1998; Zhu, 1998).

## 2.2 Non-competitiveness of the Old Paradigm

On an industrial scale, the major challenge to the old approach is that herbal medicines are susceptible to degradation which can render the product unsuitable for consumption, or at least make them visually unappealing for consumers. This is generally not a problem for small-scale producers who harvest, process and distribute the products within days of processing. However, it is a concern for larger scale producers who cannot sell or process the entire materials before degradation begins giving rise to non-competitive products.

Research has indicated the constraints leading to these as:

- Poor agricultural and collection practices
- Poor post-harvest handling
- Poor quality control procedures
- Lack of current good manufacturing practices
- Inadequate data for product development

- Low technical know-how and equipments
- Poor yields arising from inefficient processing

As a result of the foregoing, each of the many hundreds of medicinal plant fractions used in traditional medicine has an associated traditional processing procedure. According to Bensky and Gamble (1993), processing has these specific medicinal purposes:

- To increase the potency,
- To minimize side effects, and/or
- To alter medicinal properties for a particular clinical use.

The principle of traditional herbal medicines processing is thus that medicines would be produced, dispensed and administered in small scales by practitioners who are able to identify exact plant species from traditional knowledge. However, production and dispensing of herbal medicines is shifting from practitioners to commercial ventures operated by owners of herbal drug stores who lack traditional medical knowledge surrounding the practice. As a result, there is no guarantee of the authenticity and quantity of plant material used in herbal preparations.

## 2.3 Quality Non-compliance

In a study by Okunlola (2007), to investigate the pharmaceutical and microbial qualities of 21 different Herbal Medicinal Products (of various dosage forms) sourced from some traditional medicine sales outlets and retail pharmacy outlets in southwestern Nigeria, the following were observed:

- Twelve (57.1 per cent) of the products had their manufacturing and expiry dates stated,
- Only nine (42.9 per cent) products have been registered by the Nigerian National Agency for Food, Drug Administration and Control (NAFDAC)
- Ten (47.6 per cent) did not have their content stated but had their therapeutic claims indicated on the container.
- The tablet formulations showed acceptable crushing strength and friability but failed the test for disintegration time.
- The angle of repose of the powdered dosage forms were considerably high showing that the powders were highly cohesive and not free flowing.
- The microbial load of the products varied considerably.
- Ten (47.6 per cent) of the samples were contaminated by *E. coli*,
- Seven (33 per cent) were contaminated by *Salmonella spp*,
- Fifteen (71.4 per cent) were contaminated by *Staphylococcus aureus* and
- Twelve (57.1 per cent) were contaminated by fungi

The nature of medicinal and aromatic plants as herbal raw materials underscores in some ways the difficulties experienced in dealing with them. While the role of the food crops depends on the primary products of photosynthesis–the carbohydrates, proteins and triglycerides (fats and oils) and in the case of the wood and fiber crops, (cellulose and lignin), herbal medicines derive from the secondary products of metabolism–such as the alkaloids, terpenoids and flavonoids–which evolves as responses of plants to stress, predation and competition. Thus it is usually extracts, not the plants themselves (or parts of them such as seeds, grains, fruits or leaves) that are used for herbal medicines.

Therefore, the quality of herbal medicines in the market varies widely and they may not even be effective. Earlier, safety issues of herbal medicines were highlighted (Editorial AJTCAM, 2004; Fennel, 2004). The consumer is unlikely to be duped for much longer by the natural product that contains an ineffective 'whiff' of herbal extracts. The concern is the exaggerated properties put on some of these products by some herbal vendors. Thus, there is a strong move towards standardization of active chemicals derived from or found in herbal medicines.

## 3.0 Best Practices in Herbal Medicine Production

### 3.1 Post-harvest Handling and Handling Methods

There are basically three ways raw fauna and flora can provide new medicines or preventative healthcare tonics.

- They may be sold as dried or raw materials
- As refined extracts or
- Used as models for synthesizing new drugs.

In each of these instances post harvest handling is a key determinant of commercial competitiveness. Post-harvest handling and material management methods are numerous, but are economically challenging to producers in developing countries. A process as simple as drying is difficult to achieve because standard drying methods and energy sources are scarce resources in most developing countries. According to a united nation report, (*Our planet*), 1.6 billion people have no access to electricity while 2.4 billion rely on charcoal, dung or wood as principal source of energy. Majority of these people live in developing countries.

Another critical challenge of plant collection and extraction is that they are labour intensive and expensive. Collectors gather plant materials in the field, sort, clean, dry and comminute them. Extracts are removed from these materials with solvents and then screened for medicinal effects. An extract with medicinal applications will be then partially purified and given a crude check for its efficacy, modified to improve effectiveness and reduce toxicity and given an extensive battery of tests for safety before being placed on the world markets.

To solve the problem of slow processing of entire plants (drying and grinding them up, and extracting component chemicals), researchers have developed the methods of tissue culture. Several thousand species of plant cells are grown in test tubes, from which 'active ingredients' are directly produced and extracted. Plant samples from the wild can cost up to 100 times as those produced from cell cultures (Economist, 1998), and working with plant cells facilitates the second technique–employing stressors to coax plants to produce chemicals they would not ordinarily produce in the wild, or if they are picked at the wrong time. Thus before constituent chemicals are extracted, plants are sometimes, baked, frozen, injected with hormones and subjected to extremes of light and darkness. This technique has paid off in some cases.

## 3.2 Material Management and Process Flow

Production of Herbal medicines should follow a progressively sophisticated processing of medicinal plants in stages such as:

- Identification/Harvesting of authentic herbal materials
- Drying/Dry extracts
    - Comminuting of herbal raw materials
    - Packaging as powders, capsules and teas
    - Production of medicinal wines, syrup, tinsers and mixtures
- Aqueous extraction
    - Preparation of standardized liquid and extracts such as mixtures, tablets, capsules, gels and ointments
    - Production of medicinal wines, syrup, tinsers and mixtures
- Fractionation/isolation of extracts for bio-prospecting pharmaceuticals

Care should be taken when drying herbs not to cause extreme losses of heat sensitive properties. Therefore, they must be dried at low temperatures for longer periods of time resulting in large power requirements for dryer operation.

A widely used method for preserving herbal materials is dehydration. This involves the use of heat to increase surrounding air temperature of the herbal material. Thermal energy is used to evaporate moisture at the material surface causing a vapour pressure gradient between the material surface and interior. This gradient causes moisture to diffuse from the interstices of the herbal material to the surface. These designs are based on criteria of final product quality, capital cost, power requirements, and simplicity, operating cost, capacity, safety and environmental issues.

With the right dehydration parameters, this process can yield a stable product with a prolonged shelf life and little losses in the value of the herbal material. It is noteworthy that poor dehydration parameters will give rise to excessively high temperatures, causing losses of medicinal, culinary, visual, and nutraceutical properties, resulting in poor and unstable product yield. Tabil *et al.* (2001) suggested that material size and shape affect drying rate. Stems will take longer to dry than leaves. So it is important to sort leaves and stems before drying process.

## 3.3 Shifting the Processing Paradigm

It is obvious that traditional methods have some disadvantages, which could be corrected by selecting suitable research based technologies. This is imperative since ethno-medical methods were dependent on the needs and status of technology that was available at that time. It can be modified and improved by using research based technologies available today to make them more effective, stable, reproducible, controlled and in dosage forms that can easily be delivered to the site of action while at the same time being bio-available. There is a need then to select proper and appropriate technologies for the industrial production of herbal medicines such that the efficacies of the preparations are maintained.

### 3.4 Natural Product Chemistry to the Rescue

Current knowledge of natural product chemistry offers us tools and opportunities for maximizing the use of herbal raw materials for producing quality herbal medicines that will not only be efficacious and stable but will be highly competitive in the global market. Adopting the golden age principles of natural product chemistry, processing of herbal materials into medicines for internal and or external use would involve simple methods such as hot or cold-water extraction, expression of juice after crushing, powdering of dried material, formulation of powder into pastes via such a vehicle as water, oil or honey, and even fermentation after adding a sugar source.

An extract produced by soaking dried plant or animal material in an appropriate solvent under controlled conditions is the raw material for formulation of dosage forms and bio prospecting. If we were to produce known pure herbal medicines to be used in modern medicine, more processing stages from the crude extracts and sophisticated machinery would be required. Furthermore, safety and toxicity aspects can now, more than any time in research history, be totally evaluated. New formulations need to be given a sound development study, particularly on account of the nature of the processed products. Plant extracts are difficult to granulate, sensitive to moisture and prone to microbial contamination. Hence the types of excipients to be used and the processing parameters have to be extensively studied.

Processed products (galenicals) from plants could be standardised fluid/solid extracts or powders or tinctures. With adequate standardisation, some of these galenicals could be formulated for incorporation into modern dosage forms. Standardised extracts of many plants (*e.g. Aloe* species, *Atropa belladonna*, *Cassia angustifolia*, *Capsicum annuum*, *Centella asiatica*, *Cephaelis ipecacuanha*, *Digitalis* species, *Commiphora mukul*, *Panax ginseng*) have been widely used in health care.

### 3.5 The Importance of Pilot Production Plant

In addition to the creative and innovative technologies needed for new herbal medicine development, manufacturing herbal medicines presents another challenge– that Medicinal herbs could be likened to a synthetic laboratory, which produces and contains a number of chemical compounds in a matrix. Hence herbal medicines depend on combinations of ingredients for their therapeutic properties.

Pharmaceutical companies have avoided this challenge by concentrating on isolating single active compounds whose mechanisms may be understood with respect to a specific disease or pathology. This isolation and pharmacological evaluation is the distinction between pharmaceuticals and herbal medicines. In general the former is based on a single "active ingredient" from, say, a plant.

The foregoing emphasizes the need for Pilot Scale Production plants, which would be at the interphase of research and industry. Development of process parameters carried out at such plants would allow for research findings to be up-scaled to industrial production. Pilot scale production facilities have been so grossly neglected in many developing countries such that R&D efforts remain perpetually at the level of basic research with very little commercial value since such findings can not translate to industrial products. Further, the absence of commercialized research results stifle research as revolving research fund can not be generated nor could any reasonable patent be obtained for simple basic research. In the same vein, industry demanded researches are unknown hence neglected.

### 3.6 Standardisation as a Global Measure of Herbal Medicines Quality

There is a trend internationally to standardize extracts from herbal medicinal products in terms of a single ingredient as a measure of its quality. Standardization of herbal medicines is the process of concentrating an herb so that one or more of its key phytochemicals or other ingredients is present in a defined amount. For example, the level of Hypericine contents determines St. John's wort. Standardization also ensures that some ingredients are not present or are kept below a maximum tolerable level.

The identification of biologically active compounds in herbs is an essential requirement for quality control and dose determination of plant-based drugs. To be compliant to FDA and other regulatory authorities therefore, herbal processing should involve 'herb-to-pill' and 'batch-to-batch' standardization of complex crude extracts.

For example, according to Holm (1998), Wild-crafted valerian root contains low percentages of valerinic acid, while milk thistle usually contains high levels of silymarin. Studies have shown that the optimally effective valerian extracts contain 0.8 per cent valerinic acid while extracts of milk thistle have been standardized at around 80 percent because this was found to be the most effective level. In another example, kava is standardized to contain 75 mg. of kavalactones. The pills come in varying strength, from 100 to 250 mg, and the amount of kavalactones also varies. For example, a 250-mg. pill of 30 per cent extract will contain 75 mg. of kavalactones, which is in accordance with Kommission E's recommendation of 60 to 120 mgs daily of kavalactones for stress and anxiety.

Although herbalists and physicians who believe that therapeutic effects of herbal reparations arise from a synergistic blend of many organochemicals oppose standardization on a single "active ingredient", but standardization and near pharmaceutical-grade production methods would be the only logical practice of the herbal medicine industry in the 21st century. This is not to suggest that synergy is of no significance. A wide array of research report suggests synergy as a key mechanism for herbal drug effects (Keung, 1996; Onawumi, 1984; Buterweck, 1998).

While it is desirable by scientists to know the entire chemical structure of the plant materials, which actually yields, observed therapeutic effects, ethnopharmacology emphasizes the synergistic action of natural products. The scientific merit of non-standardised herbal remedies is therefore a subject of continuing controversy hence a need to adapt approaches that increases acceptability of the products universally.

From the marketing point of view, bulk buyers demand a certificate of analysis to be submitted with samples, even with wild-crafted samples, although many buyers will accept wild-crafted materials without the certificate and just perform their own analysis on samples. Although most herbal products manufacturers are deeply concerned with product quality and accuracy of standardization claims, others will sell practically anything, and hence the instances in which concentration levels of ingredients does not match label claims.

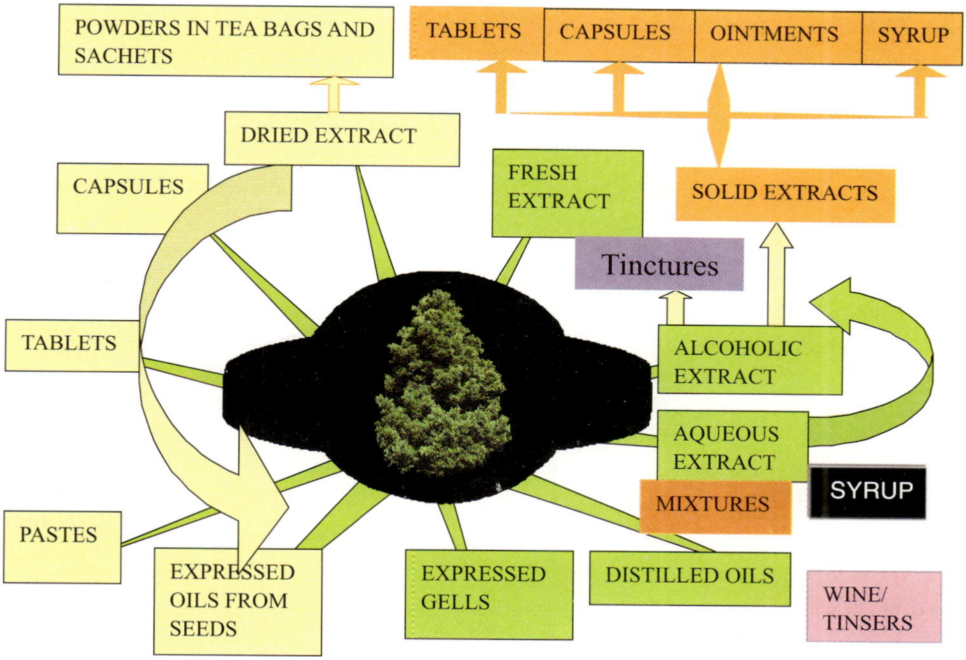


**Model Scheme for Material Processing**

## 3.7 General Quality Management

Quality has to be built into the entire production operations beginning from the selection of propagation material to the final product reaching the consumer if herbal medicines are to attain status of scientific repute. The quality requirements for medicinal plant preparations are stringent in terms of content of active principles and toxic materials. Whereas the production of herbal medicines for local use does not require such stringent standards, International Standard Specifications exist for some processed products and some countries and buyers have their own requirements.

The entire production process is important, from planting or sowing to harvesting. And even before sowing, the selection of the soil, of the genetic material to be planted and of the geographical location, will undoubtedly have a significant impact on the final outcome, on the quality of the raw material, and of the finished product. The quality of the raw material is critical to the fulfilment of the goals of processing and preservation of herbal medicines, and also determines the level of profit. The quality of a finished product essentially depends on the quality of the raw material. The material must therefore be of good quality and its industrial performance must be high. In addition to this, the raw material must be of certain basic microbiological purity. Test for contaminants such as microbes, metals, and pesticides, can also "fingerprint" samples using HPLC to compare an extract with others.

With respect to sourcing and purchasing requirements, most manufacturers source herbal materials from growers rather than wild crafters, and the main requirements for purchase involves species identification and correct drying, colour, texture, odour and taste, and sometimes certificates of analysis which indicate strength of active ingredients, in addition to completed testing for contaminants.

High performance liquid chromatography (HPLC) and GC-MS are efficient industry standards for the determination of the levels of specific required chemicals in bulk material, so the product manufacturer can concentrate active ingredients for the most optimal levels of human consumption.

## 4.0 Conclusion

Although the traditional paradigm of herbal medicine production has afforded science the foundation upon which to build the study of modern medicines, it is obvious that traditional production methods have many disadvantages. The time has come to apply the right paradigm with regard to herbal medicine processing. Modern research based methods should be used to improve and make them more stable, effective, and reproducible and in appropriate dosage forms.

Herbal medicine researches in most developing countries are government based hence slow. The economic rate of return on private research investment is generally greater than that of government research. The absence of commercialized research results stifle research, as revolving research fund cannot be guaranteed. Governments of developing countries should devise public-private partnerships (PPP) programmes to address this research incentive problem.

The necessity for Pilot scale production plants to inter-phase research and industry is most critical now than ever as developing countries struggles to evolve accurate process parameters, enhance the localization of process technologies, stimulate local design of equipments and translate research findings to industrial products to redress the burgeoning health and economic problems.

## References

AACHRD, 2002. Enhancing research into traditional medicine in the African region: a working document prepared for the 21st session of the African advisory committee for health research and development (aachrd) Port Louis, Mauritius; pp. 22-25

Adenike, Okunlola, Babatunde, A. Adewoyin and Oluwatoyin, A. Odeku, 2007. Evaluation of Pharmaceutical and Microbial qualities of Some Herbal Medicinal Products in South Western Nigeria Tropical Journal of Pharmaceutical Research, March (6 (1); pp. 661-670

Balick, M. J. and Cox, P.A., 1996. Plants, People and Culture: the science of ethnobotany. The Scientific American Library, New York.

Bensky, D. and A. Gamble. 1993. Chinese herbal medicine: Materia Medica. Rev. ed. Eastland Press, Inc., Seattle, WA; pp. 13–17.

Botanic Gardens Conservation International Fact Sheet. 'Plants as medicine'. Botanic Gardens Conservation International/British Airways/International Centre for Conservation Education.

Borman, S., 1993. Quoted in Chemical and Engineering News, September.

Butterweck, V., Petereit, F., Winterhoff, H., and Nahrsted, A., 1998. Solubilised hypericin and pseudohypericin from hypericum perforatum exert antidepressant activity in the forced swimming test. Planta Medica (64); pp. 291-294

Cannell, R. J. P., 1998a. Follow-up of natural product isolation. Methods Biotechnol (4) (Natural Products Isolation); pp. 425–463.

Cannell, R. J. P., 1998b. How to approach the isolation of a natural product. In R. J. P. Cannell (Ed.), Methods in Biotechnology (4): Natural Products Isolation. Humana, Totowa, NJ; pp. 1–51.

Cole, D., and Lombard, C., 2000. 'The sustainably harvested Devil's Claw project in Namibia: some primary producer issues'. The Centre for Research Information and Action in Africa, Windhoek

Cragg, G. M., Newman, D. J., 2001a. Natural product drug discovery in the next millennium. Pharmaceut. Biol. (39) (Suppl.); pp. 8–17.

Cragg, G. M., Newman, D. J., 2001b. Natural products drug discovery and development at the United Sates National Cancer Institute. In L. Yuan (Ed.), Drug Discovery and Traditional Chinese Medicine: Science, Regulation, and Globalization, [International Conference on Traditional Chinese Medicine: Science, Regulation and Globalization], 1st, College Park, MD, August 30–September 2, 2000 (2001) (meeting Date 2000). Kluwer Academic, Hingham, MA; pp. 19–32.

Economist May 30, 1998.

Economist, October 5th 2006. Herbal medicine: African genesis (A pharmacopoeia for Africa).

Editorial, 2004. Safety of Traditional Medicines, Complementary and Alternative Medicines in Africa. Afr. J. Trad. Comp. Alt. Med. (1); pp. 1–3.

Fennell, C.W., Lindsey, K. L., McGaw, L. J., Sparg, L. G., Stafford, G. I. Elgorashi, E. E., Grace, O. M. and van Staden, J., 2004. Assessing African medicinal plants for efficacy and safety: pharmacological screening and toxicology. J. Ethnopharmacol. (94); pp. 205-217.

Holm, W. and D. MacGregor, 1998. Processing Guide for Specialty Crops. A report published by the Science Council of BC–Okanagan.

Holt, G. A., Chandra, A., 2002. Herbs in the modern healthcare environment– An overview of uses, legalities, and the role of the healthcare professional. Clin. Res. Regulatory Affairs (USA), (19); pp. 83–107.

Huang, S. *et al.*, 1995. Inhibition of the integrase of human immunodeficiency virus (HIV) type 1 by anti-HIV plant proteins MAP30 and GAP31. Proceedings of the National Academy of Science (92); pp. 8818-8822.

Keung, W. *et al.*, 1995. Daidzin suppresses ethanol consumption by Syrian golden hamsters without blocking acetaldehyde metabolism. Proceedings of the National Academy of Science (92); pp. 8990-8993.

Keung, W., Lazo, O., Kunze, L., and Vallee, BL., 1996. Potentiation of the bioavailability of daidzen by an extract of Radix puerariae. Proceedings of the National Academy of Science, USA (93); pp. 4284-4288.

Newman, D. J., Cragg, G. M., Snader, K. M., 2000. The influence of natural products upon drug discovery. Nat. Prod. Repts. (17); pp. 215–234.

Onawumi, G. O., Yisak, W., and Ogunlana, EO., 1984. Antibacterial constituents in the essential oil of cymbopogon citrates (DC.) Stapf. Journal of Ethnopharmacology (12); pp. 279-286.

Our planet, a magazine published by the United Nations Environmental Programme

Tabil, L.G., M. Kashaninejad and B. Crerar, 2001. Drying characteristics of Purslane (*Portulaca oleraceae* L.). Department of Agricultural and Bioresource Engineering, University of Saskatchewan. Saskatoon, SK.

Tyler, V., 1999. Six man-loving herbs that really work. Prevention, April

Yang, Shou-Zhong, 1998. Translator The divine farmer's materia medica. Blue Poppy Press, Boulder, CO.

Zhu, Y., 1998. Chinese materia medica: Chemistry, pharmacology, and applications. Harwood Academic Publ., Amsterdam

*Chapter 2*

# Factors Influencing Secondary Metabolism and Therapeutic Efficacy of Medicinal Plants

***P. Pushpangadan* and Varughese George*****

*Amity Institute for Herbal and Biotech Products Development, Peroorkada, Trivandrum – 5, India*

*E-mails: *palpuprakulam@yahoo.co.in, **gerogedrv@yahoo.co.in*

## ABSTRACT

Medicinal plants constitute main resource base of almost all the traditional healthcare systems. Most of the herbal drugs produced currently in majority of the developing countries lack proper quality specification and standards. Herbal drugs used in Traditional Medicine (TM) may contain a single herb or combinations of several different herbs believed to have complementary and/or synergistic effects. Both the raw drugs and the finished herbal products manufactured contain complex mixtures of organic compounds, such as fatty acids, sterols, alkaloids, flavonoids, polyphenols, glycosides, saponines, tannins, terpenes etc (Pushpangadan and Govindarajan, 2006). The quality of the finished product is based on the quality of the raw materials. As many as 35 per cent of the medicinal plants used in Indian systems of medicine are highly cross pollinated which indicate the existence of a wide range of genetic variability in the populations of these medicinal plant species which in turn reflected in the variations in the composition of secondary metabolites. Ecological and edaphic as well as seasonal variations also cause changes in the chemical composition of medicinal plants. These facts have to be considered while developing quality parameters/standards of medicinal plants and their finished products.

The traditional medicines used to be an individual based treatment regime wherein the traditional physicians used hand picked plant materials to prepare drugs/formulations to treat their patients (Pushpangadan 2006). The prescription and preparation of the drugs or remedies were also used to be person specific and based on the constitutional nature of the patient called 'Prakriti' as per the 'Tridosha' concept of Ayurveda/Siddha. A well-experienced traditional physician in the past used to have specific knowledge about the therapeutically active plants. There were also specially trained medicinal plant collectors who go to the forest and collect the medicinal plants from certain specific habitat in specific seasons. These traditional medicinal plant collectors had intimate knowledge of plant species and could identify therapeutically effective plants from a population of a species and collect it from the right place, in the right season at the right growth and developmental stage of the medicinal plants. With such unique expertise they were able to maintain certain level of standards in the therapeutic quality of the herbal drugs. But the transformation of traditional medicine from such an individualized system to a commercial manufacturing system has resulted in great deterioration in the whole procedure and process of traditional medicine. Indeed, quality of the drugs became the casualty in this transformation.

The Traditional Indian Systems of Medicine like Ayurveda, Siddha, Unani, Amchi etc. provided specific instructions for collection by indicating location/ edaphic conditions, habitat, seasonal and even the stage of the plant growth and developmental stage. Scientific investigations now provide ample evidence to the fact that there is a flux of change in the chemical constituents, particularly those of the secondary metabolites, in such varied conditions described above. Therefore, it is extremely important to establish quality parameters of the medicinal plants by undertaking extensive and intensive study of the traditional treatise of the classical medicines or traditional practices, combined with the modern scientific knowledge and using the latest analytical and computational tools.

The emergence of system biology and metabolomics etc. now opens up the possibility of developing precise parameter and references specifications etc. required for standardization and quality control of medicinal plants and medicinal/ herbal products.

*Keywords: Medicinal plants, Herbal drugs, Poly herbals, Secondary metabolites, Quality control standardization, System biology, Metabolomics.*

## 1.0 Introduction

The use of plants for medicine can be traced back to the history and development of human race. The effort to alleviate pain, discomfort and to have better health and to feel comfortable prompted humans to search for therapeutic or health promoting agents in the environment. Medicinal plants and their preparations were being used as a part of treatment, which later became the major and effective means of treating ailments and diseases. Plant based medicines used to be the main therapeutic aid for the whole humankind till 18th century. Plant based medicines faced a declining trend and also disappeared by 19th century in most developed countries. During the turn of the 19th century, technological developments in chemistry, particularly phytochemistry, medicinal chemistry and development of biological screening methods for toxicological and efficacy evaluation led to extraction of active principles and isolation of single biologically active compounds. Further advancements in the pharmaceutical chemistry led to development of a wide range of synthetic and semisynthetic derivatives from these single biologically active compounds, which were used for therapeutic purposes. This system of medicine, known as Modern medicine or Allopathy won instant popularity due to the rapid and targeted action of the drugs that offered quick relief of symptoms associated with the disease. Modern medicine made rapid strides in the 19th and 20th century with the spectacular advancements made in the biological, chemical and pharmaceutical sciences. By the end of the 20th century modern medicine replaced traditional medicine in most of the developed countries in the world.

The turn of the 20th century however saw a revival of plant based health care. WHO in 2003, recognized the intrinsic importance of plant based traditional medicine and emphasized the strategic role of traditional medicines in providing primary health care needs of the rural population in the world. By the end of 20th century plant based medicines also found its resurgence in the developed countries causing an ever increasing demand for medicinal plants. Almost 80 per cent of the medicinal plants required for herbal remedies are met from wild resources. But the increasing demand has led to over exploitation as well as unscientific extractions threatening the fast extinction of many rare medicinal plants. Therefore, there was an erosion of quality of medicinal plants which is reflected in the finished products.

## 1.1 Developmental Quality Parameters, Prevedic and Vedic Parameters

During the prehistoric period the humans living in different agro climatic conditions selected medicinal plants to treat various ailments by a process of trial, error, experimentation and using the intuitive power of some innovative members of the community. Ancient humans explored his surroundings–first the plants, then animals and even minerals. The prehistoric humans selected his therapeutic agents, mainly plants by instinct followed by his keen observation of the behaviour of other wild animals. The early humans might have tried a wide range of plants and in this process many might have sacrificed their lives. Those medicinal plants remedies found clinically useful were freely shared with the society.

During the vedic period cooking of medicine might have gained importance. But complex formulations did not however develop even during this period. Simple single herbal preparations in the form of fresh juice, paste or decoction or fermented wines were the main form of drug administration. Animal products, minerals and metals were also slowly incorporated into pharmaceuticals during 'Samhita' period. The main resource base of all the traditional systems of medicine like Ayurveda, Siddha however continued to be medicinal plants. The most impressive development of Indian medicine during 'Samhita' period is the systematic classification of medicinal plants, accurate methods of collection, post harvest handling of raw drugs, its storage and processing into finished formulations. Concept of compatibility and incompatibility of ingredients to be incorporated in polyherbal formulations etc. were dealt in detail. The 'Samhita' period is also marked for the authentic compilations or treatises. Theoretical foundation for Ayurvedic Chemistry, Pharmacy and Pharmacology are all dealt in these treatises.

## 2.0 What is a Medicinal Plant?

Medicinal plant contains certain chemical components that have therapeutic action (to alleviate pain or cure or manage various disorders/discomforts/diseases and promote or enhance better health etc.) in organisms and in the present context in the human kind.

## 2.1 Secondary Metabolites

While in food plants our main interest is the carbohydrate/sugars, proteins, fats and other vitamins, in medicinal plants we look for therapeutically useful chemicals which are generally termed as secondary metabolites which are not that essential for the normal growth and development of the plants/organisms. Plants synthesize these compounds to protect themselves *i.e.* to adjust, adapt or defend/offend, from the hostile organisms or diseases or the environment. Secondary metabolites that are useful in medicine are mostly polyphenols, alkaloids, glycosides, terpenes, flavonoids, coumarins, tannins etc. The production of secondary metabolites although controlled by genes but their specific expression is greatly influenced by various factors including biotic and abiotic environments such as climate and edaphic factors or other associated living organisms. During the course of evolution plants have evolved various physical and chemical mechanisms to protect themselves from the vagaries of nature (drought, heat, rain, flood, etc.) and also to defend or offend the predators or to protect from predators and pathogens. The most successful adaptation of plants while developing various physiological mechanisms is through the production of a variety of phytochemicals by which they were able to face both biotic and abiotic stresses and threats. In this process of defence/offence from abiotic stress or the invading diseases causing organisms or the predators (animals, birds, insects and herbivorous animals), the plant synthesize a variety of chemical compounds. Apparently plants produce many antioxidants for protecting themselves from the oxidative stress. These compounds are in general stored in the leaves or other parts such as, bark, hardwood, fruits, etc., so that the predators or the disease causing organisms can be either knocked down or paralyzed or even get killed. In many cases, the production of the secondary metabolites in plant also depends on the association of other living organisms, more particularly, the plant or soil microbes. Such differential expressions of therapeutically active principles in plant on account of the above said factors appears to have known and well understood by the ancient Ayurvedic scholars, when they gave specific instructions in the procurement of medicinal plants.

The classical texts of Ayurveda and Siddha give detailed directions with various dos and don'ts in collection and processing of medicinal plants. They insisted collecting certain medicinal plants in certain specific seasons from specific ecosystems and also during certain particular stage of growth and development of the plants. There is increasing evidence to show that the varieties, ecosystems and stage of plant growth development etc. influence the production of secondary metabolism in many medicinal plants. Almost 35 to 40 per cent of the medicinal plants found in tropical regions are cross-pollinated species and there exists extensive genetic variability particularly, in the secondary metabolites in these species (Pushpangadan 2006). Therefore, in a given population of a medicinal plant species there may be many plants, which may not have the desired therapeutically active constituents and only a few of them may have the desired therapeutically active constituents. There used to be highly experienced medicinal plants collectors ('Bhishagwaras') in the past who were able to identify the plants with the right therapeutic property and collect them. It is believed that the plant collectors of the Samhita period possessed even some kind of intuitive knowledge, so that they were able to pick up the right plants from populations of a species having variations in their therapeutic contents. It is even stated in certain classical texts of Ayurveda that those few plants having the therapeutic property in a large population would speak to those well-experienced medicinal plant collectors with intuitive knowledge that "I am the one who has the therapeutic ability and therefore collect me". We don't have now such intuitive persons who can understand the language of plants! What we have today is the scientific expertise with sophisticated analytical tools. We have to use them appropriately.

## 2.2 Expression of Secondary Metabolites

We know now that the presence of or absence of certain secondary metabolites in medicinal plants are influenced by a variety of factors, which include climate/season, edaphic conditions or the association of other plants and other living organisms. Another factor that influenced the production of secondary metabolites in plants are the inter relationship between plants and the insect flora. It is now generally accepted that the flora and the insect flora in a tropical ecosystem have been co-evolving and co-adapting. Many of the medicinal plants are cross-pollinated and they need the help of pollinators. In an open area the wind could do the function, but in a canopied forest many of the shrubs and herbs growing under the big trees cannot get wind to pollinate. These plants are thus heavily depending upon the insects or even the birds to pollinate them. To attract the insects or birds the plants develop pleasant aroma (essential oils) and provide honey and pollen as food to these pollinators. Many flowers contain honey or pollen, which are the normal food of many insects and birds. The insects like bees and butterflies visit flowers after flowers, and take honey or pollen or both. During this process they also carry pollen on their body part, which then help in pollinating while visiting other plants. Many flowers have structurally evolved flower parts to effect such pollinations by insects. These insects also multiply on plants. They lays millions of eggs and the larvae that emerge from these eggs then feed on leaves of the plants, sometimes destroying the plants altogether by over feeding. During the course of evolution the plants began to synthesize certain toxic substance so that a good percentage of the feeding larvae could be killed. The insect on the other hand began to develop resistance so that many of the larvae could survive. The plants on the other hand again counteracted it synthesizing more and more toxic compounds. This was something like the love and hate relationship between plants and the insects, which during the course of millions of years of evolutions have resulted in the synthesis of innumerable chemical compounds, mostly the secondary metabolites in plants as well as in insects. The variability in living organisms is indeed the insurance for survival. The evolutionary origin of cross breeding was indeed a nature's device for reshuffling of genes so that new variants could be produced. Similarly, the abiotic conditions also exerted certain influence in the plants and the plants responded by developing various chemicals. In extreme drought conditions the desert exerts a kind of stress on the plants and the plants evolve by synthesizing chemicals that would help them to protect from stress induced by the desert conditions. An excellent example for this is the plant *Commiphora wightii*; an important medicinal plant used extensively in Ayurveda, Siddha and even Unani under the name 'Guggul'. The medicinal part of the plant is the gum exudates from the stem bark of living plants. This gum is traditionally collected from the desert regions of Rajasthan, Gujarat and even Afghanistan. When the senior author joined as Director of Tropical Botanic Garden and Research Institute (TBGRI), Thiruvananthapuram he found this plant growing luxuriantly at TBGRI garden. Out of curiosity the senior author collected gum from this plant and got chemically analyzed. To everyone's surprise the chemical data of this gum revealed that it do not contain most of the active compounds. A logical explanation may be that this plant growing in TBGRI botanic garden is located in a warm humid tropical forest region. It has no desert like conditions and therefore there is no question of any drought induced stress. The same plant when growing in desert has to confront drought-induced stress and the plant synthesizes the stress beating chemicals. There are many similar cases that demonstrate that certain specific climatic conditions and edaphic situations are extremely important in the production of therapeutically desirable medicinal compounds. Sandalwood is another classical example. The specific aroma of sandalwood is due to the presence of certain essential oil chemicals, mostly monoterpenes and sesquiterpenes. The production of the specific aroma chemicals is fully expressed only in those sandalwood trees that grow in certain forest regions of Karnataka. The sandalwood growing in other places in India or elsewhere in the world do not have the same kind of aroma with the corresponding chemical constituents.

## 3.0 Quality Control of Medicinal Plants and Herbal Products

The ancient Ayurvedic scholars seem to have an in-depth knowledge and understanding of this intricate behaviour of plants and therefore, they have insisted on the collection of many medicinal plants from certain specific ecosystems. They have indeed advocated for the cultivation of only a few medicinal plants, which normally do not show much variations, if cultivated and grown in different agro climates. Therefore, when it comes to the cultivation of medicinal plants the above said specific information have to be kept in mind. We need to carry out experimental studies to find out under which particular situation that the medicinal plants produce therapeutically active compounds. Only after understanding this critical aspect alone that one should venture for cultivation of medicinal plants. There used to be highly experienced plant collectors who had specific expertise to collect the medicinal plant at the right season, right stage of growth and development of the plant and thereby they were able to maintain quality of medicinal plants in batch to batch products of the herbal drugs. It was in the beginning of the 20$^{th}$ century that a few Ayurvedic pharmaceutical firms like Kottakkal Arya Vaidyasala in Kerala for the first time in Ayurvedic medical history began commercial preparation of Ayurvedic drugs and shelfable products. This transformation from the highly individualized and customized production practice to commercial production of Traditional Medicine in India confronted the issue of quality and standardization. The traditional experiential wisdom was either eroded or difficult to operate in such a commercial set up. It has also failed to imbibe the modern science and technology to overcome such shortcomings. Therefore, extensive and intensive researches are warranted in medicinal plant cultivation, harvesting, post harvest handling and processing. The Ayurveda was one of the most exact sciences developed by ancient Indians. But unfortunately there came a sudden halt in the magnificent growth of Ayurveda sometime during the 8th Century A.D.

## 4.0 System Biology Approach

The complexity of poly-herbal formulations and aspects of synergistic bioactivities in Traditional Medicine (TM) limited the analysis of quality control so far only on major components. The system biology approach a multidimensional chemical and pharmacological approach, enables linking of the complex metabolic profile of herbs with biological effects and is therefore key for quality control of herbal medicine / TM, while providing simultaneous scientific evidence for the underlying efficacy. This is very crucial for registration of herbal medicinal products under the new EU Herbal Medical Products guidelines. The approach is highlighted by a study using *Rehmannia glutinosa*, demonstrating how under controlled conditions variations can be induced and detected using herbal metabolic finger printing of herbs and extracts (Mei Wang *et al.*, 2005 and Jan Van der Greef, 2003)

Recent advances in molecular biochemistry opened up the possibility for massive profiling experiments at different biological levels such as DNA, RNA (transcriptomics), Protein (proteomics) and metabolites (metabolomics). The concept and practice of personalized medicine of Ayurveda and Siddha is now receiving considerable support and attention due to the new insights in pharmacogenomics. It is now clear that System biology can provide an important bridge function between the two complementary approaches used in TM and western medicine. System biology approach, the combination of metabolic fingerprints with bioactive assay and multivariate statistical analysis, will provide a method to involve the whole spectrum for the medical and pharmaceutical approach. Therefore, linking the biological activities with metabolomic finger printing of medicinal plants is the ultimate basis for quality control. To reach such a goal, a holistic analysis of plant metabolites is required.

Plant metabolimics start with the analysis of as many as possible detectable individual components that are in the plant material. Extracts made from individual herbs/plants and extraction or preparation methods as used in TM like Ayurveda and Siddha can be analyzed by means of different techniques such as LC-MS, GC-MS, NMR etc. resulting in total metabolite profiles.

## 5.0 Conclusion

Quality control and standardization of medicinal plants once thought to be an impossible task, now appears to be a clear possibility with the emergence of system biology and metabolomics. The complexity of ingredients and the aspects of synergistic bioactivities of poly-herbal medicines could now be well explained by system biology approach that enables linking of the complex metabolic profile of herb with biological effects.

## References

Mei Wang, Robert–Jan A.N. Lamers, Henrie A.A.J. Korthout, Joop H.J. van Neddrlrooj, Renger F. Witkamp, Rob van der Heijden, Peter J. Voshol, Louis M. Havekes, Rob Verpoorte and Jan van der Greef, 2005. Metabolomics in the context of Systems Biology: Bridging Traditional Chinese Medicine and Molecular Pharmacology. J Phytotherapy. 19 (3). pp. 173-82.

Pushpangadan, P. and Govindarajan, R. 2006. Need for scientific validation and standardization of TM to meet the Healthcare of the Third World in 21st century. *In* Herbal Medicine, phytopharmaceuticals and other Natural Products. Trends and advances. Jointly published by Centre for S&T of the Non-Aligned and other Developing Countries (NAM S&T Centre) and Institute of Chemistry, Ceylon, Sri Lanka. pp. 247-257.

Pushpangadan, P., 2006. Important Indian Medicinal Plants of Global Interest, International Conclave on Traditional Medicine. Produced and published by AYUSH and NISCAIR, CSIR, New Delhi. pp. 67-73.

Van der Greef, J., Davidow, E., Verheij, E.R., Vogles, J., van der Heijden, R., Adourian, A.S., Oresic, M., Marpe, E.W. and Naylor, S., 2003. The role of metabolomics in Systems Biology (Chapter 10) *In*: Metabolic Profiling: Its Role in Biomaker Discovery and Gene Function Analysis. Edited by Harraigan, G.G., Goodacre, R. Boston/Dordrecht/London: Kluwer Academic Publishers. pp. 70-198.

WHO, 2003. http://WWW. Who.int/mediacentre/factssheets/fs134/en

# Chapter 3

# Medicinal Plants/Traditional Medicine and IPR Protection

**P. Pushpangadan* and Varughese George****
*Amity Institute for Herbal and Biotech Products Development,*
*Peroorkada, Trivandrum – 5, India*
*E-mails: *palpuprakulam@yahoo.co.in, **gerogedrv@yahoo.co.in*

## ABSTRACT

Medicinal plants constitute the main resources base of most of the traditional systems of medicine in the world. Based on the lead from medicinal plants used in traditional systems of medicine a number of powerful molecular drugs have been developed in 19th and 20th centuries. During 20th century researchers taking lead from TM isolated biodynamic compounds and developed molecular medicines and made immense wealth. But they never shared the benefits with the providers of the initial lead. It is said that the possibility of finding the potential bioactive compound through random screening of plant samples is 1 in 10, 000 and that of hitting a marketable drug is 1 in 4. In contrast, the success rate of finding a bioactive molecule through selective screening based on ethno–botanical leads is 1 in 100 and that of discovery of a drug is 1 in 2. Many plant-derived drugs employed in modern medicine were first 'discovered' through ethnobotanical investigation. The traditional societies in India as well as in other Third World Countries (TWCs) have always considered the natural resources and the associated TK developed by them as common property to be cared and shared by all and never commodified to make personal benefits. It was with the coming of the westerners that the process of commodification and trading of bioresource and associated knowledge started.

One of the key issues involved in prospecting and commercialization of TK-derived technologies and products is the inadequacies in providing protection of TK through appropriate intellectual property laws and policy measures at national and international levels. Increasing incidences of misappropriation or misuse of TK for obtaining IPR rights without even acknowledging the role and contribution of TK holders are mounting with the recent booms in bio prospecting involving the use of genetic resources and associated TK. The turmeric, ayahausca and neem patent stories are a few examples to cite. Establishing legally binding instruments and mechanisms to ensure the Prior Informed Consent (PIC) of TK holder(s) and arriving at Mutually Agreed Terms (MAT) for benefit–sharing, third party transfers, IPR claims, and commercialization of the products or technologies derived from the use of TK associated with genetic resources are other concerns that are being discussed and debated at international forums, such as CBD, WTO-TRIPs, FAO, WIPO, UNEP, etc. Access and Benefit–Sharing (ABS) is a central issue concerned with the implementation of many of the national and international legal and policy instruments and mechanisms on biodiversity, IPR, protection of TK {including Traditional Cultural Expressions (TCE) and Folklore}, technology transfers, etc. The international conventions and treaties such as the CBD and ITPGRFA (International Treaty on Plant Genetic Resources for Food and Agriculture) now allow the Contracting Parties to have regulated access to transfer of genetic resources and biotechnologies, based on the principles of PIC and MAT. In line with CBD guidelines, several TWC members have enacted their own national laws for effective implementation of the CBD objectives.

World Trade Organization (WTO) introduced TRIPs in 1994 the monopolistic/ private rights and Intellectual Property Protection (IPR) which went against the interest of TK and contradicted what CBD has assured. It was against this background the WIPO came forward to find out a solution and established the Intergovernmental Committee on Intellectual Property and Folklore (IGC) in 2001 and it began to study the issues related to providing an international dimension to protection of TK associated with the use of genetic resources. The ongoing discussions and negotiations helped to develop two main forms of IPR related protection to TK: 1. Positive protection–*i.e.* establishing legal entitlements for TK holders, 2. Defensive protection-*i.e.* Safeguarding against illegitimate acquisition of IPR over TK or associated genetic resources. National governments have also been addressing the issue of providing IP protection to TK under the existing IP laws or *sui generis* mechanisms, so that the intellectual as well as customary rights of the TK holders are respected, recognized and rewarded.

It was India who has shown to the world that it is possible to revoke patents secured by developed countries (particularly USA), based on the indigenous biodiversity and TK of the developing countries But challenging and revoking patents are expensive and time consuming which many of the poor developing nations can not afford. It was again India who experimented the first ever benefit sharing model that recognized and rewarded the TK/TM of a forest dwelling tribe. Based on a lead received from Kani tribe of Western Ghat forest (Kerala–India) the senior author and his team developed a herbal drug which on commercialization shared the benefits (license fee+ royalty) on a 1:1 basis known as the TBGRI/Kani model or Pushpangadan's model of benefit sharing is well acclaimed in the world over and Pushpangadan received the UN-Equator Initiative Award under the Individual category in 2002 during the UN Summit at Johannesburg.

***Keywords:*** *Traditional medicine (TM), Traditional Knowledge (TK), Intellectual Protection Right (IPR).*

## 1.0 Introduction

Medicinal plants constitute an important group of plant diversity useful to mankind. The very term medicinal plants indicate that they are of therapeutical value. Man has been using medicinal plants since time immemorial to alleviate pain, discomforts and also to treat various ailments. Medicinal plants constitute the main resource base of almost all traditional systems of medicine in world over. It was from medicinal plants used in Traditional Medicine (TM) that a number of powerful modern molecular drugs developed during the 19th and 20th centuries. TM suffered a set back with the emergence of modern medicine in 18th and 19th century particularly in the developed countries. TM, however, continued to be the main source of healthcare for over 80 per cent of the people even today. Plant based medicine showed a revival of interest toward the end of 20th century. This resurgence of plant based medicine was the result of the growing awareness among the people about the harmful side effects and long term attempts caused by many modern therapeutic agents. The health hazard due to indiscriminate use of modern medicine such as antibiotics, cortico-steroids and other synthetic drugs became very clear and widely known. Modern medicine certainly has several lifesaving drugs and made unbelievable surgical advancements. Recognizing the intrinsic importance of plant based medicine/TM WHO in 1977 at its 30th World Assembly adopted a far reaching resolution urging the governments of member countries "to give adequate importance to the utilization of their traditional systems of medicine with appropriate regulations to meet their national healthcare needs". Countries where the healthcare system is based on modern (western) medicine or where traditional medicine has not been incorporated into the national healthcare system, TM is often termed as 'complementary', 'alternative' or 'non-conventional' medicine.

## 2.0 Herbal Medicine Industry in India: Opportunities and Challenges

Despite the fact that the country has a rich traditional knowledge and heritage of herbal medicine the export of herbal medicines from India is negligible. The turnover of herbal medicines in India (as over the counter product, ethical and classical formulations and home remedies of Ayurveda, Unani and Siddha Systems of medicine) is about US $ 1 billion with a mega export of about US $ 80 million. Eighty per cent of the export to developed countries are crude drugs and are not finished formulations. This leads to low revenue for the country. Moreover, most of the products developed by herbal manufacturers in India are of poor quality, obviously due to the absence of any stringent quality control measures in herbal drug manufacturing and marketing.

TK exists both in private and public domains. Most traditional medicinal knowledge is preserved by certain families or certain individuals in the community or is known to almost all members of the community. There are cases wherein the medical knowledge is known to many communities living in the same locality or in neighbouring localities/or in a particular geographical region. Ascertaining or availing the rights over their local resources and associated unique knowledge depend largely on their ability to negotiate or bargain with the takers of such knowledge for commercial ventures.

TM in many oriental countries more particularly in India runs in to two streams. The first and foremost of these two is the classical traditions of medicine like Ayurveda, Siddha, Unani and Amchi which are the written codified systems of TM with its own scientific arguments and philosophical explanations. The epistemological basis of these systems is quite different from that of the western medicine. The other stream is the oral folk stream of medicine practiced by house-wives/grandmothers, village physicians and tribal communities who transmit their knowledge orally from generation to generation and whose use is generally confined to a particular geographical region. Innovative members of the succeeding generations made incremental improvements/modifications or new addition to such medicinal practices and thus it remained a very vibrant dynamic system. The classical system on the other hand was written and documented in about 2,000 to 25,000 years back, but time and again it was redrafted to incorporate novel findings and modifications in practices. But unfortunately this dynamic aspect of modification and redrafting was discontinued on account of various reasons mainly due to the political instability resulting from the frequent invasions by foreigners. It was perhaps in 6th century AD that the last redrafting or additional innovations added to Ayurveda. This has resulted in sort of stagnation in Ayurveda and Siddha in particular. The practitioners of these systems were also became orthodox.

The oral traditions on the other hand continue to be dynamic and the innovative members of the community and thereby continuously enriched updated which impart the dynamic quality.

## 3.0 Intellectual Property Rights (IPR) and TM/TK

The Intellectual property is a class of property emanating from the activities of the human brain/intellect and just like any other property can have monopolistic ownership rights and are enforceable by legal rights developed in various jurisdictions. The IPR is essentially a concept and practice developed by industrialized western countries during the last two centuries to allow monopolistic ownership or control over intangible products. Such concept and practices are quite alien to third world nations particularly to the traditional communities. To them all the natural resources and the associated knowledge systems, innovation and practices of the indigenous and local communities are characterized as a body of knowledge integrated in a holistic world view. But in modern world where the technologically advanced countries of the world are marching fast and indiscriminately converting the resources and the associated knowledge into marketable commodities so in this process no communities in this world can escape its impact. Taking lead/s from traditional societies about the specific use of natural resources, the industrialized modern societies who are increasingly dominated by powerful corporate bodies employs researchers, inventors and technologists and manages to access the resources including TK and make marketable commodities but fail to acknowledge the traditional communities from whom they got the initial lead.

Historically the process of commoditization and trading of bioresources started about 3 centuries back when the Europeans reached the Biodiversity rich nations and colonized these countries and explored the bioresources. The colonial traders collected both the natural resources and the associated knowledge systems and with S&T intervention made value added commodities and marketed them even in the countries from where they collected the resources/raw materials. A world of trade and commerce evolved fast in the western world particularly with the discovery of coal and associated knowledge systems which made the western world richer and richer, pushing the source countries poorer and poorer. The industrial scale of production of value added products based on the raw materials and the associated knowledge of the traditional societies led to a destructive extraction of the bioresources which undermined the ecological security and stability of biodiversity rich third world nations as well as the livelihood security of the traditional communities of the Third world nations. The attractive attributes of the mass produced value added products from the factories of the developed nations attracted even the traditional communities and the efforts to procure them have driven such communities and countries into debt traps. This was the process by which the colonial powers exploited the national resources of the Biodiversity rich third world nations during the past 300 years and that made them rich driving the 3$^{rd}$ world in to poverty.

Just like any property, movable or immovable has to be protected in order to prevent from stealing the rights on the property created from the intellectual efforts are also to be protected from infringement. The results of such intellectual efforts have come to be known as Intellectual Property and the rights over them denote Intellectual Property Rights (IPR). IPR are of different types such as patents, designs, trademarks, copyrights etc. Out of these, patents are the most important and it embodies the creative strength through innovations. Medicinal knowledge can be protected by patents. For securing a patent the invention must be: (1) new and useful (novelty), (2) involve an inventive step (non obviousness) and (3) capable of industrial application (utility). Most of TM/TK may not strictly qualify these parameters for patent filing. At times TM could offer excellent leads based on which scientists could develop novel inventions and develop of novel therapeutics. Obtaining patents on medicinal plants used in TM need to satisfy the following. (1) It must be confidential information known to one person/family/community. (2) Specification about the combination of drugs (3) Mode of preparation–part used, pretreatment, if any and method of preparation and mode of presentation and application.

A patent is a grant given by the state in the form of a certificate for disclosing an invention by which certain exclusive rights are conferred on the patentee (proprietor) which can be exercised in the country which grants the rights for a limited period. Patent, therefore, is a property which like any other property, movable or immovable, may be bought, sold, assigned or licensed.

## 4.0 Misappropriation of TK/TM

The orally transmitted TK/TM is exposed to exploitation. In the absence of any written record, unscrupulous persons may access knowledge in a clandestine manner and may file patent and the patent examiner may find novelty and grant patent to individuals and the traditional knowledge holder may never come to know about it. In the case of TM/TK wherein the knowledge is documented, but not in a language known globally or published only in local language or a locally known journal or book and the patent examiner in another country is unable to access such documentation find it having novelty and may grant a patent. While the first is a case of piracy whereas the later case it is a case of granting a wrong patent. The granting of US patent to Turmeric is an instance of a wrong patent which was revoked by India's petition by providing documentary evidence on prior art on the turmeric use.

All unauthorized access to biological resources and associated TK and TM and patenting without compensation and knowledge of the knowledge holder is generally referred as bio piracy. Many instances of such bio piracies have been detected in recent times. Several examples are known where patents have been granted on applications which are based on codified TM like the Indian Systems of TM–like Ayurveda, Siddha, Unani and Amchi. It was against the above said background more particularly after the successful revoking of the US patent on Turmeric by CSIR that the Ministry of Health and Family Welfare jointly with CSIR established the Traditional Knowledge Digital Library (TKDL) in 1999. The TKDL project involve translations of the formulations involving medicinal plants included in the various citations contained in the classical text of Indian System of Medicine like Ayurveda, Siddha and Unani, into a digitized database in several international languages (English, Spanish, German, French, Japanese and Hindi). TKDL will give legitimacy to existing TK/TM and by ensuring case of retrieval of TM related information by patent examiners and thereby prevent granting of patents.

TKDL classified the entire TM related information contained in Ayurveda in a modern system as per the format of International Patent Classification (IPC) into sections, classes, subclasses, main groups and subgroups. This classification system evolved by India is known as Traditional Knowledge Resource Classification (TKRC). TKRC has been developed for Ayurveda, Unani and Siddha systems of medicine where about 8000 subgroups have been created for classifying the codified (published) TK/TM informations particularly with respect to Indian Systems of Medicine. TKRC is now recognized by the experts of IPC Union and WIPO. TKDL is a proprietary database made available to patent offices for preventing misappropriation and for collaborative research for positive protection of IP of oral tradition.

## 5.0 Protection of Innovations

Protection of all innovations through patenting or through other suitable method as per the *sui generis* model suggested in TRIPs (Article 27.3 (b)) is considered to be an important instrument for innovation and industrial development. The segments namely the government, the industry, the R and D institutions including the universities, the political system and the public are to work together to assist any country to frame law relating to the protection of IP to strike a balance between privatization of inventions to reward the inventors and concurrently to provide protection to public interest factors which in certain situations should be of paramount importance and should take dominance over inventors interest. Protection of inventions are well established instruments in industrial development, but all inventions cannot be or should not be protected due to various reasons such as strategic considerations (inventions related to countries defence etc.) or due to other reasons such as those areas which are contrary to public morale or ethics (inventions related to human body, cruelty to animals). Reasons for categorization of such areas vary from country to country and cannot be universalized. Generally, all countries exclude from patenting, the discoveries and scientific theories and laws, methods of performing mental acts, all kinds of magic, mere discovery of natural products and process of production of new substances by using essentially biological processes, aesthetic creation, carrying on or performing business by various complex but innovative methods and usually all novel processes the applications of which produce better or economically more valuable living objects. During the last 2-3 decades many countries have included patenting many of the earlier excluded patentable inventions such as patenting of microorganisms, animals and plants. The scope of ethics and morale has also been narrowed down considerably.

TRIPs would require protection of microorganisms by patents. But the definition of microorganisms would have to be settled. Microorganisms as per classical definition are independently existing single celled or multi cellular small organisms not visible to naked eye but can be seen under an ordinary microscope or electron microscope. But many countries have stretched the definition of microorganisms to cover cell lines, monoclonal cells or tissues, bits of DNA/genes isolated from higher organisms that can function independently to produce products which have industrial application. Such stretching of definitions including higher organisms like animals/humans is at best kept out of the definitions of microorganisms. Patentability of human genes and gene sequences are however, affirmed in the industrialized world provided their utility has been identified in industry and commerce.

## 6.0 Convention on Biological Diversity (CBD) and World Trade Organization (WTO)

Convention of Biological Diversity (CBD) signed by UN member countries in June 1992 at Rio for the first time agreed that Biodiversity and associated knowledge system is the sovereign properties of the nation/state and that nobody can access it without the prior approval of the competent authority of the country and its people. CBD also mandates that when utilization of knowledge, innovations and practices of local and indigenous communities leads to benefits, such benefits shall be equitably shared with the holders of such knowledge, innovations and practices.

Article 8(j) of the CBD states that Contracting parties shall:

(*i*) *Respect, preserve and maintain* knowledge, innovations and practices of indigenous and local communities embodying traditional lifestyles relevant for the conservation and sustainable use of biological diversity;

(*ii*) Promote their wider application *with the approval and involvement* of the holders of such knowledge, innovations and practices; and

(*iii*) Encourage the *equitable sharing of the benefits* arising from the utilization of such knowledge, innovations and practices.

Article 16(5) of the CBD mandates the Contracting Parties to co-operate and to ensure that IPRs are supportive of and do not run counter to the objectives of the CBD.

In their present form, IPR regimes fail to address equity, as proposed in the CBD. IPR laws proceed on a simplistic premise of the public and private domain, where the public domain, the property of none, is the common heritage for all. The vast body of specialized, community-specific traditional knowledge is considered to be in the public domain and can be used freely. The CBD attempts to redress the situation, although in the past five years, it has only led to a desperate grouping for solutions, and reams of paper of drafts and redrafts. Today, we are still far from any answer. On the other hand, the developments in the arena of IPR law and the attempt to attain certain common standards through TRIPS are progressing rapidly.

## 7.0 Conflicts Between CBD and WTO

Less than a year *i.e.*, about six months after the CBD came into force, the World Trade Organization (WTO) was established with quite different agenda. The Trade Related Aspects of Intellectual Property Rights (TRIPs) Agreement of WTO threatens to make the CBD impossible to implement. TRIPs was expressly designed to ensure that IPRs could be universally applied to all technologies, especially those which had previously been declared unsuitable for monopoly rights at the national level. These include pharmaceutical products and biological materials such as plants and microorganisms, all of which now are eligible for private property rights by IPRs. The very idea of extending patents to biodiversity was strongly resisted by developing countries during the GATT negotiations. This was based on the evidence that monopolies in the areas of food and health harm the interests of the world's poor, and efforts to conserve and make genetic resources available to present and future generations.

The new commercial opportunities opened up through the developments in biotechnology, particularly in genetic engineering have resulted engaging in a massive campaign to wrest market control over biodiversity through the patent system. The trading interest reflected in WTO has overridden two basic assumptions which are fundamental to the CBD.

The first is that the Intellectual Property is a matter of national sovereignty and policy, because it established monopolies and monopolies are, de facto, dangerous. Historically, countries have taken great care with their national IPR systems in order to protect the balance between private incentives and the public interest. The possibility of doing so is now forfeited to service the imperative of the TRIPs argument.

The second assumption is that life forms are part of the public domain. Biodiversity represents a cultural and ecological heritage, developed over generations and upon which our collective survival depends. Subjecting this heritage to a legal regime of commercial monopoly rights under TRIPs will destroy the conditions for its conservation and sustainable use, especially by the communities and thereby destroy society's access to diverse foods and medicine.

TRIPs requires countries to provide patents on products or processes from any field of technology which are new, represents an inventive step and are capable of industrial application. There are however, a few exception to this rule as provided in Article 27, 3(b) of TRIPs which states "Members may also exclude from patentability: plants and animals other than micro-organisms, and essentially biological processes for the production of plants and animals other than non-biological and micro-biological processes. However, members shall provide for the protection of 'plant varieties either by patents or by an effective "*Sui generis* system".

The relationship between the TRIPs Agreement and CBD and the multifaceted and complex Convention of Parties (COP) are now meeting to iron out the conflicts and contradictions and come out with a pragmatic solutions that will be in the best interest of the conservation of biodiversity and welfare of humankind as a whole. Since majority of the nations of the world are party to both CBD and WTO, it can work out a mutually supportive relationship between CBD and WTO and to avoid conflicts. Developing countries have expressed concern over the lack of clarity on the criteria or rationale used to determine the exclusions in Article 27.3(b). The first issue is the distinction between plants and animals (which may be excluded) and microorganisms (which may not be excluded). But now the definition microorganism is variously defined and now many developed nations consider single cells (embryo, sperm), tissues, genes, DNA etc. isolated from plants and animals including human beings are covered under micro-organisms. Also, the recent effort to develop germination control or the so called 'terminator' technologies has led to another great debate. Some corporate Hybrid seed companies in the North want to employ germination control as a method for intellectual property protection tool which then require farmers to buy new seeds every season.

Developing countries are also seeking to develop a suitable solution to implement relevant provisions of the CBD, especially those dealing with traditional knowledge and overall access to genetic resources. Developing countries are seeking intellectual property registration systems that would identify and document the sources of genetic material and also extent IPR to traditional knowledge system, particularly those of the indigenous communities in line with the Article 8(j), Article 10(c) and Article 15(7) of CBD.

In India we can be proud of having the distinction of the first country in experimenting a benefit sharing model that implemented in letter and spirit of Article 8(j) and Article 15.7 of CBD. The author and his team while at Tropical Botanic Garden and Research Institute (TBGRI) demonstrated that indigenous knowledge system merits support, recognition and fair and adequate compensation. Based on lead obtained from a Kani tribe of Kerala, the author and his co-workers developed an antifatigue, immuno-enhancing herbal formulation named 'Jeevani'. The technology of production of this drug when transferred to a pharmaceutical company on payment of license fee and a royalty of 2 per cent on the ex-factory sale of product, TBGRI resolved to share 1:1 of the license fee and royalty with the Kani tribe. Currently this model is acclaimed as a model to be emulated in similar situation elsewhere in the world. Although this model was worked out in early 1994 in full consultation with the Kani tribe it took almost 3-4 years to effect this model mainly because of the inherent inability of the 'Kani' people to receive the benefit. Finally, majority of Kani tribe resolved to form a Trust which was then registered and in February, 1999 the license fee and royalty due to them was transferred to the Trust. The trust continue to receive the royalties and the license fee accrued from the drug/s developed from their knowledge of a lesser known wild plant. [Anand (1998), Anuradha (1998), Bagla (1999), Gupta (1999), Gupta (2002), and Mashelkar (2001)]

## References

Anand, U. 1998. The Wonder Drug, UBS Publishers Ltd., New Delhi.

Anuradha, R.V. 1998. Sharing with the Kanis; a case study from Kerala, India, Benefit-Sharing case studies, Fourth Meeting of the Conference of Parties to the CBD, Bratislava, May, Secretariat of the Convention on Biological Diversity, Montreal.

Bagla, P. 1999. Model Indian deal generates payments. Science 283: 1614-1615.

Gupta, A.K. 1999. Conserving Biodiversity and Rewarding Associated Knowledge and Innovation Systems: Honey Bee Perspective. Paper presented at First Commonwealth Science Forum–Access, Bioprospecting, Intellectual Property Rights and Benefit Sharing and the Commonwealth, Goa, 23-25 September 1999.

Gupta, A.K. 2002. Value addition to local Kani tribal knowledge: patenting, licensing and benefit sharing, W.P.No. 2002-08-02, August 2002, A case study based on the data collected from kani tribe, Kerala, India.

Mashelkar, R.A. 2001. Intellectual Property Rights and the Third World, Current Science 81: 955-965.

## Chapter 4

# Regulation of Herbal Healthcare Products

**Tuley De Silva**
*Link Natural Products (Pvt.) Ltd., Sri Lanka*
*E-mail: tuleyd@hotmail.com*

## ABSTRACT

Points out that any drug has to be safe, efficacious and of good quality and in this concern Regulations have to be in place to satisfy these requirements for modern drugs. Drugs have to be registered by the Regulatory authorities of countries after evaluating dossiers submitted by the manufacturer containing a lot of valid information on tests conducted, clinical trials, quality control methods etc. Quality must be assured from the selection of propagation material to the final product and up to the time of use. Hence stringent standards have been enforced on the quality of raw materials, processes, and finished products. Here the author describes regulations and standardization of herbal healthcare products in some countries. Important information on the regulatory requirements for some countries is summarized which has been abstracted from the relevant websites.

***Keywords:*** *Natural herbal health products, Efficacy, Quality, Registration, Regulations, Standardization, Good Manufacturing Practices, Sri Lanka, Australia, Canada, United States, India, Thailand, European Union.*

## Introduction

Many Traditional medicines are complex mixtures of hundreds of compounds as they contain combined extracts of many plants. The plant source, conditions of growth, harvest time and post-harvest treatment will certainly affect the presence and concentration of bioactive constituents, which together with process technology and formulation will determine the quality and efficacy of herbal medicines.

In this context, let me define Natural Herbal Health Products (NHP) as over-the-counter products, made available for self-care and self-selection such as vitamins, herbal remedies, homeopathic medicines, traditional medicines, probiotics and other products like amino acids and essential fatty acids. Some of these are also termed Nutraceuticals and defined as:

*"Dietary supplements, as well as foods and beverages that claim or suggest to consumers specific health benefits beyond basic nutrition, including prevention of diseases."*

Nutraceuticals can be classified as being general dietary aids, performance enhancers, specific maintenance products, specific prevention products and curative supplements.

Any drug has to be safe, efficacious and of good quality. Regulations are in place to satisfy these requirements for modern drugs. Drugs have to be registered by the Regulatory authorities of countries after evaluating dossiers submitted by the manufacturer containing a lot of valid information on tests conducted, clinical trials, quality control methods etc.

Many countries do not require such detailed information for registration or licensing of herbal products. But the following are concerns that have to be considered and examined before granting licences for sale as herbal healthcare products:

- Classification of herbal medicines
- Safety of herbal medicines
- Efficacy of herbal medicines
- Quality of herbal medicines
- Substantiation of label claims
- Good Manufacturing Practices (GMP)
- Pharmacovigilance–Adverse Drug Reactions (ADR)
- Regulation & Registration system
- Manufacture, Marketing, Sale & Transport
- Control of advertisements
    - Pharmacopoeia compliance
    - Post marketing surveillance

The above stringent requirements are somewhat relaxed when applied to NHPs as these are not for cure of diseases. The efficacy has not been established through clinical trials as these products have been used as traditional medicines for several centuries. Hence much emphasis is laid on safety and quality rather than efficacy. As and Over-the-Counter (OTC) products, these have to substantiate label claims through continued use for decades. What has been strictly implemented is the reporting of adverse reactions to the authorities. The extents to which these requirements are applied vary from one regulatory authority to another. Most countries have some type of registration process and licensing.

As a safety requirement, these products should not present "a significant or unreasonable risk of illness or injury". Long traditional use without side effects of products prepared by the traditional method is sometimes accepted as safety clearance. Some times toxicity studies are required.

Quality must be assured from the selection of propagation material to the final product and up to the time of use. Hence stringent standards have been enforced on the quality of raw materials, processes, and finished products. Production and packaging have to be done in conformity with good manufacturing practices. All procedures must adhere to Standard Operating Procedures (SOP).

## Standardization

Standardization of traditional medicine or an herbal healthcare product is necessary to establish consistency and reproducibility of a particular extract to ensure guaranteed potency through acceptable levels of active compounds. This process can be carried out chemically, spectroscopically or biologically and currently involves complicated and complex procedures. Standardization will also be necessary to implement quality control, ensure batch wise consistency and uniformity of dosage, check stability for expiration dating and detect substandard or adulterated drugs and determine contaminant levels.

Good Manufacturing Practices (GMP) is a system for ensuring that products are consistently produced and controlled according to quality standards and to minimize any risks involved in any pharmaceutical production that can not be eliminated through testing the final product. GMP covers all aspects of production from the starting materials, premises and equipment to the training and personal hygiene of staff, Standard Operating Procedures, work environment, quality assurance, packaging, storage and waste disposal. There should be records to trace any product and lot or batch samples for checking stability and recall reporting.

Some of the parameters used in quality assessment are given below:

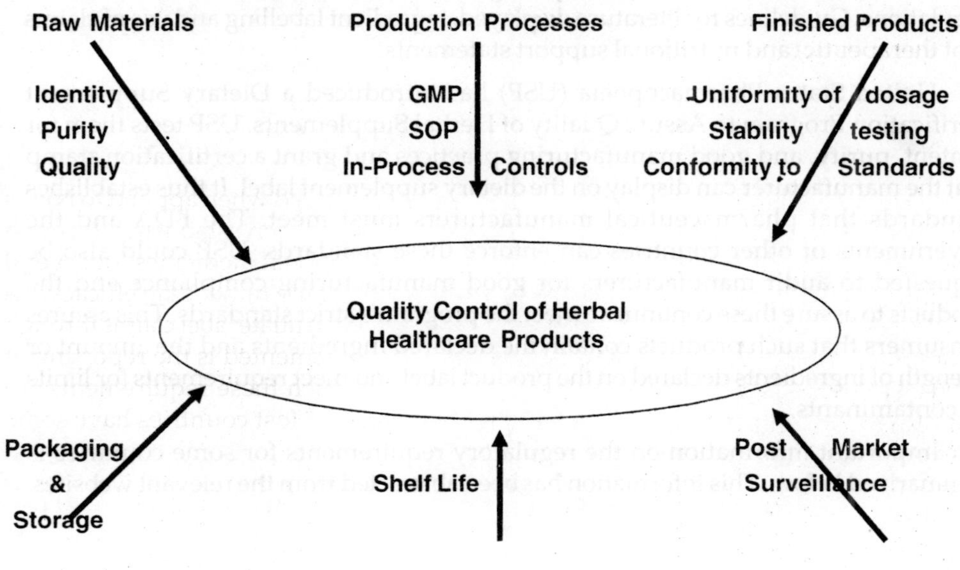

Labelling and product information of products should be in accordance with regulations and should not mislead the consumers. This requirement is strictly enforced.

The following information has to be displayed on the label panels

1. The product name.
2. The dosage form.
3. The net amount in the immediate container (by weight, volume, or number, as appropriate).
4. Identity of the product as a traditional medicine.
5. The quantities in weight of the ingredients per dosage unit
6. The product's recommended purpose or use; Must be a traditional purpose or use stated in a manner that is consistent with traditional indications and in conformity with the medical discipline in which purpose or use is established.
7. The recommended dose, including the route of administration.
8. The recommended duration of use, if any.
9. A statement that instructs consumers to seek advice from a qualified health care provider, if symptoms or conditions persist.
10. Any contraindications or warnings
11. The name and address of the marketer or manufacturer.
12. A batch or lot number.
13. A shelf life date
14. Recommended storage conditions, if any.

A framework for assuring quality and safety has to be established detailing Guidelines for Evaluation of Efficacy, Regulation for Quality of Medicines, GMP regulations, Guidelines for literature displayed, ingredient labelling and use of claims (not therapeutic) and nutritional support statements.

United States Pharmacopoeia (USP) has introduced a Dietary Supplement Verification Program to Assure Quality of Herbal Supplements. USP tests them for content, purity, and good manufacturing practices and grant a certification stamp that the manufacturer can display on the dietary supplement label. It thus establishes standards that pharmaceutical manufacturers must meet. The FDA and the governments of other countries can enforce these standards. USP could also be requested to audit manufacturers for good manufacturing compliance and the products to assure these continue to meet the program's strict standards. This assures consumers that such products contain the declared ingredients and the amount or strength of ingredients declared on the product label and meet requirements for limits on contaminants.

Important information on the regulatory requirements for some countries is summarized below. This information has been abstracted from the relevant websites.

Fōr authentic and exact requirements and more detailed information, please refer the websites, some of which have been listed at the end of this paper.

## Australia

All medicinal products are regulated through the Australian Therapeutic Goods Act of 1989. The overall objective of the Act is to ensure the quality, safety, efficacy, and timely availability of therapeutic goods. The ACT is administered by the Therapeutic Goods Administration (TGA) of the Commonwealth Department of Health and Aged Care. All therapeutic goods (TG) which includes herbal healthcare products as well, sold in Australia must be registered on the Australian Register of Therapeutic Goods (ARTG).

The Act Controls the standard of all ingredients used in manufacture, advertising and label claims for products, Registration of Product(s) on the Australian Register of Therapeutic Goods (ARTG), manufacturing and packaging conditions and controls (GMP).

### Australian Register of Therapeutic Goods (ARTG)

Registered medicines are classified as higher risk and low risk. The high risk ones are assessed individually for quality, safety and efficacy and should be manufactured under GMP. Low risk ones are called Listed medicines and contain ingredients permitted by the TGA for use in low risk medicines restricted to indication and claims relating to health maintenance, health enhancement or non-serious, self-limiting conditions. These are not assessed individually for efficacy, but must certify to the TGA they hold evidence to support all indications and claims made for their products. These too should be manufactured under Good Manufacturing Practice (GMP) as other medicines and requires Post-market regulatory activities, including reporting of adverse reactions, audit of manufacturers and laboratory testing.

LISTING and an AUSTL number is granted to products successfully satisfying the following criteria:

- Pharmacopoeial standards for starting materials.
- Compliance to GMP manufacturing requirements.
- Claims within Advertising Code guidelines.
- Formulation approval by TGA.
- Products satisfy prescribed TGOs / Aust Standards.
- Active ingredients are prescribed in the Regulations.

Though a LISTING does not specifically require submission of efficacy or stability data, TGA reserves the right to call for this data.

Australian Code of Good Manufacturing Practice for Therapeutic Goods (Medicinal Products) 1990 deals with manufacturing and packaging conditions. GMP involves attaining an acceptable standard of premises, personnel, process control and documentation.

The regulatory processes of the TGA include three key elements.

**I. Licensing and Audit of Manufacturers**

Manufacturers have to obtain a manufacturing licence, show compliance with the Australian Code of GMP which is ascertained by conducting pre-licensing audits and regular on-site audits.

**II. Pre-market Assessment**

In the pre-market assessment the following factors are considered:

- The toxicity of the ingredients
- The dosage form of the medicine
- Whether the medicine is indicated for a serious disease
- Whether for the treatment, cure, management or prevention of a disease
- Significant side effects including interactions with other medicines
- Any adverse effects from prolonged use or inappropriate self-medication.

Listed medicines may only contain ingredients that have been evaluated by the TGA to be low risk. TGA has a list of substances that may be used as active ingredients in Listed medicines. The safety of ingredients for use and Quality standards for ingredients acceptable to the TGA are given in Therapeutic Goods Orders (TGO).

The Therapeutic Goods Act 1989 requires that at the time of Listing, sponsors must certify that they hold information or evidence to support any claim that the applicant makes relating to the medicine. All indications and claims made about therapeutic goods must be capable of substantiation - that is, evidence must be held by sponsors which demonstrate the indications and claims are true, valid and not misleading.

The Australian Regulatory Guidelines for Complementary Medicines (ARGCM) contains guidance on the criteria for compositional guidelines. A *compositional guideline* is a summary of descriptions, tests and limits that defines the composition and relevant characteristics of the substance (www.tga.gov.au/docs/html/argcm.htmdvice).

These guidelines have been developed to assist sponsors in determining the appropriate evidence to support indications and claims made in relation to Listable medicines. In particular, they relate to complementary medicines, sunscreens and other Listable medicines. Where the claims/indications do not appear to be consistent with the evidence guidelines, the TGA may request the sponsors to submit full text copies of all relevant reference materials for evaluation.

Sponsors should also make reference to the Australian Regulatory Guidelines for Complementary Medicines (ARGCM) www.tga.gov.au/docs/html/argcm.htm for further advice in relation to the evidence requirements to support the indications and claims for Listable medicines. Specifically, ARGCM Part II – Listed Complementary Medicines (www.tga.gov.au/docs/html/argcm.htm#argcmp2, Section 6.2.2.)

Advice for sponsors in relation to the registration of complementary medicines is included in ARGCM Part I -Registration of Complementary Medicines www.tga.gov.au/docs/html/argcm.htm#argcmp1, Sections 4.1.3 and 7.3.

The Guidelines on levels and kinds of evidence to support claims on therapeutic goods offers advice on the level (general, medium and high) of an indication or claim and the evidence required to support it. Registered medicines can carry claims of any level, provided the TGA has evaluated the evidence to support the indication(s) and approved the indication(s) for the Registered medicine. (Guidelines for levels and kinds of evidence to support indications and claims- PDF)

**III. Post-market Regulatory Activity**

Post-market regulatory activities include targeted and random desk-based audits of Listed products, monitoring of adverse reactions to complementary medicines, targeted and random laboratory testing of products and ingredients, targeted and random surveillance in the market place, an effective, responsive and timely recalls procedure, audit of GMP, effective controls for the advertising of therapeutic goods, adverse drug reaction reporting and monitoring adverse reactions to complementary medicines.

As part of providing assurance that medicines are of high quality and safety, the TGA has a post-market monitoring program for monitoring the safety of complementary medicines. This includes monitoring reports of suspected adverse reactions, and testing of complementary medicines for quality, including heavy metal content.

Advertisements to the general public (e.g. newspapers, magazines, television and radio) must be pre-approved prior to their publication or broadcast. 'Advertisement' includes any statement, pictorial representation or design, however made, that is intended, whether directly or indirectly, to promote the use or supply of the goods (Therapeutic Goods Act 1989). Advertising should be in accordance with the Therapeutic Goods Advertising Code (TGAC) 2005 (www.comlaw.gov.au) and the supporting Regulations, Trade Practices Act 1974 and other relevant laws. This is to ensure that the marketing and advertising of therapeutic goods to consumers is conducted in a socially responsible manner that promotes the quality use of therapeutic goods and does not mislead or deceive the consumer.

Traditional Medicines such as Ayurvedic and Chinese medicines are classified as 'complementary medicines', and are generally required to meet the same standards of quality and safety as other modern medicines. In consultation with industry, the TGA has developed the Australian Regulatory Guidelines for Complementary Medicines (ARGCM) to assist sponsors of complementary medicines to meet their legislative obligations.

Once a therapeutic claim is made or implied, then the goods become therapeutic and subject to the requirements of the Australian Therapeutic Goods Act 1989. The manufacturing and packaging conditions are detailed in the Australian Code of Good Manufacturing Practice for Therapeutic Goods (Medicinal Products) 1990.

Complementary medicines in Australia are not subject to the standards and guidelines of the Codex Alimentarius Commission.

References to assist in meeting regulatory obligations in Australia

- Therapeutics Goods Act 1989 (the Act) www.comlaw.gov.au
- Therapeutic Goods Regulations 1990 (the Regulations) www.comlaw.gov.au>
- Australian Regulatory Guidelines for Complementary Medicines (ARGCM) www.tga.gov.au/docs/html/argcm.htm
- Australian Code of Good Manufacturing Practice (GMP) for Medicinal Products

  www.tga.gov.au/docs/html/gmpcodau.htm
- Substances that may be used in 'Listed' medicines in Australia
- Advertising therapeutic products
- Analytical procedure validation for complementary medicines
- Compositional guidelines
- Guidelines for levels and kinds of evidence to support indications and claims
- Labelling and packaging therapeutic products
- Pharmacovigilance and reporting adverse drug reactions
- Stability testing of Listed complementary medicines

## Canada

The Canadian Government has entrusted Health Canada to control the registration of herbal products through a body called the Natural Health Products Directorate (NHPD). The objective being to provide safe, effective and of high quality Natural Health Products (NHP) and prevent adverse effects to consumers.

NHPD assists in the development of safety standards and guidelines and regulates by conducting investigations, inspections, seizures, recalls and prosecutions. It also provides importers, manufacturers and distributors with technical information to promote safe and the responsible use of products and publishes product advisories, warnings and recalls. Post marketing surveillance is carried out on consumer products in the market.

Natural Health Product Directorate has established Natural Health Products Regulations to cover herbal remedies, homeopathic medicines, vitamins, traditional medicines, probiotics, amino acids and essential fatty acids. The regulations include provisions on Product licensing, Site licensing, GMP, Adverse Reaction reporting, Clinical trials and Labelling.

All natural health products require a product license. Information on the product, including medicinal ingredients, source, potency, non-medicinal ingredients and recommended uses has to be supplied. If a product licence number is preceded by the distinct letters NPN then the product has been reviewed and approved by Health Canada for safety and efficacy.

A Site licence is required to manufacture, package, label, and import for sale any natural health product. The manufacturing has to be done in conformity with Good Manufacturing Practices to ensure product safety and quality. GMP also includes appropriate standards and practices regarding product manufacture, storage, handling and distribution.

GMP covers specifications on premises & equipment, personnel, sanitation program, operational procedures, quality assurance, stability studies, record keeping, lot or batch sampling and recall reporting.

Adverse Drug Reaction Reporting is statutory based on risk assessment and the corresponding management of risks so that advisories, where appropriate, to the public could be issued. The Natural Health Products Regulations require that product licence holders monitor all adverse reactions and report serious adverse reactions to Health Canada.

In case of nontraditional products, Clinical trials are required to establish the product's clinical, pharmacological or pharmacodynamic effects, to identify any adverse events related to its use, to study its absorption, distribution, metabolism and excretion and to determine its safety and efficacy.

Labelling requirements are very stringent to ensure consumers can make informed choices. Label should include the product name, ingredients and the composition, quantity of product in the bottle, recommended conditions of use, health claim, dosage form, route of administration, Dose, any cautionary statements, contra-indications, ADR and storage conditions.

## Guidelines for Traditional Herbal Medicine Registration and Manufacture in Canada

- www.hc-sc.gc.ca
- Natural Health Products Regulations (SOR/2003-196) June 18, 2003 Regulations Amending the Natural Health Products Regulations (Special Access) (SOR/2004-119) June 2, 2004
- Regulations Amending Certain Regulations Made under the Food and Drugs Act–Project 1539 (SOR/2007-288) December 27, 2007
- Compliance Policy for Natural Health Products,
- Natural Health Products Compliance Guide.
- Natural Health Products Regulations

## European Union

The European Union has harmonized regulations for the marketing of herbal medicinal products and issued the Traditional Herbal Medicinal Products Directive (THMPD). The Directive allows the licensing and over-the-counter sale of herbal products that have a history of use anywhere in the world for at least 30 years, 15 of which must be in an EU Member State. The European Medicines Evaluation Agency (EMEA) issued Guideline on Specifications, Test Procedures and Acceptance, Criteria for Herbal Substances, Herbal Preparations and Herbal Medicinal Products in 2005 used to assure the quality, determined by the quality of the starting plant material, development, in-process controls, good manufacturing practice (GMP) controls, and process controls, and by specifications applied to them throughout development and manufacture.

According to the Medicines (Traditional Herbal Medicinal Products for Human Use) Regulations 2005, no traditional herbal medicinal product shall be placed on the market or distributed by way of wholesale, unless a traditional herbal registration has been obtained in accordance with the relevant Community provisions by the licensing authority.

An application for the grant of a traditional herbal registration shall include a statement indicating whether the herbal medicinal product is one that should be available only from a pharmacy or on general sale. The manufacturers will have to apply for a license for every product, and each must comply with the official published standards.

The 30-year rule also demands that traditional herbal medicinal product must be shown to have been in use for 30 years in the EU (or at least 15 years in the EU and 15 years elsewhere). Medicinal indications permitted are given in the annexes to the guidance (Medicines and Healthcare products Regulatory AgencyMHRA Website) *e.g.* "Difficulties falling asleep" is permitted but "Chronic Insomnia" is not.

## Labelling and Patient Information Leaflet (PIL)

The requirements for labelling and patient information are given in the MHRA Guidance Note 25: 'Best Practice Guidance on the labelling and packaging of medicines'. The label should include name of the product, strength, pharmaceutical form, quantity of active ingredients, posology, method of administration, indications, contraindications, excipients, shelf life and any special warnings and precautions for use etc.

Summary of Product Characteristics (SPC) : A Guideline on Summary of Product Characteristics (external link to the European Commission (Pharmaceuticals) website)

Safety and traditional use evidence from experts should be presented in a curriculum vitae format. Quality should be supported with a technical dossier covering the quality of herbal ingredients and the finished herbal product including details of all the necessary physico-chemical, biological and microbiological tests covering residual solvents, pesticide residues, microbial limits and heavy metal residues. Please see 'Guidance notes' section in the website.

A finished product specification will be required for your finished herbal products. A summary of stability studies undertaken (conditions, batches, analytical procedures) results and conclusions, the proposed storage condition and shelf life will be required. The Committee for Proprietary Medicinal Products (CPMP) guideline for stability testing of existing active substances and related finished products may assist you when considering stability aspects of your product dossier.

A finished product specification will be required for your finished herbal products and stability data of your product to support the proposed shelf life. A summary of stability studies undertaken (conditions, batches, analytical procedures) results and conclusions, the proposed storage condition and shelf life will be required. The CPMP guideline for stability testing of existing active substances and related finished products may assist you when considering stability aspects of your product dossier.

## Safety

Safety has to be established by submitting a bibliographic review of safety data together with an expert report. The expert will need to comment on both non-clinical and clinical aspects of safety. The expert can be a registered doctor, registered pharmacist, or, other scientifically qualified individual with relevant competence, for example, toxicologist, herbal practitioner who is a member of a professional body that is working towards the statutory regulation of the herbal medicine profession; or registered herbal practitioner.

## Traditional use

As covered in the 'Key requirements' section, the application will need to be accompanied by bibliographic or expert evidence that the medicinal product or a corresponding product has been in medicinal use throughout a period of 30 years. The new European Committee, the Committee on Herbal Medicinal Products (HMPC), will establish the European positive list, provided for in Directive 2004/24/EC.

### Inspections

All sites named on a wholesale dealer's licence are subject to regular inspections every three years. (MHRA Guidance Note 6, 'Notes for applicants and holders of a wholesale dealer's licence').

### Qualified Persons

All holders of a manufacturer's import licence for relevant products are required to have available the services of a Qualified Person (QP). The QP must be a resident in the UK and must be named on the manufacturer's import licence. (Article 1(2) of Directive 2004/24/EC applies Articles 49-52 of Directive 2001/83/EC to the importation of relevant products).

The EU Directive on Traditional Herbal Medicinal Products (agreed in April 2004) came into force on 30th October 2005. The Directive requires traditional, over-the-counter herbal remedies to be made to assured standards of safety and quality and in conformity with regulations so that these are standardized across Europe.

## Guidelines for Traditional Herbal Medicine Registration and Manufacture

- www.medicinescomplete.com/mc/herbals/current/1000727368.
- www.iospress.metapress.com/index/940H1FB3TXHU46HX.pdf
- www.medicinescomplete.com/mc/herbals/current/1000727368.

- www.who.int/medicinedocs
- www.medicines.mhra.gov.uk
- Guidance for Retailers, Wholesalers, Importers and Manufactures on Registering Herbal Medicine under the THMR scheme
  http://www.mhra.gov.uk/home/idcplg?IdcService=GET_FILE&dDocName=con2030651& RevisionSelectionMethod=Latest
- Consolidated Guidance on Transitional arrangements for the Directive on traditional herbal medicinal products (Directive 2004/24/EC, amending Directive 2001/83/EC) http://www.mhra.gov.uk/home/idcplg?IdcService=GET_FILE&dDocName=con009362&Revision SelectionMethod=Latest
- Guidance on regulation of unlicensed herbal medicines made up by a 3rd party for use by practitioner in a one to one consultation: arrangements pending possible reform regulation (July 2006of)

  http://www.mhra.gov.uk/home/idcplg?IdcService=GET_FILE&dDocName=con 2024066&RevisionSelectionMethod=Latest
- Guidance for Retailers, Wholesalers, Importers and Manufactures on Registering Herbal Medicine under the THMR scheme

  http://www.mhra.gov.uk/home/idcplg?IdcService=GET_FILE&dDocName=con2030651&RevisionSelectionMethod=Latest
- Traditional Herbal Medicine Registration (THMR)

  Directive 2004/24/EC of the European Parliament and of the Council of 31 March 2004 Amending, as Regards Traditional Herbal Medicinal Products, Directive 2001/83/EC on the Community Code Relating to Medicinal Products for Human Use
- Guidance on Specifications: Test Procedures and Acceptance Criteria for Herbal Substances, Herbal Preparations, and Herbal Medicinal Products/ Traditional Herbal Medicinal Products
- Guideline on Quality of Herbal Medicinal Products/Traditional Herbal Medicinal Products

## United States America

In the United States, herbal products can be marketed without FDA approval only as food supplements without specific health claims. The overall strategy is to ensure that products are safe and wholesome, their labelling is truthful and not misleading so that the consumers can make informed and appropriate health care choices.

USA passed the Dietary Supplement Health and Education Act (DSHEA) of 1994 to cover the sale of dietary health supplements. The preamble of DSHEA states.

*"There is a link between the ingestion of certain nutrients or dietary supplements and the prevention of chronic diseases such as cancer, heart disease, and osteoporosis..."*

DSHE Act authorises the Secretary of Health and Human Services, and the FDA to issue regulations on dietary supplements and current Good Manufacturing Practices (cGMPs). Companies are expected to provide truthful non-misleading scientific research of health benefits from the use of specific dietary supplements. FDA will have the authority to determine standards that firms should apply in production and labelling. Under DSHEA, manufacturers have to substantiate the safety and efficacy of the dietary ingredients, produce unadulterated and properly labelled dietary supplements, substantiate any claims made about their products by adequate evidence to show that they are not false or misleading. This requires the product to be free from microbiological, pesticide, and heavy metal contamination and adulteration. The consumers should have confidence that the dietary supplement products they purchase contain the identity, purity, quality, strength, and composition that the label claims.

The act has made provisions to:

- Define dietary supplements and dietary ingredients;
- Establish a new framework for assuring safety;
- Outline guidelines for literature displayed where supplements are sold;
- Provide for use of claims and nutritional support statements;
- Ensure ingredient and nutrition labelling;
- Grant FDA the authority to establish current Good Manufacturing Practice (cGMP) regulations

The Act provided for the appointment of a Commission on Dietary Supplements to make recommendations on the regulation of label claims and statements for dietary supplements, procedures for the evaluation of the claims how best to provide truthful, scientifically valid, and not misleading information.

The act also provided for the establishment of an Office of Dietary Supplements to explore the potential role of supplements to improve health care, to promote scientific study of supplements and their value in preventing chronic diseases, to collect and compile a database of scientific research on supplements and individual nutrients and to serve as a scientific adviser to FDA.

FDA's Proposed Rule establishes cGMPs, helps reduce risks due to adulterated or misbranded dietary supplement products, establishes manufacturing standards to ensure that dietary supplements are consistent as to identify, purity, quality, strength, and composition.

cGMPs will help prevent product quality problems relating to over doses / lower doses, wrong ingredients, contaminants (e.g., microorganisms, pesticides, heavy metals), colour variation, tablet size or size variation, foreign material, improper packaging and mislabelling.

Under the cGMP proposed rule, manufacturers would be required to:

- Employ qualified employees;
- Design and construct their physical plant in a manner to protect from becoming adulterated during manufacturing, packaging and storage;

- Use equipment and utensils that are of appropriate design and construction for the intended use;
- Establish and use a quality control unit and master manufacturing and batch production records;
- Store and distribute materials used to manufacture, package and label and finished products under proper conditions of temperature, humidity, light and sanitation
- Keep a written record of each consumer product quality complaint related to CGMPs;
- Retain records for 3 years beyond the date of manufacture of the last batch of dietary ingredients or dietary supplements

## Label Claims

In USA, Herbal products labels cannot make statements to diagnose, prevent, mitigate, treat, or cure a specific disease. E.g. product may not carry the claim "cures diabetes" or "treats arthritis," but can make claims on the nutritional value or content of the product like "good source" and approved "health claims" between an ingredient and a disease or health-related condition. Statements not authorized by FDA are effects on "structure or function" of the body or the "well-being" but if they are truthful and not misleading and the product qualifies to bear the claim e.g. calcium may reduce the risk of osteoporosis.

The label also should bear the statement "THIS STATEMENT HAS NOT BEEN EVALUATED BY THE FOOD AND DRUG ADMINISTRATION. THIS PRODUCT IS NOT INTENDED TO DIAGNOSE, TREAT, CURE, OR PREVENT ANY DISEASE."

## Quality

The products should be manufactured under cGMPs established by the FDA for dietary supplements to ensure their safety during preparation, packing, storage and transport. In addition information on identity, authenticity, purity, the amount of active ingredient, uniformity of dosage, method of standardization, stability, date of expiry are obligatory to establish the quality of the product.

Dietary Supplement and Nonprescription Drug Consumer Protection Act. S.3546, H.R.6168 (2006). This new Act requires manufacturers of dietary supplements and over-the-counter (OTC) products to submit serious adverse event reports (SAERs) to the Food and Drug Administration including contact information on the labels of their products for consumers to use in reporting adverse events. Companies must further notify the FDA of any serious adverse event reports within 15 business days of receiving such reports. Adverse "serious adverse event" would be defined as any event resulting in death, a life-threatening experience, inpatient hospitalization, a persistent or significant disability or incapacity, or a congenital anomaly or birth defect, any adverse event requiring a medical or surgical intervention to prevent one of the aforementioned conditions, based on reasonable medical judgment.

Federal Trade Commission Act (FTC) has issued a guidance document entitled, "Dietary Supplements: An Advertising Guide for Industry" which requires substantiation that labelling and advertising claims are truthful and not misleading. To substantiate claim(s) being made, relationships of the evidence to the claim, quality of the evidence and the totality of the evidence have to be detailed.

The FTC standard of competent and reliable scientific evidence (FTC case law) states "tests, analyses, research, studies, or other evidence based on the expertise of professionals in the relevant area, that has been conducted and evaluated in an objective manner by persons qualified to do so, using procedures generally accepted in the profession to yield accurate and reliable results."

## Relationship of the Evidence to the Claim

Manufacturers have to submit studies appropriately specified and measured as to the nutritional deficiency, structure/function, or general well being that is the subject of the claim. The studies have to be based on a population that is similar to that which will be consuming the dietary supplement product young adults, but the product's claims involve conditions seen only in the elderly. The claim should accurately convey to consumers the extent, nature, or permanence of the effect achieved in the relevant studies and the level of scientific certainty for that effect.

## Quality of the Evidence

The scientific quality of studies should be based on several criteria including study population, study design, conditions (e.g., presence of a placebo control), data collection (e.g., dietary assessment method), statistical analysis and outcome measures. Design factors affecting the quality of a study, bias, and other limitations are lack of appropriate randomization and blinding, the number of subjects in the protocol vs. the number of subjects who actually participated in the trial, demographics, and adequacy of primary variables, compliance, control agent, dropouts, statistical procedures, subgroup analysis, safety issues, and reproducibility of results.

Information useful as background to support a claim can be animal studies, In vitro studies, testimonials and other anecdotal evidence, review articles, comments and letters to the Editor usually focussing on a particular issue or issues from a study, presentation at a meeting etc. and Product Monographs prepared by the manufacturer to convey specific information about a product such as its specifications.

In stating the evidence to support the claim one should consider the strength of the entire body of evidence, including criteria such as quality, quantity (number of various types of studies and sample sizes), consistency, relevance of exposure, and persuasiveness. The totality of the evidence has to support the claim(s). The factors that can be considered to establish whether information would constitute "competent and reliable scientific evidence" are the extent to which each study or evidence bear a relationship to the specific claim, strengths and weaknesses of the study's or evidence, the type of study, the design of the study, analysis of the results, and peer review. In case of multiple studies, they should use reliable methodologies suggesting a particular outcome.

Factors that contribute to higher quality studies include adequacy and clarity of the design, population studied, assessment of intervention or exposure and outcomes, Data Analysis and Peer Review.

## Guidelines for Traditional Herbal Medicine Registration and Manufacture

- www.faqs.org/nutrition/Diab-Em/Dietary-Supplements
- www.cfsan.fda.gov/
- www.fda.gov/consumer/updates/dietarysupps062207
- www.hhs.gov/asl/testify/t990325e
- Dietary Supplement and Nonprescription Drug Consumer Protection Act. S.3546, H.R.6168 (2006). Available at: www.govtrack
- www.ahpa.org/03_0828_DirectFinalRule_HoC2.pdf. Ingredient labelling of dietary supplements that contain botanicals Accessed December 2, 2005
- www.functionalfoodsjapan.com/

## India

Drugs & Cosmetic Act, 1940 includes provisions relating to Ayurvedic, Unani and Siddha Drugs in addition to modern drugs. An Ayurvedic, Unani and Siddha Drugs Technical Advisory Board and the Ayurvedic, Siddha and Unani Drugs Consultative Committee controls the registration and regulation of medicines. Information on labelling, packing and limit of alcohol in ayurvedic (including siddha) or unani drugs can be obtained from the website (www.indianmedicine.nic.in/html/pharma/apmain.htm).

Good Manufacturing Practices for Ayurvedic, Siddha and Unani Medicines are notified under Drugs & Cosmetic Act 1940 on 23rd June 2000

The Good Manufacturing Practices are prescribed to ensure that:

1. Raw materials used in the manufacture of drugs are authentic, of prescribed quality and are free from contamination
2. The manufacturing process is as has been prescribed to maintain the standards
3. Adequate quality control measures are adopted
4. The manufactured drug, which is released for sale, is of acceptable quality.

## Thailand

The Food and Drug Administration (FDA), under the Ministry of Public Health (MOPH), is the main agency in charge of drug approval and registration. Its main sections relating to pharmaceutical registration are:

1. Drug Products, under the Drug Control Division;
2. Import Licenses, under the Division of Manufacturing and Import Facilities Control;
3. Product Registration, under the Food Control Division;
4. Label Registration, is also under the Food Control Division.

Both manufacturers and importers are required to get a license to produce, sell or import any pharmaceutical products into Thailand.

Some International Organizations and Regulatory bodies of countries described in this text, which could provide more information on Regulatory aspects of Herbal Healthcare products

**WHO**

- WHO guidelines on Herbal medicines, intellectual property rights, quality & safety, technical co-operation and traditional medicines
- www.who.int/medicinedocs
- www.whqlibdoc.who.int/publications/2005/9241593237_part3.pdf
- www.searo.who.int/LinkFiles/Reports_TradMed82.pdf
- www.searo.who.int/LinkFiles/Reports_TradMed82.pdf

**ICH**

International Conference on Harmonization of Technical Requirements for the Registration of Pharmaceuticals for Human Use guidelines defining quality, safety, efficacy & related aspects for developing and registering new medicinal products in Europe, Japan and the United States

www.ich.org

**Codex Alimentarius**

International food standards and guidelines adopted by the Codex Alimentarius Commission under the Joint FAO / WHO Food Standards Programme

www.codexalimentarius.net

**WTO**

World Trade Organization (WTO), the global international organization dealing with the rules of trade between nations, TRIPS

www.wto.org

**EMEA**

European Medicines Agency (EMEA), a decentralized body of the European Union headquartered in London, prescribes guidelines for herbal products and medicines

www.emea.europa.eu

**US FDA**

Regulations, guidelines, US Food and Drug Administration

www.fda.gov, www.nutraingredients-usa.com

www.ayuherbal.com/usa_regulations.htm

**TGA**

Specifications regulating medicines, medical devices, herbal products, Australia products, issued by Therapeutic Goods Administration, the Australian regulatory body

www.tga.gov.au

**MHRA UK**

News, warnings, information and publications of Medicines and Healthcare products Regulatory Agency (MHRA), responsible for ensuring efficacy and safety of medicines and medical devices

www.mhra.gov.uk

**Health Canada**

Advisories, warnings, recalls, reports, publications, activities, legislations and guidelines from Health Canada, the Federal Department responsible for health related issues.

www.hc-sc.gc.ca

**CDSCO India**

Central Drugs Standard Control Organization (CDSCO), Ministry of Health & Family Welfare, Government of India provides general information about drug regulatory requirements in India

www.cdsco.nic.in

**Thai FDA**

Thai Food and Drug Administration laws and regulations with respect to drugs, food, cosmetics and narcotics

www.fda.moph.go.th

The Ministries, Departments and Regulatory bodies from where more information on licensing and regulatory requirements could be obtained

**Australia**

Therapeutic Goods Administration

www.tga.gov.au

**Belgium**

Directorate- General Medicinal Products, Belgium (DGMP)

www.efomp.org

**Bangladesh**

Ministry of Health The Drug Administration

www.mohfw.gov.bd

**Bhutan**

Ministry of Health; The Institute of Traditional Medicine Sciences

www.rub.edu.bt

**Brazil**

Ministry of Health

www.who.int/medicinedocs

**Canada**

Health Canada, the Federal Department responsible for health related issues in Canada

www.hc-sc.gc.ca

**China**

State Food and Drug Administration

www.sfda.gov.cn/eng

**Denmark**

Danish Medicines Agency

www.dkma.dk

**Egypt**

Ministry of Health, National Centre for Medicinal Plants

www.mohp.gov.eg

**Finland**

National Agency for Medicines

www.laakelaitos.fi

**France**

Agence Francaise De Securite Sanitaire Des Produits De Sante

afssaps.sante.fr

**Greece**

National Drug Organisation

www.eof.gr

**Hungary**

Drugs Control and Traditional Medicines Division of the National Institute of Health

www.enwhp.org

**India**

Central Drugs Standard Control Organization (CDSCO), Ministry of Health & Family Welfare, Government of India

www.cdsco.nic.in

**Indonesia**

National Agency of Drug and Food Control

www.pom.go.id

**Iran**

Ministry of Health, Department of Pharmaceutical Affairs

www.mohme.gov.ir

**Ireland**

Ministry of Health, Irish Medicines Board

www.dohc.ie, www.imb.ie

**Italy**

Dipartimento per la Valutazione dei Medicinali e la Farmacovigilanza

www.farmacovigilanza.org

**Japan**

Ministry Health & Welfare (Koseisho), Pharmaceuticals and Medical Devices Agency

www.mhlw.go.jp

**Malaysia**

National Pharmaceutical Control Bureau, Malaysia NPCB

www.bpfk.gov.my

**Myanmar**

Ministry of Health, Department of Traditional Medicine

www.moh.gov.mm

**Nepal**

Ministry of Health, Department of Ayurveda

www.moh.gov.np

**Netherlands**

Medicines Evaluation Board

www.brd.agro.nl

**New Zealand**

New Zealand Medicines and Medical Devices Safety Authority.

www.medsafe.govt.nz

**Nigeria**

National agency for Food Administration and Control (NAFDAC)

www.nafdacnigeria.org

**Norway**

Norwegian Medicines Agency

www.mericon.no, www.legemiddelverket.no

**Pakistan**

Ministry of Health, Drugs Control and Traditional Medicines Division of the National Institute of Health

www.dcomoh.gov.pk

**Philippines**

Department of Health, Philippines

www.doh.gov.ph

**Portugal**

Instituto National da Farmácia e do Medicamento

www.infarmed.pt

**Saudi Arabia**

Ministry of Health

www.saudinf.com/main/c6m.htm

**Singapore**

Health Sciences Authority (HSA)

www.hsa.gov.sg

**South Africa**

Department of Health, South Africa.

www.doh.gov.za

**South Korea**

Korea Food and Drug Administration (KFDA)

www.kfda.go.kr

**Spain**

The Agencia Espaniola del Medicamento

www.esnips.com/_t_/medicamentos, www.agemed.es

**Sri Lanka**

Ministry of Indigenous Medicine, Department of Ayurveda

www.ayurveda.gov.lk

**Sweden**

Medical Products Agency

www.lakemedelsverket.se

**Switzerlan**

Swiss regulatory agency for therapeutic products

www.swissmedic.ch

**Tanzania**

Ministry of Health, Department of Curative Services
www.moh.go.tz

**Thailand**

Thai Food and Drug Administration
www.fda.moph.go.th

**Turkey**

Ministry of Health
www.saglik.gov.tr/en

**UK**

Medicines and Healthcare products Regulatory Agency (MHRA),
www.mhra.gov.uk

**USA**

US Food and Drug Administration
www.fda.gov

**Vietnam**

Ministry of Health, Department of Traditional Medicine
www.moh.gov.vn

---

**The author is a Retired Special Technical Adviser, United Nations Industrial Development Organization, Austria and a Former Professor of Chemistry, University of Sri Jayewardenepura, Sri Lanka. He is presently the President of the Pharmaceutical Society of Sri Lanka.

# Chapter 5

# Traditional Medicine in the Developing and Developed Countries and Expected Trends in Future

*Tuley De Silva*
*Link Natural Products (Pvt.) Ltd., Sri Lanka*
*E-mail: tuleyd@hotmail.com*

TRADITIONAL Medicine has been practiced through the ages in almost all countries providing valuable health care. Traditional drugs have utilized locally-available plant, animal and mineral materials and continue to provide health care to people in many developing countries. Traditional Medicine (TM) evolved with time and continued to be the primary health service of rural communities and the poorest levels of society. Presently there is increasing reliance on traditional health care by urban populations.

WHO defines traditional medicine as "diverse health practices, approaches, knowledge and beliefs incorporating plant animal and/or mineral based medicines, spiritual therapies, manual techniques and exercises, applied singularly or in combination to maintain well being as well as to treat, diagnose or prevent illness"

In Asia, there are formalized traditions/systems which have theoretical frameworks. With established traditions of training, formalized educational process, a recorded materia medica with many preparations and clinical practices with a range of preventative and therapeutic modalities, *e.g.* Traditional Chinese Medicine Ayurvedic Medicine, Traditional Vietnamese Medicine, Unani, Siddha.

In the practice of traditional medicine, illness is caused by an imbalance in the whole person and medicine is based on the harmony between physical, mental, emotional, spiritual, and environmental factors. Most of the therapies use the healing power of nature. Therapy is based on the body's inherent ability to establish, maintain, and restore health. Healing process is facilitated by the doctor who diagnoses the illness.

The cause of disease is treated, rather than merely relieving the symptoms. Practitioner educates the patient on lifestyle changes, self-care, and prevention of disease and promotion of health. Practitioner assesses risk factors and teaches the patient to improve these areas to achieve optimal health.

TM treatments for restoring balance and harmony usually involve the prescribing of herbal tea decoctions, acupuncture, specific diet counselling, massage, and other therapies including cupping, moxibustion, exercise (tai chi and qi gong) and meditation.

Many traditional medicines are complex mixtures of hundreds of compounds. The quality and efficacy of these medicines are dependent on the plant source, conditions of growth, harvest time, postharvest treatment and process technology and formulation. Hence quality must be secured from the selection of propagation material, cultivation practices to the final product and up to the time of use. This means stringent standards have to be enforced on raw materials, processes, finished products, conformity to internationally acceptable specifications, machinery and processes validation, good manufacturing practices, packaging and storage.

It is necessary to establish the consistency and reproducibility of a particular extract to ensure guaranteed potency of a traditional medicine or an herbal healthcare product. This is achieved by a process of Standardization, which can be carried out using chemical, spectroscopic or biological methods. The development of specifications is also necessary to implement quality control, ensure batch wise consistency, uniformity of dosage, stability for expiration dating and detect adulteration and determine contaminant levels.

In order to minimize any risks involved in any healthcare production that can not be eliminated through testing the final product is ensured by introducing Good Manufacturing Practices (GMP) that include all aspects of production from the starting materials, premises, equipment, Standard Operating Procedures (SOP), Clean production, training and personal hygiene of staff, work environment, quality assurance, packaging, storage and waste management.

Majority of people in developing countries seek the help of TM practitioners for their healthcare. Even urban populations who have access to modern medicine take traditional medicines for common ailments and make a first call to TM practitioners. The people in developing countries have faith in their native healers and the medicines that originate from natural sources.

## 1.0 Traditional Medicine in Developed Countries

Traditional drugs have been used in ancient times in all countries and with the development of modern medicine, their use has been drastically reduced in the developed world. Although these healthcare products had a limited use, there is a revival of interest in them due to many factors, major being the consumer demand to go natural. As a result new regulations governing the quality, efficacy and safety of these products have been introduced in the developed countries together with stringent requirements for dosage forms and manufacturing practices. These systems are called alternative/complementary systems of medicines.

In fact the EU insists on at least 15 years of use of these medicines in their countries as a requirement for licensing and sale of traditional medicines. These countries have introduced a new class of products called nutraceuticals/herbal healthcare products. Health supplements can be offered for sale with less stringent requirements only as over the counter medications without any claims for cure and prevention of disease.

Presently the major differences in the use of traditional herbal healthcare products between developed and developing countries are listed below:

| *Developed Countries* | *Developing Countries* |
|---|---|
| Ancient use no established system | Folklore and established systems |
| Treatment disease based | Treatment holistic |
| Small percentage uses TM | Many use Traditional medicines |
| Modern medicine is the first choice | Mix of Modern and Traditional |
| New regulations in force | Less regulated by governments |
| Quality control and Standard specifications | Quality and Standards variable are in place |

A survey has shown that the Percentage of the population in the developed countries which has used complementary and alternative medicine, *at least once*, as follows:

| | | |
|---|---|---|
| Australia | – | 48 per cent |
| Canada | – | 50 per cent |
| USA | – | 42 per cent |
| Belgium | – | 40 per cent |
| France | – | 75 per cent |
| United Kingdom | – | 90 per cent |

These figures are very much higher when one considers herbal healthcare products. The current sales show a significant increase in total annual sales of herbal products. More than 60 per cent of people are now using vitamins and minerals and herbal products and more than 80 per cent of GPs had referred patients to natural therapists.

Traditional medicinal drugs are not evidence-based or scientifically proven but have a history of long-term use. TM drugs are not much used as immediate cures for acute illnesses but rather for chronic ailments. It is necessary to ensure batch-to-batch consistency, quality control, safety and absence of contaminants for these products. It is also necessary to test for possible drug interactions and the delivery of health benefits that are claimed.

Herbal treatments are less expensive and safer than patented medicines. 85 per cent of the national health care bill is for treatment of chronic diseases. Many preventable health conditions are caused by dietary imbalances. According to Centre for Disease Control in US, expansion of nutrition and lifestyle-modification can control 54 per cent of heart disease, 37 per cent of cancer, 50 per cent of cerebrovascular disease and 49 per cent of atherosclerosis. Hence control of health-care costs may be achieved by emphasizing holistic and preventive medicine.

*But the current impetus for the demand for TM/Herbal healthcare products in the developed world is due to certain ground realities*:

- Green revolution resulting in the growing demand for "Naturals" in developed countries
- New concept that there is a place for TM/complementary medicines in health care
- As only 1-5 per cent of the plant chemo-diversity has been studied, there is a potential for new medicines
- Need to search for new phytopharmaceuticals to combat chronic and killer diseases
- Free market economy creating markets and demand for new resources, materials and products
- Acceptance of long human use without side effects as an indication of safety of the product
- Consumer orientation of societies and increasing affluence
- Realisation that diet and practices can prevent diseases

## 2.0 Herbal Healthcare Products

Health care products are plant or plant combinations/extracts used as is or in a formulated form for health care and can be used as preventives/protective remedies/cures and for the promotion of health, maintenance of health and restorative/rejuvenative/revitalizing effects. They are also sometimes referred to as Nutraceuticals.

Nutraceuticals include Health foods, Dietary supplements, Health supplements, Nutritional supplements, Alternative health products, Sports nutrition, Natural personal care products (Cosmeceuticals) and Performance enhancers (Figure 5.1). These should provide consumers specific health benefits beyond basic nutrition.

Most modern drugs have side effects, contraindications, iatrogenic reactions and some dose dependent toxic effects. Some bacteria become resistant to these drugs.

Whereas herbal products are used in very low concentrations, they are combined products acting at widespread sites bringing about the effects. These have been used for centuries safely without side effects. If quality standards and good manufacturing practices are maintained, these are safer than modern drugs as over the counter drugs.

The resurgence of interest in naturals is mainly due to the disillusionment with conventional medicines because of concerns about their adverse effects, absence of cures for chronic ailments and new deadly diseases and high costs. There is also a strong belief that naturals are able to assist in ageing problems and disabilities.

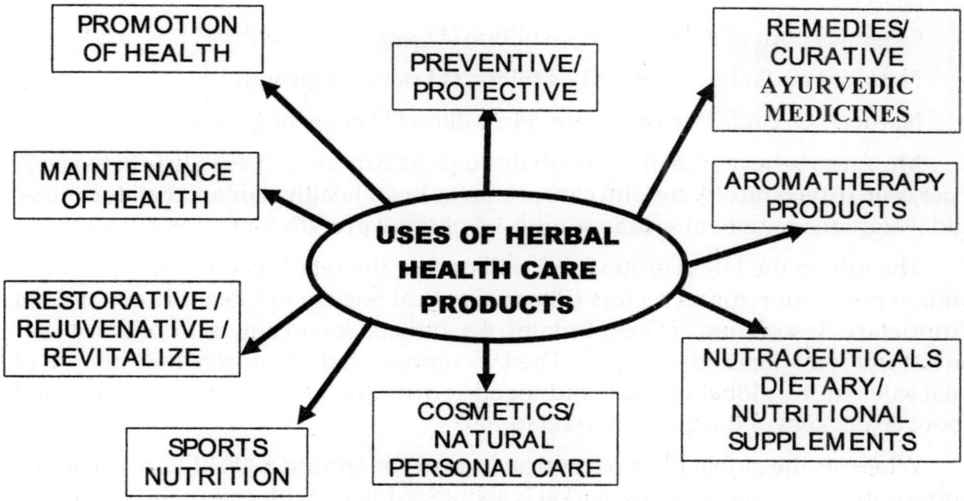


**Figure 5.1**

## 3.0 Global Scenario

Nutraceuticals augment daily diets and provide health benefits. It has been reported that there is a positive relationship between sound dietary practice and good health and there is a connection between dietary supplement use, reduced health-care expenses, and disease prevention.

The Nutrition Business Journal (2001) reports that retail sales of dietary supplement products in the U.S. was \$11.3 billion in 2000 and the two leading categories of supplements sold were for "general health" and "sports/energy/weight-loss" with \$4.4 billion and \$4.7 billion respectively. In 2004, \$5.8 billion worth of supplements were sold, the top-selling categories being for sports, energy, and weight loss (28 per cent of total market share) (Tom Aarts, Nutrition Business Journal). The categories that showed the most growth included sexual health (\$200 million), gastrointestinal health (\$424 million) and diabetes (\$508 million) with increases of 8 per cent, 10 per cent and 9 per cent respectively over 2003 sales.

The Natural Marketing Institute (NMI) revealed that retail sales of health and wellness industry reached \$79 billion in 2005. This constitutes a total growth of 15 per cent over 2004. These figures are from the NMI's annual Health and Wellness Trends Database™(HWTD) research study of 2,800+ U.S. consumer households.

Based on consumer spending by product categories and projected data, industry retail sales for 2005 are as follows:

Functional/Fortified Foods and Beverages: $29.4 billion (26 per cent growth)

Vitamins, Minerals, Herbal and Dietary Supplements: $19.6 billion (3 per cent growth)

Organic Foods/Beverages: $12.8 billion (17 per cent growth)

Natural Foods/Beverages: $12.4 billion (11 per cent growth

Natural/Organic Personal Care: $4.9 billion (22 per cent growth)

Mr. Aarts believes that the growth through 2008 in specialties will be between 7-9 per cent, driven mostly by joint care products, heart health, hair and nail formulas, and weight management solutions with 4-6 per cent growth for sports nutrition.

The sale in the UK is around £93 million (for the retail sector) and up to £240 million per annum for all sectors (Pharmaceutical Society of Great Britain and the Proprietary Association of Great Britain). Australians spend almost $1 billion a year on natural remedies and therapies. The U.S. represented 32 per cent ($21 billion) of total sales in the global market, and together with the EU and Japan represented about 86 per cent of the global market in 2007.

Where as the global pharmaceutical industry is around $300 billion a year, the nutraceuticals/cosmeceuticals market is about $86 billion with an expanding annual growth rate.

Natural medicines can also be used for health promotion, maintenance of health, relieving symptoms of chronic ailments, antiageing, rejuvenation, and holistic immune-boosting effects. They also enhance natural healing "placebo effect" and effects of modern medicine. Furthermore, they are choices for self medication, natural life styles and environment conservation. There are also new types of products as memory enhancers and adaptogens.

There are also new problems that have arisen due to population growth, ageing population, climatic change, stringent food safety requirements, higher incidence of deadly new diseases and life expectancy at birth being reduced. Hence the possible role of Herbal based therapies in the Future of Global Health will encompass treatment of several degenerative disorders and chronic conditions (where modern drugs are inadequate) and healing of conditions which are traced to social or spiritual disorder by addressing the root cause of the disease.

Human genomics have shown that no two individuals are identical in precise terms. This is more in consonance with the traditional systems where treatment was holistic and individual based.

Drug industry too has expanded its interest in herbal products due to improved drug screening techniques, biotechnology capabilities to engineer screening, advances in separation and analytical techniques, desire to rediscover ancient traditional treasures in order to satisfy consumer demand, reduce cost and to Complement/ Supplement modern drugs.

## 4.0 Future Trends

Current trend is for individual demands as custom designed "made just for me." The fear factor about tighter food and drug safety and the need for environmentally-friendly products will also contribute for the increasing demand for natural products. Another area that has an explosive expansion is in men's personal care items, mainly due to the continued expansion of health and wellness into skincare, haircare, dentalcare and bodycare products.

Over riding all these is the media influence in marketing of products. Companies want to seize the moment by developing new products for health and wellness. With greater public access to health information, consumer demand is for products that can be useful in memory enhancement, anti-ageing and longevity.

According to Global Industry Analysts INC., global nutraceuticals sales is projected to reach $187 billion by 2010 due to rising sales in the U.S. and the European Union (EU), and in emerging markets like China and India. In addition to branding and marketing, successful companies will have to become global and has to have economy of scale and be competitive to survive.

One future growth trend for nutraceutical companies is the formation of international joint ventures to harness the best country sources of supply, manufacturing and consumers. There is a tendency for more joint ventures with Chinese companies.

Another important aspect in the industry will involve intellectual property protection as it is essential for increasing revenue. This will be possible only by conducting more research and validation through clinical trials. Where there is intellectual property protection, there also will be more venture capital available.

*Natural Marketing Institute (NMI) in US has listed the following* factors that will contribute to growth of herbal healthcare products.

- Serious side-effects of conventional products, leading to regulatory concessions on natural medicine development
- Acceptance of herbal strategy by some of the major pharmaceutical firms
- Evidence of increasing resistance to over-prescribed conventional drugs
- AIDS epidemic leading to political pressure to allow herbal drugs and other alternative therapies
- Agreement by state insurance and sickness funds to reimburse patients receiving alternative treatment
- Transfer of technology from the East to the West bringing effective treatment for chronic and other conditions
- Growth of the 'green' movement in the West
- Disenchantment among doctors and patients alike with the side-effects of modern medicines

## 5.0 Challenges

There are a number of challenges that have to be overcome in order to successfully introduce herbal healthcare products such a raw material sourcing, trained R&D staff, development of new innovative products and the speed at which products are introduced to the market. In addition one has to take into account Regulatory changes and Non tariff barriers that may be introduced.

Traditional medicines do not easily lend themselves to the vigorous testing protocols used for modern drugs mainly because these are mixtures of compounds of sometimes still unknown constituents and composition acting together in a complex manner and of the difficulty of evaluating scientifically the fundamental concepts and principles on which the traditional medical systems are based. Furthermore, there are no suitable animal models to simulate the holistic approach to the use of these medicines including the psychosomatic involvement and the accompanying exercises/practices and dietary requirements.

But there is a possibility of combining traditional medicines with modern medicines for better healthcare. Given below are some valid reasons for pursuing combined therapies in the future:

- Recipes of constituents in TM/Herbal drugs have already demonstrated the use of multicomponent drugs. Modern practitioners too have begun to prescribe multicomponent drugs expecting either combined effects or for enhancing bioavailability
- TM has a treatment regimen consisting of Drugs, Diet and Practices. There is a trend for using this combination for modern healthcare practices. Hence here too a combination or complementation is possible
- TM Treatment consists of pretreatment, treatment and post treatment. More and more of these practices are being introduced to the modern treatment regimen. Post treatment is vital to bring the patient to normalcy after a debilitating illness
- Transdermal absorption has been a major route of administration using specific vehicles in TM. Modern transdermal patches are a technological improvement of these. Hence a combination of TM with modern with respect to this route of administration may be a future possibility
- In Ayurveda, a type of rejuvenation therapy called Panchakarma is practiced. Panchakarma is a cleansing, purification, balancing, healing and rejuvenation programme for the body, mind and consciousness that involves a series of specialized of therapeutic treatments. It can restore your natural state of health and wellness by cleansing your body of toxins, bringing balance into your system and improving bodily functions. This type of practices is being introduced to the modern practices as well.

Future therefore could be a scenario where both systems would deliver complementary effects to relieve cure and prevent diseases and promote health more effectively, quickly and at a lower cost

All components of a multicomponent traditional medicine may not directly affect the mechanism of action but could influence other effects such as bioavailability, delayed metabolism, improvement of the stability of the active components, synergism, additive or potentiating effect, excretion of the active component and reduction of side effects.

Consumers with more information will use herbal products as preventives, promoters, rejuvenators, performance enhancers, antioxidants, adaptogens, antiageing drugs and immunostimulants.

## 6.0 Role of Developing Countries

There are some key activities that the developing countries should undertake to supply the products in demand.

- Develop herbal healthcare products of quality that could be subjected to clinical evaluation and toxicity clearance
- Exploit the vast plant resources without affecting the environment and restoring biodiversity conservation
- Develop specifications for testing the quality of raw materials and finished products
- Follow GMP guidelines strictly
- Clearly label products without misleading the consumers
- Follow any adverse reactions or interaction with modern drugs
- Manufacture products that are safe, efficacious and of good quality

Drugs that will be in demand that have to be developed are for diseases where no cures are available, chronic conditions, new disease conditions, promotion of health antiaging, rejuvenation etc. Drugs for prevention of diseases, replacement of drugs that have side effects and those for which resistance have also to be developed. There may be a consumer demand for weight reduction or gain, products that will aid recovery after surgery and to address ill health and improve the quality of life.

## References

American-Herbal-Products-Association (www.articlesbase.com/health-articles)

Dietary Supplement Health and Education Act (www.fda.gov/opacom/laws/dshea.html#sec3)

Dietary Supplements: Office of Dietary Supplements (ODS (http://ods.od.nih.gov)

FDA (www.cfsan.fda.gov/~dms/ds-info.html)

Global Industry Analysts Inc, Market Research Reports, Inc. (2008) www.strategyr.com/showgsbr.asp?ind=PACK and Pageview=Execute

Global Industry Analysts Reports (www.marketresearch.com), www.strategyr.com

Global Nutraceuticals Market (ww1.prweb.com/releases/nutraceuticals_dietary)

Global Strategic Business Report by Global Industry Analysts Inc (2008) (www.strategyr.com/Nutraceuticals_Market_Report.asp

Health and Wellness Trends Report (HWTR) (www.nmisolutions.com/r_hwt.html) (www.the-infoshop.com/study/nmi51026-wellness.html)

Herbal Gram: The Journal of the American Botanical Council (www.herbalgram.org/abc/herbalgram), (www.herbalgram.org)

International Food Information Council (http://ific.org/index.cfm)

Institute of Food Technologists (www.ift.org/cms)

NMI Reports 2005 Health and Wellness Industry Sales. (www.npicenter.com/anm/templates/newsATemp.aspx?articleid)

Natural Marketing Institute–Health and Wellness Trends Report (April 1, 2007) (www.marketresearch.com/product/display.asp?productid)

Nutrition Business Journal (NBJ) (www.nutritionbusiness.com)

The Global Report on Nutraceuticals (2003), Clare Harman, ABOUT Publishing Ltd.

The Natural Marketing Institute (NMI) (www.nmisolutions.com/lohasd_workshop.html).

*Part II*

# Phytochemistry

*Chapter 6*

# New and Interesting Compounds from Some Medicinal Plants of Bangladesh

**Choudhury M. Hasan**
*Bangladesh Council of Scientific and Industrial Research (BCSIR), Dhaka, Bangladesh*
*E-mail: cmhasan@citechco.net*

## ABSTRACT

Extensive chemical studies with 52 medicinal plants, belonging to 30 families, have resulted in the isolation and characterization of 156 compounds, including 44 new molecules. Terpenoids were the major constituents among the isolated compounds. The crude extracts and several purified compounds obtained from some of these plants demonstrated significant *in vitro* antibacterial and antifungal activities.

*Keywords: Bangladesh medicinal plants, Terpenoids, Antibacterial, Antifungal.*

## 1.0 Introduction

Bangladesh being a subtropical country is a good repository of plants. There are around 5,000 angiosperms distributed among 200 families. Approximately 500 of these are being used in the traditional medicines for the treatment of different types of diseases. Here, we describe the chemistry and antimicrobial activity of some of the isolated constituents from 48 medicinal plants of Bangladesh.

## 2.0 Methodology

The chemical investigation of a plant involved collection and proper identification of the plant materials, extraction, fractionation, purification and isolation

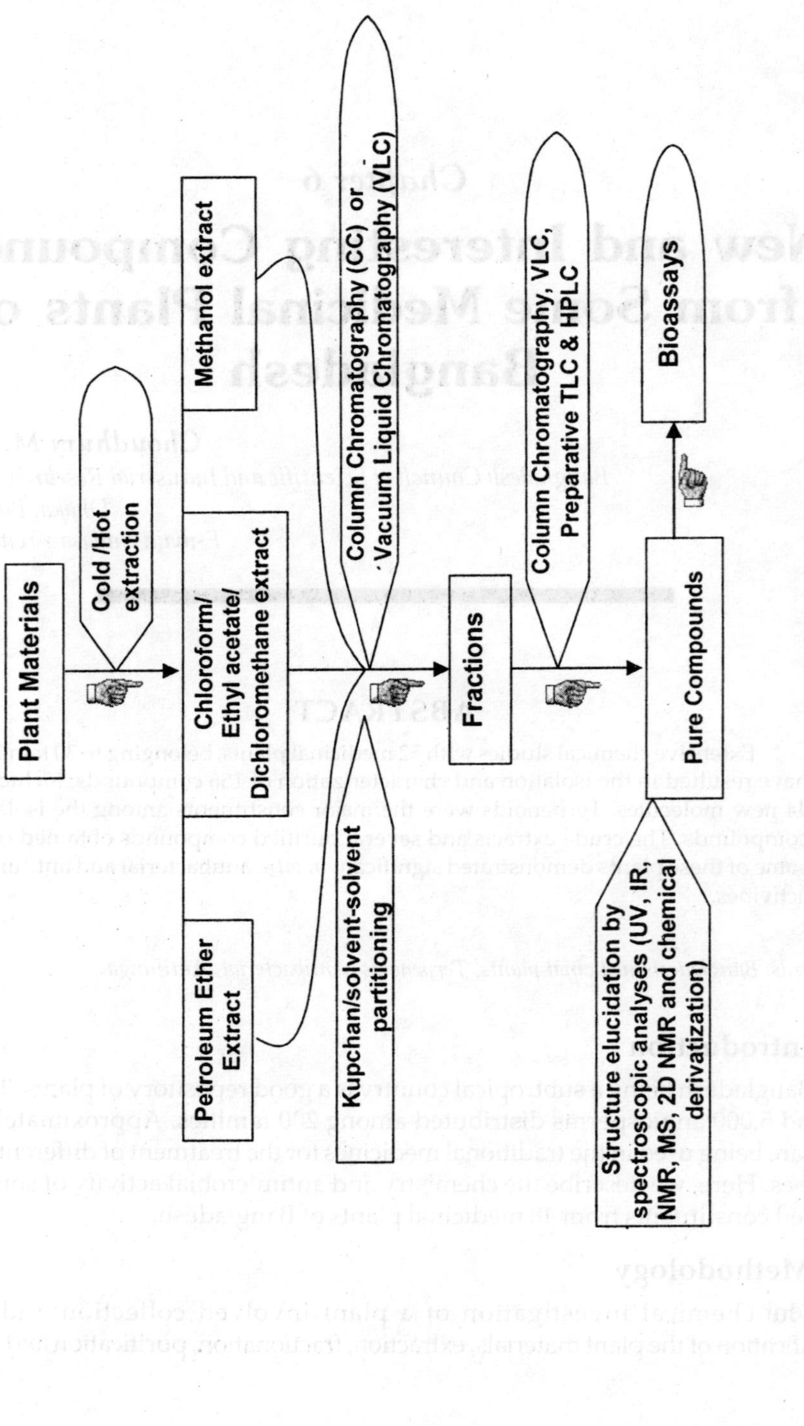


**Figure 6.1: Extraction and Analysis of Plant Materials**

of compounds and structural characterization of the purified compounds (Figure 6.1). Various chromatographic techniques were utilized for isolation and purification of the plant constituents. On the other hand, the structures of the purified compounds were determined by extensive analyses of UV, IR, NMR and mass spectroscopic data as well as by chemical derivatization, when needed. The whole process can be explained in the following way:

## 3.0 Results and Discussion

Extensive chromatographic separation and purification of the extracts obtained from 49 medicinal plants of Bangladesh afforded a total of 137 pure chemical entities, including 37 new molecules. The structures of these compounds were elucidated by spectroscopic studies and chemical derivatization wherever needed. Some of the isolated compounds exhibited significant antibacterial and antifungal activities, when subjected to antimicrobial screening by disc diffusion technique. The structures of some of the isolated compounds are shown in Figure 6.2.

**Figure 6.2: Structures of Some Isolated Compounds**

**Sesquiterpenes from *Amoora rohituka* (Meliaceae)**
**(Chowdhury, Hasan and Rashid, 2003)**

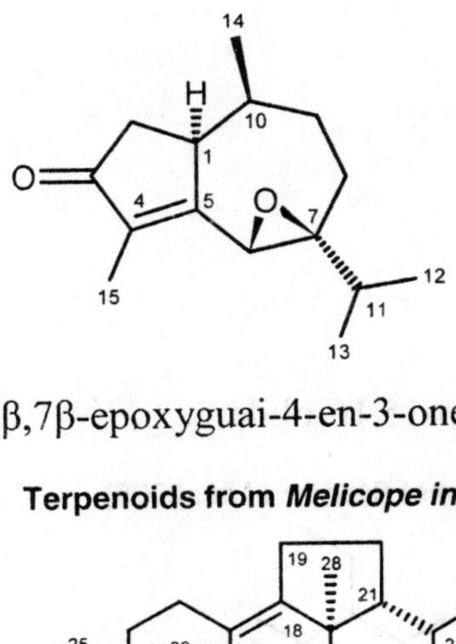

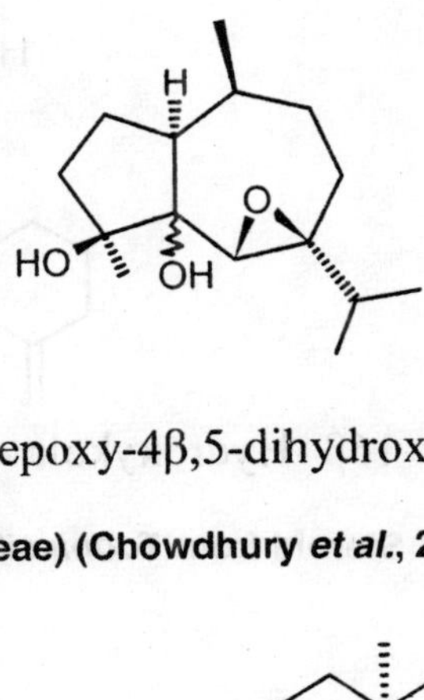

6β,7β-epoxyguai-4-en-3-one   6β,7β -epoxy-4β,5-dihydroxyguaiane

**Terpenoids from *Melicope indica* (Rutaceae) (Chowdhury *et al.*, 2003)**

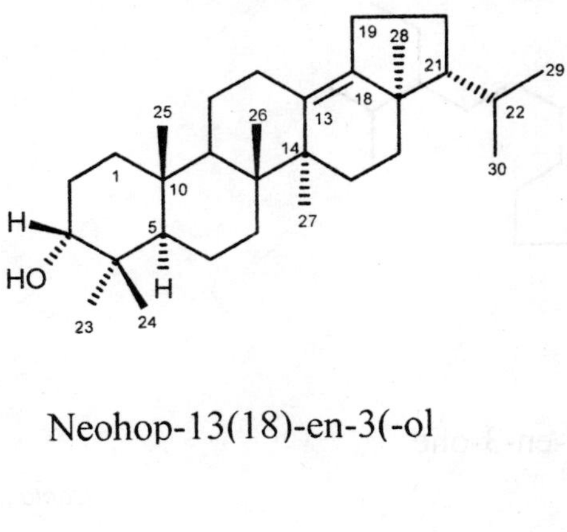

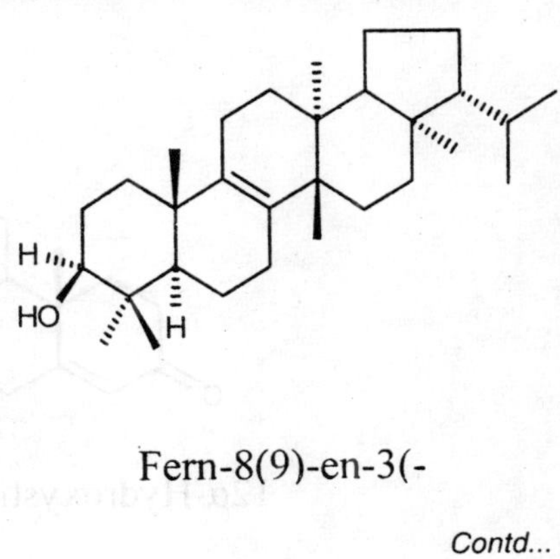

Neohop-13(18)-en-3(-ol   Fern-8(9)-en-3(-

*Contd...*

**Figure 6.2–Contd...**

**Steroids A and B from *Artabotrys odoritissimus* (Connolly *et al.*, 1994) and *Desmos longiflorus* (Datta *et al.*, 2002) (Annonaceae) respectively**

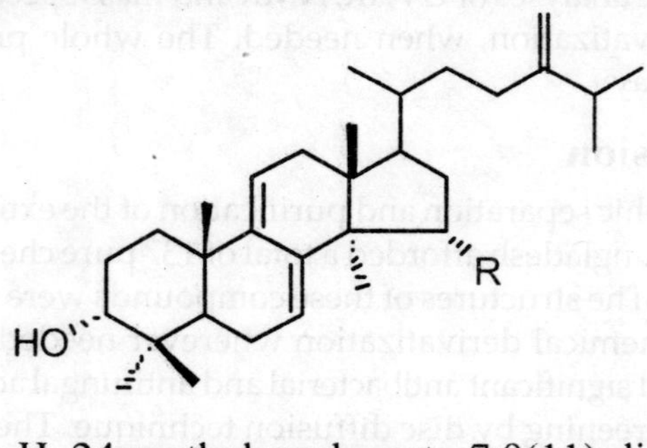


(A) R = H, 24-methylene-lanosta-7,9(11)-dien-3β-ol

(B) R = OH, 15α-hydroxy-24-methylene-lanosta-7,9(11)-dien-3-one

**Diterpene from *Polyalthia longifolia* var. *pendulla* (Annonaceae) (Farruque *et al.*, 2003)**

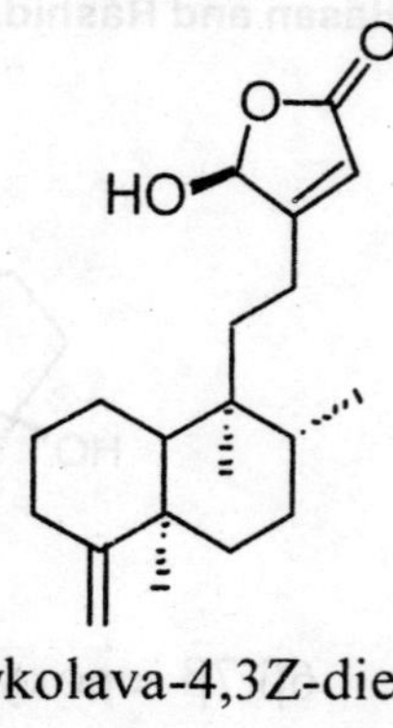


16β-Hydroxykolava-4,3Z-dien-15,16-olide

**Steroid from *Toona ciliata* (Meliaceae) (Haque *et al.*, 2006)**

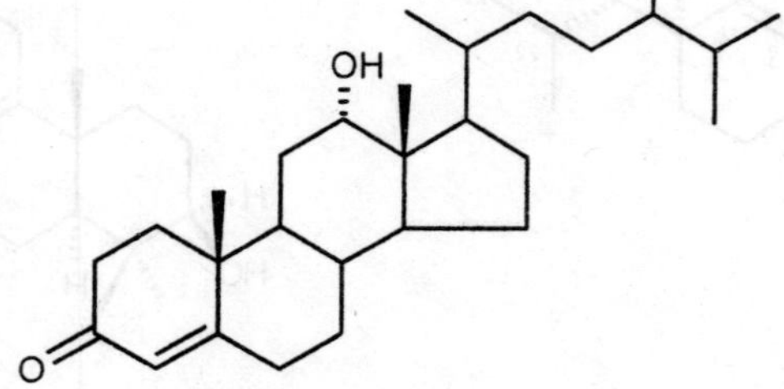


12α-Hydroxystigmast-4-en-3-one

*Contd...*

**Figure 6.2–Contd...**

**Triterpene glycosides *Corchorus capsualris* (Tiliaceae)**
**(Hasan *et al.*, 1984; Hasan, Hossain and Rashid, 1995)**

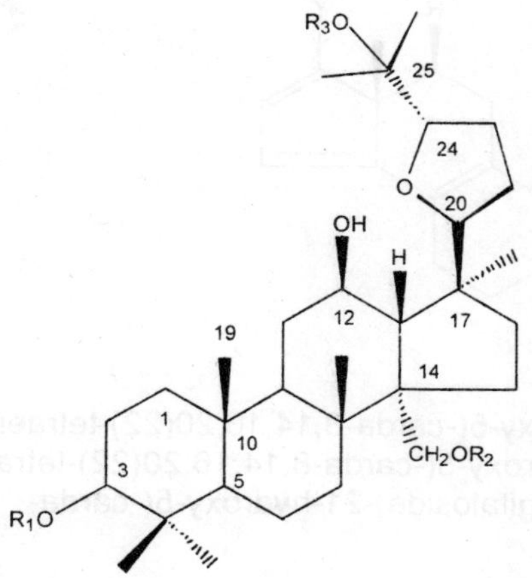

R1 = R2 = R3 = H; capsugenine
R1 = R3 = H, R2 = glucose; capsugenine-30-O-β -glucopyranoside
R1 = H, R2 = R3 = glucose; capsugenine-25, 30-O-β-glucopyranoside

**Steroids from *Nerium oleander* (Apocynaceae)**
**(Hasan *et al.*, 1995; Hasan, Mia`and Rashid, 1996)**

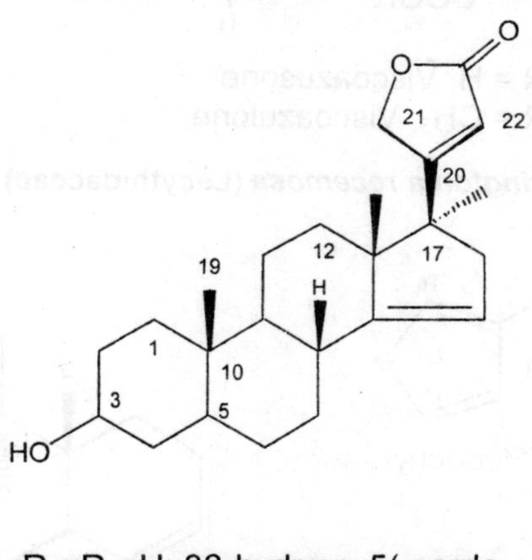

$R_1$=$R_2$=H; 3β-hydroxy-5(-carda-14(15),20(22)-dienolide

*Contd...*

**Figure 6.2–Contd...**

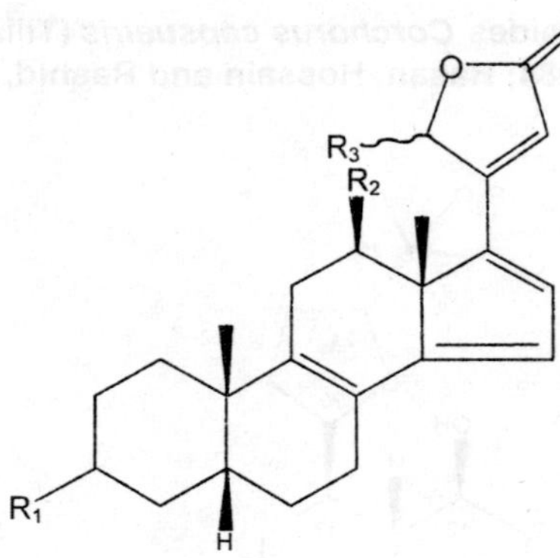

$R_1$=OH, $R_2$=$R_3$=H; 3β-hydroxy-5(-carda-8,14,16,20(22)-tetraenolide
$R_1$=$R_3$=H, $R_2$ = OH; 12(-hydroxy-5(-carda-8,14,16,20(22)-tetraenolide
$R_1$=glu, $R_2$=H, $R_3$=OH; 3(-digitaloside)-21-hydroxy-5(-carda-8,14,16,20(22)-tetraenolide

**Terpenoids from *Polygonum viscosum* (Polygonaceae) (Hasan *et al.,* 2000)**

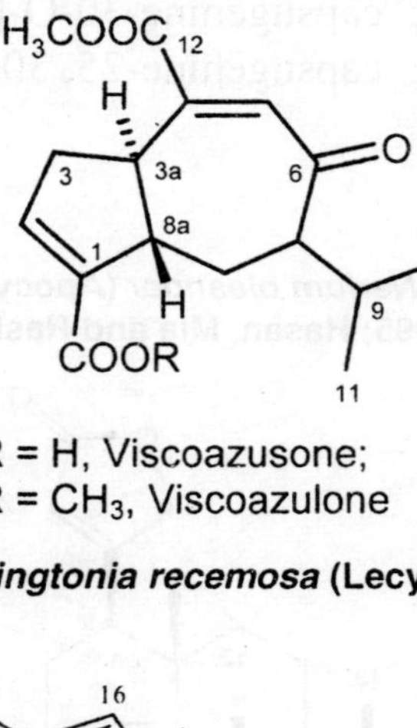

R = H, Viscoazusone;
R = $CH_3$, Viscoazulone

**Diterpenoids from *Barringtonia recemosa* (Lecythidaceae) (Hasan *et al.,* 1994)**

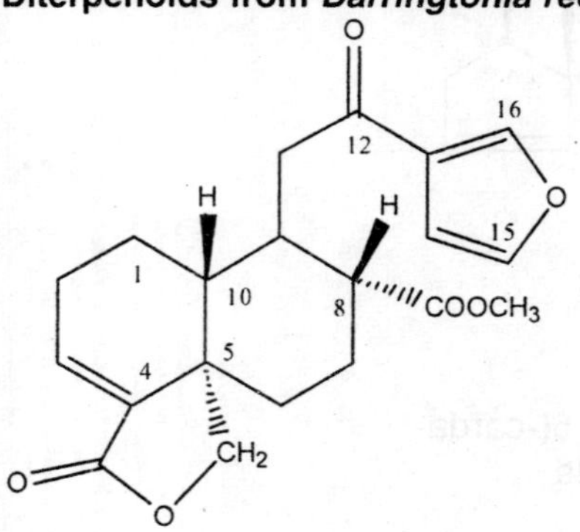

Nasimalun A

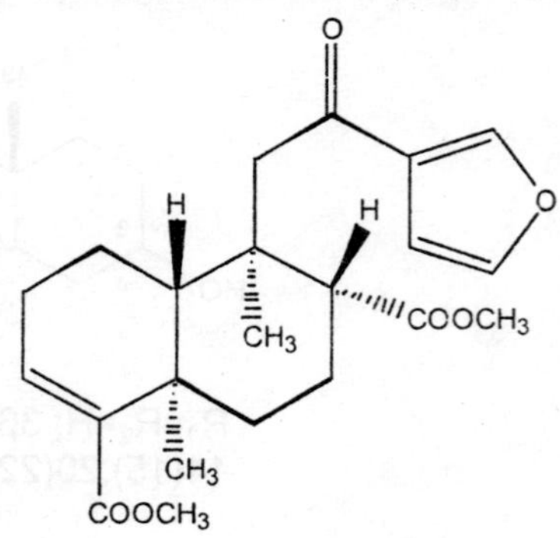

Nasimalun B

*Contd...*

**Figure 6.2–Contd...**

**Terpenoids from *Coffea bengalensis* (Rubiaceae) (Hasan *et al.*,1987)**

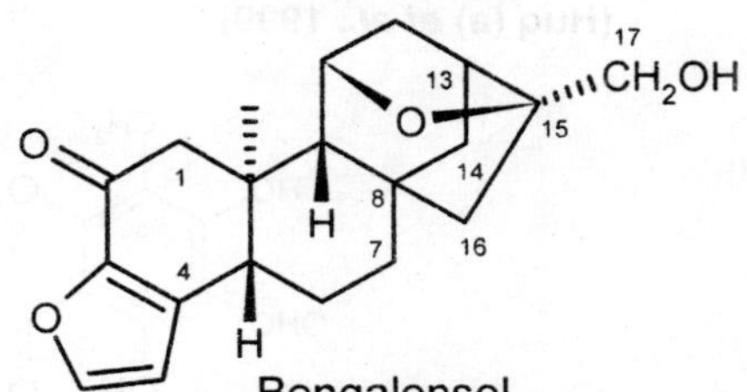

Bengalensol

**Coumarins (Lunamarins A-C) from *Claussena heptaphylla* and *Micromelum minutum* (Rutaceae) (Huq *et al.*, 1999)**

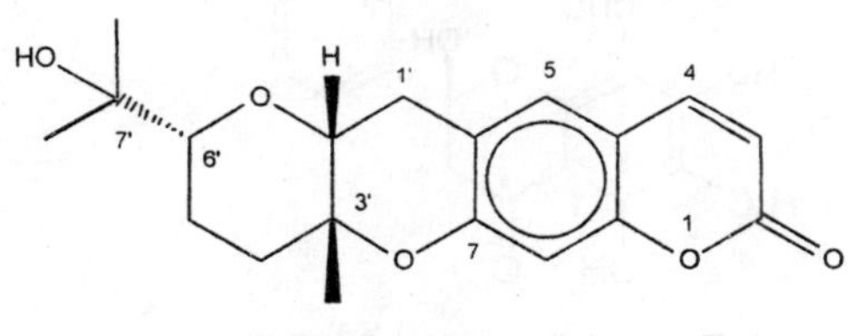

Lunamarin A

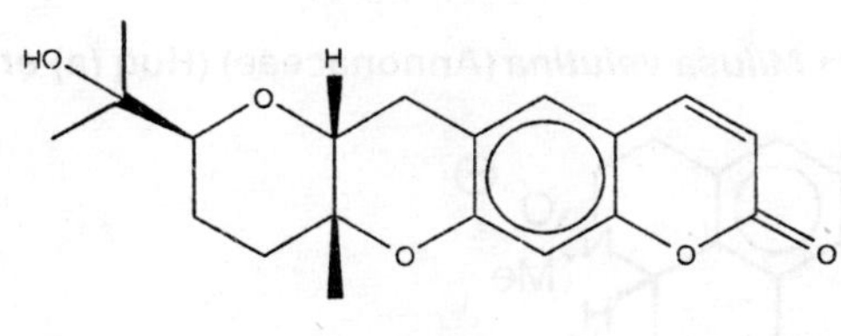

Lunamarin B

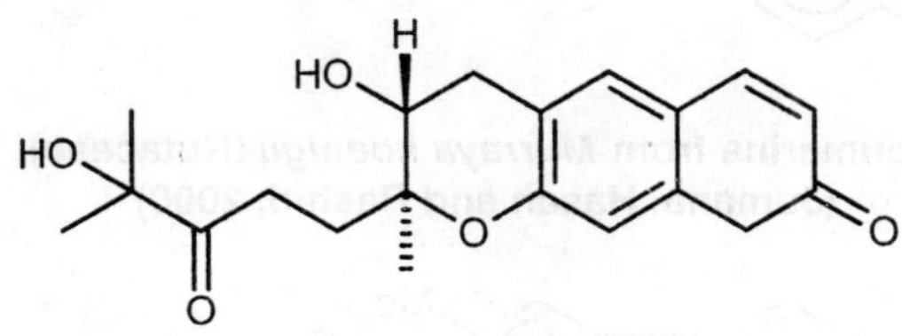

Lunamarin C

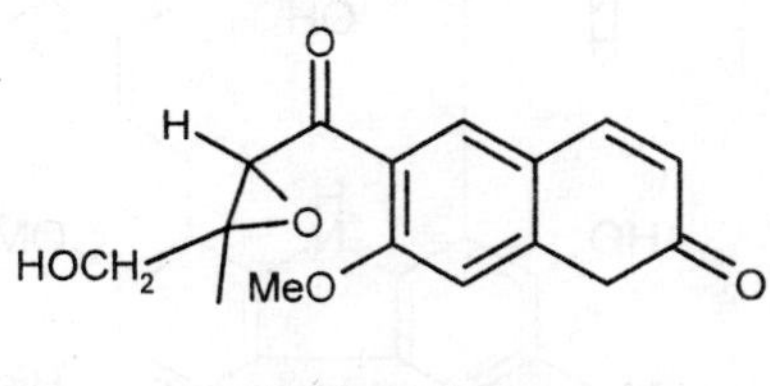

Hopeyhopol

*Contd...*

**Figure 6.2–Contd...**

**Flavonoids from *Unona discolor/Uvaria chinensis* (Annonaceae) (Huq (a) *et al.*, 1999)**

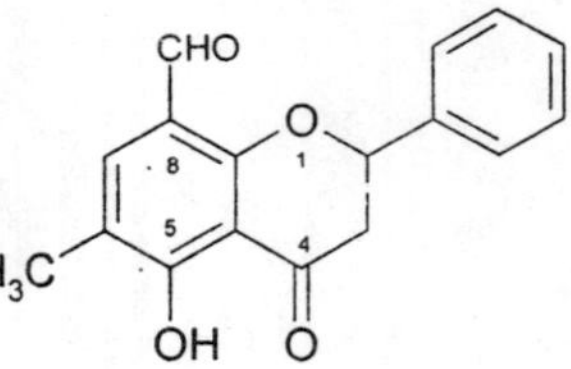

8-Formyl-6-methyl-5-hydroxyflavone

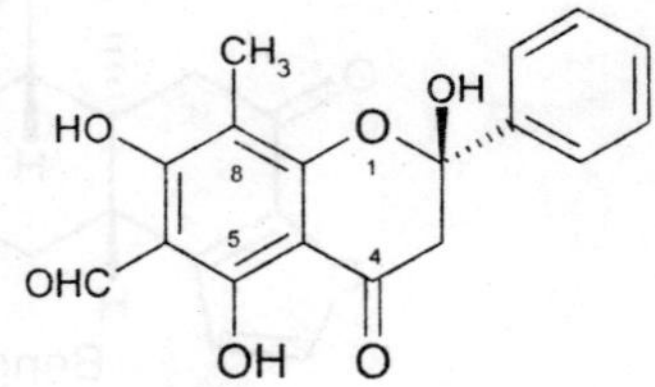

6-Formyl-8-methyl-2β,5,7-trihydroxyflavanone

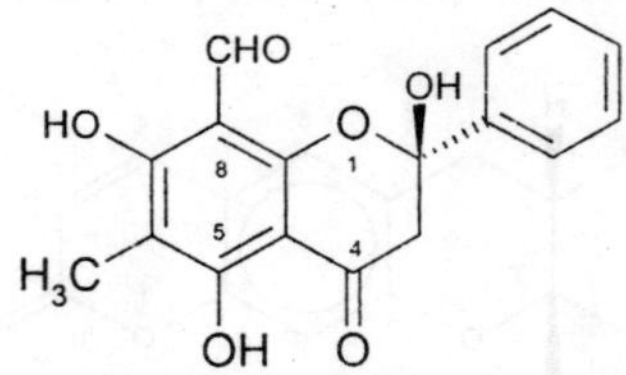

8-Formyl-6-methyl-2β,5,7-trihydroxyflavanone

**Alkaloid from *Milusa velutina* (Annonaceae) (Huq (a) *et al.*, 1999)**

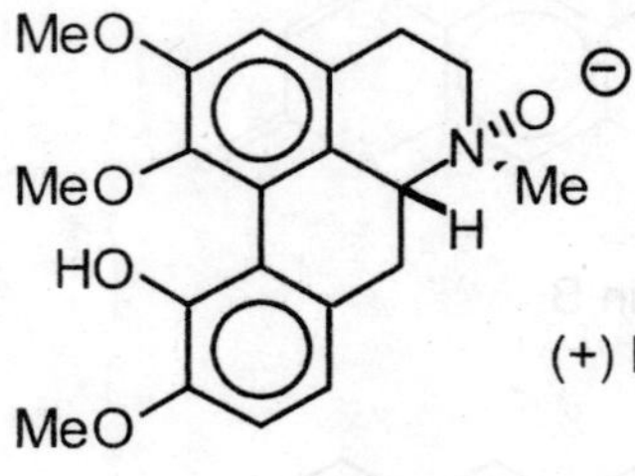

(+) Isocorydine-*N*-oxide

**Coumarins from *Murraya koenigii* (Rutaceae) (Jumana, Hasan and Rashid, 2000)**

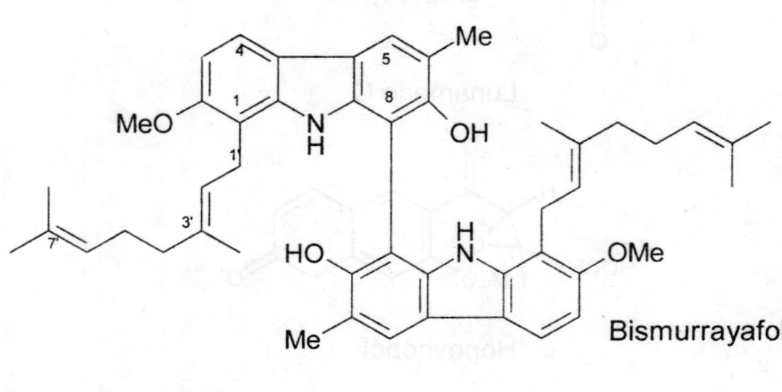

Bismurrayafoline

*Contd...*

**Figure 6.2–Contd...**

**Acetogenins from *Goniothalmus sesquipedalis* (Annonaceae)**
**(Nutun, Hasan and Rashid, 1999)**

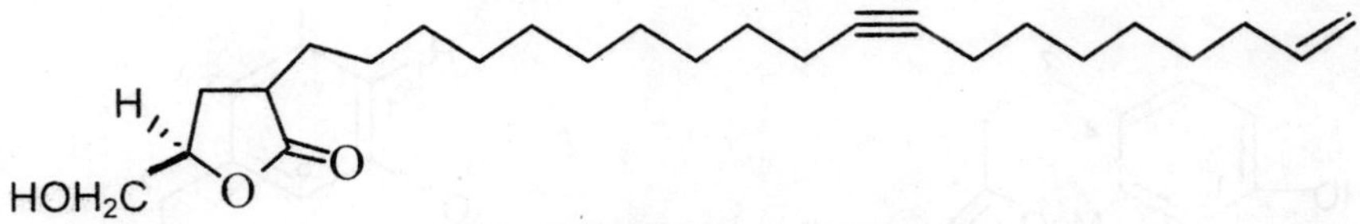


Isogoniothalamusin (B)

**Styryl lactone from *Goniothalmus sesquipedalis* (Annonaceae)**
**(Quader *et al.*, 1987)**

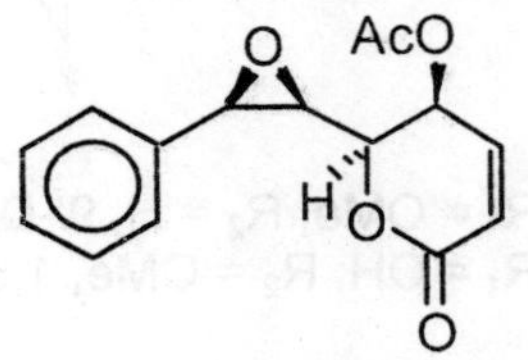


5-Acetoxyisogoniothlamine oxide

**Anthraquinones and napthaquinones from *Stereospermum chelonoides***
**(Bignoniaceae) (Rahman *et al.*, 2001)**

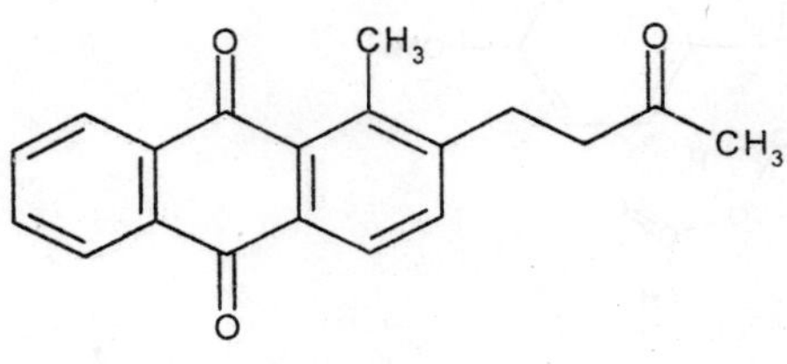


Stereochenol A

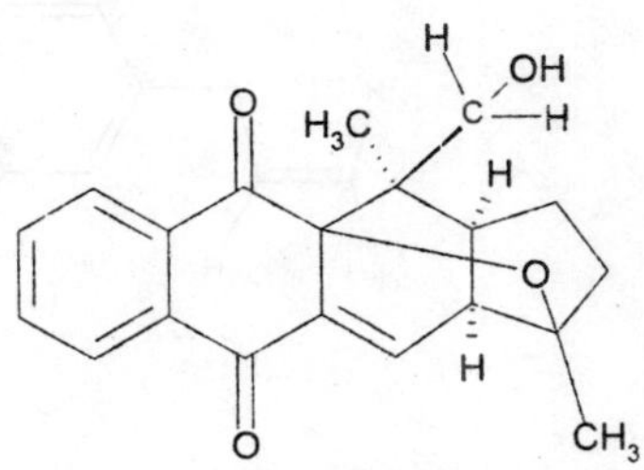


Stereochenol B

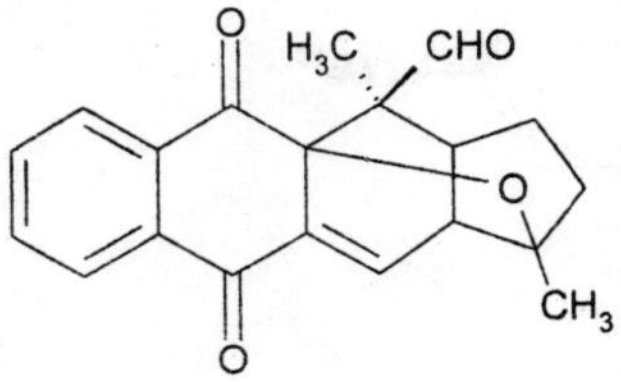


Sterekunthal B

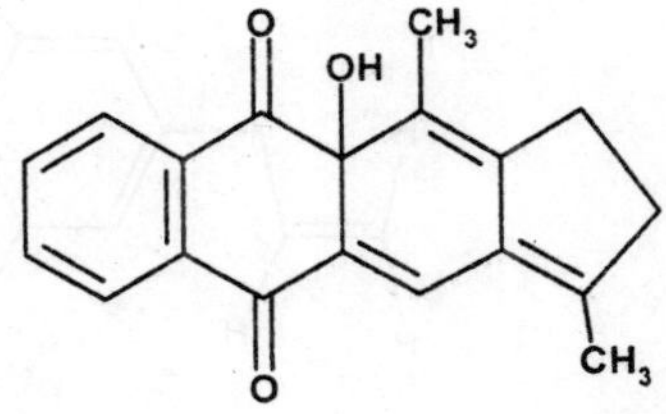


Sterequinone C

*Contd...*

**Figure 6.2–Contd...**

**Diarylheptanoids from *Garuga pinnata* (Burseraceae) (Sohrab *et al.*, 2002)**

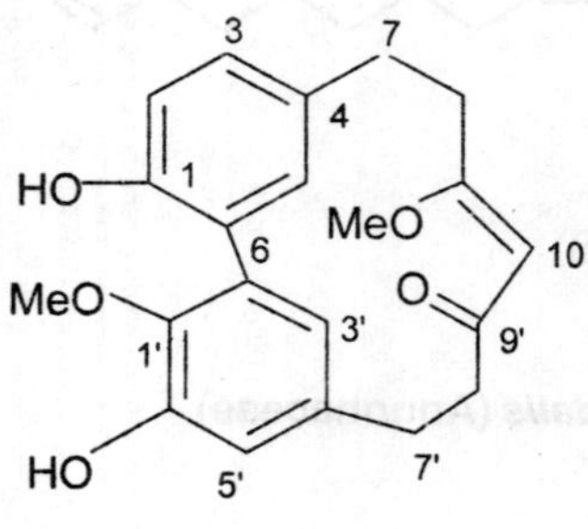

6'-Hydroxygaruganin V

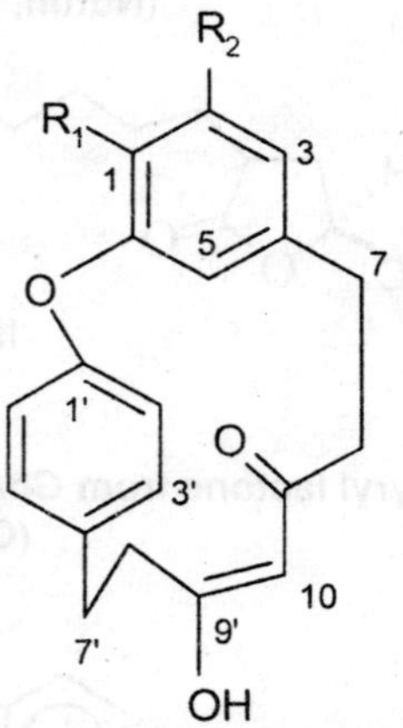

$R_1$ = OMe; $R_2$ = H, 9'-Desmethylgarugamblin
$R_1$ = OH; $R_2$ = OMe, 1,9'-Didesmethylgaruganin

**Neolignans from *Quisqualis indica* (Combreataceae)**

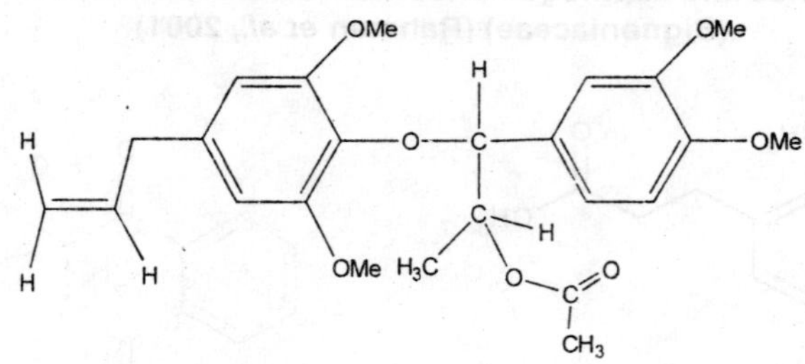

QI-6

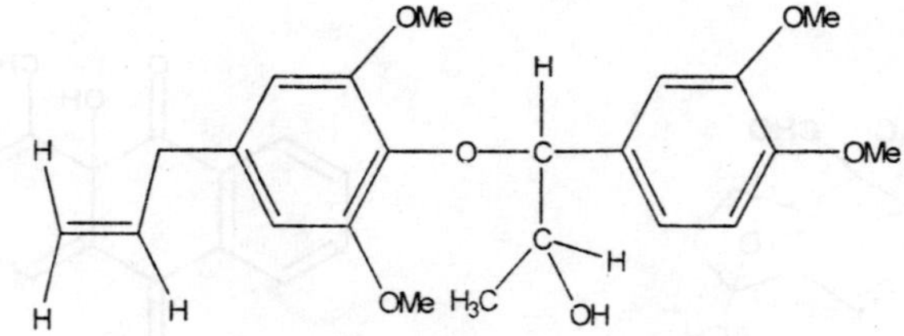

QI-5

*Contd...*

**Figure 6.2–Contd...**

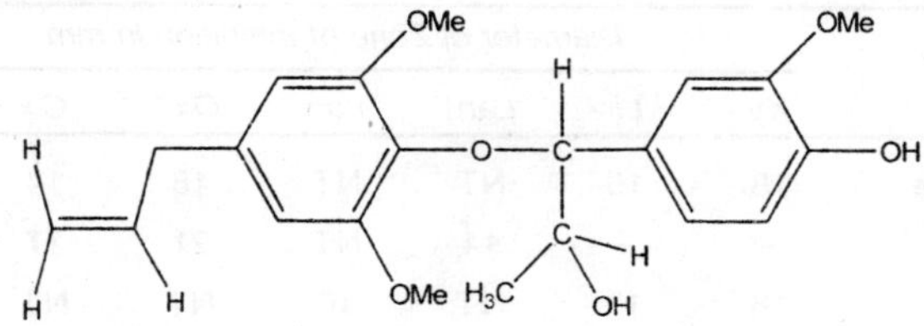

QI-7

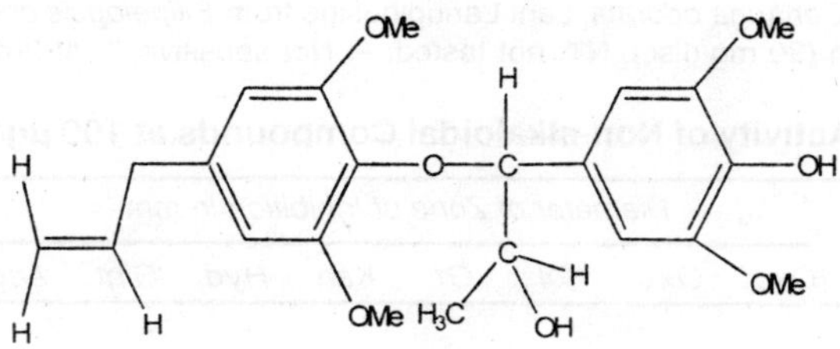

QI-11

The compounds isolated from different plant were screened for antibacterial and antifungal activities. The results of those screenings are shown in the following tables:

**Table 6.1: Antibacterial Activity of Purified Alkaloids at 100 μg/disc**

| *Name of Bacteria* | *Diameter of Zone of Inhibition in mm* | | | | | | |
|---|---|---|---|---|---|---|---|
| | *Xy* | *Lir* | *Lan** | *Lan* | *Ox** | *Ox* | *Am* |
| **Gram positive** | | | | | | | |
| *Bacillus cereus* | 15 | 14 | 16 | 12 | 21 | 16 | – |
| *B. subtilis* | 19 | 15 | 19 | 14 | 10 | 16 | 15 |
| *B. megaterium* | 12 | 15 | NT | NT | NT | NT | 10 |
| *B. polymyxa* | 13 | 13 | NT | NT | NT | NT | – |
| *Streptococcus β-haemolyticus* | 17 | 12 | NT | NT | NT | NT | – |
| *Staphylococcus aureus* | – | – | 15 | 11 | 20 | 15 | 20 |
| *Sarcina lutea* | 16 | 17 | NT | NT | NT | NT | – |
| **Gram negative** | | | | | | | |
| *Escherichia coli* | 18 | 17 | NT | NT | 20 | 17 | – |
| *Shigella boydii* | NT | NT | NT | 11 | NT | NT | – |
| *Sh. dysentriae* | 17 | 16 | 16 | NT | NT | 18 | – |
| *Sh. flexneri* | 17 | 16 | NT | 12 | NT | NT | 18 |
| *Sh. sonnei* | – | – | NT | NT | NT | NT | – |

*Contd...*

**Table 6.1–Contd...**

| *Name of Bacteria* | *Diameter of Zone of Inhibition in mm* | | | | | | |
|---|---|---|---|---|---|---|---|
| | *Xy* | *Lir* | *Lan** | *Lan* | *Ox** | *Ox* | *Am* |
| *Pseudomonas aeruginosa* | 18 | 15 | NT | NT | 18 | 14 | 33 |
| *Salmonella typhi* B | – | – | 14 | NT | 21 | 17 | 27 |
| *Sal. paratyphi* A | 18 | 17 | NT | 10 | NT | NT | 21 |
| *Sal. paratyphi* B | 18 | 16 | 15 | NT | 18 | 14 | – |

Xy: Xylopine, Lir: Liriodenine from *Cananga odorata*, Lan: Lanuginosine from *Ellipeiopsis cherrevensis*, Ox: Oxostephanine; Am: Ampicillin (30 mg/disc), NT: not tested; –: Not sensitive; *: at 200 mg/disc.

**Table 6.2: Antibacterial Activity of Non-alkaloidal Compounds at 100 µg/disc**

| *Bacterial Strain* | *Diameter of Zone of Inhibition in mm* | | | | | | | | |
|---|---|---|---|---|---|---|---|---|---|
| | *Oxc** | *Oxc* | *Kol* | *Gt* | *Kan* | *Hyd* | *Gigt* | *Acg* | *Am* |
| **Gram positive** | | | | | | | | | |
| *Bacillus cereus* | 14 | 12 | 11 | 18 | 14 | 15 | 15 | 18 | – |
| *B. subtilis* | 25 | 18 | 13 | 15 | 15 | 18 | 25 | 22 | 15 |
| *B. megaterium* | 20 | 18 | 10 | 18 | 15 | 16 | NT | NT | 10 |
| *B. polymyxa* | 27 | 20 | 12 | 12 | 14 | 22 | NT | NT | – |
| *Streptococcus β-haemolyticus* | 22 | 21 | 10 | – | 19 | 18 | NT | NT | – |
| *Staphylococcus aureus* | 16 | 13 | NT | 11 | 23 | – | 19 | 17 | 20 |
| *Sarcina lutea* | 20 | 18 | – | 11 | 18 | 18 | 23 | 15 | – |
| **Gram negative** | | | | | | | | | |
| *Escherichia coli* | 11 | 12 | NT | 14 | 14 | 13 | 16 | 14 | – |
| *Shigella boydii* | 30 | 27 | 12 | 18 | 14 | 25 | NT | NT | – |
| *Sh. dysentriae* | 17 | 13 | 10 | 17 | 15 | 15 | 25 | 12 | – |
| *Sh. sonnei* | 22 | 19 | – | 15 | 10 | – | 23 | 12 | 18 |
| *Sh. shiga* | 21 | 27 | 12 | 12 | 17 | 18 | NT | NT | – |
| *Pseudomonas aeruginosa* | 20 | 11 | NT | 20 | 22 | 14 | 6 | – | NT |
| *Salmonella typhi*–A | 19 | 16 | 11 | 18 | 19 | 14 | 24 | 10 | 29 |
| *Salmonella typhi*–B | 17 | 14 | NT | 20 | 14 | 16 | NT | NT | – |
| *Sal. Typhi* B–52 | 16 | 14 | NT | 12 | 22 | 17 | NT | NT | NT |
| *Sal. Typhi* B–56 | 12 | 12 | NT | 12 | 21 | 21 | NT | NT | NT |
| *Sal. Typhi* B–62 | 21 | 19 | 10 | 14 | 18 | 19 | NT | NT | NT |
| *Vibrio cholerae* | 21 | 15 | NT | – | NT | 18 | NT | 19 | 27 |

Oxc-1: 16-oxocleroda-3,13E-dien-15-oic-acid from *Polyalthia longifolia* var. *pendulla*, Kol: Kolavenic acid from *Polyalthia longifolia* var. *pendulla*, Gt: Goniothalamin from *Goniothalamus sesquipedalis*, Hyd: 16β-hydroxycleroda-3,13-dien-15,16-olide from *Polyalthia longifolia* var. *pendulla*, Gigt: Gigantetrocin, Gigp: Giganpetocin, Acg: 5-Acetoxygoniothalaminoxide from *Goniothalamus sesquipedalis*, Kan: Kanamycin (30µg/disc), Am: ampicillin (30µg/disc), NT: Not tested; –: not sensitive, *: at 200 µg/disc.

**Table 6.3: Antifungal Activity of Isolated Alkaloidal Compounds at 100 μg/disc**

| *Name of Fungi* | *Diameter of Zone of Inhibition in mm* | | | | | | | |
|---|---|---|---|---|---|---|---|---|
| | *Xy* | *Lir* | *Lan* | *Gri* | *Oxoc* | *Kol* | *Hyd* | *Kan* |
| *Rhizopus oryzae* | 12 | – | 12 | – | NT | NT | NT | NT |
| *R. oligosporous* | NT | NT | 11 | – | NT | NT | NT | NT |
| *Aspergillus niger* | 16 | 17 | – | – | NT | NT | NT | NT |
| A. *Fumigatus* | 18 | 22 | NT | – | 18 | – | 13 | – |
| *Candida albicans* | – | – | – | – | 10 | – | 8 | – |
| A. *Krusii* | – | – | – | – | NT | NT | NT | NT |
| *Trichoderma sp.* | NT | NT | 13 | – | NT | NT | NT | NT |
| *Saccharomyces cerevisiae* | 12 | – | NT | – | 11 | 9 | 13 | – |
| *S. rosea* | NT | NT | NT | NT | 12 | – | 13 | 11 |
| *S. caulbequence* | NT | NT | NT | NT | 11 | 10 | 12 | – |

Xy: Xylopine, Lir: Liriodenine, Lan: Lanuginosine, Oxoc: 16-oxocleroda-3,13-*E*-dien-15-oic-acid, Kol: Kolavenic acid, Hyd: 16β-hydroxycleroda-3,13-dien-15,16-olide, Gri: Grisofulvin, Kan: Kanamycin (30 μg/disc), NT: Not tested; –: not sensitive

## 5.0 Conclusion

A total of 52 plant species have been investigated. Many structurally unique and diversified compounds having interesting biological activities were isolated from these plants. Our studies show that Bangladeshi plants can be a promising source of novel drug candidates.

## Acknowledgements

I wish to express my sincere thanks to my co-workers and students who actually did the main laboratory works. I am also grateful to the organizer for inviting me and providing me with the local hospitality.

## References

Ara, K., Rahman, A.H.M.M., Hasan, C.M., Iskander, M.N., Asakawa, Y., Quang, D.N. and Rashid, M.A., 2006. Macrocyclic diarylheptanoids from *Garuga pinnata*. Phytochem, 67, pp. 2659-2662.

Chowdhury, R., Hasan, C.M. and Rashid, M.A., 2003. Guaiane Sesquiterpenes from *Amoora rohituka*. Phytochem, 62, pp. 1213-1216.

Chowdhury, R., Rashid, R. B., Sohrab, M.H., Hasan, C.M., 2003. 12α-hydroxystigmast-4-en-3-one: a new bioactive steroid from *Toona ciliata* (Meliaceae). Pharmazie 58, pp. 272-273.

Connolly, J.D., Hoque, M.E., Hasan, C.M. and Haider, S.S., 1994. Constituents of the stem bark of *Artabotrys odoritissimus*. Fitoterapia, 65, pp. 92-93.

Datta, B.K., Datta, S.K., Rashid, M.A., Kundu, J.K., Hasan, C.M., and Sarker, S.D., 2002. Furhter sequiterpenes from *Polygonum viscosum* (Polygonaceae). Nat. Prod. Lett., 16, pp. 143-148.

Farruque, R., Chowdhury, R., Sohrab, M. H., Hasan, C. M. and Rashid, M.A., 2003. Triterpene constituents from the leaves of *Melicope indica*. Pharmazie, 58, pp. 518-520,.

Haque, M.R., Rahman, K.M., Iskander, M.N., Hasan, C.M. and Rashid, M.A., 2006. Stereochenols A and B, two quinones from *Stereospermum chelonoides*. Phytochem, 67, pp. 2663-2665.

Hasan, C.M., Islam, A., Ahmed, M., Ahmed, M. U. and Waterman, P.G., 1984. Capsugenin, a dammarane triterpene from *Corchorus capsularis*. Phytochem, 23, pp. 2583-2587.

Hasan, C.M., Hossain, M.A. and Rashid, M.A., 1995. Clerodane diterpenoids from *Polyalthia longifolia* var. *pendulla*. Biochem. Syst. Ecol., 23, pp. 331-332.

Hasan, C.M., Huda, Q., Lavaud, C., Connolly, J.D. and Huq, M.E., 1995. Bengalensol, A new 16-epicafestol derivative from the leaves of *Coffea bengalensis*. Nat. Prod. Lett, 4, pp. 55-60.

Hasan, C.M., Mia, M.Y. and Rashid, M.A., 1996. A new acetogenin from *Goniothalamus sesquipedalis* (Annonaceae). Dhaka Univ. J. Biol. Sci., 5, pp. 99-102.

Hasan, C.M., Khan, S., Jabbar, A. and Rashid, M.A., 2000. Two novel neoclerodane diterpenes from *Barringtonia recemosa*. J. Nat. Prod., 63, pp. 411-412.

Hasan, C.M., Mia, M.Y., Rashid, M.A. and Connolly, J. D., 1994. 5-Acetoxyisogoniothalamin oxide, a new epoxystyryl lactone from *Goniothalamus sesquipedalis* (Annonaceae). Phytochem, 37, pp. 1763–1764.

Hasan, C.M., Shahanz, S., Ilias, M., Gray, A.I. and Waterman, P.G., 1987. Chemistry in the Annonaceae, XXIII. 24-Methylene-lanosta-7,9(11)-dien-3$\beta$-ol from *Artabotrys odorotissimus* stem bark. J. Nat. Prod. 50, pp. 762-763.

Huq, M.M., Jabbar, A., Rashid, M.A., Hasan, C.M., 1999. A novel antibacterial and cardiac steroid from the roots of *Nerium oleander*. Fitoterapia, 70, pp. 5-9.

Huq, M.M (a)., Jabbar, A., Rashid, M.A., Hasan, C.M., Ito, C. and Furukawa, H., 1999. Steroids from the roots of *Nerium oleander*. J. Nat. Prod ., 62, pp. 1055-1057.

Jumana, S., Hasan, C.M. and Rashid, M.A., 2000. (+) Isocorydine-$\alpha$-N-oxide: A new aporphine alkaloid from *M. velutina*. Nat. Prod. Lett., 14, pp. 393-397.

Nutun, M.T.H., Hasan, C.M. and Rashid, M.A., 1999. Bismurrayafoline E: a new dimeric carbazole alkaloid from *Murraya koenigii*. Fitoterapia, 70, pp. 130–133.

Quader, M.A., Ahmed, M.U., Hasan, C.M. and Waterman, P.G., 1987. A new glycoside from the leaves of *Corchorus* capsularies. J. Nat. Prod., 50, pp. 479-481.

Rahman, S., Hasnat, A., Hasan, C. M., Rashid, M. A. and Ilias, M., 2001. Pharmacological evaluation of Bangladeshi medicinal plants–a review. Pharmaceutical Biol 39, pp. 1-6.

Sohrab, M.H., Begum, B, Hasan, C.M. and Rashid, M.A., 2002. Antimicrobial screening of the leaf of *Micromelum pubescens*. Bangladesh J. Microbiology, 16, pp. 203-205-574.

# Chapter 7

# Xanthone Derivatives from *Cratoxylon cochinchinense* Blume

***Ha Viet Son*, Hoang Thanh Huong and Nguyen Huu Khoi***

*Institute of Natural Products Chemistry,*
*Vietnamese Academy of Science and Technology,*
*18 Hoang Quoc Viet, Cau Giay, Hanoi, Vietnam*
**E-mail: havietson@yahoo.fr*

## ABSTRACT

Two xanthones, named cratoxanthone A and cratoxanthone B, were isolated from the crude methanolic extract of *Cratoxylon cochinchinense*. Their structures were primarily elucidated by spectroscopic analysis including $^1$H-NMR, $^{13}$C-NMR, DEPT, COSY, HSQC, HMBC and ESI MS. The known xanthones, pancixanthone B and mangiferin were also isolated and characterized.

***Keywords**: Cratoxylon cochinchinense, Cratoxanthone A, Cratoxanthone B, Xanthones, Pancixanthone B, Mangiferin, Methanolic extract.*

## 1.0 Introduction

*Cratoxylon cochinchinense* (Lour.) Blume is a traditional medicine in Vietnam. People used it to treat fever, cough, diarrhoea, itch, ulcer (Chi, 1996). The crude methanolic extract of its leaves showed on bioassay abroad spectrum of antifungal and antibacterial activity. The following fractionation of this by repeated chromatography afforded successively the four-xanthone derivatives 1, 2, 3, 4. The structures of these were deduced from their respective spectral data to quote ESI MS and $^1$H-NMR, $^{13}$C-NMR, DEPT, COSY, HSQC, HMBC among others. 1,2 were identified by literature comparison as the known pancixanthone B (Ito, 1996) and mangiferin (Fujita, 1982). 3, 4 were recognized however as two new ones. They were then named cratoxanthone A (3) and B (4) respectively in consideration of their plant origin.

## 2.0 Experimental Procedure

### 2.1 Plant Material

Leaves of *Cratoxylon cochinchinense* (Lour.) were collected May 2005 in National Park Cuc Phuong (Ninh Binh). The voucher specimen was identified by the taxonomist on the Park–Bs. Vu Van Can, and now deposited in the Herbarium of INPC.

### 2.2 Extraction and Fractionation

Chopped, dried leaves of *Cratoxylon cochinchinense* (7.2 kg) were ultrasonically extracted with methanol in 12 hours. The MeOH was then removed in vacuum, $H_2O$ (1000ml) added, the whole sequentially extracted with n-hexane, $CHCl_3$, EtOAc and n-butanol. Further removal of these solvents in vacuum afforded the n-hexane extract, the $CHCl_3$ extract, the EtOAc extract and the n-butanol extract respectively. Since this time, every chromatographic separation, CC and TLC was performed on corresponding RP-18, silica gel Merck. EtOAc extract (7 g) was subjected to CC over silica gel (63-100μm) using chloroform-methanol (gradient) as eluents to give fractions $A_1$-$A_{18}$. Fraction $A_8$ (812.3mg) was subjected to silica gel column and eluted with chloroform: methanol (100:6) to give fractions $A_8$A (109.9mg), $A_8$B (68.7mg), $A_8$C (118.1mg), $A_8$D (182.5mg). Repeated chromatography of fraction $A_8$A (67mg) on silica gel column using chloroform: methanol (100:6) as mobile phase yielded the yellow solid 1 (8.1 mg). Fraction $A_8$D (91mg) was separated by CC over silica gel and eluted with chloroform: methanol (100:8) to give the white solid 3 (8.7mg). Fraction $A_9$ (308.5mg) was subjected to silica gel column and eluted with chloroform: methanol (10:3) to give the white solid, purified by TLC of silica gel G eluted by acetone yielded 4 (11.4 mg). Fraction $A_{14}$ (108.9mg) was subjected to RP-18 column and eluted with methanol to give the yellow solid, purified by TLC of silica gel G eluted by acetone yielded 2 (9.4 mg).

### 2.3 Compound Characterization

Melting points were measured on a BOETIUS and optical rotations on a POLATRONIC D Schmidt + Haensch. UV data were obtained with a JASCO V530 and IR data with an IMPACT 410-Nicolet. ESI-MS was recorded on a LC/MSD Trap Agilent Series 1100 and 1D-, 2D–NMR on a BRUKER Avance 500 MHz.

1. Yellow solid, $[\alpha]_D$ +3 (c, 0.1 in $CHCl_3$). UV (MeOH) $\lambda_{max}$ (nm): 215; 238 (sh); 246; 256 (sh); 320; 362. IR (KBr) $\nu_{max}$ ($cm^{-1}$): 3284 (br); 1648. MS (m/z, per cent): 312 ($M^+$, 35); 297(100); 282(17); 269(23). For $^1H$ NMR ($CD_3OD$) and $^{13}C$ NMR ($CD_3OD$) spectroscopic data, see Tables 7.1, 7.2.
2. Yellow solid; $[\alpha]_{32}{}^D$ +32 (EtOH). M.p. 278-280. UV (MeOH) $\lambda_{max}$ (nm): 240; 241; 257; 315; 316; 364; 365. IR (KBr) $\nu_{max}$ ($cm^{-1}$): 3392 (br); 3366; 3195; 2964; 1650. MS (m/z): 423 $[M+H]^+$. For $^1H$ NMR (DMSO) and $^{13}C$ NMR (DMSO) spectroscopic data, see Tables 7.1, 7.3.

3. White solid, m.p. 276-277. UV (MeOH) $\lambda_{max}$ (nm): 213; 231 (sh); 246; 253 (sh); 318; 355. IR (KBr) $\nu_{max}$ (cm$^{-1}$): 3210 (br); 1688; 1470. MS (m/z): 329 $[M+H]^+$, 327 $[M-H]^+$. For $^1$H NMR ($CD_3OD$) and $^{13}$C NMR ($CD_3OD$) spectroscopic data, see Tables 7.1, 7.4.
4. White solid, m.p. 274-275. IR (KBr) $\nu_{max}$ (cm$^{-1}$): 3318 (br); 1658. MS (m/z): 327 $[M-H]^+$; 351 $[M+Na]^+$. For $^1$H NMR ($CD_3OD$) and $^{13}$C NMR ($CD_3OD$) spectroscopic data, see Tables 7.1, 7.5.

## 3.0 Results and Discussion

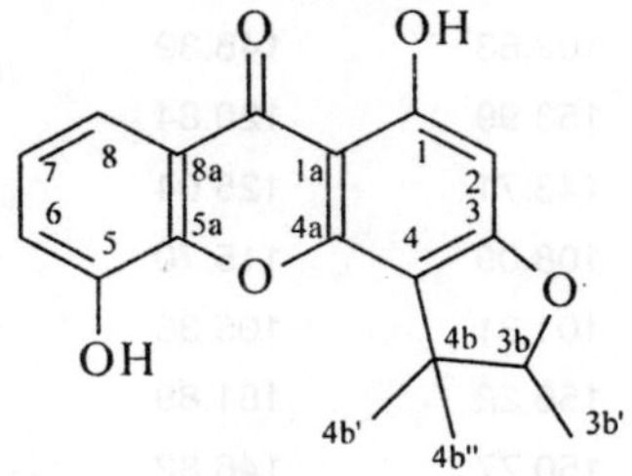

(1)

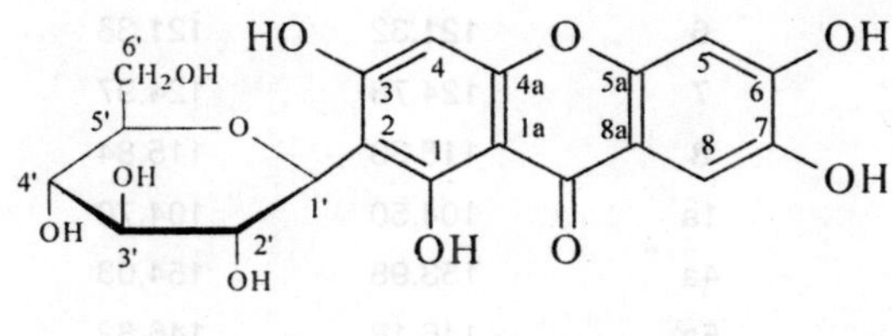

(2)

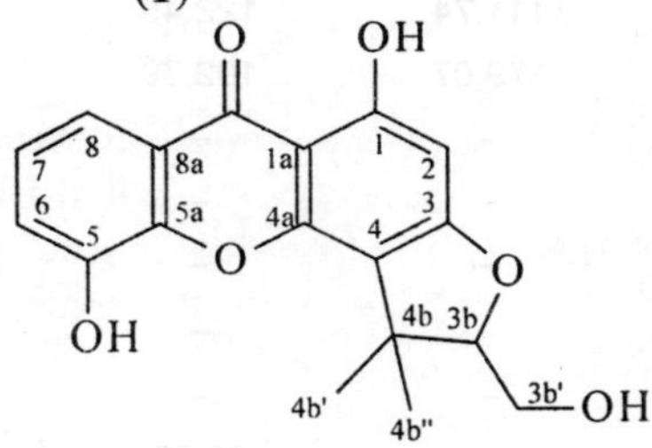

(3)

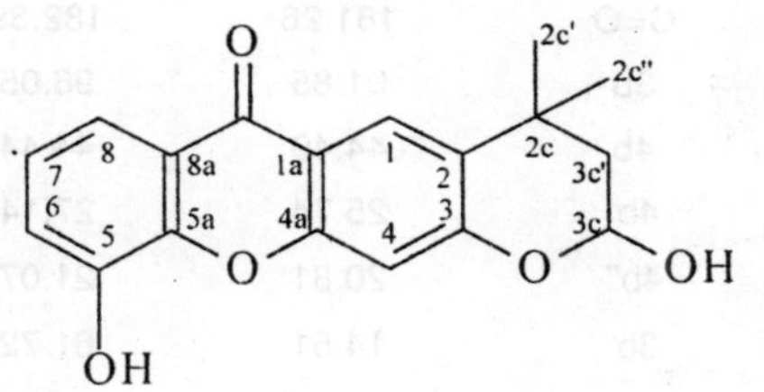

(4)

Compound 1 was obtained as a yellow solid having $[\alpha]_D$ +3 ($CHCl_3$). From the mass spectrum data molecular formula was determined to be $C_{18}H_{16}O_5$. The UV and IR spectrum showed absorptions characteristic of a 1,3,5-trioxygenated-xanthone derivative (Dharmaratne, 1997). The IR spectrum also showed a broad band at $\nu_{max}$ 3284 (br)(OH) and 1648 cm$^{-1}$ due to hydroxyl and carbonyl groups. In the $^1$H NMR spectrum, alone 1H singlet at $\delta_H$ 6.19 and three aromatic protons at $\delta_H$ 7.67 (dd, $J$ = 8.1, 1.5 Hz); 7.37 (dd, $J$ = 8.1, 1.5 Hz), 7.25 (dd, $J$ = 8.1, 8.0 Hz) ascribable to the C-2, C-8, C-6 and C-7 protons of the xanthone nucleus (Bennett, 1988; Ito, 1996), respectively. The observation of two 3H-singlets ($\delta_H$ 1.63 and $\delta_H$ 1.34), a 3H-doublet ($\delta_H$ 1.41, $J$ = 6.6Hz) and a 1H-quartet ($\delta_H$ 4.60, dd, $J$ = 6.6, 5.0 Hz) suggested the presence of 2,3,3-trimethyldihydrofuranring. An angular orientation of the furan ring in the molecule was indicated by the appearance of C-H long-range correlations in the HMBC spectrum between the oxygenated methane carbon at $\delta_C$ 91.85 and two methyl protons at $\delta_H$ 1.63 and 1.34, which further correlated to an aromatic carbon at $\delta_C$ 114.00 and a quaternary carbon at $\delta_C$ 44.49, and also between the C-2 aromatic carbon at $\delta_C$ 94.04 and a hydroxy signal at $\delta_H$ 13.25. From the above results and in comparison with those given in the literature, compound 1 was identified to be pancixanthone B.

**Table 7.1: $^{13}$C-NMR Spectroscopic Data of Xanthone Derivatives from *C. cochinchinense***

| *C–position* | $\delta_C$ *(ppm)* | | | |
|---|---|---|---|---|
| | *1* | *3* | *2* | *4* |
| 1 | 165.24 | 167.58 | 161.77 | 100.19 |
| 2 | 94.04 | 94.35 | 107.60 | 110.98 |
| 3 | 165.70 | 165.44 | 163.82 | 162.14 |
| 4 | 114.00 | 114.26 | 93.32 | 157.13 |
| 5 | 147.17 | 148.49 | 102.63 | 148.39 |
| 6 | 121.32 | 121.38 | 153.99 | 120.84 |
| 7 | 124.73 | 124.97 | 143.71 | 125.04 |
| 8 | 116.33 | 115.84 | 108.09 | 115.70 |
| 1a | 104.50 | 104.70 | 101.31 | 105.36 |
| 4a | 153.98 | 154.03 | 156.22 | 161.89 |
| 5a | 146.18 | 146.82 | 150.77 | 146.82 |
| 8a | 121.84 | 122.68 | 111.74 | 122.45 |
| C=O | 181.26 | 182.39 | 179.07 | 182.79 |
| 3b | 91.85 | 96.05 | – | – |
| 4b | 44.49 | 44.44 | – | – |
| 4b' | 25.74 | 27.14 | – | – |
| 4b" | 20.81 | 21.07 | – | – |
| 3b' | 14.51 | 61.72 | – | – |
| 2c | – | – | – | 33.35 |
| 3c | – | – | – | 94.23 |
| 3c' | – | – | – | 47.25 |
| 2c' | – | – | – | 29.13 |
| 2c" | – | – | – | 28.92 |
| Glucose | | | | |
| 1' | – | – | 73.08 | – |
| 2' | – | – | 70.63 | – |
| 3' | – | – | 78.98 | – |
| 4' | – | – | 70.25 | – |
| 5' | – | – | 81.55 | – |
| 6' | – | – | 61.48 | – |

Compound 2: The $^{13}$C NMR and UV absorption spectrum are characteristic of 1,3,6,7-tetraoxygenated xanthone C-glycosides. The IR spectrum also showed a broad band at $\nu_{max}$ 3392 (br), 3366 due to hydroxyl and 1650 cm$^{-1}$ and due to carbonyl groups. From the mass spectrum, the molecular formula of 2 was determined to be $C_{19}H_{18}O_{11}$. This compound gave a positive Gibbs test, indicating that an aromatic

proton is located para to a phenolic hydroxyl group and that glucose is linked at C-2. The [1]H NMR spectrum showed the signals of three aromatic protons ($\delta_H$ 6.37, 6.86 and 7.38, each 1H, s) ascribable to the C-4, C-5 and C-8 protons of the xanthone nucleus, respectively, on the basic of known data (Fujita, 1982). This compound was obtained as a yellow solid having $[\alpha]_{32}^{D}$ +32 (EtOH) and melting point at 278-280°C. From the above results and in comparison with those given in the literature, the structure of 2 was identified to be mangiferin.

**Table 7.2: The ¹H-NMR and HMBC Spectroscopic Data of 1**

| *H-position* | *Compound 1* | |
|---|---|---|
| | *$\delta_H$ (ppm)* | *HMBC* |
| 2 | 6.19(1H, s) | C-4, C-1a |
| 6 | 7.37 (1H, dd, *J* = 8.1, 1.5 Hz) | C-8, C-5a |
| 7 | 7.25 (1H, dd, *J* = 8.1, 8.0 Hz) | C-8a, C-5 |
| 8 | 7.67 (1H, dd, *J* = 8.1, 1.5 Hz) | C-5a, C-6, C = O |
| 3b | 4.60 (1H, dd, *J* = 6.6, 5.0 Hz) | C-4b', C-4b'', C-3b' |
| 4b' | 1.63 (3H, s) | C-3b, C-4, C-4b |
| 4b'' | 1.34 (3H, s) | C-3b, C-4, C-4b |
| 3b' | 1.41 (3H, d, *J* = 6.6 Hz) | C-3b, C-4b |

**Table 7.3: The ¹H-NMR and HMBC Spectroscopic Data of 2**

| *H-position* | *Compound 2* | |
|---|---|---|
| | *$\delta_H$ (ppm)* | *HMBC* |
| 4 | 6.37 (1H,s) | C-2, C-9a |
| 5 | 6.86 (1H,s) | C-7, C-8a |
| 8 | 7.38 (1H,s) | C-6, C-5a, C = O |
| Glucose | | |
| 1' | 4.59 (1H,d, *J* = 9.8 Hz) | C-2, C-3, C-2', C-3', C-5' |
| 2' | 4.04 (1H, t, *J* = 9.4 Hz) | |
| 3' | 3.20 (1H, t, *J* = 8.6 Hz) | |
| 4' | 3.11 (1H, t, *J* = 9.2 Hz) | |
| 5' | 3.16 (1H, m) | |
| 6' | 3.68 (1H,dd, *J* = 12.0, 1.8 Hz) | |
| | 3.40 (1H,dd, *J* = 12.0, 1.8 Hz) | |

Compound 3 was obtained as a white solid having melting point 276-277 °C. The UV and IR spectrum showed absorptions characteristic of a 1,3,5-trioxygenated xanthone derivative (Ito, 1996). The IR spectrum also showed a broad band at $\nu_{max}$ 3210 (br) and 1688 cm$^{-1}$ due to hydroxy and carbonyl groups, respectively. From the mass spectrum, the molecular formula was determined to be $C_{18}H_{16}O_6$. From the above results and NMR spectrums (Tables 7.1, 7.4), combined with the mass spectrum and compared with those of Pancixanthone B, 3 was identified to be 3b′-hydroxy pancixanthone B. This structure has one hydroxyl group (linked with C-3b′) more than Pancixanthone B. The presence additional of this hydroxyl group at position 3b′ was ascertained by the resonances at $\delta_H$3.90/ $\delta_C$61.72 (H-3b′, C-3b′) and $\delta_H$4.51/ $\delta_C$96.05 (H-3b, C-3b).

**Table 7.4: The ¹H-NMR and HMBC Spectroscopic Data of 3**

| H-position | Compound 3 | |
|---|---|---|
| | $\delta_H$ (ppm) | HMBC |
| 2 | 6.24 (1H, s) | C-4, C-1a |
| 6 | 7.26 (1H, dd, *J* = 8.0, 1.5 Hz) | C-8, C-5a |
| 7 | 7.21(1H, dd, *J* = 8.0, 8.0 Hz) | C-8a, C-5 |
| 8 | 7.63 (1H, dd, *J* = 8.0, 1.5 Hz) | C-5a, C-6, C = O |
| 3b | 4.51 (1H, dd, *J* = 6.5, 5.0 Hz) | C-4b′, C-4b″, C-3b′ |
| 4b′ | 1.71 (3H, s) | C-3b, C-4, C-4b |
| 4b″ | 1.46 (3H, s) | C-3b, C-4, C-4b |
| 3b′ | 3.90 (1H, d, *J* = 6.5 Hz) | C-3b, C-4b |
| | 3.90 (1H, d, *J* = 5.0 Hz) | C-3b, C-4b |

**Table 7.5: The ¹H-NMR and HMBC Spectroscopic Data of 4**

| H-position | Compound 4 | |
|---|---|---|
| | $\delta_H$ (ppm) | HMBC |
| 1 | 6.21(1H, s) | C-3, C-4a, C = O, C-2, C-2b |
| 6 | 7.27 (1H, dd, *J* = 8.0, 1.5 Hz) | C-5a, C-8 |
| 7 | 7.23 (1H, dd, *J* = 8.0, 8.0 Hz) | C-5, C-8a |
| 8 | 7.63 (1H, dd, *J* = 1.5, 8.0 Hz) | C-6, C = O, C-5a |
| 3c | 5.44 (1H, dd, *J* = 5.5, 5.5 Hz) | C-3c′, C-2c |
| 3c′ | 1.92-1.97 (2H, brd) | C-2c′, C-2c″, C-3c′ |
| 2c′ | 1.73 (3H, s) | C-3c′, C-2c″ |
| 2c″ | 1.62 (3H, s) | C-3c′, C-2c′ |

Compound 4 was obtained as a white solid having melting point 274-275°C. The IR spectrum also showed a broad band at $\nu_{max}$ 3318 (br) and 1658 cm$^{-1}$ due to hydroxy and carbonyl groups, respectively. The ¹H NMR spectrum showed the signals of four aromatic protons at $\delta_H$ 6.21(1H, 1s); 7.27 (1H, dd, *J* = 8.0, 1.5 Hz); 7.23 (1H, dd, *J* = 8.0, 8.0 Hz); 7.63 (1H, dd, *J* = 1.5, 8.0 Hz)) ascribable to the C-1, C-6, C-7 and C-8 protons of the xanthone nucleus, respectively (Ampofo, 1986; Ito, 1996). The observation of two 3H-singlets ($\delta_H$ 1.73 and $\delta_H$ 1.62), a 2H-doublet ($\delta_H$ 1.92-1.97) and a 1H-quartet ($\delta_H$ 5.44, dd, *J* = 5.5, 5.5 Hz) suggested the presence of 2-hydroxy-4, 4-

dimethyldihydropyranring. The presence of the pyran ring in the molecule was indicated by the appearance of C-H long-range correlations in the HMBC spectrum between the methylene carbon at $\delta_C$ 47.25 and two methyl protons at $\delta_H$ 1.73 and 1.62, which further correlated to an aromatic carbon at $\delta_C$ 110.98, and also between a methine carbon at $\delta_C$ 94.23 and a methylene proton signal at $\delta_H$ 1.92, between an aromatic proton at $\delta_H$ 6.21 and a quaternary carbon at $\delta_C$ 33.35. From the above results, 4 were identified to be a new xanthone, named cratoxanthone B.

## Acknowledgement

We are grateful to Mr. Vu Van Can of Cuc Phuong national forest for identification of the plant.

## References

Ampofo, S.A., Waterman, P.G., 1986. Xanthones and neoflavonoids from two Asian species of *Calophyllum*. Phytochem, 25 (11): pp. 2617–2620.

Bennett, G.J., Lee, H.H., 1988. Xanthones from *Guttiferae*. Phytochem, 28 (4): pp. 967–998.

Chi, V. V., 1996. Glossary of Medicinal Plants in Vietnam. Y hoc Publisher, Vietnam: pp. 1135.

Dharmaratne, H.R.W., Wijesinghe, W.M.N.M., 1997. A trioxygenated diprenylated chromnxanthone from *Calophyllum moon2*. Phytochem, 46 (7): pp. 1293–1295.

Fujita, M., Inoue, T., 1982. Studies on the constituents of *Iris florentina* L. 2. C-glucosides of xanthones and flavones from the leaves. Chem. Pharm. Bull. 30(7): pp. 2342–2348.

Ito, C., Miyamoto, Y., Rao, K. S., Furukawa, H., 1996. A novel Dibenzofuran and Two New Xanthones from *Calophyllum panciflorum*. Chem. Pharm. Bull. (44): pp. 441–443.

Rukachaisirikul V., Kaewnok W., Koysomboon S., Phongpaichit S., Taylor W.C., 2000. Caged–tetraprenylated xanthones from *Garcinia scortechin2*. Tetrahedron (56): pp. 8539-8543.

# Chapter 8

# Flavonoids from *Belamcanda sinensis*

**Le Minh Ha[1]*, Nguyen Van Hoan[1] and Tran Cam Son[2]**

[1]*Institute of Natural Products Chemistry, Vietnamese Academy of Science and Technology, Hanoi, Vietnam*

[2]*Hanoi University of Technology, Hanoi, Vietnam*

**E-mail: halm2vn@gmail.com*

## ABSTRACT

*Belamcanda sinensis* (Iridaceae family) of Vietnam has been studied for its on chemical constituents and biological activity. Two isoflavonoids: tectorigenin (1), iristectorin A (2) and one flavonol rhamnocitrin (3) have been isolated from the rhizomes of *B. sinensis*. Their structures were elucidated by spectroscopic methods. Compound 1 was obtained as a main compound, 0.078 per cent from the dry rhizomes.

***Keywords:*** *Belamcanda sinensis, Dry rhizmomes, Tectorigenin, Tristectorin A, Rhamnocitrin, Vietnamese traditional medicine.*

## 1.0 Introduction

*Belamcanda sinensis* is a perennial shrub belonging to Iridaceae family. It is widely distributed in the cold and wet hillsides in Vietnam. The dried rhizomes have been used in Vietnamese traditional and folk medicine as an anti-inflammatory, antitussive, and expectorant agent as well as against throat trouble (Loi, 1991). With regard to the chemical constituents of the plant, the occurrence of iridal-type triterpenoids and isoflavonoids in the rhizomes, and phenol, benzoquinones and benzofurans in the seed was reported (Woo, 1993 and Takahaski, 2000). In Vietnam, *B. sinensis* has not been investigated for its chemical constituents and biological activity.

In this report, we describe the isolation and structural elucidation of two isofiavonoids: tectorigenin (1), iristectorin A (2) and one flavonol rhamnocitrin (3) isolated from the rhizomes of *B. sinensis*.

## 2.0 Materials and Methods

### 2.1 Plant Material

The rhizomes of *B. sinensis* was collected in Tamdao National Botanical Garden, Vietnam, in February 2007 and identified by biologist Ngo Van Trai. A voucher specimen is deposited in the Herbarium of Institute of Natural Products Chemistry, Vietnamese Academy of Science and Technology.

### 2.2 General Experimental Procedures

NMR spectra were recorded on a Bruker AM500 FT-NMR spectrometer (500MHz for $^1$H and 125MHz for $^{13}$C) in $CD_3OD$ and $CDCl_3$, using TMS as internal standard. ESI-MS spectra were obtained from an AGILENT spectrometer. The following adsorbents were used for purification: TLC normal phase Kieselgel 60 $F_{254}$ (Merck 5554, 0.2 mm), CC: normal phase Si gel (Merck, 0.063-0.200 mm). The TLC chromatogram were visualized under UV at 254 and 368 nm and sprayed with solution of $Ce(SO_4)_2$ in $H_2SO_4$ 65 per cent.

### 2.3 Extraction and Isolation

2kg of air-dried powdered rhizomes of *B. sinensis* were soaked successively in *n*-hexane three times at room temperature to yield a *n*-hexane extract. The residue was further extracted with MeOH. The methanolic concentrated solution was diluted with $H_2O$ and extracted successively with ethyl acetate and *n*-BuOH. After removal of the solvents *in vacuo* to give ethyl acetate and *n*-BuOH extracts. The ethyl acetate extract was subjected to column chromatography over silica gel using a solvent system $CHCl_3$-MeOH (99:1 to 90:10) in stepwise gradient mode. The eluate with $CHCl_3$-MeOH (95:5) was further purified by repeated column chromatography over silica gel using $CHCl_3$-MeOH (95:5 to 90:10) to afford tectorigenin (1), iristectorin A (2) and rhamnocitrin (3).

**Tectorigenin (1)**

Pale yellow plates (1560mg, 0.078 per cent from the dry rhizomes), mp.235-236°C, $C_{16}H_{12}O_6$, ESI-MS *m/z* 299 [M-H]$^+$.

$^1$H-NMR ($CD_3OD$ and $CDCl_3$): $\delta$ (ppm) 3.87 (3H, s, $OCH_3$-6), 6.41 (1H, s, H-8), 6.84 (2H, dd, J = 8.5, 1.5Hz, H-3′, 5′), 7.35 (2H, dd, J = 8.5, 1.5Hz, H-2′, 6′), and 7.99 (1H, s, H-2).

$^{13}$C-NMR ($CD_3OD$ and $CDCl_3$): $\delta$ (ppm) 60.9 ($OCH_3$-6), 94.9 (C-8), 106.6 (C-10), 116.2 (C-2′,6′), 123.1 (C-3), 124.1 (C-1′), 131.3 (C-3′, 5′), 132.7 (C-6), 154.4 (C-5), 154.7 (C-7), 154.8 (C-2), 158.5 (C-9), 158.6 (C-4′), and 182.4 (C-4).

**Iristectorin A (2)**

Pale yellow amorphous powder (120mg, 0.006 per cent from the dry rhizomes), mp.237-238°C, $C_{17}H_{14}O_7$, ESI-MS *m/z* 329 [M-H]$^+$.

$^1$H-NMR ($CD_3OD$ and $CDCl_3$): δ (ppm) 3.89 (3H, s, $OCH_3$-6), 3.90 (3H, s, $OCH_3$-4′), 6.46 (1H, s, H-8), 6.88 (1H, d, J = 8.0Hz, H-2′), 6.96 (1H, dd, J = 8.0, 2.0Hz, H-6′), 7.14 (1H, J = 2.0Hz, H-5′), and 8.06 (1H, s, H-2).

$^{13}$C-NMR ($CD_3OD$ and $CDCl_3$): δ (ppm) 56.4 ($OCH_3$-4′), 60.9 ($OCH_3$-6), 94.9 (C-8), 106.6 (C-10), 113.8 (C-5′), 116.1 (C-2′), 122.7 (C-6′), 123.5 (C-3), 124.2 (C-1′), 132.7 (C-6), 147.7 (C-3′), 148.6 (C-4′), 154.4 (C-5), 154.7 (C-7), 154.8 (C-2), 158.6 (C-9), and 182.4 (C-4).

**Rhamnocitrin (3)**

Yellow amorphous powder (40mg, 0.002 per cent from the dry rhizomes), mp.221-223°C, $C_{16}H_{12}O_6$, ESI-MS *m/z* 299 $[M-H]^+$.

$^1$H-NMR ($CD_3OD$ and $CDCl_3$): δ (ppm) 3.89 (3H, s, $OCH_3$), 6.54 (1H, s, H-8), 6.56 (1H, s, H-6), 6.93 (2H, dd, J = 8.5, H-3′, 5′), and 7.82 (2H, dd, J = 9.0Hz, H-2′, 6′).

$^{13}$C-NMR ($CD_3OD$): δ (ppm) 60.9 ($OCH_3$-7), 92.1 (C-8), 104.3 (C-10), 115.6 (C-3′,5′), 135.6 (C-3), 121.8 (C-1′), 129.5 (C-2′, 6′), 97.6 (C-6), 160.3 (C-5), 164.8 (C-7), 147.4 (C-2), 156.3 (C-9), 159.5 (C-4′), and 176.8 (C-4).

## 3.0 Results and Discussion

Compound 1 was obtained as a main compound (0.078 per cent from the dry rhizomes) with pale yellow plates, mp.235-236°C. The presence of an isoflavone skeleton was suggested from the UV spectrum (max 259, 320nm). Its molecular formula $C_{16}H_{12}O_6$ was determined by electrospray ionization mass spectrometer ESI-MS with *m/z* 299 $[M-H]^+$. The $^1$H-NMR spectrum of 1 showed signals of two sets of *ortho*-coupled aromatic protons at $\delta_H$ 7.35 (2H, dd, J = 8.5, 1.5Hz, H-2′, 6′) and 6.84 (2H, dd, J = 8.5, 1.5Hz, H-3′, 5′) together two singlet at $\delta_H$ 6.41 (1H, s, H-8), 7.99 (1H, s, H-2) and one methoxyl group at δ 3.87 ppm (3H, s, $OCH_3$-6). These features are characteristic of a 7,5,4′-trihydroxyisoflavone derivative. These data are in good agreement with those reported for 4′, 5, 7–trihydroxy-6 methoxyisoflavone. Therefore, compound 1 was identified as tectorigenin (Agrawal, 1989). It is reported that tectorigenin possess anti-inflammatory activity *in vivo*. Shin *et al.* (1999) examined the effects of tectorigenin and tectoridin on $PGE_2$ production in rat peritoneal macrophages stimulated by TPA. Tectorigenin inhibited $PGE_2$ production with the $IC_{50}$ values of 3μM, 10 times more potent than that of tectoridin ($IC_{50}$: 30μM). These results suggested that tectorigenin is very rich in Vietnamese *B. sinensis* and this compound may be a potential lead for application against inflammation

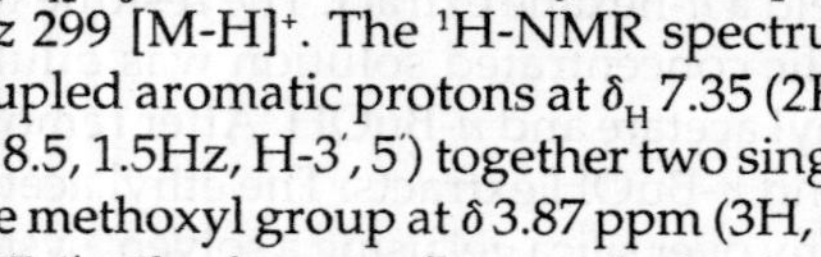

1

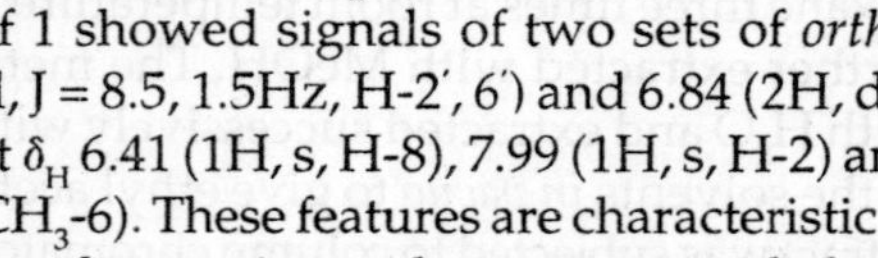

2

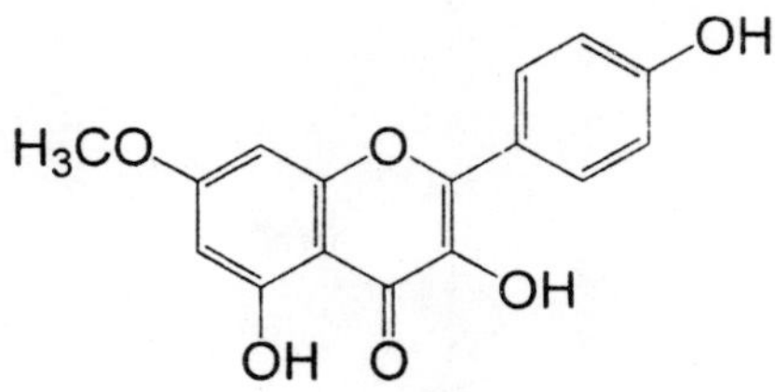

**3**

Compound 2 was obtained as a pale yellow amorphous powder mp.237-238°C. Its molecular formula $C_{17}H_{14}O_7$ was determined by electrospray ionization mass spectrometer (ESI-MS) with *m/z* 329 [M-H]$^+$. The UV, $^1$H–and $^{13}$C-NMR spectra of 2 were similar to those of 1 confirming the isoflavonoid skeleton. Comparison between the $^1$H-NMR spectrum of 1 and 2 indicated that 2 differed for the presence of an additional methoxyl proton resonances at $\delta_H$ 3.90 ppm (3H, s, $OCH_3$-4′) and the hydroxyl group of 2 allocated to the C-3′ position ($\delta_C$ 147.7ppm) instead of the C-4′ position of 1. On the basis of these data, compound 2 was characterized as iristectorin A or (3′, 5, 7–trihydroxy–4′, 6 dimethoxyisoflavone) (Agrawal, 1989).

Compound 3 was obtained as a yellow amorphous powder, mp.221-223° and gave a mass spectrum with a [M-H]$^+$ peak at *m/z* 299 consistent with the formula $C_{16}H_{12}O_6$, which was confirmed by $^{13}$C-NMR and DEPT experiments. The UV spectrum showed absorption maxima at 255, 269nm (band II) and 365nm (band I) typical of a flavonol skeleton. The bathochromic shifts of band I with $AlCl_3$/HCl is characteristic of a 3,5-dihydroxyflavone. The $^1$H-NMR spectrum confirmed of the above and, in addition, revealed the presence of one methoxy group at $\delta_H$ 3.32ppm (3H, s, $OCH_3$). The site of methylation of C-7 was downfield at $\delta_C$ 164.9ppm. Therefore, compound 3 was identified as rhamnocitrin (or kaempferol 7-methyl ether) (Barabera *et al.*, 1986).

## References

Agrawal, P.K., 1989. Carbon–13 NMR of flavonoids, Elsevier Science Publishers B.V., pp. 203.

Barabera, O., Sanz, J.F. and Parareda, J.S., 1986. Further flavonol glycosides from *Anthyllis onobrychioides*. Phytochemistry (25), 2361-2365.

Loi, D. T., 1991. Vietnamese Traditional Medicine Plants, Hanoi Scientific and Technology Publisher, Hanoi, pp. 63.

Shin, Kuk Hyun, Kim, Yong Pil, Lim, Soon Sung, Lee, Sanghyun, Ryu, Nama, Yamada, Masateru and Ohuchi, Kazuo, 1999. Inhibition of Prostaglandin $E_2$ production by the isoflavones tectorigenin and tectoridin isolated from the rhizomes of *Belamcanda chinensis*, Planta Med. (65), pp. 776-777.

Takahashi, K., Hoshino, Y., Suzuki, S., Hano Y., 2000. Iridals from *Iris tectorum* and *Belamcanda chinensis*. Phytochemistry (53), pp. 925-929.

Woo, W. S., Woo E. H., 1993. An isoflavone noririsflorentin from *Belamcanda chinenesis*. Phytochemistry (33), pp. 939-940.

# Chapter 9

# Peroxygenases: New Extra-cellular Mushroom Enzymes which Oxygenate Aromatic Compounds

*René Ullrich[1], Dau Hung Anh[1,4], Matthias, Kinne[1], Martin Kluge[1], Christian Dolge[2], Mandy Starke[2], Christiana Liers[1], Katrina Scheibner[3], Do Hue Nghi[4], Le Mai Huong[4] and Martin Hofrichter[1]**

[1]*International Graduate School of Zeta, Unit of Environmental Biotechnology, Markt 23, 02763 Zittau, Germany*

[2]*University of Applied Sciences Zittau/Görlitz, Biotechnology Group, Theodor-Koerner-Allee 16, 02763 Zittau, Germany*

[3]*Lausitz University of Applied Sciences Senftenberg, Department of Biotechnology, Post Box 101548, 01958 Senftenberg, Germany*

[4]*Institute of Natural Products Chemistry, Vietnamese Academy of Science and Technology 18 Hoang Quoc Viet Rd., Hanoi, Vietnam*

**E-mail: hofrichter@ihi-zittau.de*

## ABSTRACT

Agaric mushrooms of the families Bolbitiaceae and Coprinaceae secrete a novel type of heme enzyme into their microenvironment when growing on nitrogen-rich substrates. The enzyme is a functional hybrid of peroxidases and cytochrome P450 monooxygenases and capable of catalyzing the following reactions: aromatic oxygenation/hydroxylation, *O*-dealkylation, aromatic bromination, aromatic side-chain oxygenation as well as phenol oxidation. It was discovered in *Agrocybe aegerita* (Black poplar mushroom) and first described as *Agrocybe aegerita* peroxidase (AaP); later also other *Agrocybe* as well as *Coprinus* species have been found to produce similar enzymes. They are all highly glycosylated heme-thiolate proteins and use hydrogen peroxide as co-substrate that acts as the primary electron acceptor and oxygen source. Due to their exceptional biochemical properties, mushroom peroxygenases could become a versatile biotechnological tool in organic synthesis.

***Keywords***: *Peroxidase, P450, Agrocybe, Coprinus, Hydroxylation, O-dealkylation.*

## 1.0 Introduction

Heme-thiolate proteins are versatile biocatalysts (P450s, haloperoxidases) transferring, amongst others, oxygen to various substrates and, certain P450s can also catalyze *O*-dealkylation. For more than 40 years, chloroperoxidase (CPO) from the ascomycete *Caldariomyces fumago* ("sooty mold") has been the only known peroxidase of this type. CPO was found to oxygenate aliphatic and cyclic dienes (but no aromatic substrates) (Hofrichter and Ullrich, 2006), chlorinate and cleave non-phenolic lignin model compounds, depolymerize synthetic guaiacyl lignin (Ortiz *et al.*, 2003) and catalyzes other interesting reactions. We have recently discovered a second fungal heme-thiolate peroxidase in the alkaliphilic basidiomycete *Agrocybe aegerita* (Black poplar mushroom) that shares spectral and catalytic properties both with P450 enzymes and CPO and can therefore be regarded as a functional hybrid of both enzyme types (Ullrich and Hofrichter, 2007). It was first designated as AaP (*Agrocybe aegerita* peroxidase) but is nowadays also referred to as haloperoxidase-peroxygenase or simply peroxygenase, since it is found in other mushrooms (*e.g. Coprinus* spp.) as well and shows both peroxygenating, oxidative and halogenating activities. Here we report on several AaP-catalyzed reactions, which may be relevant for the chemical modification and degradation of aromatic compounds by mushrooms.

## 2.0 Materials and Methods

*Agrocybe aegerita* was isolated from a bark–and straw-containing compost pile in Jena (Germany), and its peroxidase (AaP) has routinely been produced in culture flasks (500 to 1000 ml) and stirred-tank bioreactors (5 to 10 liters) using complex media based on soy beans (Ullrich *et al.*, 2004). The enzyme was purified to homogeneity by several ultrafiltration and chromatography steps (fast protein liquid chromatography) involving strong cation and anion exchangers (*e.g.* Mono Q and Mono S columns). In the same way, the peroxygenase (CrP) of the coprophilous ink cap *Coprinus radians* (nowadays named *Coprinellus radians*) that had been isolated from dung, was produced and purified (Anh *et al.*, 2007).

*In-vitro* oxygenation/oxidation, dealkylation and halogenation tests with the purified enzyme were performed in phosphate buffers at neutral or acidic pH. The AaP co-substrate $H_2O_2$ was directly added or continuously generated by glucose oxidase or a pump system. Among the substrates tested were various aromatic compounds including aryl ethers, alcohols and aldehydes, alkyl benzenes, polycyclic aromatic hydrocarbons, pyridine and non-phenolic lignin model compounds ($\beta$-O-4 dimers). Following analytical methods and techniques were used to characterize peroxygenases and their reactions: FPLC, SDS-PAGE, IEF, HPLC, LC-MS, GC-MS,

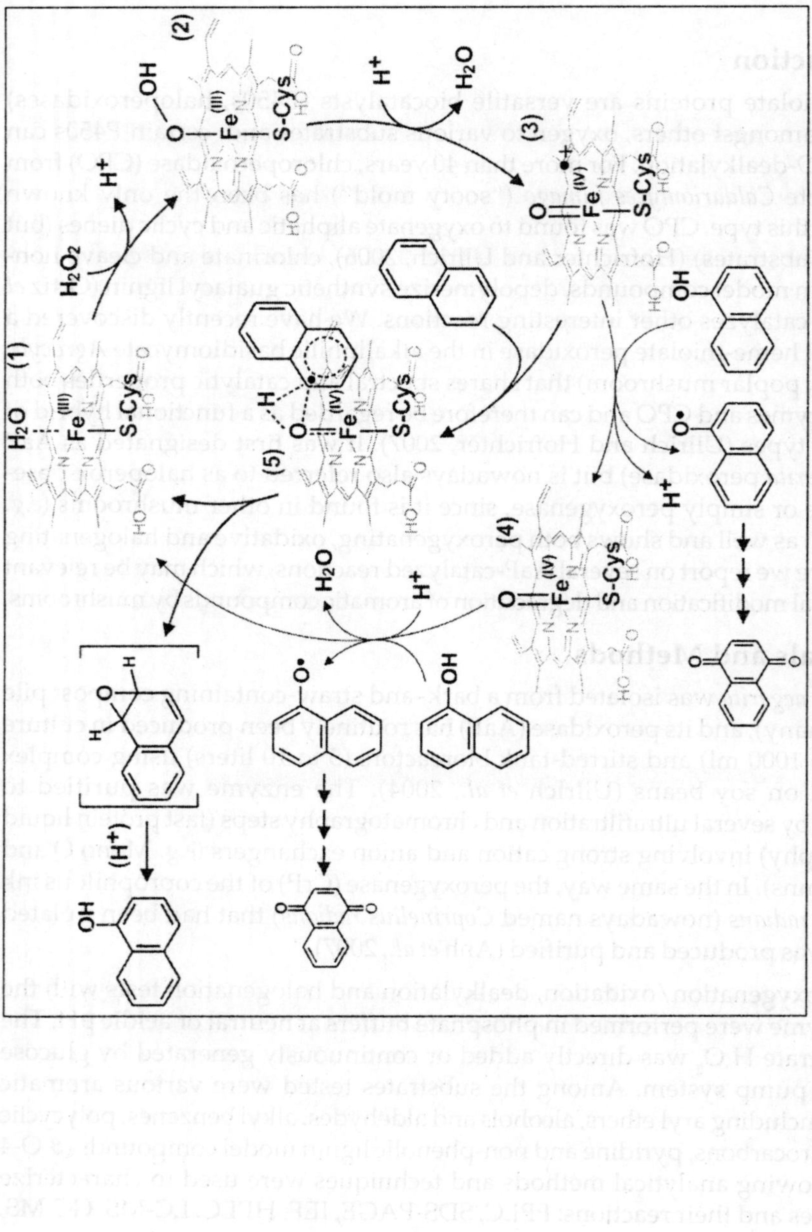


**Figure 9.1: Hypothetical Catalytic Cycle of Aromatic Peroxygenases (e.g. AaP) Illustrated by the Oxygenation/Hydroxylation and Oxidation of Naphthalene (modified according to Hofrichter and Ullrich, 2007 and Kluge *et al.* 2007) 1–native enzyme, 2–Compound 0, 3–Compound I, 4–Compound 2 Naphthalene is oxygenated to instable naphthalene 1, 2-oxide that hydrolyzes to 1-naphthol as major product. The latter in turn is oxidized to the corresponding phenoxy radical that disproportionates to 1,4-naphthoquinone**

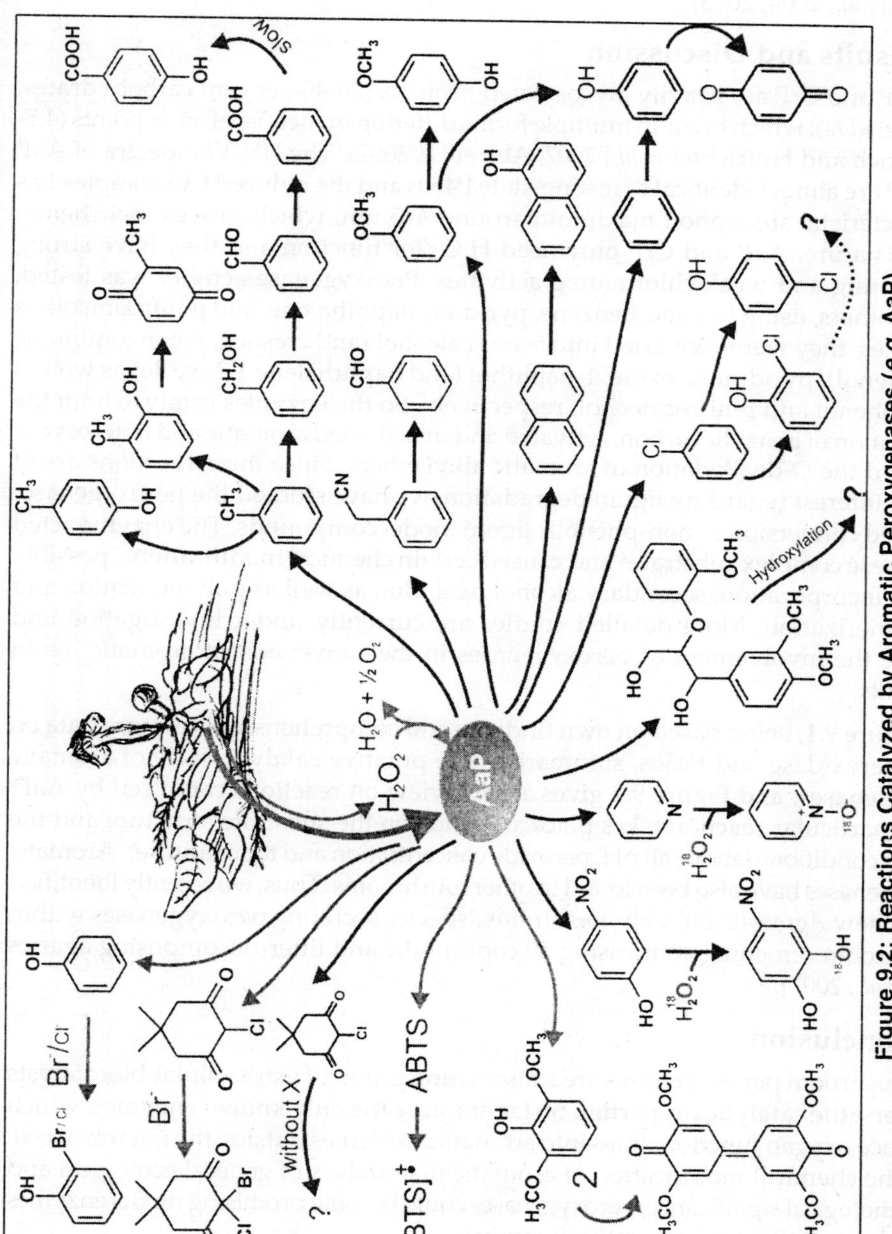


**Figure 9.2: Reactions Catalyzed by Aromatic Peroxygenases (*e.g.* AaP). Among them are halogenations (preferably brominations), classic peroxidase reactions (*e.g.* phenol oxidation), aryl alcohol and aldehydes oxidation as well as several oxygenation/hydroxylation reactions (modified according to Hofrichter 2006).**

HPSEC (high performance size exclusion chromatography) and UV-Vis spectroscopy (Ullrich *et al.*, 2004, 2005).

## 3.0 Results and Discussion

AaP and CrP are heavily glycosylated proteins (20-40 per cent carbohydrates, $M_w$ 43-46 kDa), which occur in multiple forms differing in their isoelectric points (4.5-5.5; Ullrich and Hofrichter *et al.*, 2007; Abh *et al.*, 2007). The UV-Vis spectra of AaP and CrP are almost identical to resting-state P450s and the reduced CO-complex has a characteristic absorption maximum around 445 nm, which proves their heme-thiolate nature. AaP and CrP only need $H_2O_2$ for function and they have strong brominating and weak chlorinating activities. Peroxygenase activity was tested, among others, using toluene, benzene, pyridine, naphthalene, and *p*-nitroanisole as substrates; they were converted into benzyl alcohol (and cresols), *p*-benzoquinone (and phenol), pyridine *N*-oxide, 1-naphthol (and naphthalene 1,2-oxide) as well as *p*-nitrophenol and *p*-nitrocatechol, respectively. So the enzymes catalyze both the oxygenation of benzylic carbon, activated and unactivated aromatic and heterocyclic rings and the *O*-dealkylation of aromatic alkyl ethers. Since these reactions are of general interest regarding lignin degradation, we have studied the peroxygenase-catalyzed conversion of non-phenolic lignin model compounds. The enzyme acted on all these complex substrates and caused certain chemical modifications, possibly oxygen incorporation, secondary alcohol oxidation as well as polymerization and depolymerization. More detailed studies are currently under investigation and indicate the involvement of peroxygenases in the conversion of aromatic lignin fragments.

Figure 9.1, being based on own findings and comprehensive literature data on chloroperoxidase and P450s, summarizes the putative catalytic cycle of aromatic peroxygenases, and Figure 9.2 gives an overview on reactions catalyzed by AaP. Which particular reaction takes place, depends on the substrate structure and the reaction conditions (above all pH, peroxide concentration and temperature). Aromatic peroxygenases have also been found in other mushrooms. Thus, we recently identified several new *Agrocybe* and *Coprinus* strains/species secreting peroxygenases within a mushroom screening comprising 50 coprophilic and litter-decomposing agarics (Anh *et al.*, 2007).

## 4.0 Conclusion

Mushroom peroxygenases are a fascinating group of extracellular biocatalysts with versatile catalytic properties. So far, they are the only known enzymes, which introduce oxygen functionalities into aromatic molecules outside the microbial cell. Since the chemical modification of aromatic materials is of general ecological and biotechnological significance, peroxygenases could become promising model enzymes for biodegradation and biosynthesis studies.

## Acknowledgements

Financial support by the European Union (integrated project BIORENEW), the German Ministry for Education and Research (BMBF; projects 0313433D, VNM 05/

003), the German Environmental Foundation (DBU; Az 13225–32 ChemBioTec) and the German Academic Exchange Service (DAAD; projects A/04/20213, D/05/11714) is gratefully acknowledged. We thank C. Liers, M. Kluge (Inge), M. Kinne (Konrad), M. Brandt, and U. Schneider for technical and scientific assistance.

## References

Anh *et al.*, 2007. The coprophilous mushroom *Coprinus radians* secrete a haloperoxidase that catalyzes aromatic peroxygenation. Appl. Environ. Microbiol. (73): pp. 5477-5485.

Hofrichter, M., Ullrich, R., 2006. Heme-thiolate haloperoxidases: versatile biocatalysts with biotechnological and environmental significance. Appl. Microbiol. Biotechnol. (71): pp. 276-288.

Hofrichter, M., Ullrich, R., Steffen, K., 2007. Application of fungi and their versatile biocatalysts in sustainable technologies. In: Filho, W.L., Greif, D., Delakowitz, B. (eds.) Sustainable chemistry and biotechnology–a contribution to rivers' management, Peter Lang, Frankfurt A.M.: pp. 137-150.

Kluge, M., Ullrich, R., Scheibner, K., Hofrichter, M., 2007. Spectrophotometric assay for detection of aromatic hydroxylation catalyzed by fungal haloperoxidase-peroxygenase. Appl. Microbiol. Biotechnol. (75): pp. 1473-1478.

Ortiz-Bermúdez, P., Srebotnik, E., Hammel, K. 2003. Chlorination and cleavage of lignin structures by fungal chloroperoxidases. Appl. Environ. Microbiol. (69): pp. 5015-5018.

Ullrich, R., Hofrichter, M., 2005. The haloperoxidase of the agaric fungus Agrocybe aegerita hydroxylates toluene and naphthalene. FEBS Lett. (579): pp. 6247-6250.

Ullrich, R., Hofrichter, M., 2007. Enzymatic hydroxylation of aromatic compounds. Cell. Mol. Life Sc1. (67): pp. 271-293.

Ullrich, R., Nüske, J., Scheibner, K., Spantzel, J., Hofrichter, M., 2004. Novel haloperoxidase from the agaric basidiomycete *Agrocybe aegerita* oxidizes aryl alcohols and aldehydes. Appl. Environ. Microbiol. (70): pp. 4575-4581.

Ullrich, R., Huong, L.M., Dung, N.L., Hofrichter, M., 2005. Laccase from the medicinal mushroom *Agaricus blazei*: production, purification and characterization. Appl. Microbiol. Biotechnol. (67): pp. 357-363.

## Abbreviations

AaP: *Agrocybe aegeriata* peroxidase; CPO: chloroperoxidase; CrP: *Coprinus radians* peroxidase; FPLC: Fast protein liquid chromatography; GC: MS–gas chromatography mass spectrometry; HPLC: high performance liquid chromatography; HPSEC: High performance size exclusion chromatography: IEF: Isoelectric focussing; LC-MS: Liquid chromatography mass spectrometry: $M_w$: Molecular mass; P450: Cytochrome P450; SDS-PAGE: Sodium dodecyl sulphate polyacryl amide gel electrophoresis.

# Chapter 10

# A New Flavan from the Stems of *Dracaena cambodiana*

**Tran Thu Huong[1], Nguyen Hai Dang[2], Phan Van Kiem[2] and Chau Van Minh[2]***

[1]*Faculty of Chemical Technology, Hanoi University of Technology, 1st Dai Co Viet, Hai Ba Trung, Hanoi, Vietnam*

[2]*Institute of Natural Products Chemistry, Vietnam Academy of Science and Technology, 18 Hoang Quoc Viet, Caugiay, Hanoi, Vietnam*

**E-mail: cvminh@fpt.vn*

## ABSTRACT

A new flavan (-)-7,5'-dihydroxy-3'-methoxy-8-methylflavan (1) along with five known compounds (-)-7,4'-dihydroxy-8-methylflavan (2), *N-p*-coumaroyltyramine (3), 1,2-dihydroxyallylbenzene (4), 1-*O*-$\beta$-D-glucopyranosyl-2-hydroxy-4-allylbenzene (5), and 4$\alpha$-methyl-5$\alpha$-cholest-7-en-3$\beta$-ol (6) have been isolated from the methanol extract of the stems of *Dracaena cambodiana*. Spectroscopic evidences elucidated their structures. Compounds 1-5 exhibited antifungal activities against *Asp. niger* with the MICs of 50 μg/ml. Compounds 2 and 3 exhibited antifungal activities against *F. oxysporum* with the MICs of 50 μg/ml.

***Keywords**: Dracaenaceae, Dracaena cambodiana, Flavan, (-)-7,5'-dihydroxy-8-methyl-3'-methoxylflavan*

## 1.0 Introduction

The "Dragon blood" (*Dracaena cambodiana*) belongs to the genus *Dracaena* (Dracaenaceae), which is found in the North of Vietnam. It has been used in traditional medicine for treatment of menoschesis, ostealgia and anti ulcer remedy (Bich, 2006; Chi, 1997; Loi, 2001). Phytochemical studies on *Dracaena* species led to the isolation of several phenolic compounds, flavonoids, steroidal sapogenins and steroidal saponins (Gonzalez, 2004; Mimaki, 1998; Tran, 2001). These compounds usually showed antioxidant, antimicrobial and anti-tumour activities (Yokosuka, 2000; Wu, 1995). Recent studies have shown that the chloroform extract, ethyl acetate extract, and *n*-butanol of extract *D. cambodiana* exhibited strong growth inhibitory activity on B16 cells and SMMC-721 cells in a MTT assay system. Among which, the chloroform extract was the most active (Mei, 2005).

In our course of study on the bioactive components from the stems of *D. cambodiana*, we have isolated a new flavan and five known compounds. Their structures were established by the means of MS, 1D–and 2D-NMR studies.

## 2.0 Materials and Methods

### 2.1 General Experiment Procedures

The $^{1}$H-NMR (500MHz) and $^{13}$C-NMR (125MHz) spectra were recorded on a Bruker AM500 FT-NMR spectrometer. Chemical shifts are referenced to $\delta$ using tetramethylsilan (TMS) as an internal standard. The Electron Spray Ionization (ESI) mass spectrum was obtained using an AGILENT 1100 LC-MSD Trap spectrometer. Column chromatography (CC) was performed on silica gel 230-400 mesh (0.040-0.063 mm, Merck) or YMC RP-18 resins (30-50 µm, Fujisilisa Chemical Ltd.). Thin layer chromatography (TLC) was performed on DC-Alufolien 60 $F_{254}$ (Merck 1.05715) or $RP_{18}$ $F_{254s}$ (Merck) plates.

### 2.2 Plant Material

The stems of *D. cambodiana* were collected in Hoa Binh province, Vietnam in January 2006 and identified by Dr. Tran Huy Thai, Institute of Ecology and Biological Resources, VAST, Vietnam. An authentic sample was deposited at the Institute of Natural Products Chemistry, VAST, Vietnam.

### 2.3 Extraction and Isolation

The dried stems of *D. cambodiana* (4 kg) were extracted with MeOH three times (7 days each time) and then concentrated under low pressure to obtain 150 g MeOH extract. The MeOH extract was suspended in water and partitioned with hexane, $CHCl_3$ and BuOH to obtain fractions hexane (60 g), $CHCl_3$ (35 g), and BuOH (65 g). The $CHCl_3$ fraction was then chromatographed on silicagel column eluting with $CHCl_3$-MeOH gradient (from 10:1 to 1:1 v/v) to give fractions C1 (16 g), C2 (11 g), and C3 (7 g). C1 fraction was chromatographed on a silica gel column using $CHCl_3$-EtOAc (3:1) as eluent to give subfractions C3A (6.5 g), C3B (3.4 g), C3C (6.0 g). The C3A subfraction (2.5 g) was chromatographed on an YMC RP-18 column using a MeOH-$H_2O$ (4:1 v/v) system as eluent yielded 1 (20.5 mg) and 2 (9 mg) as yellow amorphous powders. The C3B subfraction (3.4 g) was chromatographed on an YMC RP-18 column using MeOH-$H_2O$ (5:2 v/v) system as eluent to give 3 (50 mg) as white amorphous powder. The C3C sub-fraction (6.0 g) was chromatographed on a silica gel column using a $CHCl_3$-MeOH (3:1 v/v) system as eluent yielded 4 (20 mg) and 5 (15 mg) as brown oils. Compound 6 (65 mg) was recrystalised from hexane fraction using *n*-hexanhexane-acetone solvent system. The structures of compounds 1–6 are shown in Figure 10.1.

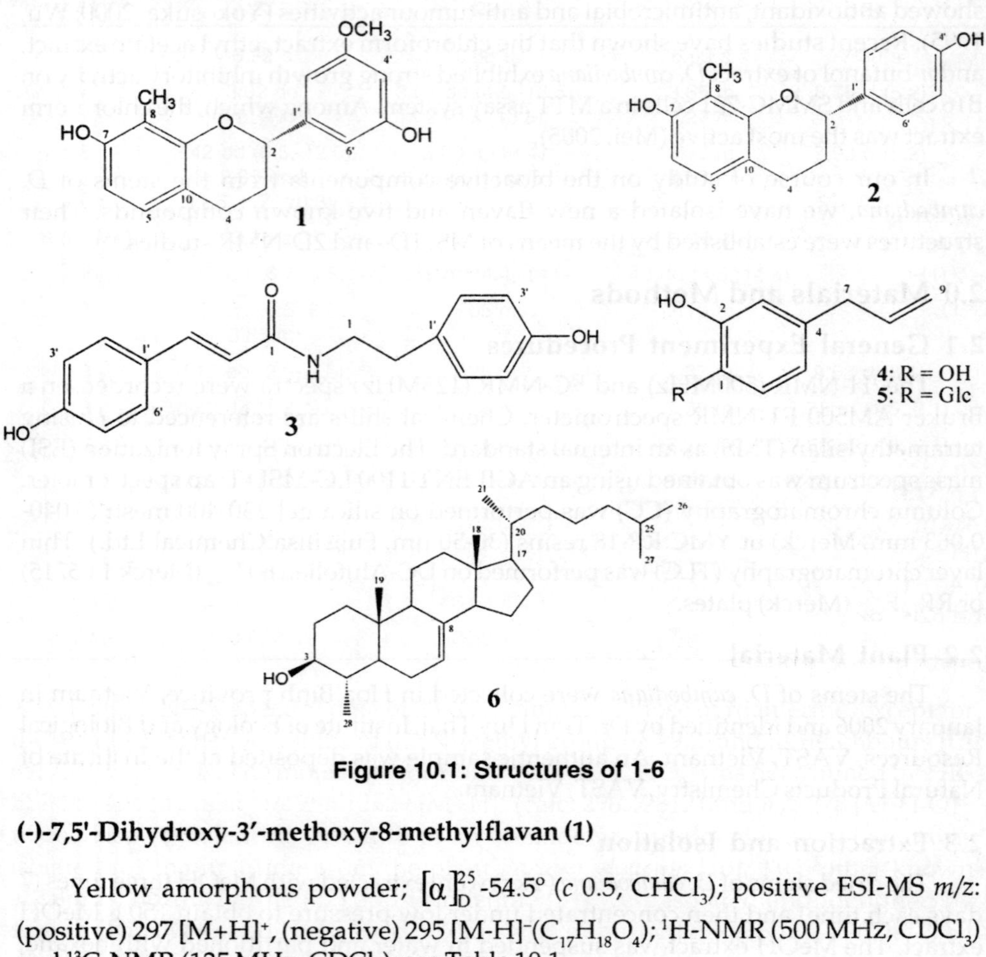

**Figure 10.1: Structures of 1-6**

**(-)-7,5'-Dihydroxy-3'-methoxy-8-methylflavan (1)**

Yellow amorphous powder; $[\alpha]_D^{25}$ -54.5° (*c* 0.5, $CHCl_3$); positive ESI-MS *m/z*: (positive) 297 $[M+H]^+$, (negative) 295 $[M-H]^-$($C_{17}H_{18}O_4$); $^1$H-NMR (500 MHz, $CDCl_3$) and $^{13}$C-NMR (125 MHz, $CDCl_3$): see Table 10.1.

**(-)-7,4'-Dihydroxy-8-methylflavan (2)**

Yellow amorphous powder; $[\alpha]_D^{25}$ -49.2° (*c* 0.12, $CHCl_3$); positive ESI-MS *m/z*: 257.0 $[M+H]^+$; $^1$H-NMR (500 MHz, $CDCl_3$) $\delta$: 5.00 (q, *J* = 2.5, 10.5 Hz, H-2), 2.14-1.94 (m, H-3), 2.88-2.69 (m, H-4), 6.78 (d, *J* = 8.0 Hz, H-5), 6.37 (d, *J* = 8.0 Hz, H-6), 2.12 (s, $\underline{C}H_3$-8), 7.29 (dd, *J* = 3.0, 6.0 Hz, H-2', H-6'), and 6.83 (dd, *J* = 2.5, 6.5 Hz, H-3', H-5'); $^{13}$C-NMR (125 MHz, $CDCl_3$) $\delta$: 77.2 (C-2), 30.1 (C-3), 24.9 (C-4), 126.6 (C-5), 107.2 (C-6), 152.7 (C-7), 111.4 (C-8), 153.7 (C-9), 113.9 (C-10), 8.1 ($\underline{C}H_3$-8), 134.5 (C-1'), 127.3 (C-2', C-6'), 115.2 (C-3', C-5'), and 155.0 (C-4').

***N-p*-Coumaroyltyramine (3)**

White powder; positive ESI-MS *m/z*: 283.9 $[M+H]^+$, 305.9 $[M+Na]^+$; negative ESI-

MS *m/z*: 282.0 $[M-H]^-$; $^1$H-NMR (500 MHz, $CD_3OD$) δ: tyramine moiety 3.46 (d, *J* = 7.5 Hz, H-1), 2.75 (d, *J* = 7.5 Hz, H-2), 7.41 (dd. *J* = 2.0, 8.5 Hz, H-2', H-6'), 6.80 (dd, *J* = 2.0, 8.5 Hz, H-3', H-5'), coumaroyl moiety 6.38 (d, *J* = 16.0 Hz, H-2), 7.45 (d, *J* = 16.0 Hz, H-3), 7.06 (dd, *J* = 2.0, 8.5 Hz, H-2', H-6'), and 6.73 (dd, *J* = 2.0, 8.5 Hz, H-3', H-5'); $^{13}$C-NMR (125 MHz, $CD_3OD$) δ: tyramine moiety 35.8 (C-1), 42.5 (C-2), 131.3 (C-1'), 130.5 (C-2', C-6'), 116.3 (C-3', C-5'), 156.9 (C-4'), coumaroyl moiety 169.3 (C-1), 118.5 (C-2), 141.8 (C-3), 127.8 (C-1'), 130.7 (C-2', C-6'), 116.7 (C-3', C-5'), and 160.5 (C-4').

**1,2-Dihydroxyallylbenzene (4)**

Brown oil; negative ESI-MS *m/z*: 149.1 $[M-H]^-$; $^1$H-NMR (500 MHz, $CD_3OD$) δ: 6.62 (d, *J* = 2.0 Hz, H-3), 6.49 (dd, *J* = 2.0, 8.0 Hz, H-5), 6.68 (d, *J* = 8.0 Hz, H-6), 3.22 (d, *J* = 7.0 Hz, H-7), 5.89 (m, H-8), and 4.98 (m, H-9); $^{13}$C-NMR (125 MHz, $CD_3OD$) δ: 144.5 (C-1), 146.2 (C-2), 116.7 (C-3), 132.9 (C-4), 120.8 (C-5), 116.3 (C-6), 40.6 (C-7), 139.5 (C-8), and 115.2 (C-9).

**1-*O*-β-D-glucopyranosyl-2-hydroxy-4-allylbenzene (5)**

Brown oil; negative ESI-MS *m/z*: 311.1 $[M-H]^-$; $^1$H-NMR (500 MHz, $CD_3OD$) δ: 6.70 (d, *J* = 2.5 Hz, H-3), 6.61 (dd, *J* = 2.5, 8.0 Hz, H-5), 7.11 (d, *J* = 8.0 Hz, H-6), 3.28 (d, *J* = 6.5 Hz, H-7), 5.92 (m, H-8), 5.01 (m, H-9), 4.72 (d, *J* = 7.5 Hz, 1-Glc), 3.50 (m, 2-Glc), 3.41 (m, 3-Glc), 3.42 (m, 4-Glc), 3.48 (m, 5-Glc), and 3.72-3.89 (m, 6-Glc); $^{13}$C-NMR (125 MHz, $CD_3OD$) δ: 145.2 (C-1), 148.4 (C-2), 119.1 (C-3), 117.3 (C-4), 121.0 (C-5), 119.2 (C-6), 40.6 (C-7), 139.0 (C-8), 115.8 (C-9), Glc 104.8 (1), 74.9 (2), 78.3 (3), 71.3 (4), 77.7 (5), and 62.4 (6).

**4α-Methyl-5α-cholest-7-en-3β-ol (6)**

Colourless needles; positive ESI-MS *m/z*: 401.1 $[M+H]^+$, 383.2 $[M-H_2O+H]^+$; $^1$H-NMR (500 MHz, $CDCl_3$) δ: 3.12 (m, H-3), 5.18 (d, *J* = 5.18 Hz, H-7), 0.53 (s, H-18), 0.84 (s, H-19), 0.98 (s, H-21), 0.86 (d, *J* = 6.5 Hz, H-26), 0.85 (d, *J* = 6.5 Hz, H-27), and 0.91 (d, *J* = 6.5 Hz, H-28); $^{13}$C-NMR (125 MHz, $CDCl_3$) δ: 36.5 (C-1), 31.4 (C-2), 76.0 (C-3), 40.7 (C-4), 47.1 (C-5), 27.1 (C-6), 117.8 (C-7), 139.6 (C-8), 50.1 (C-9), 35.3 (C-10), 21.8 (C-11), 39.5 (C-12), 43.8 (C-13), 55.4 (C-14), 23.3 (C-15), 28.4 (C-16), 56.6 (C-17), 12.2 (C-18), 14.1 (C-19), 36.6 (C-20), 19.2 (C-21), 37.4 (C-22), 24.3 (C-23), 39.9 (C-24), 28.4 (C-25), 23.2 (C-26), 22.9 (C-27), and 15.5 (C-28).

## 3.0 Results and Discussion

Compound 1 was obtained as yellow amorphous powder from the $CHCl_3$ fraction. The molecular formula was suggested as $C_{17}H_{18}O_4$ from the ESI-MS at *m/z* 287.0 $[M+H]^+$ in the positive mode and at *m/z* 285.1 $[M-H]^-$ in the negative mode. The NMR spectra of 1 displayed the signals due to the resonances of 17 carbons including 1 methyl, 1 methoxyl, 2 methylene, 6 methine, 4 quaternary, and 3 oxygenated tertiary carbons. The $^1$H-NMR spectrum of 1 showed the signals of two doublets at $\delta_H$ 6.78 (*J* = 8.0 Hz) and 6.37 (*J* = 8.0 Hz) typical for aromatic protons at ring A. Besides, a singlet methyl signal at δ 2.13 was assigned to the methyl in the ring A. The signals of two multiples at $\delta_H$ 1.98 and 2.72 and a doublet of doublet at $\delta_H$ 5.00 (*J* = 2.0, 10.0 Hz) suggested the presence of an oxygenated methine and two methylene groups in the ring C. Three singlet signals observed at δ 6.92, 6.92, and 6.98 corresponded to three meta protons in the ring B at C-2', C-4', and C-6'. The [13]C-NMR data of the carbons in the ring A and C were similar to those of published data (Coxon, 1980; Ioset, 2001). These results led to the suggestion that 1 bare a flavan structure. Moreover, the HMBC spectrum of 1 exhibited the correlations of the methyl proton ($\delta_H$ 2.13) to C-7, C-8, and C-10, a hydroxyl proton ($\delta_H$ 4.61) to C-6, C-7, and C-8. These evidence demonstrated the attachments of the hydroxyl group to C-7 and the methyl group to C-8 in the ring A. Similarly, the correlations observed from the HMBC spectrum between the methoxyl proton ($\delta_H$ 3.90) and C-3' ($\delta_C$ 146.5), a hydroxyl proton ($\delta_H$ 5.60) and C-5' ($\delta_C$ 145.1) confirmed the location of these groups. The H-C correlations observed in HMBC and HSQC spectra of 1 are summarized in Table 10.1. Furthermore, the ESI-MS spectrum of 1 exhibited the quasi-molecular ion peaks at *m/z*: (positive mode) 297 $[M+H]^+$, (negative mode) 295 $[M-H]^-$corresponding to the molecular formula of $C_{17}H_{18}O_4$. Thus, 1 was defined as (-) 7,5'-dihydroxy-8-methyl-3'-methoxylflavan. To the best of our knowledge, this is the first report of this compound from the nature.

**Table 10.1: NMR Data of 1**

| *Position* | $\delta_C$ [a,b] | $\delta_H$ [a,c] *mult. (J, Hz)* | *HMBC (H to C)* |
|---|---|---|---|
| | 77.6 | 5.00 dd (2.0, 10.0) | C-4, C-1', C-2', C-6' |
| 1 | 30.3 | 1.98 m; 2.15 m | C-2 |
| 2 | 25.0 | 2.72 m; 2.88 m | C-3, C-5, C-9, C-10 |
| 3 | 126.6 | 6.79 d (8.0) | C-4, C-7, C-9 |
| 4 | 107.3 | 6.37 d (8.0) | C-8, C-10 |
| 5 | 152.7 | | |
| 6 | 111.3 | | |
| 7 | 153.7 | | |
| 8 | 113.9 | | |
| 1' | 134.3 | | |
| 2' | 118.8 | 6.92 s | C-1', C-3', C-6' |
| 3' | 146.5 | | |
| 4' | 114.2 | 6.92 s | C-6' |
| 5' | 145.1 | | |
| 6' | 108.5 | 6.98 s | C-2, C-1', C-2', C-5' |
| $CH_3$-8 | 8.1 | 2.13 s | C-7, C-8, C-9 |
| $OCH_3$ | 55.9 | 3.90 s | C-3' |
| OH-7 | | 4.61 s | C-6, C-7, C-8 |
| OH-5' | | 5.61 s | C-4', C-5' |

[a] Measured in $CDCl_3$; [b] 125 MHz; [c] 500 MHz, Chemical shift (δ) in ppm.

The NMR data of 2 were closed similar to those of 1 except for the lost of the methoxyl signals. The [1]H-NMR spectrum of 2 showed 1 methyl singlet at $\delta_H$ 2.12, 2 doublets at $\delta_H$ 6.78 and 6.37 assigned to H-5 and H-6, two 2-proton doublets of doublet at $\delta_H$ 7.29 and 6.83 assigned to H2'/H4' and H3'/H5', respectively. The quartet signal at $\delta_H$ 5.0 observed in $^{1}$H-NMR spectrum of 2 was assigned to the H-2 proton. The $^{13}$C-NMR data of 2 were compared with those of published data and found to match. The molecular formula corresponded to $C_{16}H_{16}O_3$ by the appearance of the ion peak at *m/z*: 257.0 $[M+H]^+$ in the ESI-MS (positive ion mode). Therefore 2 was identified as (-)-7,4'-dihydroxy-8-methylflavan. Recently, this compound has been noted to exhibit strong radical scavenging activity (Coxon, 1980; Ioset, 2001).

Compound 3 was obtained as amorphous powder. Its molecular weight of 283 was established from the appearance of the ion peak at *m/z*: 283.9 $[M+H]^+$ and 305.9 $[M+Na]^+$ in the positive mode ESI-MS. By investigating the $^{1}$H–and $^{13}$C-NMR spectra of 3, its structure was clarified. The $^{1}$H-NMR spectrum of 3 displayed the signals of eight aromatic, two methylene, and two methine carbons. The $^{13}$C-NMR spectrum of 3 displayed the resonances due to the signals of a ketone group and two hydroxylated carbons. Together with the suggested molecular weight by ESI mass spectrum, the NMR data of 3 showed the appearance of a nitrogen atom in its structure. By comparison with the published data, the structure of 3 was deduced as *N-p*-coumaroyltyramine (Zhao, 1992). Remarkably, this compound exhibited a complete inhibitory effect on the aggregation of rabbit platelets induced thrombin, arachidonic acid, collagen and PAF at concentration of 60 µM. Moreover, the potent cytotoxic activity against P-388 cell line of 3 was also demonstrated (Wu, 1995).

The spectroscopic data of 5 were very similar to those of 4 except for the signals supposed to an addition of a sugar moiety to the aglycon of 5. The NMR data of 4 and 5 were in good agreement with those in the literature. Furthermore, the correlations established from their HSQC and HMBC spectra confirmed the 2-hydroxy-4-allylbenzen structure of the aglycon of these compounds. Thus, the structures of 4 and 5 were elucidated to be 1,2-dihydroxyallylbenzene and 1-*O*-$\beta$-D-glucopyranosyl-2-hydroxy-4-allylbenzene, respectively (Ly, 2002). By carrying out the same methods on structural elucidation using spectroscopy in comparison with the reported data, compound 6 was identified as 4$\alpha$-methyl-5$\alpha$-cholest-7-en-3$\beta$-ol (Chitwood, 1991).

Compounds 1–6 were evaluated for antifungal activities. Remarkably, 1–5 exhibited considerable antifungal activities against *Aspergillus niger* with the MICs of 50 µg/ml. Moreover, 2 and 3 exhibited the inhibitory activities against *Fusarium oxysporum* with the MICs of 50 µg/ml. Notably, 3 with various reported bioactivities should be considered as a potential agent for the development of new pharmaceuticals.

## References

Bich, D. H., Chung, D. Q., Chuong, B. X., Dong, N. T., Dam, D. T., Hien, P. V., Lo, V. N., Mai, P. D., Man, P. K., Nhu, D. T., Tap, N., Toan, T., 2006. "Medicinal Animals and Plants in Vietnam". Hanoi Science and Technology Publishing House, Vol. 1.

Chi, V. V., 1997, "Vietnamese Medical Plant Dictionary". Hanoi Medicinal Publishing House.

Chitwood, D. J., Lusby, W. R., 1991. Metabolism of plant sterols by nematodes. Lipids (26), pp. 619-627.

Coxon, D. T., O'Neill, T. M., Mansfield, J. W., Porter, A. E. A., 1980. Identification of three hydroxyflavan phytoalexin from daffodil bulbs. Phytochemistry (19), pp. 889-891.

Gonzalez, A. G., Leon, F., Hernandez, J. C., Padron, J. 1., Pinto, L. S., Barrera, J. B., 2004. Flavan of dragon's blood from *Dracaena draco* and *Dracaena tamaranae*. Biochem. Syst. Ecol. (32), pp. 179-184.

Ioset, J. A., Marston, A., Gupta, M. P., Hostettmann, K., 2001. A methylflavan with free radical scavenging properties from *Pancratium littorale*. Fitoterapia, 72, pp. 35-39.

Loi, D. T., 2006. "Glossary of Vietnamese Medicinal Plants". Hanoi Science and Technology Publishing House.

Ly, T. N., Yamauchi, R., Shimoyamada, M., Kato, K., 2002. Isolation and structural elucidation of some glycosides from the rhizomes of smaller galangal (*Alpinia officinarum* Hance). J. Agric. Food Chem. (50), pp. 4919-4924.

Mei, W., Dai, H., Wu, J., Zhuang, L., Hong, K., 2005. Study on the new use of antitumor of *Dracaena cambodiana*. Zhong Yao Cai (28), pp. 871-873.

Mimaki, Y., Koruda, M., Takaashi, Y., Sashida, Y., 1998. Steroidal saponins from the stem of *Dracaena concinna*. Phytochemistry (47), pp. 1351-1356.

Tran, Q. L., Tezuka, Y., Banskota, A. H., Tran, Q. K., Saiki, 1., Kadota, S., 2001. New spirostanol steroids and steroidal saponins from stems and rhizomes of *Dracaena angustifolia* and their antiproliferative activity. J. Nat. Prod. (64), pp. 1127-1132.

Wu, C. H., Chang, G. Y., Ko, F. N., Teng, C. M., 1995. Bioactive constituents from the stems of *Annona montana*. Planta Med. (61), pp. 146-149.

Yokosuka, A., Mimaki, Y., Shashida, Y., 2000. Steroidal saponins from *Dracaena surculosa*. J. Nat. Prod. (63), pp. 1239-1243.

Zhao, G., Hui, Y., Rupprecht, K., McLaughlin, J., 1992. Additional bioactive compounds and trilobacin, a novel highly cytotoxic acetogenin, from the bark of *Asimisia triloba*. J. Nat. Prod. (55), pp. 347-356.

## Chapter 11

# Genetic Diversity of *Andrographis paniculata* (Burm. f.) Nees of Brunei Darussalam Determined by RAPD and PCR-RFLP Analyses

*Kui Hong Chua[1]*, C.G. Li[1], C.L. Xue Charlie[1] and E.C.K. Pang[2]*

[1]*Chinese Medicine Research Group, School of Health Sciences, Royal Melbourne Institute of Technology, P.O. Box 71, Bundoora, Melbourne, Victoria-3083, Australia*

[2]*Biotechnology and Environmental Biology, School of Applied Sciences, Royal Melbourne Institute of Technology, P.O. Box 71, Bundoora, Melbourne, Victoria-3083, Australia*

*E-mail: kuihongchua@hotmail.com*

## ABSTRACT

The genetic diversity of nine accessions of *Andrographis paniculata (Burm. f.) Nees*, an important medicinal plant of Brunei Darussalam was determined by Random Amplified Polymorphic DNA (RAPD) and Restriction Fragment Length Polymorphism (PCR-RFLP) analyses. The genetic dissimilarity matrix was generated using POPGENE and the diversity dendrogram was constructed using MEGA2 with Unweighted Pair Group Method of Arithmetic Mean (UPGMA). The accessions from Brunei Darussalam formed two main clusters with a maximum dissimilarity of 10 per cent between nine accessions, indicating that these accessions were closely related to each other. The polymorphisms generated using RAPD analysis demonstrated that it could be effectively used to survey the genetic diversity of *Andrographis paniculata (Burm. f.) Nees* species which will be beneficial in the characterisation and authentication of this medicinal plant. However, the PCR-RFLP analysis did not generate any polymorphisms and failed to demonstrate any distinction between the nine accessions of *Andrographis paniculata (Burm. f.) Nees* Brunei Darussalam.

***Keywords:*** *Andrographis paniculata (Burm. f.) Nees, Daun pahit, King of Bitters, RAPD, PCR-RFLP.*

## 1.0 Introduction

It is known that the world's population relies upon plants as the primary source of medicine for the treatment of diseases. Worldwide, more than 80 per cent of the world population use botanical preparations, as medicines, and herbalism are experiencing resurgence. The U.S. market amounts to about $1.5 billion per year (Marwick, 1995); the European market amounts to three times that of U.S. (Brevoort, 1996).

DNA profiling can specifically identify herbal varieties/species or cultivar, to ensure the quality if there is any linkage of its genetic identity with either their chemical constituents or bioactivities and to ascertain the genetic uniformity of herbal materials. Therefore, continued research on the establishment of the correlations between the genetic diversity profile and the chemical constituents and compositions of medicinal plants used by the communities' at large need to be supported.

Brunei Darussalam has a wealth of natural plant resources with great potential for molecular analyses to conserve the genetic diversity and consequently provides avenues for studies on phytochemical contents and bioactivities of the medicinal plants. All communities in Brunei Darussalam use herbal remedies, they are within easy reach and the crude medicines are readily available in the markets. However, at present there is a lack of documentation and study on the genetic diversity of the medicinal plants.

Brunei Darussalam is situated on the northwest coast of the island of Borneo and lies in the heart of South East Asia. It is close to the equator between east longitudes 114° 04' and 11° 23' and north latitudes 04° 00' and 05° 05'. It has a total land area of 5,765 square kilometres and a coastline of about 161 kilometres and bounded on the north by the South China Sea, on the other sides by the Malaysian state of Sarawak. It comprises of four districts namely the Brunei-Muara, Tutong, Kuala Belait and Temburong. Therefore, this study on *Andrographis paniculata* is of paramount importance for the future research and development of the genetic diversity and variability study on medicinal plants, which are of clinical potential in the health care system.

An estimated 5,000 native species have been found in the tropical rain forests, which constitute 80 per cent of the total land area. Ethno botanical surveys recorded 340 species with 160 species were positively identified (Department of Agriculture, 2000). Out of these species, *Andrographis paniculata* is a widely used medicinal plant in Asia in particularly India, China and South East Asia including Brunei Darussalam for many disease conditions. It is a popular plant from the *'Acanthaceae'* family used by the communities to lower high blood pressure, managing diabetes and to relieve abdominal pains. In addition to the existing active components, Andrographolide, Dehydroandrographolide, Deoxyandrographolide and Neo-andrographolide, Pramanick *et al.* (2005) isolated newer *ent*-labdane type diterpenoids from the leaves of *Andrographis paniculata*, which are now being investigated for their bioactivities. Studies on the genetic diversity information of these species or varieties are gaining popularity worldwide in the authentication of this important plant species with the aim to identify superior genotype(s). Therefore, the genetic profile of genus *Andrographis* collected from different geographical distributions need to be assessed in order to provide important correlations between genetic markers and their metabolic compounds or chemotypes.

In view of its wide use and important active components of beneficial clinical implications, our study aimed at examining the genetic diversity of the genotypes of the *Andrographis paniculata* known as '*Daun pahit*' from Brunei Darussalam. Currently, there is no documented genetic diversity profile of *Andrographis paniculata* of Brunei Darussalam. To the best of our knowledge, this is the first study conducted. Literature search reported that the genus *Andrographis* also known as '*King of Bitters; Kalmegh of Ayurveda*' is of potential significance to India as 25 out of 28 species in the world are distributed mainly in India with 23 of them occurring in the peninsular region. As a result of its popular demand by the Asian communities, more research is now focusing on studying the content of its active components from the *Andrographis paniculata* leaves collected from different geographical locations in Asia (Padmesh *et al.*, 1999; Sabu *et al.*, 2001).

These different species and varieties of *Andrographis paniculata* are used interchangeably as herbal remedies worldwide. *Andrographis paniculata* has also been listed as herbal medicines in the Chinese Pharmacopoeia Volume II 2000, the British Pharmaceutical Codex 1911 and Therapeutic Goods Administration (TGA), Australia 2004 for its medicinal benefits.

RAPD and PCR-RFLP analyses have become a popular means for the identification and authentication of natural products such as plant and animal species. For instance, they have been used to characterise species such as *Epimedium* species (Nakai *et al.*, 1996) and to examine the genetic relationships within genera of herbal species (Kim *et al*,. 2004a; Roser *et al.*, 2001). Interspecies variation studies on various genera of *Glycyrrhiza* (Yamazaki *et al*,. 1994), *Echinaceae* (Kapteyn *et al.*, 2002), *Curcuma* (Chen *et al.*, 1999) were also conducted. Wang *et al.* (2004) revised the phenotypic relationship between 20 species from the subgenus *Yulania* based on RAPD technique. The significant genetic distance between the species derived from different geographical locations of Asia and America were investigated among 17 species of subgenus *Yulania* using RAPD analysis that generated high levels of polymorphisms. In general, RFLP markers are much less polymorphic, more expensive and labour intensive compared to RAPD. The aim of this study was to use RAPD and PCR-RFLP at 5S-rRNA region to determine the intra specific genetic variability of nine genotypes of *Andrographis paniculata* collected from three districts of Brunei Darussalam.

## 2.0 Materials and Methods

### 2.1 Plant Material

Brunei Darussalam has a tropical climate with uniform temperature of 22°C-28°C with high humidity and annual rainfall ranges from around 2,790 millimetres (Department of Information, 2003). Tropical rainforest covers 80 per cent of the country's total land area, which may have some medicinal plants with unique characteristics of active metabolites.

The Department of Agriculture, Ministry of Industry and Primary Resources, Brunei Darussalam authenticated the plant materials. The reference control Chuan Xin Lian (CXL) leaves were authenticated by the Chinese Medicine Clinic of RMIT University, Bundoora West Campus, Melbourne, and Victoria.

Using a PCR-based DNA fingerprinting technique (Sun *et al.*, 2004) for the identification of air-dried fresh leaves materials from nine accessions of *Andrographis paniculata* obtained from the three districts of Brunei Darussalam such as Bandar Seri Begawan from the Brunei/Muara district designated as AP2, AP4, AP6, AP8, AP11, AP14, AP15; Kuala Belait district designated as K.B.; Temburong district designated as T from Brunei Darussalam compared to Chuan Xin Lian (CXL) imported from China by the Chinese Medicine Clinic, Chinese Medicine Division of Royal Melbourne Institute of Technology for treating patients.

In a related study, Chua *et al.* (2006, unpublished) attempted to obtain the correlation between the polymorphisms of three genotypes CXL, T and K.B. and the levels of per centw/w Andrographolides (A) and per cent w/w Dehydroandrographolides (D). Their genetic differences and the medicinally active principles were analysed quantitatively using HPLC to study their phytochemical diversity from different geographical locations. In addition to the cluster analysis, principal component analysis of the similarity coefficient was performed and the diagram of the components extracted was constructed as illustrated in Figure 11.1. The HPLC analysis of three accessions CXL, T and K.B. accumulating significant concentrations of per cent w/w Andrographolide were 1.14 per cent, 3.43 per cent and 0.67 per cent and per cent w/w Dehydroandrographolide were 0.66 per cent, 0.12 per cent and 0.24 per cent respectively may be potentially useful for breeding and cultivar development. The results of the dendrogram and principal component analysis were in agreement with the overall representation of relationships among the genotypes studied.

Total DNA from air-dried fresh leaves was extracted using the DNeasy Plant Mini Kit (Qiagen). Thirty four random oligonucleotide primers-10mer (Operon Technologies Inc.) and 5S-rRNA sequences using primers-20mer 5SP1 (forward) (5'-GTG CTT GGG CGA GAG TAG TA-3') and 5SP2 (reverse) (5'-TTA GTG CTG GTA TGA TCG CA-3') purchased from Geneworks were designed for Random Amplified Polymorphic DNA (RAPD) and Restriction Fragment Length Polymorphism (PCR-RFLP) analysis respectively.

## 2.2 RAPD Analysis

The RAPD analysis was modified from that described in published literature (Cui *et al.*, 2003, Shaw and But, 1995). The 25µl PCR mixture comprised of 40ng of template DNA, 2.5µl of 10xPCR buffer (100mM Tris-HCl, 500mM KCl, 0.01 per cent gelatin, Invitrogen, Australia), 0.75µl of 50mM $MgCl_2$, 6µl of 1mM dNTP, 1µl of 10µM primer and 1 unit Taq Polymerase (Invitrogen, Australia). PCR reaction consisted of 3 min at 94°C, followed by 15 seconds at 94°C (denaturing), 1 min at 40°C (annealing), 1 min at 72°C (extension) for 35 cycles, and terminating with 5 minutes at 72°C for RAPD analysis by Px2 Thermal Cycler (Thermal Electron Corporation, UK). Each

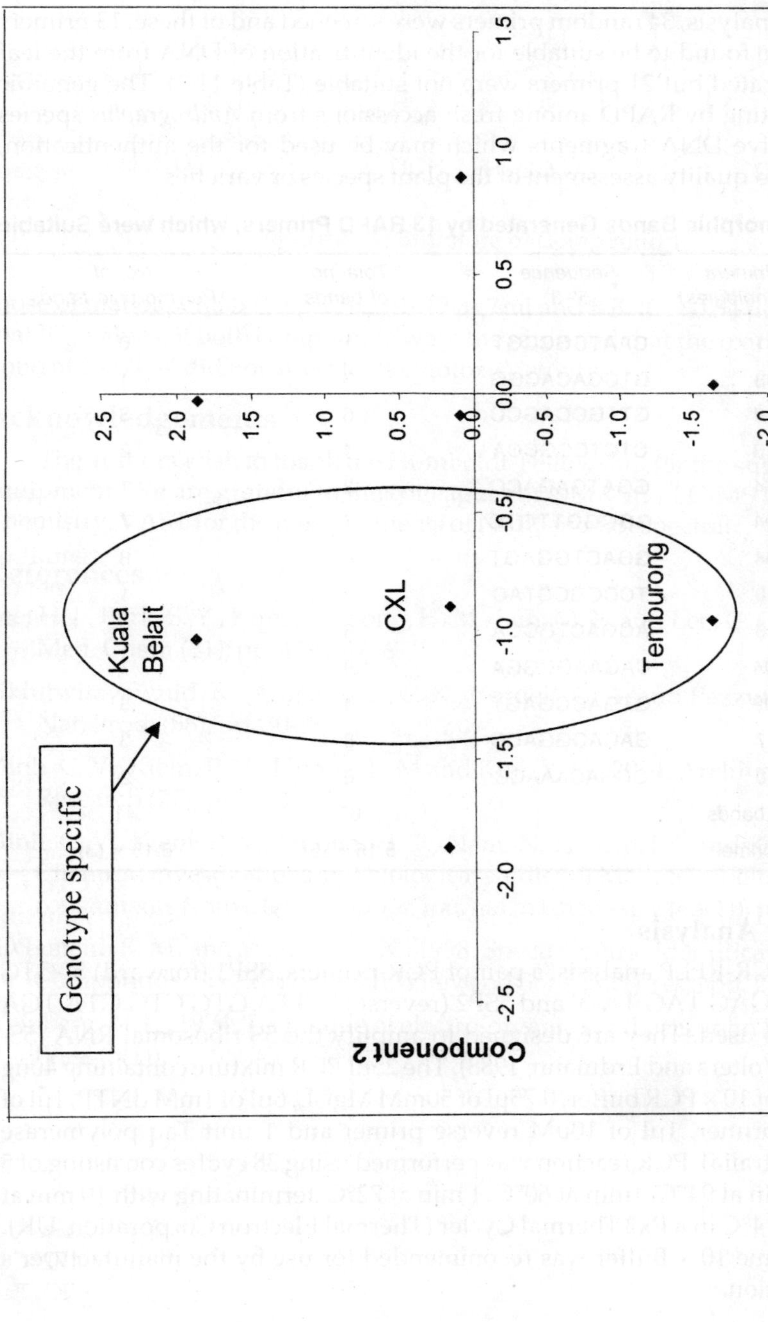


**Figure 11.1: Principal Component Diagram Based on RAPD Analysis**

PCR product was electrophoresed in 1.5 per cent agarose gel and visualized by ethidium bromide staining. The Discovery Series Quantity One 1-D Analysis Software (BioRad, Australia) was used for imaging the electrophoresis gels.

For RAPD analysis, 34 random primers were screened and of these, 13 primers (Table 11.1) were found to be suitable for the identification of DNA from the leaf samples investigated but 21 primers were not suitable (Table 11.2). The genomic DNA fingerprinting by RAPD among fresh accessions from *Andrographis* species showed distinctive DNA fragments which may be used for the authentication, identification and quality assessment of the plant species or varieties.

**Table 11.1: Polymorphic Bands Generated by 13 RAPD Primers, which were Suitable**

| *13 RAPD Primers (Operon Technologies)* | *Sequence 5'–3'* | *Total no. of bands* | *No. of Polymorphic bands* |
|---|---|---|---|
| OPA-11 | CAATCGCCGT | 1 | 0 |
| OPB-08 | GTCCACACGG | 3 | 1 |
| OPC-19 | GTTGCCAGCC | 6 | 3 |
| OPG-13 | CTCTCCGCCA | 4 | 2 |
| OPG-14 | GGATGAGACC | 2 | 1 |
| OPM-04 | GGCGGTTGTC | 7 | 7 |
| OPN-04 | GGACTGGAGT | 8 | 8 |
| OPP-10 | TCCCGCCTAC | 3 | 1 |
| OPT-13 | AGGACTGCCA | 6 | 3 |
| OPW-04 | CAGAAGCGGA | 9 | 7 |
| OPW-09 | GTGACCGAGT | 4 | 3 |
| OPX-17 | GACACGGACC | 8 | 3 |
| OPZ-10 | CCGACAAACC | 6 | 2 |
| Total no. of bands | | 67 | 41 |
| Mean per primer | | 5.15 ≈ (5) | 3.15 ≈ (3) |

## 2.3 PCR-RFLP Analysis

As for the PCR-RFLP analysis, a pair of PCR-primers, 5SP1 (forward) 5'-GTG CTT GGG CGA GAG TAG TA-3' and 5SP2 (reverse) 5'-TTA GTG CTG GTA TGA TCG CA-3' were used. They are designed to amplify the 5S ribosomal RNA (5S-rRNA) spacer (Wolters and Erdmann, 1988). The 25µl PCR mixture containing 40ng leaf DNA, 2.5µl of 10 × PCR buffer, 0.75µl of 50mM $MgCl_2$, 6µl of 1mM dNTP, 1µl of 10µM forward primer, 1µl of 10µM reverse primer and 1 unit Taq polymerase (Invitrogen, Australia). PCR reaction was performed using 38 cycles consisting of 5 min at 94°C, 1 min at 94°C, 1min at 60°C, 1 min at 72°C, terminating with 10 min at 72°C and hold at 4°C in a Px2 Thermal Cycler (Thermal Electron Corporation, UK). Restriction enzyme 10 × Buffer was recommended for use by the manufacturer's product information.

**Table 11.2: List of 21 RAPD Primers which were Not Suitable**

| | |
|---|---|
| OPZ-02 | CCTACGGGGA |
| OPZ-04 | AGGCTGTGCT |
| OPZ-12 | TCAAGGGGAC |
| OPZ-16 | TCCCCATCAC |
| OPAW-03 | CCATGCGGAG |
| OPAW-05 | CTGCTTCGAG |
| OPV-06 | ACGCCCAGGT |
| OPU-03 | CTATGCCGAC |
| OPT-17 | CCAACGTCGT |
| OPT-03 | TCCACTCCTG |
| OPA-07 | GAAACGGGTG |
| OPB-18 | CCACAGCAGT |
| OPB-17 | AGGGAACGAG |
| OPB-12 | CCTTGACGCA |
| OPB-07 | GGTGACGCAG |
| OPB-06 | TGCTCTGCCC |
| OPB-04 | GGACTGGAGT |
| OPB-03 | CATCCCCCTG |
| OPA-14 | TCTGTGCTGG |
| OPZ-06 | GTGCCGTTCA |
| OPZ-08 | GGGTGGGTAA |

Briefly, 4μl of the PCR products from the 5S-rRNA gene were then digested with the 13 restriction enzymes in purified BSA 100x (New England Biolabs, USA) were incubated at 37°C for 2hr (Lin *et al*,. 2001) and out of these, *HinfI, MnlI, MspI, HaeIII, NlaIV, Tsp* 509I were found to be suitable (Table 11.3). Each PCR products was fractionated in 2.0 per cent agarose gel and visualized by Ethidium Bromide staining. The Discovery Series Quantity One 1-D Analysis Software (BioRad, Australia) was used for imaging the electrophoresis gels. Only clear, coherent and consistent banding patterns revealed by RAPD analysis were scored. RAPD bands were scored as present (1) or absent (0) for each genotype.

## 2.4 Data Analysis

On the basis of Nei's coefficient, a matrix of genetic distances estimation between the accessions of *Andrographis paniculata* from different districts of Brunei Darussalam based on dissimilarity ($D=1-S_{XY}$) indices was obtained by POPGENE version 1.31, a Microsoft Window-based free software for population genetic analysis (Yeh *et al.*, 1999). The Molecular Evolutionary Genetics Analysis 2 (MEGA 2) was used for reconstruction and comparing the genetic distances between all individuals by an Unweighted Pair Group Method with Arithmetic Mean (UPGMA) method (Kumar *et al*,,2001). The linearised tree was expressed as percentage of the dissimilarity indices.

**Table 11.3: Results from the Restriction Endonuclease Digestions of the 5SP1 and 5SP2 PCR Products Amplified for all Genotypes**

| *Restriction Enzymes* | *Number/Colour of Buffer* | *Sequence (Promega Technologies)* | *Length of Amplifications of the 5S-rRNA Region* |
|---|---|---|---|
| *Hinf*I | No. 2/Blue Buffer | G-ANT C<br>C TNA-G | 150bp<br>250bp |
| *Mnl*I | No. 2/Blue Biolab | $CCTC(N)_7^-$<br>$GGAG(N)_6^-$ | 70bp<br>100bp<br>220bp |
| *Msp*I | No.2/Blue Buffer | C-CG G<br>G GC-C | 100bp<br>125bp<br>150bp |
| *Nla*IV | No.4/Green Buffer | GGN-NCC<br>CCN-NGG | 200bp<br>200bp |
| *Hae*III | No.2/Blue Buffer | GG-CC<br>CC-GG | 70bp<br>70bp<br>100bp<br>150bp |
| *Tsp* 509I | No.1/Yellow Buffer | -AATT<br>TTAA- | 180bp<br>220bp |
| *Hha*I | No.4/Green Buffer | G CG-C<br>C-GC G | Restricted amplicon into two equal fragment |
| *Alu*I | No.2/Blue Buffer | AG-CT<br>TC-GA | No restriction |
| *Bsa*JI | No.2/Blue Buffer | C-CNNG G<br>G GNNC-C | No restriction |
| *Bst*XI | No.3/Red Buffer | CCAN NNN-NTGG<br>GGTN-NNN NACC | No restriction |
| *Dde*I | No.3/Red Buffer | C-TNA G<br>G ANT-C | No restriction |
| *Apo*I | No.3/Red Buffer | A-AATT T<br>T TTAA-A | No restriction |
| *Mse*I | No.2/Blue Buffer | T-TAA<br>AAT-T | No restriction |

## 3.0 Results and Discussion

There was a considerable level of polymorphism among the genotypes investigated. Of the total 67 loci scored, 61 per cent were polymorphic with an average of 3 bands per primer (Table 11.1). The number of bands produced per primer ranged from 1 (OPA-11) to 9 (OPW-04) with an average of 5 bands per primer and the products ranged in size from 280bp to 3000bp. The maximum genetic distance was 0.3545 between accessions AP6 and CXL. The minimum genetic distance was 0.0303 between accessions AP15 and AP6 as shown in Table 11.4.

**Table 11.4: Dissimilarity Matrix of Nine Accessions of *Andrographis paniculata***

| | *CXL* | *T* | *KB* | *AP2* | *AP4* | *AP6* | *AP8* | *AP11* | *AP14* | *AP15* |
|---|---|---|---|---|---|---|---|---|---|---|
| CXL | 1.0000 | | | | | | | | | |
| T | 0.2729 | 1.0000 | | | | | | | | |
| KB | 0.2729 | 0.1616 | 1.0000 | | | | | | | |
| AP2 | 0.3129 | 0.0938 | 0.1974 | 1.0000 | | | | | | |
| AP4 | 0.1793 | 0.2157 | 0.1793 | 0.2534 | 1.0000 | | | | | |
| AP6 | 0.3545* | 0.0938 | 0.2344 | 0.0616 | 0.2927 | 1.0000 | | | | |
| AP8 | 0.3129 | 0.0938 | 0.1272 | 0.1616 | 0.1442 | 0.1974 | 1.0000 | | | |
| AP11 | 0.2157 | 0.0776 | 0.2157 | 0.1103 | 0.1616 | 0.1103 | 0.1793 | 1.0000 | | |
| AP14 | 0.3335 | 0.1103 | 0.1793 | 0.0458 | 0.2729 | 0.0458 | 0.1793 | 0.1272 | 1.0000 | |
| AP15 | 0.3129 | 0.0938 | 0.2344 | 0.0616 | 0.2927 | 0.0303# | 0.1974 | 0.1103 | 0.0458 | 1.0000 |

*: Greatest dissimilarity; #: Least dissimilarity.

Nine genotypes were grouped into two main clusters based on the maximum dissimilarity of 10 per cent between genotypes as illustrated in Figure 11.2. Chuan Xin Lian (CXL) from China (Family: *Acanthaceae*, Species: *Andrographis paniculata*, Genus: *Andrographis*) as reference control, was found to be the most genetically distant from all other accessions where the greatest dissimilarity was between CXL and AP6 (15 per cent). Cluster I consisted of AP8, KB, AP4 and Cluster II consists of AP11, T, AP2, AP14, AP15 and AP6 (Table 11.5).

**Table 11.5: Clusters I * and Cluster II**
**(% Dissimilarity of nine accessions of *Andrographis paniculata*)**

| | | *Cluster I** | | | | | *Cluster II* | | | |
|---|---|---|---|---|---|---|---|---|---|---|
| | | * | * | * | | | | | | |
| | *CXL* | *AP8* | *KB* | *AP4* | *AP11* | *T* | *AP2* | *AP14* | *AP15* | *AP6* |
| CXL | 100% | 8% | 8% | 6% | 10% | 10% | 11% | 12% | 13% | 13% |

The finding of the close genetic distances between all the nine accessions from Brunei Darussalam and Chuan Xin Lian (CXL) are in agreement with the other studies on lotus (Campose *et al.*, 1994), sweet potato (Cannoly *et al*,. 1994), and *Andrographis paniculata* of India (Padmesh *et al.*, 1999) which suggest that RAPD is more appropriate for the analysis of genetic diversity in closely related genotypes.

Chuan Xin Lian (CXL) is about 4 per cent dissimilar from all the Brunei Darussalam accessions by combining Clusters I and II together as one major group. On an individual basis, CXL is 6 per cent dissimilar to Cluster I and 9 per cent to Cluster II. This finding is in agreement with the RAPD analysis in the study by Padmesh *et al.* (1999) on the intraspecific genetic diversity of *Andrographis paniculata* where the genetic dissimilarity is at 0.51 between AP-29 from Assam and AP48 from Thailand. The nine accessions of *Andrographis paniculata* in the current study were

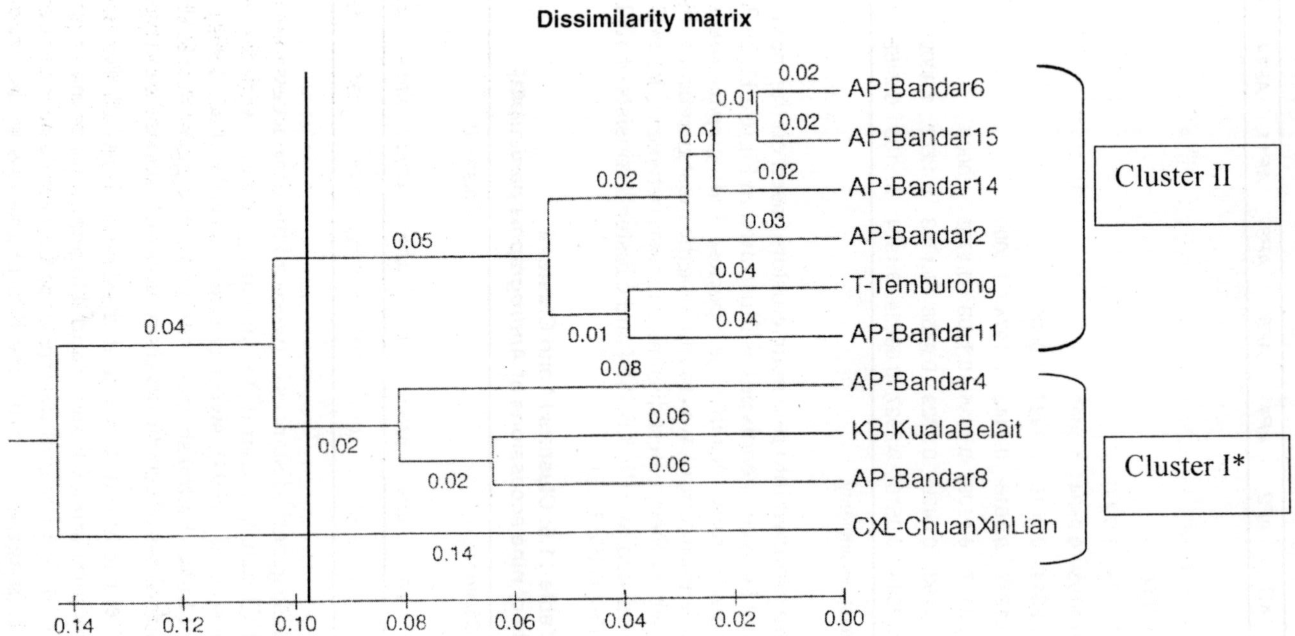


**Figure 11.2: A Dendrogram Showing Genetic Relationship of the Nine Accessions of *Andrographis paniculata* from Brunei Darussalam Compared to the Reference Control Chuan Xin Lian (CXL) (matrix scale is expressed as percentage x100)**

collected from Brunei Darussalam, whereas the accessions in previous studies were obtained from different parts of India, Thailand, Malaysia and Indonesia.

It is possible that the genotypes from different distantly geographical regions can be genetically similar to genotypes with immediate spatial relationships association which may be attributed to the unique, broad genetic base combinations, seed movement and gene flow since *Andrographis paniculata (Burm. f.) Nees* is an introduced species into Thailand and Brunei Darussalam. This species is also reported from Hongkong, Borneo, Sulawesi, Jamaica, Barbados, Bahamas and Christmas Island in Indian Ocean but there is no precise data with regards to the introduction and naturalisation of *Andrographis paniculata* in these countries. As this study focused on the intraspecific genetic diversity of the species, the future study of interspecific variability of the different species of *Andrographis paniculata* from different near and distant geographical locations may be useful and lead to better understanding of these existing findings.

PCR amplification using the 5S-rRNA primers produced a 400bp amplicon. Restriction enzyme digestion using six endonucleases revealed that all the restriction fragments were identical among all genotypes (Table 11.3). This suggested that the nine accessions of *Andrographis paniculata* from Brunei Darussalam were closely related. There are different varieties of *Andrographis* in India, the native homeland of the plant, which has always been the interest of researchers to analyse them genetically. At present, no information is available whether the different varieties have arisen due to more than one introduction to Brunei Darussalam or as a result of genetic mutation.

PCR-RFLP digestion can be a useful tool for resolving subspecies taxonomic status, but in this analysis the 5S-rRNA region is not variable enough for taxonomic comparison. However, future study using a larger number of restriction enzymes may possibly uncover differences in the taxonomic pattern. Although in this section PCR-RFLP was not a useful diagnostic tool, PCR-RFLP's was reported to be useful for deciphering phylogenetic relationships between two varieties of *Imperata cylindrica L. Beauv.* (*Congograss*). (Chou and Tsai, 1999)

In contrast, the RAPD analysis potentially explores genetic polymorphism across the entire genome therefore may potentially reveal greater genetic diversity with higher degree of polymorphism (Lynch and Milligan, 1994). Such characteristic features of the RAPD are useful for the identification of medicinal plants despite the weakness of RAPD method with low reproducibility and high sensitivity of contaminants during the hash processing of DNA (Penner *et al.*, 1993). The PCR-RFLP of multi copy genes, such as 5S-rRNA, may perhaps be more appropriate for the differentiation and authentication of medicinal plants as in it's application in differentiating four medicinal *Codonopsis* species from their related adulterants, *Campanumoea javania* and *Platycodon grandiflorus* (Joshi *et al.*, 2004).

The findings of this study using RAPD and PCR-RFLP of 5S-rRNA region of the phylogenetic diversity of nine accessions samples collected from the three districts namely Bandar Seri Begawan from the Brunei/Muara district (AP2, AP4, AP6, AP8, AP11, AP14, AP15), Kuala Belait district (K.B.), Temburong district (T) and Chuan

Xin Lian (CXL) from China constituted as the first report on the genetic diversity study on *Andrographis paniculata* from Brunei Darussalam. *Andrographis paniculata* populations are genetically and moderately different in Brunei Darussalam on the basis of RAPD analysis.

The two main principal components extracted from the PCA were plotted and analysed. The first component accounted for 59.55 per cent and the second component was 26.60 per cent of the total variance. The combined cumulative was 86.14 per cent among the genotypes studied. Three clusters of genotype-specific RAPD markers were identified from the PCA plot as shown in Figure 11.2. These markers may be employed in future studies to identify these genotypes, but additionally may be useful as predictors of Andrographolide and Dehydroandrographolide levels in accessions of *Andrographis paniculata*. However, further studies are required to confirm the linkages of these RAPD polymorphisms with the gene loci responsible for Andrographolide production.

## Acknowledgements

We acknowledged the help and support of the Ministry of Health, Brunei Darussalam and also the Department of Agriculture, Ministry of Industry and Primary Resources Brunei Darussalam. This PhD candidature is supported by scholarship from His Majesty's Government of Brunei Darussalam.

## References

Brevoort, P., 1996. The U.S. Botanical Market: an overview. Herbalgram (36): pp. 49-57.

Campose, L.P., *et al.*, 1994. Genome relationship among lotus species based on random Amplified polymorphic DNA (RAPD). Theoretical and Applied Genetics (88): pp. 417-422.

Cannoly, A.G., *et al.*, 1994. Interpretation of random amplified polymorphic DNA marker data for fingerprinting sweet potato (*Ipomoea batatas L.*). Theoretical and Applied Genetics (88): pp. 332-336.

Chen, Y.S., *et al.*, 1999. Random amplified polymorphic DNA analysis on *Curcuma wenuujin* and *sichuanensis*. Zhongguo Zhong Yao Za Zhi (Chinese) (24(3)): pp. 131-133.

Chou, C.H. and Tsai, C.C., 1999. Genetic variation in the intergenic spacer of ribosomal DNA of *Imperata cylindrical (L.) Beauv.var.major* (*Cogongrass*) populations in Taiwan. Botanical Bulletin of Academia Sinica (40): pp. 319-327.

Chua *et al.*, 2006. Inhibition of iNOS mediated relaxations by Andrographolide, Dehydroandrographolide and *Andrographis paniculata* of Brunei Darussalam in the rat aorta (paper submitted).

Cui, X.M., *et al.*, 2003. Authentication of Panax notoginseng by 5S-rRNA Spacer Domain and Random Amplified Polymorphic DNA (RAPD) Analysis. Planta Med (69): pp. 584-586.

Department of Information (2003). Brunei Darussalam In Brief. Publication Division, Prime Minister's Office, Brunei Darussalam.

Department of Agriculture (2000). Medicinal Plants of Brunei Darussalam, Ministry of Industry and Primary Resources, Brunei Darussalam.

Joshi, K., *et al.*, 2004. Molecular markers in herbal drug technology. Curr Sci (87(2)): pp. 159-165.

Kapteyn, J., *et al.*, 2002. Genetic relationships and diversity of commercial relevant *Echinaceae*. Theoretical and Applied Genetics (105(2-3)): pp. 369-376.

Kim, Y.D., *et al.*, 2004. Taxonomic and phytogeographic implication from ITS phylogeny in *Berberis* (*Berberidaceae*). J.Plant Res. (117): pp. 175-182.

Kumar, S., *et al.*, 2001. MEGA2: molecular evolutionary genetics analysis software. Bioinformatics (17): pp. 1244-1245.

Lin, T., *et al.*, 2001. Genetic heterogeneity of *Borrelia burgdorferi sensu lato* in the southern United States based on restriction fragment length polymorphism and sequence analysis. J Clin Microbiol (39): pp. 2500-2507.

Lynch, M. and Milligan, B.G., 1994. Analysis of population genetic structure with RAPD Markers. Mol Ecol (3): pp. 91-99.

Marwick, C.H., 1995. Growing use of medicinal botanicals forces assessments by drug Regulators. JAMA (273): pp. 607-609.

Nakai, R., *et al.*, 1996. Genetic Characterization of *Epimedium* species using random amplified Polymorphic DNA (RAPD) and PCR-restriction fragment length polymorphism DNA (RFLP) diagnosis. Biol. Pharm. Bull. (19): pp. 67-70.

Padmesh, P., *et al.*, 1999. The use of RAPD in assessing genetic variability in *Andrographis paniculata Nees*, a hepatoprotective drug. Curr Sci (76): pp. 833-835.

Penner, G.A., *et al*,. 1993. Reproducibility of random amplified polymorphic DNA (RAPD) Analysis among laboratories. PCR Methods Appl (2): pp. 341-345.

Pramanick, S., *et al.*, 2005. Andrographolide and Isoandrographolide. Minor Diterpenoids from *Andrographis paniculata:* Structure and X-ray Crystallographic Analysis. J Nat. Prod.

Roser, M., *et al.*, 2001. Molecular diversity and physical mapping of 5S rDNA in wild and cultivated oat grasses (*Poaceae Aveneae*). Mol. Phylogen. Evol (21): pp. 198-217.

Sabu, K.K., 2002. Intraspecific variations in *Andrographis paniculata Nees*. PhD. thesis. Kerala University, Thiruvananthapuram, India.

Shaw, P.C., and But, P.P., 1995. Authentication of *Panax* species and their adulterants by Random primed polymerase chain reaction. Planta Med (61): pp. 466-469.

Sun, Y., *et al.*, 2004. Characterization of medicinal *Epimedium* species by 5S rRNA gene Spacer sequencing. Planta Med (70): pp. 287-288.

Wang, Y.L., *et al.*, 2004. Studies on Classification of Subgenus *Yulania* by RAPD Analysis. Bio X.

Wolters, J. and Erdmann, V.A., 1988. Compilation of 5S rRNA and 5S-rRNA gene sequences. Nucleic Acids Res. (16) Suppl: pp. 70

Yamazaki, M., *et al.*, 1994. Genetic relationships among *Glycyrrhiza* plants determined by RAPD and RFLP analyses. Biol. Pharm. Bull. (17(11)): pp. 1529-1531.

Yeh, F., *et al.*, 1999. POPGENE Version 1.31.

# Chapter 12

# Improvement of the Method for Simultaneous Determination of Indirubin and Indigo by UV-Visible Spectrophotometry

***Bui Huu Tai and Nguyen Manh Cuong****

*Institute of Chemistry, Vietnam Academy of Science and Technology, 18 Hoang Quoc Viet Road, Caugiay, Hanoi, Vietnam*

**E-mail: nmcuong@ich.vast.ac.vn*

## ABSTRACT

A direct quantitative method has been improved for the simultaneous determination of indigo and indirubin using UV-visible spectrophotometry. The method is based on the measurements of the sulphated derivatives of indigo and indirubin at wavelengths of 610 nm and 541 nm, respectively. Calibration curves show excellent linearity ($r^2$>0.9998 for indigo at 610 nm) and ($r^2$>0.9996 for indirubin at 541 nm) in the range of 0.6–20.8 $\mu$g/ml. The method has high precision with the standard deviation of 0.410 and 0.057, and the relative standard deviation of 1.63 per cent and 0.76 per cent for indigo and indirubin, respectively. The accuracy of method is good with recoveries greater than 99 per cent. The proposed method is high precision, rapid and inexpensive. Application of this method to a natural indigo powder produced from the leaves of *Strobilanthes cusia*, resulted in indigo and indirubin contents of 35.4 per cent and 15.6 per cent, respectively.

***Keywords:** Indirubin, Indigo, UV-Vis spectrophotometry, Quantitative determination.*

## 1.0 Introduction

Natural indigo, a dark blue powder is prepared from the leaves of *Polygonum tinctorium* Ait. (Polygonaceae), *Isatis indigotica* Fort. (Brassicaceae), *Indigofera suffrutticosa*

Mill. (Fabaceae), *Indigofera tinctoria* Linn. (Fabaceae) and from *Baphicacanthus cusia* Brem, which has synonymous name of *Strobilanthes cusia* (Nees.) O. Kuntze (Acanthaceae) in Thailand and Vietnam. Indigo was known throughout the ancient world for its ability to colour fabrics a deep blue. Egyptian suggests that indigo was employed as early as 1600 B.C. and it has been found in Africa, India, Indonesia, and China. In Vietnam, indigo powder, produced from the leaves of *Strobilanthes cusia*, has been used as a natural dye and in folklore medicine. It is recommended for the treatment of wounds, ulcers, tumours and various inflammatory ailments (Bich, 2004).

The chemical investigation showed that indigo powder containing two major components of indigo (blue pigment) and indirubin (red isomer pigment). Their quantity in indigo powder affects directly to colour of the natural dye. High performance liquid chromatographic method was reported for determination of indigo and indirubin (Nittaya, 2002; Peng, 2007; Qian, 2005). The method needs the expensive instruments and is complicated due to low solubility of indigo and indirubin in organic solvents. Some other quantitative determination procedures based on titrimetric, chromatographic and electrochemical methods were reported (Eogenio, 2004). The spectrophotometric method was applied for the determination of indigo by absorption measurement of its sulphated derivative at wavelength of 610 nm (Pharmacopoeia, 2000). However, the method could only give total content of indigoids calculated as indigo. No official procedure has been given so far in other pharmacopoeias for simultaneous determination of indigo and indirubin by using UV-VIS spectrophotometric method. In previous report, we described the procedure for determination of indigo and indirubin by simultaneous measurements at two wavelengths 541 nm and 610 nm (Tai, 2007).

This paper reports the improvement of the method in terms of their equation system and also the higher accuracy and better repeatability in simultaneous determination of indirubin and indigo in indigo powder.

## 2.0 Experimental

### 2.1 Apparatus

Absorption was recorded in 1 cm quartz cells using on Cintra 4.0 double-beam UV-visible spectrophotometer (AIR Analytical Instrument Recycle, Inc., USA).

### 2.2 Isolation of Indigo and Indirubin from Indigo Powder

The dried powder of indigo powder was extracted with ethyl acetate at boiling temperature of the solvent. The extract to which was added an amount of silica gel and was evaporated in vacuum to dried residue. The residue was subjected to column chromatography on silica gel, eluting with $CHCl_3$ to furnish 2 fractions which were combined according to TLC monitoring. The solvent was evaporated to obtain pure indigo (blue solid powder) and indirubin (red solid), respectively. Both pure indirubin and indigo were used as standard compounds in quantity of indigoids.

## 2.3 Preparation of the Standard Solutions

An accurately weighed amount of the pure indigo and indirubin (1.5 mg for indigo and 2.6 mg for indirubin, respectively) was sulphated in a flask by adding 2 ml of concentrated sulphuric acid slowly at 80°C on a water bath. Mixture was stirred gently for 30 minutes. Then, the mixture was cooled to 25 °C, transferred into a 100 ml volumetric flask and diluted to volume with distilled water to have the stock solutions of 1.5 mg/100ml of indigo (57.2519 $\mu$M) and 2.6 mg/100ml of indirubin (99.2366 $\mu$M), respectively. The solution was filtered through a 0.45 $\mu$m filter. The standard solutions in 25-ml volumetric flasks containing seven specified concentrations of the sulphated indigo (0.6–12.0 $\mu$g/ml) and indirubin (1.04–20.8 $\mu$g/ml) were prepared from the stock solutions by appropriate dilution with 0.368 M $H_2SO_4$ solution.

## 2.4 Determination of Absorption Wavelength for Sulphated Indigo and Indirubin

UV spectra of the standard solutions of the sulphated indigo and indirubin were measured in the range of 400–700 nm at 1 nm interval in scanning mode-spectrum measurement to determine appropriate wavelength for each compound. Blank cell contains 0.368 M $H_2SO_4$ solution.

## 2.5 Analysis of Indigo Powder

Dried indigo powder (2-3 mg) was mixed with 2 ml of concentrated sulphuric acid as described above. The mixture was transferred into a 100 ml volumetric flask to which was added distilled water to volume. The sample solution was measured at 541 and 610 nm, and the concentrations of indigo and indirubin were calculated.

# 3.0 Results and Discussion

The UV spectroscopic method is popularly applied for quantitative determination of organic compounds in general and coloured compounds in particular. The analysis of multi-absorbers is possibly determined by using the Beer-Lambert law, in which the total absorbance is given by:

$$A_\lambda = \log (Io/I) = (\varepsilon_1 C_1 + \varepsilon_2 . C_2 + ..).B$$

A: Absorbance or optical density at a particular wavelength

$I_0$: Incident light intensity of blank cell

I: Incident light intensity of sample cell

$\varepsilon_i$: Molar absorption coefficient of analyte i ($mol^{-1}.cm^{-1}.l$)

$C_i$: Molar concentration of material in solution of analyte (mol/l).

B: The absorption path length (cm).

In the case of the indigo powder, assumed that it contains mostly indigo and indirubin at suitable wavelength, two calibration curves of the sulphated indigo and indirubin are constructed and their concentrations could be calculated from the system of two regression equations.

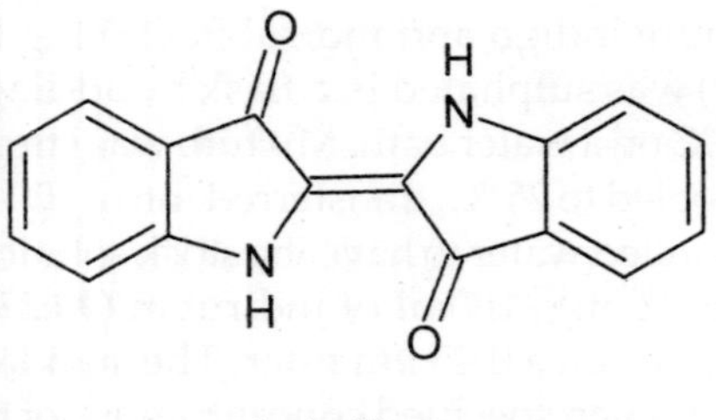

1. indigo

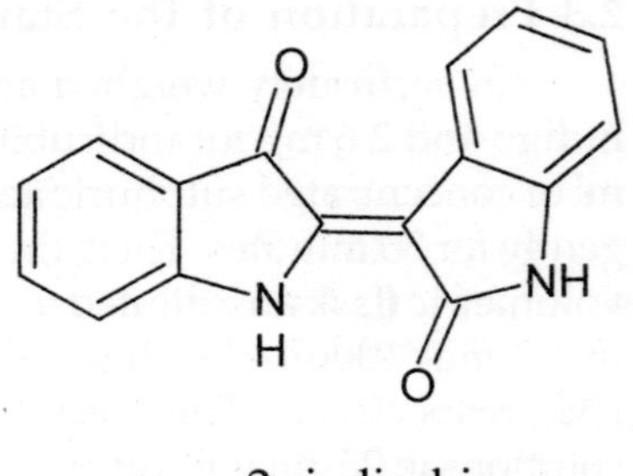

2. indirubin

### 3.1 Maximum Absorption Wavelength of Sulphated Indigo and Indirubin

Measurement of a series of indigo samples in scan mode showed that the maximum absorption wavelength of indigo is around 610 nm. Similarly, the maximum absorption wavelength of indirubin at 541 nm is determined.

### 3.2 Construction of Calibration Curves

The calibration curve of indigo (IG) and indirubin (IR) at wavelengths of 541 nm and 610 nm was constructed by plotting the obtained absorbance *versus* seven given concentrations of the standard solutions.

Figure 12.1 shows the calibration curves of indigo at wavelength of 541 nm (a) and 610 nm (b). Calibration curves of indirubin at wavelength of 541 (c) and 610 (d) nm are presented in Figure 12.2. These calibration curves showed good linearity with the relative coefficient $R^2$ (0.9991–0.9998) in the 0.6–20 $\mu$g/ml range of indigo and indirubin. The slopes of graphs were molar absorption coefficient of indigo and indirubin at the specified wavelength. Thus, the molar absorption coefficient of indigo at $\lambda_1$ = 541 nm was $\varepsilon_1 = 3432$ $mol^{-1}.cm^{-1}.l$ and at $\lambda_2$ = 610 nm was $\varepsilon_2 = 11070$ $mol^{-1}.cm^{-1}.l$. The molar absorption coefficient of indirubin at $\lambda_1$ = 541 nm was $\varepsilon'_1 =$ 9528 $mol^{-1}.cm^{-1}.l$ and $\lambda_2$ = 610 nm was 1566 $mol^{-1}.cm^{-1}.l$, respectively.

The system of equations is established as belows:

$$\begin{cases} 3432.C_{IG} + 9528.C_{IR} = A^{541} \\ 11070.C_{IG} + 1566.C_{IR} = A^{610} \end{cases}$$

In which, $C_{IG}$, $C_{IR}$ were concentration of indigo and indirubin in analytic material, respectively. $A^{541}$ and $A^{610}$ were absorbance measured at two wavelength $\lambda_1$ = 541 nm and $\lambda_2$ = 610 nm.

### 3.3 Repeatability of Method

The repeatability of the proposed methods was evaluated by measuring the quantity of indigo and indirubin in one sample at three different concentrations (low, medium and high). The results are summarized in Table 12.1.

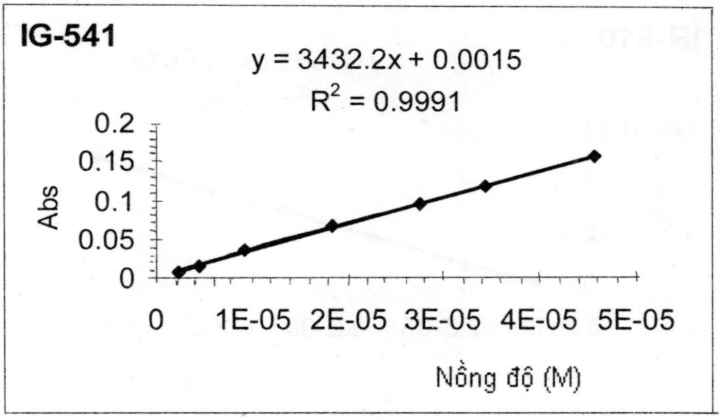


**(a)**

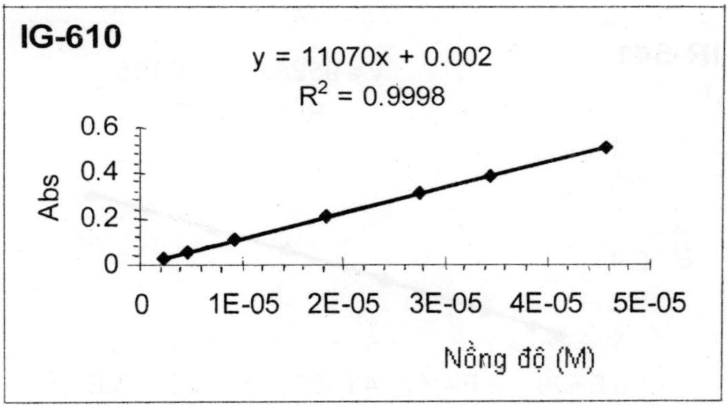


**(b)**

**Figure 12.1: Calibration Curves of Indigo at Wavelengths of 541 nm (a) and 610 nm (b)**

**Table 12.1: Repeatability Data of Determination of Indigo and Indirubin**

| *Sl.No.* | *Con. (μg/ml)* | *Abs.* | | *% IR* | *% IG* |
|---|---|---|---|---|---|
| | | *541 nm* | *610 nm* | | |
| 1. | 34 | 0.205 | 0.378 | 7.483 | 25.254 |
| 2. | 44 | 0.262 | 0.478 | 7.494 | 24.651 |
| 3. | 55 | 0.335 | 0.616 | 7.587 | 25.435 |
| | | | | $\%\overline{IR}$ = 7.522 | $\%\overline{IG}$ = 25.113 |
| | | | | S = 0.057 | S= 0.410 |
| | | | | RSD = 0.76% | RSD = 1.63% |

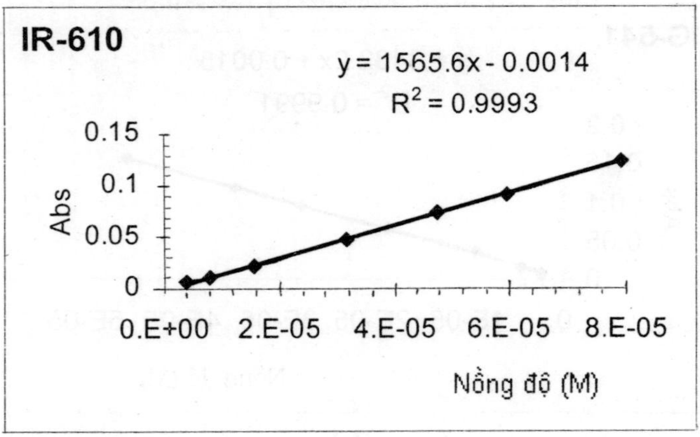


(c)

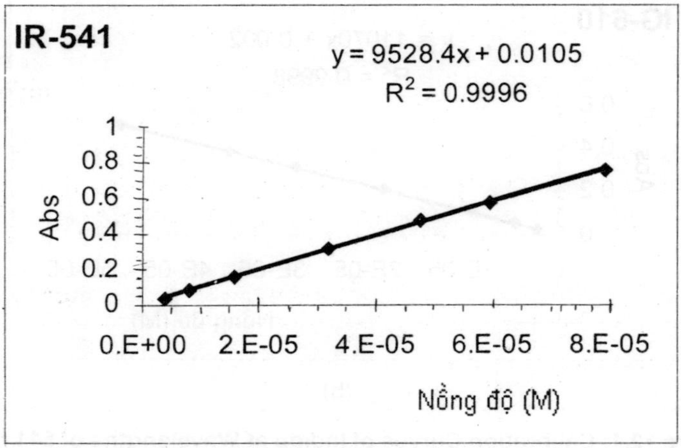


(d)

**Figure 12.2: Calibration Curves of Indirubin at Wavelengths of 610 nm (c) and 541 nm (d)**

The method showed high repeatability with the standard deviations (S) of 0.410 and 0.057, and the relative standard deviation (RSD) of 1.63 per cent and 0.76 per cent for indigo and indirubin, respectively.

## 3.4 Accuracy

In order to determine the accuracy of the method, recovery studies were carried out by standard addition method. An accurate quantity of pure indirubin was added to pre-analyzed formulations and the mixtures were analyzed following the procedure. The total to amount of the indirubin was then determined and the amount of the added indirubin was calculated by difference. Results were given in Table 12.2.

**Table 12.2: Accuracy Data of the Method**

| *Sl.No.* | *IR in Sample (μg/ml)* | *$IR_{added}$ (μg/ml)* | *$IR_{found}$ (μg/ml)* | *$IR_{recovery}$ (μg/ml)* | *$IR_{recovery}$ (%)* |
|---|---|---|---|---|---|
| 1. | 2.625 | 4.000 | 6.597 | 3.972 | 99.28 |
| 2. | 2.835 | 4.000 | 6.815 | 3.980 | 99.48 |
| 3. | 2.562 | 4.000 | 6.500 | 3.938 | 98.43 |
| | | | | | $\overline{IR}_{re.}$ = 99.06 |
| | | | | | S = 0.569 |
| | | | | | RSD =0.575% |

The method showed good accuracy with the average percentage of recoveries of 99.06 per cent for added indirubin, as well as the standard deviation of 0.569 and the relative standard deviation of 0.575 per cent.

### 3.5 Application of the Proposed Methods

The proposed method was successfully applied for the determination of indirubin and indigo in indigo powder. Three different samples of indigo powder were analyzed and results were showed in Table 12.3. The proposed method allowed determining indigo and indirubin contents as well as total indigoid contents. Table 12.3 shows that the concentration of indigo calculated by the measurement at one wavelength (610 nm) as described in [6] may give wrong results if the sample contains significant amount of indirubin.

**Table 12.3: Concentration of Indigo and Indirubin in Some Indigo Powders**

| *Sl.No.* | *ABS* | | *IR (%)* | *IG (%)* | *Indigoids (%)* | *Indigo (%)** |
|---|---|---|---|---|---|---|
| | *541 nm* | *610 nm* | | | | |
| IP1 | 0.464 | 0.715 | 15.6 | 35.4 | 51.0 | 37.5 |
| IP2 | 0.175 | 0.384 | 4.8 | 26.1 | 30.9 | 26.6 |
| IP3 | 0.363 | 0.606 | 13.4 | 35.9 | 49.3 | 37.6 |

*: The content of indigo in indigo powder determined by one wavelength method.

## 4.0 Conclusion

From the results of this study it can be concluded that the UV-visible spectrophotometric method can be used for simultaneous determination of indigo and indirubin. This method is high precision, rapid and inexpensive.

## Acknowledgement

This investigation was funded by grants from the National Science Council of Vietnam (Project No. 511406) and Vietnam Academy of Science and Technology (2007-2008).

## References

Bich, D.H., Chung D.Q., Chuong B.X., Dong N.T., Dam D.T., Hien P.V., Lo V.N., Mai P.D, Man P.K., Nhu D.T., Tap N., Toan T., 2004. Medicinal plants and animals in Vietnam. Science and Technology Publishing House (1); pp. 401.

Eogenio O. Reyes-Salas, José A. Manzanilla-Cano, Manuel H. Barceló–Quintal, Juan Ramírez–Balderas, 2004. Direct electrochemical determination of indigo in dimethylsulfoxide. Analytical Letters (37(3)); pp. 463-472.

Nittaya Chanayath, Sorasak Lhieochaiphant, Suree Phutrakul, 2002. Pigment extraction techniques from the leaves of *Indigofera tinctoria* Linn. and *Baphicacanthus cusia* Brem. and chemical structure analysis of their major components. Chiang Mai University Journal (1(2)); pp. 149-160.

Peng Zou and Hwee Ling Koh, 2007. Determination of indican, isatin, indirubin and indigotin in *Isatis indigotica* by liquid chromatography / electrospray ionization tandem mass spectrometry. Rapid Commun. Mass Spectrom. (21); pp. 1239–1246.

Pharmacopoeia of the People's Republic of China, Indigo Naturalis, English Edition 2000 (I); pp. 126.

Qian, B., Panichayayupakaranant, P., Sirikatitham, A., Zhang, R., Guo, Y., Ywu, Y. 2005. Quantitative HPLC determination of indigotin and indirubin in indigo naturalis. Ars Pharmaceutica (46(4)); pp. 429-438.

Tai Bui Huu, Ha Nguyen Viet, Cu Luu Dam, Thao Nguyen Thi Phuong, Chien Nguyen Quyet, Cuong Nguyen Manh, 2007. Quantitative determination of indigo and indirubin by UV-VIS method. Journal of Science and Technology (45 (1B)); pp. 174-180 (in Vietnamese).

# Chapter 13

# Study on Chemical Constituents of *Ophiopogon confertifolius*

**Nguyen Thi Vinh Hue[1], Nguyen Duy Thuan[2], Nguyen Trong Thong[3], Chau Van Minh[4] and Phan Van Kiem[4]***

[1]*Traphaco Joint Stock Company, Ministry of Health, Hanoi, Vietnam*
[2]*National Institute of Medicinal Materials, Ministry of Health, Hanoi, Vietnam*
[3]*Hanoi Medical University, Ministry of Health, Hanoi, Vietnam*
[4]*Institute of Natural Products Chemistry, Vietnamese Academy of Science and Technology, 18 Hoang Quoe Road, Caugiay, Hanoi, Vietnam*
**E-mail: phankiem@yahoo.com*

## ABSTRACT

Six new compounds named ophiofolius A-F (1-6) and four known (7-10) were isolated from the methanolic extract of the roots of *Ophiopogon confertifolius* N. Tanaka (*Convallariaceae*). The new structures were elucidated as 6,8-dimethyl-4'methoxy-3',5',5,7–tetrahydroxyflavanone (1), 3-eudesmene-1$\alpha$,11-diol (2), 7-oxo-3$\alpha$,4,10$\beta$-trihydroxycarotane-1(2)-en (3), 3-*O*-$\beta$-D-arabinopyranosyl-25(*S*)-ruscogenin-1$\beta$,3$\beta$-diol 1-*O*-[$\alpha$-L-rhamnopyranosyl-(1$\rightarrow$2)-$\beta$-D-fucopyranoside] (4), 26-*O*-$\beta$-D-glucopyranosyl-1$\beta$,3$\beta$,16$\alpha$,26-tetrahydroxycholest-5-en-22-one 1-*O*-$\alpha$-L-rhamnopyranosyl-(1$\rightarrow$2)-$\beta$-D-arabinopyranoside sulphate (5), and 22-*O*-methyl-26-*O*-$\beta$-D-glucopyranosyl-25(*R*)-furost-5-ene-1$\beta$,3$\beta$,22$\xi$,26-tetraol 1-*O*-[$\alpha$-L-ramnopyranosyl-(1$\rightarrow$2)-$\beta$-D-arabinopyranoside] (6), and the known compounds were determined to be 6,8-dimethyl-3',4',5'-trimethoxy-5,7-dihydroxyflavanone (7), and 6-methoxy-5,7-dihydroxyflavanone (8), cholest-5-ene-3$\beta$-22(*R*)-diol (9), and $\beta$-sitosterol (10) by the spectroscopic evidences (1D NMR, 2D NMR, EI-MS, and ESI-MS).

*Keywords: Ophiopogon confertifolius, Convallariaceae, Ophiofolius A, B, C, D, E, F.*

## 1.0 Introduction

"Cao cang", a traditional medicinal plant of the people who lives in some mountainous areas of Bac Giang province. It has been used to treat osteocopic pain, rheumatic, analgesic, backache, rickets, dispel swelling and blood clotting in ecchymosis, renal failure. The scientific name of this plant has been identified as *Ophiopogon confertifolius* N. Tanaka (Convallariaceae). This is a new species of Vietnamese flora (Do, 2007). *Ophiopogon* genus is a rich source of steroidal glycosides with the ruscogenin skeleton (Asano, 1993; Yu, 1996). However, up to date, no studies on the chemical and bioactivities of this plant were carried out. As a part of our study on this plant, we report herein the isolation and the structural elucidation of six new compounds named ophiofolius A-F (1-6) and four known compounds (7-10) from the methanolic extract of the roots. Their structures were elucidated by the spectroscopic experiments.

## 2.0 Experimental

### 2.1 Plant Material

The roots of *Ophiopogon confertifolius* N. Tanaka (Convallariaceae) were collected in Yen The, Bac Giang province, Vietnam and was identified by Dr Nguyen Thi Do, Institute of Ecology and Biological Resources, Vietnam Academy of Science and Technology for the plant identification. The voucher of specimen was deposited at National Institute of Medicinal Materials, Ministry of Health.

### 2.2 General Experimental Procedures

Melting points were determined using an Electro Thermal IA-9200. The IR spectra were obtained on a Hitachi 270-30 type spectrometer with KBr discs. Optical rotations were determined on a Jasco DIP-1000 KUY polar meter. The electrospray ionization (ESI) mass spectra were obtained using an AGILENT 1100 LC-MSD Trap spectrometer. The $^{1}$H-NMR (500 MHz) and $^{13}$C-NMR (125 MHz) spectra were recorded on a Bruker AM500 FT-NMR spectrometer and TMS was used as an internal standard. Column chromatography (CC) was performed on silica gel (Kieselgel 60, 70-230 mesh and 230-400 mesh, Merck) and YMC RP-18 resins.

### 2.3 Extraction and Isolation

Dried roots of *O. confertifolius* were needles and then extracted three times with MeOH. The MeOH extract (50 g) was suspended in water and partitioned in turn with *n*-hexane, chloroform, ethyl acetate, and *n*-BuOH to obtain *n*-hexane (5.8 g), chloroform (10,2 g), ethyl acetate (20 g), and *n*-BuOH fractions (13,0 g). The ethyl acetate fraction (20 g) was chromatographed on silica gel column using $CHCl_3$-MeOH-$H_2O$ (80:20:2) and on YMC column using MeOH-$H_2O$ (3:1) to yield compounds 1 (75 mg), 7 (15 mg), and 8 (21 mg) as yellow crystals. The chloroform fraction (10.2 g) was combined chromatographed on silica gel column and then on YMC column to yield compounds 2 (14 mg) and 3 (8.5 mg), 9 (17 mg) and 10 (34 mg) as colourless crystals. The *n*-BuOH fractions (13.0 g) was chromatographed on silica gel column using $CHCl_3$-MeOH-$H_2O$ (60:40:5) to give five sub fractions [SFr. A(1.3 g), B (2.5 g), C (1.8 g),

D (3.5 g) and E (3.0 g)]. The sub fraction B (2.5 g) was then chromatographed on YMC column using MeOH-$H_2O$ (2:1) to yield compounds 4 (13 mg) and 5 (13 mg). The sub fraction D (3.5 g) was chromatographed on YMC column using MeOH-$H_2O$ (1.5:1) to yield 6 (18 mg) colourless needles.

**6,8-Dimethyl-4'methoxy-3',5',5,7-tetrahydroxyflavanone (ophiofolius A, 1)**

Yellow crystals; mp. 223-224°C; IR (KBr) $\nu_{max}$ $cm^{-1}$: 3400 (OH), 1716 (C=O), 1445 (C=C); ESI-MS *m/z*: 347 $[M+H]^+$; 345 $[M-H]^-$ ($C_{18}H_{18}O_7$); $^1$H-NMR (500 MHz, DMSO-$d_6$) and $^{13}$C-NMR (125 MHz, DMSO-$d_6$): see Table 13.1.

**Table 13.1: NMR Data of 1, 7 and 8**

| C | *1* | | *7* | | *8* | |
|---|---|---|---|---|---|---|
| | $\delta_C$ | $\delta_H$ | $\delta_C$ | $\delta_H$ | $\delta_C$ | $\delta_H$ |
| 2 | 77.58 | 5.34 dd (3.0, 12.5) | 77.92 | 5.36 dd (3.0, 12,0) | 80.54 | 5.42 dd (3.0, 12.0) |
| 3 | 42.06 | 2.76 dd (3.0, 17.00) 3.02 dd (12.5, 17.0) | 42.19 | 2.70 dd (3.0, 17.00) 3.12 dd (12.5, 17.0) | 44.19 | 2.78 dd (3.0, 17.00) 3.08 dd (12.0, 17.0) |
| 4 | 196.51 | – | 196.56 | – | 198.05 | – |
| 5 | 158.34 | – | 158.46 | – | 160.85 | – |
| 6 | 103.21 | – | 103.37 | – | 130.53 | – |
| 7 | 162.39 | – | 162.47 | – | 159.98 | – |
| 8 | 102.54 | – | 102.62 | – | 96.27 | 6.02 s |
| 9 | 157.09 | – | 157.15 | – | 140.38 | – |
| 10 | 101.74 | – | 102.62 | – | 103.52 | – |
| 1' | 135.25 | – | 134.61 | – | 140.38 | – |
| 2' | 105.33 | 6.43 s | 107.40 | 6.64 s | 127.32 | 7.38–7.50 |
| 3' | 150.70 | – | 153.19 | – | 130.53 | 7.38–7.50 |
| 4' | 134.36 | – | 136.2 | – | 129.60 | 7.38–7.50 |
| 5' | 150.70 | – | 150.57 | – | 130.53 | 7.38–7.50 |
| 6' | 105.33 | 6.43 s | 101.75 | 6.64 | 127.32 | 7.38–7.50 |
| 6–Me | 7.55 | 1.95 s | 7.59 | 1.96 s | | |
| 8–Me | 8.26 | 1.98 s | 8.29 | 1.99 s | | |
| 4'–OMe | 59.63 | 3.68 s | 55.75 | 3.68 s | | |
| 3'–OMe | | | 55.89 | 3.79 s | | |
| 6–OMe | | | | | 60.99 | 3.80 s |
| 5–OH | | 12.33 | | 12.35 | | |

[a]125 MHz, [b]500 MHz, [c]In DMSO-$d_6$, [d]In $CD_3OD$. Chemical shifts are given in ppm; coupling constant *J* (in parentheses) in Hz.

**3-Eudesmene-1α,11-diol (ophiofolius B, 2)**

Colourless crystals; mp. 175-176°C; IR (KBr) $\nu_{max}$ cm$^{-1}$: 3340 (OH), 2985-2890 (CH), 1445 (C=C); EI-MS (70 eV) *m/z* (per cent): 220 [M-$H_2O$]$^{+\cdot}$ ($C_{15}H_{26}O_2$), (54.6), 203 (55.4), 187 (14.2), 177 (98.4), 159 (46.6), 147 (28.3), 107 (44.3), 91 (40.1), 81 (43.7), 59 (100.0); $^1$H-NMR (500 MHz, $CDCl_3$) and $^{13}$C-NMR (125 MHz, $CDCl_3$): see Table 13.2.

**Table 13.2: NMR Data of 2**

| C | $\delta_C$ | DEPT | $\delta_H$ | $^1$H-$^1$H COSY | ROESY | HMBC H to C |
|---|---|---|---|---|---|---|
| 1 | 74.52 | CH | 3.40 br s, $H_{eq}$ | H–2 | H–15 | C–3 |
| 2 | 31.30 | $CH_2$ | 2.47 dm (16.5), $H_{ax}$<br>2.05 dm (16.5), $H_{eq}$ | H–1, H3<br>H–1, H–3 | | C–3, C–4 |
| 3 | 119.10 | CH | 5.83 br s | H–2 | H–14 | C–1, C–5, C–14 |
| 4 | 135.40 | – | – | | | |
| 5 | 39.57 | CH | 2.16*, $H_{ax}$ | H–6 | | |
| 6 | 24.18 | $CH_2$ | 1.95 dd (13.5, 2.5), $H_{ax}$<br>1.38 dd (13.5, 4.5), $H_{eq}$ | H–5, H–7<br>H–5, H–7 | $H_{eq}$–7,$H_{ax}$–8, $H_{eq}$–9<br>H–13 | C–4, C–5, C–7<br>C–4, C–5, C–7 |
| 7 | 44.68 | CH | 1.16*, $H_{eq}$ | H–6, H–8 | $H_{ax}$–6, $H_{ax}$–8 | |
| 8 | 22.32 | $CH_2$ | 1.61 ddd (12.5, 6.0, 3.0), $H_{ax}$<br>1.29 dd (12.5, 3.5), $H_{eq}$ | H–7, H–9<br>H–7, H–9 | $H_{ax}$–6, $H_{eq}$–7, H–15<br>H–12 | C–7, C–9 |
| 9 | 31.32 | $CH_2$ | 1.26*, $H_{ax}$<br>1.40 dd (12.5, 3.5), $H_{eq}$ | H–8<br>H–8 | $H_{ax}$–6 | |
| 10 | 36.29 | – | – | | | |
| 11 | 72.77 | – | – | | | |
| 12 | 26.93 | $CH_3$ | 1.18 s | | $H_{eq}$–8 | C–7, C–11 |
| 13 | 27.05 | $CH_3$ | 1.19 s | | $H_{eq}$–6 | C–7, C–11 |
| 14 | 21.66 | $CH_3$ | 1.70 s | | H–3 | C–3, C–4, C–5 |
| 15 | 22.09 | $CH_3$ | 1.11 s | | H–1, $H_{ax}$–8 | C–1, C–5, C–9, C–10 |

[a]125 MHz, [b]500 MHz, [c]In $CDCl_3$. Chemical shifts are given in ppm; coupling constant *J* (in parentheses) in Hz, *Overlapped signals.

**7-Oxo-3α,4,10β-trihydroxycarotane-1(2)-en (ophiofolius C, 3)**

Colorless crystals; mp. 191-192°C; ESI-MS *m/z* (per cent): 269 [M+H]$^+$ (positive), 267 [M-H]$^-$ (negative), ($C_{15}H_{24}O_4$); $^1$H-NMR (500 MHz, $CDCl_3$) and $^{13}$C-NMR (125 MHz, $CDCl_3$): see Table 13.3.

**3-*O*-β-D-arabinopyranosyl-25(*S*)-ruscogenin-1β,3β-diol 1-*O*-[α-L-ramnopyranosyl-(1→2)-β-D-fucopyranoside] (ophiofolius D, 4)**

Colourless needles; mp. 248-249°C; ESI-MS *m/z*: 855 [M+H]$^+$ ($C_{44}H_{70}O_{16}$); $^1$H-NMR (500 MHz, $CD_3OD$) and $^{13}$C-NMR (125 MHz, $CD_3OD$): see Table 13.4.

**Table 13.3: NMR Data of 3**

| C | $\delta_C$[a,b] | DEPT | $\delta_H$[a,c] | $^1H$-$^1H$ COSY | ROESY | HMBC H to C |
|---|---|---|---|---|---|---|
| 1 | 138.95 | – | – | | | |
| 2 | 137.00 | CH | 6.34 dd (1.5, 6.5) | H–3 | H–14 | C–4, C–14 |
| 3 | 70.31 | CH | 4.08 d (6.5) | H–2 | H–15 | C–1, C–2, C–4, C–5 |
| 4 | 75.20 | – | – | | | |
| 5 | 41.94 | – | – | | | |
| 6 | 53.55 | $CH_2$ | 2.51 d (13.5), $H_a$<br>2.83 d (13.5), $H_b$ | | $H_b$<br>$H_a$ | C–1, C–4, C–5, C–7<br>C–1, C–4, C–5, C–7 |
| 7 | 204.33 | – | – | | | |
| 8 | 36.23 | $CH_2$ | 1.26 m | H–9 | | C–10 |
| 9 | 23.62 | $CH_2$ | 1.86 m | H–8 | | C–4, C–5 |
| 10 | 79.06 | – | – | | | |
| 11 | 29.84 | CH | – | H–12, H–13 | | |
| 12 | 19.61 | $CH_3$ | 1.15 d (7,0) | H–11 | | C–10, C–11 |
| 13 | 19.05 | $CH_3$ | 1.10 d (7,0) | H–11 | | C–10, C–11 |
| 14 | 21.95 | $CH_3$ | 1.92 s | | H–2 | C–1, C–2, C–7 |
| 15 | 21.72 | $CH_3$ | 1.16 s | | H–3 | C–4, C–5, C–6, C–8 |

[a]125 MHz, [b]500 MHz, [c]In $CDCl_3$. Chemical shifts are given in ppm; coupling constant $J$ (in parentheses); In Hz, *Overlapped signals.

**Table 13.4: NMR Data of 4**

| C | $\delta_C$[a,c] | $\delta_H$[b,c] | H–H COSY | HMBC (H to C) |
|---|---|---|---|---|
| 1 | 84.55 | 3.40* | | |
| 2 | 35.78 | 1.83 m; 2.18 m | | |
| 3 | 75.42 | 3.43* | | |
| 4 | 41.18 | 1.20*; 1.69* | | |
| 5 | 138.29 | – | | |
| 6 | 126.44 | 5.60 d (5.5) | H–7 | 4, 5, 8, 10 |
| 7 | 32.87 | 2.00*; 1.32* | H–6, H–8 | |
| 8 | 34.02 | 1.56* | H–7 | |
| 9 | 51.50 | 1.26* | | |
| 10 | 43.52 | – | | |
| 11 | 24.78 | 1.46 dt (3.5, 13.5) | | |
| 12 | 40.09 | 2.29 m | | |
| 13 | 41.14 | – | | |
| 14 | 57.97 | 1.16* | | |

*Contd...*

**Table 13.4–Contd...**

| *C* | $\delta_C$[a,c] | $\delta_H$[b,c] | *H–H COSY* | *HMBC (H to C)* |
|---|---|---|---|---|
| 15 | 32.71 | 1.72*; 2.00* | | |
| 16 | 82.19 | 4.40 dd (7.5, 15.0) | | |
| 17 | 64.01 | 1.75* | | 16 |
| 18 | 17.08 | 0.83 s | | 12, 13, 14, 17 |
| 19 | 15.19 | 1.11 s | | 1, 5, 8, 10 |
| 20 | 42.91 | 1.93 m | H–21 | |
| 21 | 14.80 | 1.02 d (6.5) | H–20 | 17, 20, 22 |
| 22 | 110.60 | – | | |
| 23 | 32.44 | 1.57*; 1.72* | H–24 | |
| 24 | 29.89 | 1.45*; 1.66* | H–23, H–25 | |
| 25 | 31.44 | 1.32*; 1.53* | H–24, H–26, H–27 | |
| 26 | 67.84 | 3.32*; 3.47* | H–25 | 24, 25, 27 |
| 27 | 17.47 | 0.81 d (6.5) | H–27 | 24, 25, 26 |
| **Fuc** | | | | |
| 1' | 101.15 | 4.30 d (7.0) | H–2' | 1, 2', 3' |
| 2' | 76.85 | 3.43* | H–1', H–3' | |
| 3' | 80.09 | 3.44* | H–2', H–4' | |
| 4' | 73.96 | 3.42* | H–3', H–5' | |
| 5' | 69.98 | 3.71 m | H–4', H–6' | |
| 6' | 17.98 | 1.30 d (6.5) | H–5' | 4', 5' |
| **Rha** | | | | |
| 1" | 101.40 | 5.40 d (1.5) | H–2" | 2' |
| 2" | 72.37 | 3.80 dd (3.5, 1.5) | H–1", H–3" | |
| 3" | 72.37 | 3.70* | H–2", H–4" | |
| 4" | 74.08 | 3.42* | H–3", H–5" | |
| 5" | 69.64 | 4.12 m | H–4", H–6" | |
| 6" | 18.32 | 1.26 d (6.5) | H–5" | 4", 5" |
| **Ara** | | | | |
| 1''' | 100.67 | 4.85* | H–2''' | 3, 2''', 3''' |
| 2''' | 72.12 | 3.69* | H–1''', H–3''' | |
| 3''' | 72.69 | 3.77 dd (3.0, 1.5) | H–2''', H–3''' | |
| 4''' | 71.70 | 3.48* | H–3''', H–5''' | |
| 5''' | 67.20 | 3.15 dd (10.0, 11.5) | | |
| | | 3.86 dd (5.0, 11.5) | H–4''' | 3''', 4''' |

[a]125 MHz, [b]500 MHz, [c]In $CD_3OD$. Chemical shifts are given in ppm; coupling constant *J* (in parentheses) in Hz; *Overlapped signals.

**26-*O*-β-D-Glucopyranosyl-1β,3β,16α,26-tetrahydroxycholest-5-en-22-one 1-*O*-α-L-rhamnopyranosyl-(1→2)-β-D-arabinopyranoside sulphate (ophiofolius E, 5)**

Colourless needles; mp. 256-257°C; ESI-MS *m/z*: 991.3 $[M+Na]^+$; 967.5 $[M-H]^-$ (C44H$_{72}$SO21); 1H-NMR (500 MHz, $CD_3OD$) and $^{13}C$-NMR (125 MHz, $CD_3OD$): see Table 13.5.

**Table 13.5: NMR Data of 5 and 6**

| *C* | *5* | | | *6* | | | |
|---|---|---|---|---|---|---|---|
| | $\delta_C^{a,b}$ | $\delta_H^{a,c}$ | *HMBC H to C* | $\delta_C^{a,b}$ | $\delta_H^{a,c}$ | *H–H COSY* | *HMBC H to C* |
| 1 | 84.52 | 3.38* | | 84.58 | 3.37* | 2 | |
| 2 | 37.16 | 1.72 m; 2.12 m | 1, 3 | 37.26 | 1.70 m, 2.10 m | 2, 1 | |
| 3 | 69.14 | 3.37 m | | 69.17 | 3.37 m | 3 | |
| 4 | 43.21 | 2.25 m, 1.90 m | 2, 3, 5, 6 | 43.34 | 2.25 m, 1.97 m | | 5, 6 |
| 5 | 139.40 | – | | 139.49 | – | | |
| 6 | 125.99 | 5.57 d (5.5) | 7, 10 | 125.96 | 5.57 d (5.5) | 7 | 7 |
| 7 | 32.42 | 1.50*; 1.97 dd (12.0, 4.5) | 5, 6, 9 | 32.65 | 1.52*, 2.00* | 6 | |
| 8 | 34.04 | 1.50* | | 35.01 | 1.56* | 9, 14 | |
| 9 | 51.28 | 1.27* | | 51.45 | 1.25* | 8 | |
| 10 | 43.33 | – | | 43.35 | – | | |
| 11 | 24.73 | 1.50*; 2.45 dd (12.0, 3.0) | | 24.81 | 1.46 m, 2.49 dd (12.0, 3.0) | | |
| 12 | 41.38 | 1.26*; 1.82* | | 41.12 | 1.69*, 2.21* | | |
| 13 | 42.41 | – | | 41.55 | – | | |
| 14 | 55.79 | 1.00* | | 57.94 | 1.15 m | 8, 15 | |
| 15 | 35.62 | 1.62 dt (13.5, 4.5) | 16 | 32.90 | 1.30*, 1.98* | 14, 16 | |
| 16 | 80.11 | 4.65 m | 13 | 82.45 | 4.38 dd (13.5, 7.5) | 15, 17 | 13, 20 |
| 17 | 57.97 | 1.87* | 16, 21 | 65.33 | 1.74* | 16 | |
| 18 | 14.02 | 0.95 s | 12, 13, 14, 17 | 17.16 | 0.86 s | | 12, 13, 14, 17 |
| 19 | 15.17 | 1.10 s | 1, 5, 9, 10 | 15.25 | 1.10 s | | 1, 5, 9, 10 |
| 20 | 44.26 | 3.04 m | | 41.19 | 1.19* | | |
| 21 | 16.97 | 1.09 d (6.5) | 17, 20, 22 | 16.16 | 1.03 d (6.5) | | 17, 20, 22 |
| 22 | 217.42 | – | | 114.03 | – | | |
| 23 | 40.20 | 2.74 m; 2.83 m | 22, 24 | 31.41 | 1.66*, 1.86 dt (5.0, 12.0) | | |
| 24 | 27.83 | 1.49*, 1.72* | | 28.98 | 1.17*, 1.62* | | |
| 25 | 33.96 | 1.78 m | | 34.05 | 1.57* | | |
| 26 | 76.04 | 3.40*, 3.75* | 24, 27, 1' | 76.01 | 3.42*, 3.77* | | |
| 27 | 17.16 | 0.97 d (6.5) | 24, 25, 26 | 17.28 | 0.97 d (6.5) | | 24, 25, 26 |

*Contd...*

**Table 13.5–Contd...**

| C | 5 | | | 6 | | | |
|---|---|---|---|---|---|---|---|
| | $\delta_C$ [a,b] | $\delta_H$ [a,c] | HMBC H to C | $\delta_C$ [a,b] | $\delta_H$ [a,c] | H–H COSY | HMBC H to C |
| | | | **Gluc** | | | | |
| 1' | 104.54 | 4.29 d (7.5) | 26, 2'' | 104.60 | 4.25 d (7.5) | 2' | 26, 2'' |
| 2' | 75.21 | 3.20 dd (7.5, 8.0) | 1'' | 75.19 | 3.22 dd (7.5, 8.0) | 1', 3' | 1'' |
| 3' | 78.06 | 3.40* | 2'' | 78.16 | 3.37* | 2', 4' | 2'' |
| 4' | 71.69 | 3.33* | | 71.69 | 3.30* | 3', 5' | |
| 5' | 77.80 | 3.28* | | 77.90 | 3.28* | 4', 6' | |
| 6' | 62.75 | 3.70*; 3.87* | | 62.84 | 3.68*, 3.88* | 5' | |
| | | | **Ara** | | | | |
| 1'' | 101.03 | 4.32 d (7.5) | 1 | 101.08 | 4.31 d (7.5) | 2'' | 1 |
| 2'' | 77.35 | 3.42* | | 77.35 | 3.42* | 1'', 3'' | |
| 3'' | 79.96 | 3.45 dd (8.5, 3.0) | | 79.99 | 3.46* | 2'', 4'' | |
| 4'' | 71.69 | 3.47 m | | 71.74 | 3.46* | 3'', 5'' | |
| 5'' | 67.10 | 3.16 dd (12.0, 3.5) 3.86* | | 67.11 | 3.16*, 3.86 dd (12.0, 5.0) | 4'' | |
| | | | **Rha** | | | | |
| 1''' | 101.44 | 5.37 d (1.5) | 2'' | 101.48 | 5.36 d (1.5) | 2''' | 2'' |
| 2''' | 72.07 | 3.71* | | 72.33 | 3.80 dd (1.5, 9.5) | 1''', 3''' | |
| 3''' | 72.30 | 3.91* | | 72.11 | 3.70* | 2''', 4''' | |
| 4''' | 74.08 | 3.43* | | 74.11 | 3.43* | 3''', 5''' | |
| 5''' | 69.67 | 4.10 m | | 69.68 | 4.10 m | 4''', 6''' | |
| 6''' | 18.37 | 1.28 d (6.5) | 4''', 5''' | 18.39 | 1.26 d (6.5) | 5''' | 4''', 5''' |
| OMe | | | | 47.62 | 3.16 s | | 22 |

[a]125 MHz, [b]500 MHz, [c]In $CD_3OD$. Chemical shifts are given in ppm; coupling constant *J* (in parentheses) in Hz; *Overlapped signals.

**22-*O*-Methyl-26-*O*-β-D-glucopyranosyl-25(*R*)-furost-5-ene-1β,3β,22ξ,26-tetraol 1-*O*-[α-L-ramnopyranosyl-(1→2)-β-D-arabinopyranoside] (ophiofolius F, 6)**

Colourless needles, mp. 212-213°C; ESI-MS *m/z*: 925.3 $[M+Na]^+$; 901.5 $[M-H]^-$ ($C_{45}H_{74}O_{18}$); $^1$H-NMR (500 MHz, $CD_3OD$) and $^{13}$C-NMR (125 MHz, $CD_3OD$): see Table 13.5.

**6,8-dimethyl-3′,4′-dimethoxy-5,7,5′-trihydroxyflavanone (7)**

Yellow crystals, mp. 234-235°C; ESI-MS *m/z*: 361 $[M+H]^+$; 359 $[M-H]^-$($C_{19}H_{20}O_7$); $^1$H-NMR (500 MHz, DMSO-$d_6$) and $^{13}$C-NMR (125 MHz, DMSO-$d_6$): see Table 13.1.

**6-Methoxy-5,7-dihydroxyflavanone (8)**

Yellow crystals; mp. 176-177°C; ESI-MS *m/z*: 287 $[M+H]^+$; 285 $[M-H]^-$($C_{16}H_{14}O_5$); $^1$H-NMR (500 MHz, $CD_3OD$) and $^{13}$C-NMR (125 MHz, $CD_3OD$): see Table 13.1.

**Cholest-5-ene-3β-22*R*-diol (9):**

White crystalline, $[\alpha]^{25}_{D}$–36° ($CHCl_3$, c 1.0) EI-MS *m/z*: 402 $[M]^+$ ($C_{27}H_{46}O_2$); $^1$H-NMR (500 MHz, $CDCl_3$) δ (ppm): 1.07 (m, Ha-1), 1.84 (m, Hb-1), 1.52 (m, Ha-2), 1.83 (m, Hb-2), 3.52 (m, H-3), 1.69 (m, Ha-4), 2.25 (m, Hb-4), 5.34 (br s, H-6), 1.47 and 1.98 (H-7), 1.96 (H-8), 0.95 (H-9), 0.91 and 1.53 (H-11), 1.19 and 2.02 (H-12), 1.00 (H-14), 1.13 and 1.60 (H-15), 1.20 and 1.38 (H-16), 1.14 (H-17), 0.70 (s, H-18), 1.10 (s, H-19), 2.21 (m, H-20), 0.90 (d, J = 6.5 Hz, H-21), 3.61 (br d, J = 8.5 Hz, H-22), 1.17 and 1.41 (H-23), 1.39 and 1.71 (H-24), 1.45 (m, H-25), 0.89 (d, J = 6.5 Hz, H-26) and 0.88 (d, J = 6.5 Hz, H-27); $^{13}$C-NMR (125 MHz, $CDCl_3$) δ (ppm): 37.28 (C-1), 31.67 (C-2), 71.77 (C-3), 42.30 (C-4), 140.83 (C-5), 121.60 (C-6), 31.91 (C-7), 31.96 (C-8), 50.17 (C-9), 36.52 (C-10), 21.10 (C-11), 39.79 (C-12), 42.65 (C-13), 56.37 (C-14), 24.40 (C-15), 27.46 (C-16), 53.21 (C-17), 11.87 (C-18), 19.39 (C-19), 42.36 (C-20), 12.45 (C-21), 74.10 (C-22), 36.14 (C-23), 27.69 (C-24), 28.19 (C-25), 22.47 (C-26), and 22.95 (C-27).

## 3.0 Results and Discussion

Compound 1 was isolated as yellow crystals from the ethyl acetate fraction suggesting a flavonoid compound. The $^1$H-NMR spectrum of 1 showed only a singlet at δ 6.43 (2H) of the aromatic ring suggesting that the A ring was full substituted, and the B ring was substituted at C-1, C-3, C-4, C-5 positions. The signals at δ 5.34 (dd, *J* = 3.0, 12.5 Hz), 2.76 (dd, *J* = 3.0, 12.5 Hz) and 3.02 (dd, *J* = 12.5, 17.0 Hz) confirming the presence of a flavanone compound (Kamperdick, 2002), two methyl groups resonance at δ 1.98 (3H, s) and 1.95 (3H, s) suggested that they were directly attached to the A ring. In addition, the signal at δ 12.33 displayed the hydroxyl group at C-5 (Agrawal, 1989) and a methoxyl group was at δ 3.68 (3H, s).

The $^{13}$C-NMR of 1 displayed signals of 18 carbon atoms, including 15 signals of the flavonoid and 3 signals of the two-methyl groups (δ 7.55 and 8.26) and of the methoxyl group at 59.63. The carbonyl group was assigned at δ 196.51; the flavanone compound was confirmed by the signals of the oxymethine at δ 77.58 and of the methylene group at δ 42.06. In the HSQC spectrum, protons at δ 6.43, 5.34, 3.68, 1.98 and 1.95 had cross-peaks to carbons at δ 105.33, 77.58, 59.63, 8.26 and 7.55, respectively. While protons at δ 2.76 and 3.02 had cross-peaks to carbon at δ 42.06. In the HMBC, proton H-2' at δ 6.43 correlated with carbon C-2 (δ 77.58)/C-1' (δ 135.25)/C-3' (δ 150.70) and carbon C-4' (δ 134.36), methoxyl proton at δ 3.68 correlated with C-4' (δ 134.36), methyl proton at δ 1.98 correlated with C-7 (δ 162.39)/C-8 (δ 102.54)/C-9 (δ 157.09), methyl proton at δ 1.95 correlated with C-5 (δ 158.34)/C-6 (103.21)/C-6 (162.39). This evidence confirmed the position of the two hydroxyl groups at C-3' and C-5', and methoxyl group at C-4', and two methyl groups at C-6 and C-8 of the A ring. In addition, H-C long-range correlations were observed between H-2 (δ 5.34) and C-1' (δ 135.25)/C-3 (δ 42.06)/C-4 (δ 196.51), between proton H-3 (δ 2.67/3.02) and carbons C-2 (δ 77.58)/C-4 (δ 196.51) in the HMBC confirming again the flavanone skeleton of 1. Comparing the chemical shifts ($\delta_C$ and $\delta_H$) and proton coupling-constants (*J*) at C-2 and C-3 of 1 ($J_{H\text{-}2/Ha\text{-}3}$ = 12.5 Hz, $J_{H\text{-}2/Hb\text{-}3}$ = 3.0 Hz, $J_{H\text{-}3gem}$ = 17.0 Hz) with those naringerin (Shen, 1993) led to determine the absolute configuration at C-2 as *R*. Furthermore, the ESI-MS spectrum of 1 exhibited the quasi ion peaks at *m/z* 347 $[M+H]^+$ (positive) and 345 $[M-H]^-$(negative), corresponding to the molecular formula of $C_{18}H_{18}O_7$. From the above data, compound 1 was determined to be new natural product 8-dimethyl-4'methoxy-3',5',5,7-tetrahydroxyflavanone, which we named ophiofolius A.

The NMR data of 7 were very similar to those of 1 except for the additional signals of one methoxyl group at $\delta_C$ 59.89/$\delta_H$ 3.79. This suggested that compound 7 was a methoxyl derivative of 1 with the suggested molecular formula as $C_{19}H_{20}O_7$, which was further confirmed by the appearance of the quasi ion peaks at *m/z* 361 $[M+H]^+$ (positive) and 359 $[M-H]^-$(negative) in the ESI-MS spectrum. To determine the position of the additional methoxyl group, the HSQC and HMBC spectra were taken. All the NMR data of this compound were summarized in Table 13.1. Consequently, the structure of 7 was determined as 6,8-Dimethyl-3',4',5'-trimethoxy-5,7-dihydroxyflavanone, which was isolated from Alluaudiposis marnieriana. However, this is the first report of 7 from *Ophiopogon* species, and the NMR data (1D and 2D) of this compound have been reported here for the first time.

The $^{13}$C-NMR spectrum of 8 displayed the resonances of 16 carbon atoms including a benzene ring (B ring) and a methoxyl group at $\delta_C$ 60.99/$\delta_H$ 3.80. The signals at $\delta$ 80.54 (CH) and 44.19 ($CH_2$) suggesting a flavanone compound. In the $^1$H-NMR, signal at $\delta$ 5.42 (1H, dd, $J$ = 3.0, 12.0 Hz), 2.78 (1H, dd, $J$ = 3.0, 17.0 Hz) and 3.08 (1H, dd, $J$ = 12.0, 17.0 Hz) suggesting the 2*R* configuration of 8 (Shen, 1993) as 1. The position of the methoxyl and the two hydroxyl groups were determined from the analysis of the HSQC and HMBC as shown in Table 13.1. In addition, the ESI-MS spectrum of 8 showed the quasi in peaks at *m/z* 287 $[M+H]^+$ (positive) and 285 $[M-H]^-$ (negative) corresponding to the molecular formula of $C_{16}H_{14}O_5$. Thus, compound 8 was determined to be 6-methoxy-5,7-dihydroxyflavanone, which was the first isolated from *Ophiopogon* species. To the best of our knowledge, the NMR data (1D and 2D) of this compound have been reported here for the first time.

Compound 2 was isolated as colourless crystals from the chloroform fraction. The $^1$H-NMR spectrum of 2 showed a broad singlet signal of the three-substituted double bond at $\delta$ 5.33, four methyl singlet signals at $\delta$ 1.11, 1.18, 1.19 and 1.70, in which proton resonance at $\delta$ 1.17 suggesting that this methyl group must be attached to the double bond. A proton of the methine bearing oxygen atom was assigned at $\delta$ 3.40 as a broad singlet. Two other methine proton were assigned at $\delta$ 2.16 and 1.16, and eight protons of four methylene groups were at 2.47 (dm, $J$ = 16.5 Hz, $H_{ax}$-2), 2.05 (dm, $J$ = 16.5 Hz, $H_{eq}$-2), 1.95 (dd, $J$ = 13.5, 2.5 Hz, $H_{ax}$-6), 1.38 (dd, $J$ = 13.5, 4.5 Hz, $H_{eq}$-6), 1.61 (ddd, $J$ = 12.5, 6.0, 3.0 Hz, $H_{ax}$-8), 1.29 (dd, $J$ = 12.5, 3.5 Hz, $H_{eq}$-8), 1.26 (overlapped, $H_{ax}$-9), and 1.40 (dd, $J$ = 12.5, 3.5 Hz, $H_{eq}$-9) deduced from the DEPT, HSQC and ROESY spectra. The $^{13}$C-NMR spectrum of 2 exhibited signals of 15 carbon atoms suggesting a sesquiterpene structure, including four methyl ($\delta$ 27.05, 26.93, 22.09, and 21.66), four methylene ($\delta$ 31.32, 31.30, 24.18, and 22.32), four methine (119.10, 74.52, 44,68, and 39.57), two quaternary carbons ($\delta$ 135.40 and 36.29), and one tertiary carbon at $\delta$ 72.77, which were further deduced from the DEPT 90° and DEPT 135° spectra. In the heteronuclear single quantum coherence (HSQC) spectrum, H-3 proton at $\delta$ 5.33 had a cross peak with carbon at $\delta$ 119.10, H-1 proton at $\delta$ 3.40 had cross peak with carbon at $\delta$ 74.52. Other cross peaks between protons linking to corresponding carbons was elucidated from the HSQC as shown in Table 13.1. The partial structures of 2 were carefully deduced from the $^1$H-$^1$H correlation spectroscopy ($^1$H-$^1$H COSY), In the $^1$H-$^1$H COSY spectrum, H-2 ($\delta$ 2.47 and 2.05) correlated with H-1 ($\delta$ 3.40) and with H-3 ($\delta$ 5.33), H-6 ($\delta$ 1.95 and 1.38) correlated with H-5 ($\delta$ 2.16) and with H-7 ($\delta$ 1.16), as well as H-8 ($\delta$ 1.29 and 1.61) correlated with H-7 ($\delta$ 1.16) and with H-9 ($\delta$ 1.40 and 1.26). Comparing the NMR data of 2 with those of 3-eudesmene-1$\beta$,11-diol and of 7-epi-$\gamma$-eudesmol (Su, *et. al.* 1995) suggesting the 3-eudesmene skeleton with the H-7 configuration as *equatorial* (H$\beta$-7). The carbon chemical shifts at $\delta$ 119.10 (CH) and 135.4 (C) together with the results of $^1$H-$^1$H COSY spectrums confirmed the location of the double bon at C-3 and C-4 (Su, *et. al.* 1995). The suggesting chemical structure of 2 was shown in Figure 13.1. The chemical shifts at C-5, C-6, C-7, C-8, C-11, C-12, and C-13 of 2 and 3-eudesmene-1$\alpha$,11-diol differed. This evidence suggested that their C-7 absolute configurations differed with the H$\beta$-7 of 2 and H$\alpha$-7 of 3-eudesmene-1$\alpha$,11-diol. This was further confirmed by the ROESY spectrum.

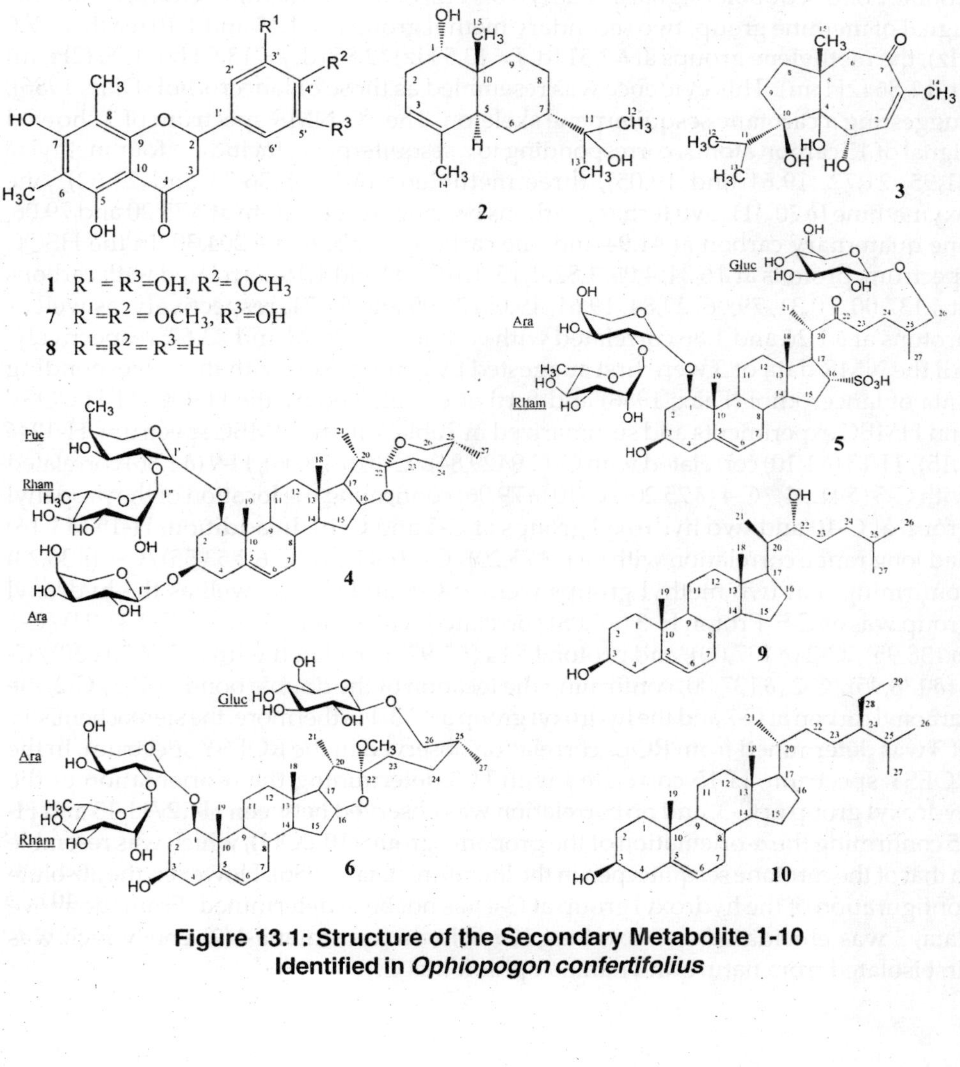


**Figure 13.1: Structure of the Secondary Metabolite 1-10 Identified in *Ophiopogon confertifolius***

In the ROESY spectrum, H-15 methyl protons at δ 1.11 correlated with H-1 proton (δ 3.40) and $H_{ax}$-8 (δ 1.61) confirming that they are β-configuration. $H_{ax}$-8 proton (δ 1.61) correlated with $H_{eq}$-7 at δ 1.16 further confirming the β-configuration of H-7. All the absolute configuration of 2 was carefully deduced and shown in Table 13.2. In addition, H-C long-range correlation between H-14 (δ 1.70) and C-3 (δ 119.10)/C-4 (δ 135.4)/C-5 (39.57), between H-2 (δ 2.47/2.05) and C-1 (δ 74.52)/C-3 (δ 119.10)/C-4 (135.40)/C-10 (δ36.29), between H-13 (δ 1.19)/H-12 (δ 1.18) and carbon C-11 (δ 72.77)/ C-7 (δ 44.68), and between H-6 (δ 1.95/1.38) and C-5 (39.57)/C-7 (δ 44.68) were observed in the HMBC spectrum of 2. This evidence confirmed the 3-eudesmene-1α,11-diol structure of 2. Furthermore, the exhibition of the quasi ion peak at *m/z* 220 $[M-H_2O]^+$ in the EI-MS spectrum of 2 correspond to the molecular formula of $C_{15}H_{26}O_2$. From the above data, the structure of 2 was determined to be a new nature product as 3-eudesmene-1α,11-diol and named ophiofolius B.

The $^1$H-NMR of 3 exhibited signal at δ 6.34 (dd, J = 6.5, 1.5 Hz) of the tri-substituted double bond, a doublet signal at 4.08 (J = 6.5 Hz) of the oxymethine group, a multiple signal of methine group, two secondary methyl group at δ 1.15 and 1.10 (each, J = 7.0 Hz), the methylene groups at δ 2,51 (d, *J* = 13,5 Hz)/2,85 (d, *J* = 13,5 Hz), 1,26 (2H, m) and 1,86 (2H, m). This evidence was resembled as those of lancerodiol (Diaz, 1986), suggesting a carotane sesquiterpene skeleton. The $^{13}$C-NMR spectrum of 3 showed signal of 15 carbon atoms, corresponding to a sesquiterpene, including four methyl (δ 21,95, 21,72, 19,61 and 19,05), three methylene (δ 53,55,36,23 and 23,62), one oxymethine (δ 70.31), two tertiary carbons bearing oxygen atom at δ 75.20 and 79.06, one quaternary carbon at 41.94 and one carbonyl carbon at δ 204.30. In the HSQC spectrum, protons at δ 6,34, 4,08, 1,82, 1,15, 1,10, 1,92 and 1,16 correlated with carbons at δ 137,00, 70,31, 79,06, 29,84, 19,61, 19,05, 21,95 and 21,71, respectively, as well as protons at δ 1.26 and 1.86 correlated with carbons at δ 36.23 and 23.62, respectively. All the NMR data of 3 were first suggested by comparison with the corresponding data of lancerodiol (Diaz, 1986) and further established by the HSQC, H-H COSY and HMBC experiments and summarized in Table 3. In the HMBC spectrum, H-12 (δ 1,15)/H-13 (δ 1,10) correlated with C-11 9δ 29,84)/C-10 (δ 79,06), H-9 (δ 1,86) correlated with C-5 (δ 41,94)/C-4 (δ 75,20)/C-10 (δ 79,06) confirming the location of the propanyl group at C-10 and two hydroxyl groups at C-5 and C-10. In addition, H-15 (δ 1.16) had long range correlation with C-4 (δ 75,20)/C-5 (δ 41,94)/C-6(δ 53,55)/C-8 (δ 36,23) confirming that two methyl groups were at C-6 and C-8, as well as the hydroxyl group was at C-5. Proton H-3 (δ 4,08) correlated with C-4 (δ 75,20)/C-5 (δ 41,94)/C-1 (δ 138,95)/C-2 (δ 137,00), and proton H-14 (δ 1,92) correlated with C-7 (δ 204,30)/C-1 (δ 138,95)/C-2 (δ 137,00) confirming the location of the double bond at C-1/C-2, the carbonyl carbon at C-7 and the hydroxyl group at C-3. Furthermore, the stereochemistry of 3 was determined from ROEs correlation observed in the ROESY spectrum. In the ROESY spectrum, H-15 correlated with H-3 determining the α-orientation of the hydroxyl group at C-3, and no correlation was observed between H-12/H-13 and H-15 confirming the α-orientation of the propanyl group (10-βOH), which was resemble to that of the carotane sesquitecpen in the literature (Diaz, 1986). However, the absolute configuration of the hydroxyl group at C-4 has not been determined. From the above data, 3 was elucidated as 7-oxo-3α,4,10β-trihydroxycarotane-1(2)-ene, which was first isolated from nature and named ophiofolius C.

The $^{13}$C-NMR spectrum of 4 showed signals of 44 carbon atoms including three sugar units identified from the anomeric carbon signals at δ 101.15, 101.40 and 100.47, and 27 carbon signals of the steroidal skeleton comparison with those of steroidal compounds from *O. japonicus* (Asano, 1993), including four methyl, nine methylene, ten methine, three quaternary carbons, and one tertiary carbon bearing oxygen atom determined by the DEPT 90° and DEPT 135° spectra. The carbon chemical shifts were at δ 84.55 (CH), 82.19 and 75.42 (CH) suggesting three methine carbons bearing oxygen atoms at C-1, C-16 and C-3, and the δ values of 138.99 (C) and 126.44 (CH) suggested the presence of a tri-substituted double bond at C-5 and C-6 of the aglycon (Asano, 1993). In addition, the tertiary carbon bearing oxygen atom was assigned at δ 110.60 and all the carbon chemical shifts of carbons from C-23 to C-27 differed from that of LS-10 (with *axial* configuration of the methyl group at C-27) and were in good agreement with those of ophiopogonin B and D (Asano, 1993), confirming the *equatorial* configuration of the methyl group at C-27 of 4. Comparing to the NMR data of the aglycon of 4 with the corresponding data of LS-10, ophiopogonin B and D led to identify the aglycon structure of 4 as shown in Fig. 1, which was further confirmed by the HSQC, H-H COSY and HMBC spectra and summarized in Table 13.4. The higher δ value 75.42 (C-3) of 4 comparing with value δ 68.4 of LS-10 and with the value δ 74.4 of lirioprolisoside A suggested that one sugar linked to C-3 by ether linkage (Yu, 1996). Three sugar units were identified as β-D-fucopyranoside, β-D-arabinopyranoside and α-L-ramnopyranoside by comparing the NMR data with those in literature (Asano, 1993; Yu, 1996; Yoshimitsu, 2000).

The $^{1}$H-NMR spectrum of 4 exhibited an olefinic proton at δ 5.60 (d, $J$ = 5.5 Hz), three anomeric protons at δ 4.30 (d, $J$ = 7.0 Hz) and 3.43 (overlapped with solvent signal), and at δ 5.40 (d, $J$ = 1.5 Hz), two tertiary methyl groups were assigned at δ 1.11 and 0.83, and three secondary methyl groups at 0.81 (d, $J$ = 6.5 Hz), 1.02 (d, $J$ = 6.5 Hz), and 1.26 (d, $J$ = 6.5 Hz, H-$6_{rha}$). Furthermore, in the HMBC spectrum, proton H-1' (δ 4.30) correlated with C-1 (δ 84.55), proton H-1'' (δ 5.40) correlated with C-2' (δ 76.85), as well as proton H-1''' (δ 4.85) correlated with C-3 (δ 75.42) confirming that the arabinopyranosyl unit attached to C-3, the fucopyranosyl unit attached to C-1 and the rhamnopyranosyl attached to C-2' of the fucose by ether linkages. In addition, the sugar NMR data were further assigned by the detailed analysis of the H-H COSY as summarized in Table 13.4. Meanwhile, the ESI-MS spectrum of 4 gave the quasi ion peaks with at $m/z$ 855 [M+H]$^+$, corresponding to the molecular formula of $C_{44}H_{70}O_{16}$. From the above evidence, the structure of 4 was concluded to be 3-*O*-β-D-arabinopyranosyl-25(*S*)-ruscogenin-1β,3β-diol 1-*O*-[α-L-ramnopyranosyl-(1→2)-β-D-fucopyranoside] and named as ophiofolius D.

The $^{13}$C-NMR spectrum of 5 showed signals of 44 carbon atoms including three sugar units identified from the anomeric carbon signals at δ 104.54, 101.44 and 101.03, and 27 carbon signals of the steroidal skeleton comparing with those of steroid compounds from *O. japonicus* (Asano, 1993), and with those of cholestane glycosides from *Solanum abutiloides* (Yu, 1996). The carbon chemical shifts were at δ 84.52 (CH) and 69.14 (CH) suggesting two methine carbons bearing oxygen atoms at C-1 and C-3, and the δ values of 139.40 (C) and 125.99 (CH) suggested the presence of a tri-substituted double bond at C-5 and C-6 of the cholestane (Asano, 1993). In addition, the carbonyl group was assigned at δ 217.42 and all the carbon chemical shifts of the side chain were in good agreement with those of abutiloside G (Yoshimitsu, 2000), including a methylene group bearing oxygen atom at C-26. Comparing to the NMR data of 5 and abutiloside G (Yoshimitsu, 2000) led to identify their aglycon structures are similar except for the double bond at C-5/C-6. However, the carbon chemical shifts at C-14, C-15, C-16 and C-17 of 5 and abutiloside G differed. The higher δ value (80.11) of 5 compared to δ value (75.9) of abutiloside G and to the related sulphate compound suggesting the appearance of a sulphate group attached to C-16 with α-configuration (Yoshimitsu, 2000; Minale, 1991). The $^{1}$H-NMR spectrum of 5 exhibited an olefinic proton at δ 5.57 (d, *J* = 5.5 Hz), two anomeric protons with the *axial* configuration at δ 4.29 (d, *J* = 7.5 Hz) and 4.32 (d, *J* = 7.5 Hz), and the other anomeric proton with the *equatorial* configuration at 5.37 (d, *J* = 1.5 Hz), two tertiary methyl groups were at δ 1.10 and 0.95, and two secondary methyl groups at 0.97 (d, *J* = 6.5 Hz) and 1.28 (d, *J* = 6.5 Hz). Further analysis of the sugar NMR data of 5 in comparison with the literature (Asano, 1993; Yu, 1996; Agrawal, 1992) showed that compound 5 had the β-D-glucopyranosyl, α-L-rhamnopyranosyl, and β-D-arabinopyranosyl units (*see* Table 13.5). All the NMR assignment of 5 was first deduced from the comparison of the NMR data of 5 with the corresponding data of abutiloside G (Yoshimitsu, 2000), then further confirmed by the HSQC and HMBC experiments and summarized in Table 13.5. In the HMBC spectrum, proton H-1' (δ 4.29) correlated with C-26 (δ 76.04), as well as proton H-26 (δ 3.40/3.75) correlated with C-1' (δ 104.54) confirming that the glucopyranosyl unit attached to C-26. The H-C long-range correlations between H-1'' (δ 4.32) and C-1 (δ 84.52), between H-1''' (δ 5.37) and C-2'' (δ 77.35), between H-19 (δ 1.10) and carbons C-1 (δ 84.52)/C-5 (δ 139.40)/C-9 (51.28)/C-10 (δ 43.33), and between H-2 (δ 1.72/2.12) and C-1 (δ 84.52)/C-3 (δ 69.14) were also observed in the HMBC spectrum of 5. This evidence confirmed that the rhamnopyranosyl linked to C-2'' of the arabinopyranosyl, this arabinopyranosyl linked to C-1 of the aglycon by ether linkages, and that the other hydroxyl group was at C-3. Furthermore, the H-C long-range correlations between H-16 (δ 4.65) and C-13 (δ 42.41) and between H-20 (δ 3.04) and C-16 (δ 80.11) were observed in the HMBC spectrum confirming the location of the sulphate group at C-16. The good agreements of the NMR data at C-1, C-2, C-3, C-4, C-5, and C-10 of 5 (δ 84.52, 37.16, 69.14, 43.21, 139.40 and 43.33, respectively) with those of ophiopogonin B (δ 84.3, 38.4, 68.6, 44.3, 139.7, and 43.4, respectively) (Asano, 1993) confirmed the β-configuration of the hydroxyl groups at C-1 and C-3. Meanwhile, the ESI-MS spectrum of 5 gave the quasi ion peaks at *m/z* 991.3 $[M+Na]^+$ and 967.5 $[M-H]^-$ corresponding to the molecular formula of $C_{44}H_{72}SO_{21}$. From the above evidence, the structure of 5 was concluded to be 26-*O*-β-D-glucopyranosyl-1β,3β,16α,26-tetrahydroxycholest-5-en-22-one 1-*O*-α-L-rhamnopyranosyl-(1→2)-β-D-arabinopyranoside sulphate and named as ophiofolius E.

The $^{13}$C-NMR of 6 displayed signals of 45 carbon atoms, including 27 signals of the furost skeleton type and 17 signals of the three sugar units, and a methoxyl group (Kanmoto, 1994). Comparison the NMR data of 6 and 5 (Table 13.5) suggesting that they had the same partial structure from C-1 to C-14, with two methine carbons bearing oxygen atoms at C-1 and C-3, and the double bond at C-5 and C-6. Further comparison of the NMR data from C-11 to C-27 of 6 with the corresponding data of 22-*O*-methyl-26-*O*-β-D-glucopyranosyl-25(*R*)-furost-5-ene-3β,22ξ,26-triol 3-{*O*-β-D-glucopyranosyl-(1→2)-*O*-[β-D-xylopyranosyl-(1→3)]-*O*-β-D-glucopyranosyl-(1→4)-β-D-galactopyranoside} (Kanmoto, 1994) suggested the other partial structure of 6. Furthermore, analysis the NMR data of the sugar units of 6 in comparison with those of 5 confirmed that they had the same sugar units with a β-D-glucopyranosyl attached to C-26, rhamnopyranosyl linked to C-2'' of the arabinopyranosyl, this arabinopyranosyl linked to C-1 of the aglycon by ether linkages. The structure of 6 and its NMR assignments were established from the above comparison and further confirmed by HSQC, H-H COSY, and HMBC experiments and summarized in Table 13.5. In addition, the ESI-MS spectrum of 6 gave the quasi ion peaks at m/z 925.3 $[M+H]^+$ and 901.5 $[M-H]^-$, corresponding to the molecular formula of $C_{45}H_{74}O_{18}$. From the above evidence, the structure of 6 was determined to be 22-O-methyl-26-*O*-β-D-glucopyranosyl-25(*R*)-furost-5-ene-1β,3β,22ξ,26-tetraol 1-*O*-[α-L-ramnopyranosyl-(1→2)-β-D-arabinopyranoside], a new nature product and named as ophiofolius F.

Compound 9 was obtained from the methanolic extract of the roots of *O. confertifolius*. The $^1$H-NMR spectrum of 9 showed a olefinic signal at δ 5.34 (br s), singlet of two tertiary methyl groups at δ 1.10 and 0.70, doublets of the three secondary methyl groups at δ 0.90 (J = 6.5 Hz), 0.88 (J = 6.5 Hz) and 0.89 (J = 6.5 Hz), two signals of the protons of methine carbons bearing oxygen atoms at δ 3.52 and 3.61. The $^{13}$C-NMR spectrum of 9 exhibited signal of 27 carbon atoms, including five methyl, ten methylene, nine methine, and three quaternary carbons, confirming by the DEPT 90° and DEPT 135°, suggesting the presence of a sterol compound. A tri-substituted double bond was assigned at δ 140.83 (C) and 121.60 (CH), two oxymethine carbons were at δ 71.77 and 74.10, five methyl carbons were at δ 22.95, 22.47, 19.39, 12.45 and 11.87. All the NMR assignments were confirmed by HMQC, and HMBC experiments. In the HSQC spectrum, protons at δ 5.34, 3.61 and 3.52 correlated with carbons at 121.60, 74.10 and 71.77, respectively. While protons at δ 1.10, 0.70, 0.90, 0.89 and 0.88 correlated with carbons at 19.39, 11.87, 12.45, 22.47 and 22.95, respectively. In the HMBC spectrum, proton H-5 (δ 5.34) had long-range correlations with carbon C-4 (δ 42.3)/C-5 (δ 140.83)/C-8 (δ 31.96), proton H-3 (δ 3.52) correlated with C-5 (δ 140.83)/C-1 (δ 37.28) confirming the location of the hydroxyl group at C-3 and the double bond at C-5/C-6. Furthermore, H-C long-range correlations were observed between H-21 (δ 0.90) and carbons–17 (δ 53.21)/C-20 (δ 42.36)/C-22 (δ 74.10). This evidence confirmed that the other hydroxyl group was at C-22. All the NMR data of 9 were in good agreement with those of cholest-5-ene-3β-22*R*-diol (Dunoau, 1996). Interestingly, the absolute configuration of C-20 was (*R*), which was differed with almost nature steroids. In addition, the EI-MS spectrum of 9 exhibited a molecular ion peak at m/z 402 [M]+·, corresponding to the molecular formula of $C_{27}H_{46}O_2$. From the above data, compound 9 was identified as cholest-5-ene-3β-22*R*-diol, which was for the first time isolated from Convallariaceae family.

## References

Agrawal, P. K., 1989. Carbon 13 NMR of flavonoids. Elsevier Science Publishers B. V.

Asano, T., Murayama, T., Hirai, Y., and Shoji, J., 1993. Comparative studies on the constituents of Ophiopogonis tuber and its congeners. V3. Studies on the glycosides of the subterranean part of *Ophiopogon japonicus* Ker-Gawler cv. Nanus. Chem. Pharm. Bull. (41), pp.566-570.

Diaz, J. G. Fraga, B. M., Gonzalez, A. G., Hernander, M. G., and Prrales, A., 1986. Carotane sesquiterpenes from *Ferula linkii*. Phytochemistry (25), pp. 1161-1163.

Do, N. T., Hue, N. T. V., Thuan, N. D., Trai, N. V., Thin, N. N., 2007. "Cao cang" *Ophiopogon confertifolius* N. Tanaka (*Convallariaceae*), a new *species of* Vietnamese flora. Vietnamese Journal of Pharmacy (369), pp. 19-21.

Dunoau, C., Belle, R., Oulad-Ali, A., Anton, R., and David, B., 1996. Triterpenes and sterols from *Rusus aculeatus*. Planta Medica (62), pp. 189-190.

Kamperdick, C., Van, N. H., Sung, T. V., 2002. Constituents from *Miliusa balansae* (Annonaceae). Phytochemistry (61), pp.991-994.

Kanmoto, T., Mimaki, Y., Sashida, Y., Nikaido, T., 1994. Steroidal constituents from the underground part of *Reineckea carnea* and their inhibitory activity on cAMP phosphodietherase. Chem. Pharm. Bull. (42), pp. 926-931.

Minale, L., Riccio, R., Rinaldo, G., Zollo, F., 1991. Novel marine polyhydroxylated steroids from the starfish *Myxoderma platyacanthum* ether finamore, J. Org. Chem. (56), pp. 1146-1153.

Shen, C. C., Chang, Y. S., and Ho, L. K., 1993. Nuclear magnetic resonance studies of 5,7-dihydroxy flavonoids. Phytochemistry (340, pp.843-845.

Su, W. C., Fang, J. M., and Cheng, Y. S., 2002. Sesquiterpenes from leaves of *Cryptomeria japonica*. Phytochemistry (61), pp.991-994.

Yoshimitsu, H., Nishida, M., and Nohara, T., 2000. Cholestane glycosides from *Solanum abutiloides*. 3. Chem. Pharm. Bull. (48), pp.556-558.

Yu, B. Y., Qiu, S. X., Zaw, K., Xu, G. J., Hirai, Y., Shoji, J., Fong, H. H. S., and Kinghorn, A. D., 1996. Steroidal glycosides from the subterranean parts of *Liriope spicata* var. *prolifera*. Phytochemistry (43), pp.201-206.

## Chapter 14

# Isostephaoxocanine: A New Dihydroisoquinoline Alkaloid from the Roots of *Stephania brachyandra* Diels.

***Nguyen Quoc Huy[1], Pham Thanh Ky[1], Tran Van On[1], Chau Van Minh[2] and Phan Van Kiem[2]****

*[1]Hanoi University of Pharmacy, 13-15 Le Thanh Tong, Hanoi, Vietnam*

*[2]Institute of Natural Products Chemistry, Vietnam Academy of Science and Technology, 18 Hoang Quoc Viet, Caugiay, Hanoi, Vietnam*

**E-mail: phankiem@vast.ac.vn*

## ABSTRACT

A new dihydroisoquinoline named isostephaoxocanine (1) was isolated from the roots of *Stephania brachyandra* Diels by using combinations of various chromatography methods. Its structure was established on the basis of the physicochemical and spectroscopic data.

***Keywords:*** *Stephania brachyandra Diels., Isostephaoxocanine, Dihydroisoquinoline.*

## 1.0 Introduction

*Stephania brachyandra* Diels. belongs to family Menispermaceae and is distributed in the Northern of Vietnam (Bich, 2004; Loi, 1997; Chi, 2006). This is a Vietnam herb that has been used primarily as a relaxant and sleep aid but more recently its anti melanoma properties are being discovered. The plant is a very rare tuber that is found at high altitudes in the forest as in Sapa, Lao Ca1. A large number of studies on the isolation and structure elucidation of hundred alkaloids from *Stephania* genus have been carried out (Kunitomo, 1981; Tanahashi, 2000; Pharadai, 1985, Patra, 1980;

Nishiyama, 2004; etc.). However, only dehydrodicentrine was found in *S. brachyandra* Diels. up to date. As part of our current interest in the *Stephania* genus, we report herein the isolation and structure elucidation of a new dihydroisoquinoline named isostephaoxocanine from the roots of *S. brachyandra* Diels. Its structure was elucidated by the analysis of NMR spectral data including 2D techniques and ESI-mass spectrometry.

## 2.0 Experimental

### 2.1 Plant Material

The roots of *Stephania brachyandra* Diels. were collected in Sapa (Lao Cai Provice) in August 2006 by one of the authors Nguyen Quoc Huy, and was identified by Bachelor Nguyen Chieu, National Institute of Medicinal Materials. A voucher of specimens was deposited at National Institute of Medicinal Materials and at Hanoi University of Pharmacy.

### 2.2 General Experimental Procedures

Melting points were determined using an Electro thermal IA-9200. The IR spectra were obtained on a Hitachi 270-30 type spectrometer with KBr discs. Optical rotations were determined on a Jasco DIP-1000 KUY polar meter. The electrospray ionization (ESI) mass spectra were obtained using an AGILENT 1100 LC-MSD Trap spectrometer. The $^{1}$H-NMR (500 MHz) and $^{13}$C-NMR (125 MHz) spectra were recorded on a Bruker AM500 FT-NMR spectrometer and TMS was used as an internal standard. Column chromatography (CC) was performed on silica gel (Kieselgel 60, 70-230 mesh and 230-400 mesh, Merck) and YMC RP-18 resins.

### 2.3 Extraction and Isolation

Dried roots of *Stephania brachyandra* Diels. were powdered and then extracted three times with 5 per cent AcOH in MeOH. After removal the solvent, the extract (55 g) was suspended with 10 per cent AcOH in water (pH = 4.0) and partitioned in turn with *n*-hexane, chloroform, ethyl acetate, and *n*-BuOH to obtain *n*-hexane, chloroform, ethyl acetate, and *n*-BuOH fractions. The water layer was neutralized with $NH_4OH$ (pH = 9) and then partitioned with chloroform to give the chloroform extract (35.0 g). The chloroform extract (35.0 g) was chromatographed on a silica gel column and then on an YMC column to yield compounds 1 (13 mg) as colourless fine needles.

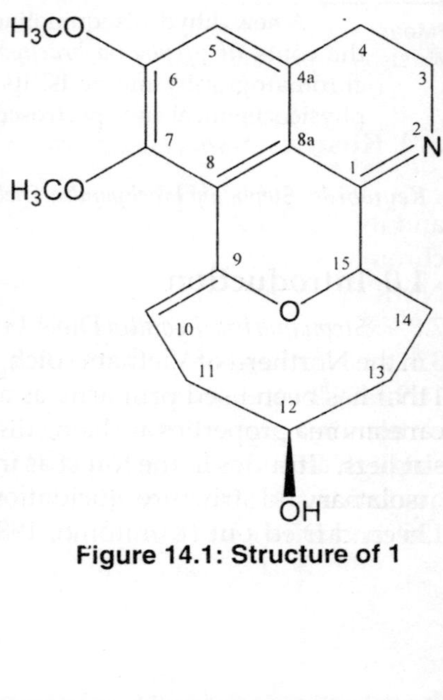

**Figure 14.1: Structure of 1**

**Isostephaoxocanine (1)**

Colorless fine needles, mp. 176-177°C; $[\alpha]^{25}_{D}$–55°; ESI-MS *m/z*: 316 $[M+H]^+$; 314 $[M-H]^-$, ($C_{18}H_{21}NO_4$); $^{1}$H-NMR (500 MHz, $CDCl_3$) and $^{13}$C-NMR (125 MHz, $CDCl_3$): see Table 14.1.

**Table 14.1: NMR Data of 1**

| C | $\delta_C$ [a,c,#] | 1 | | | | |
|---|---|---|---|---|---|---|
| | | $\delta_C$ [a,c] | DEPT | $\delta_H$ [a,b] mult. (J. Hz) | H–H COSY | HMBC (H–C) |
| 1 | 162.29 | 162.40 | – | – | | |
| 3 | 46.95 | 46.87 | $CH_2$ | 3.62 ddd (15.9, 11.0, 7.3)<br>3.89 ddd (15.9, 7.0, 7.3) | H–4 | 1, 4, 4a, 8a<br>1, 4, 4a, 8a |
| 4 | 25.18 | 25.21 | $CH_2$ | 2.77 ddd (15.9, 11.0, 7.0)<br>2.65 ddd (15.9, 7.0, 7.3) | H–3 | 3, 4a, 5, 8a<br>3, 4a, 5, 8a |
| 4a | 133.20 | 133.24 | – | – | | |
| 5 | 110.45 | 110.55 | CH | 6.63 s | | 4, 4a, 6, 7, 8 |
| 6 | 155.14 | 155.30 | – | – | | |
| 7 | 142.89 | 142.91 | – | – | | |
| 8 | 126.26 | 126.31 | – | – | | |
| 8a | 115.94 | 115.30 | – | – | | |
| 9 | 145.55 | 144.46 | – | – | | |
| 10 | 117.13 | 116.38 | CH | 6.19 dd (7.8, 7.8) | H–11 | 8, 9, 11 |
| 11 | 31.52 | 34.41 | $CH_2$ | 2.88 ddd (11.0, 11.0, 7.8)<br>2.29 m | H–10, H–12 | 9, 12, 13<br>9, 12, 13 |
| 12 | 71.20 | 73.38 | CH | 3.51 tt (11.0, 3.0) | H–11, H–13 | |
| 13 | 33.76 | 36.02 | $CH_2$ | 1.89 m<br>2.14 br t (10.7) | H–12, H–14 | |
| 14 | 23.21 | 26.55 | $CH_2$ | 1.81 m<br>1.89 m | H–13, H–15 | 12, 13, 15<br>12, 13, 15 |
| 15 | 83.56 | 81.69 | CH | 4.62 dd (11.9, 4.5) | H–14 | 9 |
| 6–$OCH_3$ | 56.00 | 56.02 | $CH_3$ | 3.91 s | | 6 |
| 7–$OCH_3$ | 60.35 | 60.38 | $CH_3$ | 3.80 s | | 7 |

[a]Measured in $CD_3OD$ [b]125 MHz, [c]500 MHz, Chemical shift ($\delta$) in ppm; *Overlapped signals; $\delta^{\#}$: stephaoxocanine.

## 3.0 Results and Discussion

The MeOH extract of the roots of *Stephania brachyandra* Diels. was fractionated, and the alkaloid-containing fraction was separated by combination of the column chromatography to afford isostephaoxocanine (1) as colorless fine needles. The $^1$H-NMR spectrum of 1 showed a singlet at $\delta$ 6.63 and a doublet of doublet at $\delta$ 6.19 ($J$ = 7.8, 7.8 Hz) of two olefinic protons, five methylene groups resonance at $\delta$ 2.77/2.65, 3.62/3.89, 2.29/2.88, 1.89/2.14, and 1.81/1.89 (1H, each), two signals at 4.62 (dd, $J$ = 11.9, 4.5 Hz) and 3.51 (tt, $J$ = 11.0, 3.0 Hz) were assigned to two protons of the methine carbons bearing oxygen atoms, and two methoxyl groups were at $\delta$ 3.91 and 3.80 as singlets. The $^{13}$C-NMR spectrum exhibited signals of 18 carbons, including 7 quaternary, 4 methine, 5 methylene, and 2 methyl carbons deduced from the DEPT 135° and DEPT 90° spectra. Two methoxyl groups were at $\delta$ 56.02 and 60.38, two methine carbon bearing oxygen atoms were assigned at δ 81.69 and 73.88. The signal at δ 46.87 of the methylene carbon ($CH_2$) and signal at δ 162.40 (C) suggested that they were linked to nitrogen atom. The heteronuclear single quantum coherence (HSQC) spectrum led to determine the protons attached to their corresponding carbons and these results were summarized in Table 14.1. The partial structures of 1 were connected from the detailed analysis of the $^1H$-$^1H$ chemical shift correlation spectroscopy (COSY). In the H-H COSY spectrum, H-3 (δ 3.62/3.89) correlated with H-4 (δ 2.77/2.65), H-11 (δ2.29/2.88) correlated with H-10 (δ 6.19) and H-12 (δ 3.51), H-13 (δ 1.89/2.14) correlated with H-12 and H-14 (δ 1.81/1.89), and H-14 correlated with H-15 (δ 4.62). Comparing to the NMR data of 1 with those of stephaoxocanine, a alkaloid from *Stephania cepharantha* Hayata and Yamamoto (Kashiwaba, 1996) found that almost the NMR data of 1 were in good agreement with the corresponding data of stephaoxocanine, except for the NMR data from C-11 to C-15 (*see* Table 14.1). This evidence suggested that the stereochemistry of the hydroxyl group at C-12 of compound 1 and stephaoxocanine differed.

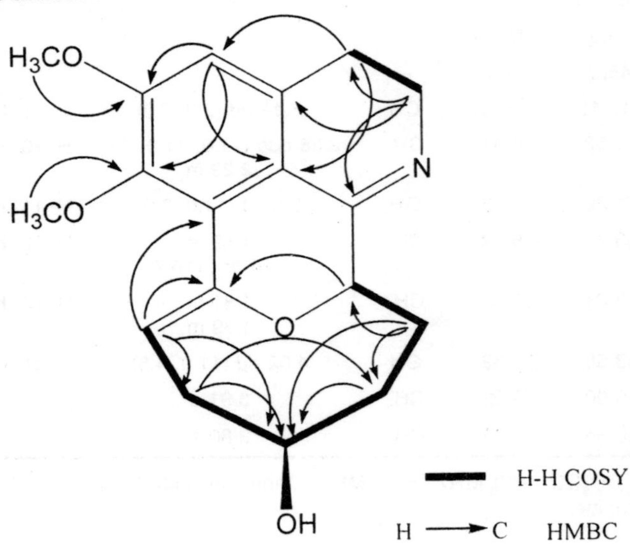


**Figure 14.2: Selected the H-C Long Range Correlations in the HMBC of 1**

Furthermore, the H-C long range correlations were observed between H-10 and C-8/C-9/C-11, between H-11 and C-9/C-12/C-13, and between H-14 and C-12/C-13/C-15 in the heteronuclear multiple-bond correlation (HMBC) spectrum. This evidence confirmed the location of the hydroxyl group at C-12, as well as the double bond was at C-9/C-10. All the HMBC correlations were analyzed and shown in Table 14.1 and Figure 14.2. In addition, the ESI-MS spectrum of 1 exhibited the quasi ion peaks at m/z 316 $[M+H]^+$ (positive) and m/z 314 $[M-H]^-$(negative), corresponding to the molecular formula of $C_{18}H_{21}NO_4$. From the above data, compound 1 was proposed for isostephaoxocanine, a new compound from nature.

## References

Bich, D. H., Chung, D. Q., Chuong, B. X., Dong, N. T., Dam, D. T., Hien, P. V., Lo, V. N., Mai, P. D., Man, P. K., Nhu, D. T., Tap, N., Toan, T., 2004. "Medicinal Plants and Animals in Vietnam". Hanoi Science and Technology Publishing House, vol. 1.

Chi, V. V., 1997, "Vietnam Medical Plant Dictionary". Hanoi Medicinal Publishing House.

Kashiwaba, N., Morooka, S., Kimura, M., and Ono, M., 1996. Staphaoxocanine, a novel dihydroisoquinoline alkaloid from *Stephania cepharantha*. J. Nat. Prod. (59), pp. 803-805.

Kunitomo, J. Oshikata, M., and Murakami, Y., 1981. 4-Hydroxycrebanine, a new 4-hydroxyaporphine alkaloid, and (R)-roemeroline from *Stephania sasakii* Hayata. Chem. Pharm. Bull. (29), pp. 2251-2253.

Loi, D. T., 2006. "Glossary of Vietnam Medicinal Plants". Hanoi Science and Technology Publishing House.

Nishiyama, Y., Moriyasu, M., Ichimaru, M., Iwasa, K., Kato, A., Mathenge, S. G., Mutiso, P. B. C., and Juma, F. D., 2004. Quaternary isoquinoline alkaloids from *Xylopia parviflora*. Phytochemistry (65), pp. 939-944.

Patra, A., Ghosh, A., and Mitra, A. K., 1980. Alkaloids of *Stephania glabra*. Planta Med. (40), pp. 333-336.

Pharadai, K., Pharadai, T., Tantisewie, B., Guinaudeau, H., Frsyer, A., and Shamma, M., 1985. (-)-O-Acetylsukhodianine and oxostephanosine: two new aporphinoids from *Stephania venosa*. J. Nat. Prod. (48), pp. 658-659.

Tanahashi, T.,Su, Y., Nagakura, N., and Nayeshiro, H., 2000. Quaternary Isoquinoline alkaloids from *Stephania cepharantha*. Chem. Pharm. Bull. (48), pp. 370-373.

Wright, C. W., Marshall, S. J., Russell, P. F., Anderson, M. M., Phillippson, J. D., Kirby, G. C., Warhurst, D. C., and Schiff, P. L., 2000. *In vitro* antiplasmodial, antiamoebic, and cytotoxic activities of some monomeric isoquinoline alkaloids. J. Nat. Prod. (63), pp. 1638-1640.

*Chapter 15*

# Gleditschiaside B and C: Two New Carbohydrate Esters of Cinnamic Acid from the Leaves of *Gleditschia australis* Hemsl.

***Nguyen Thi Hong Van[1], Phan Van Kiem[1]*, Chau Van Minh[1] and Alessandra Braca[2]***

*[1]Institute of Natural Products Chemistry, Vietnam Academy of Science and Technology, Hanoi, Vietnam*

*[2]Dipartimento di Chimica Bioorganica e Biofarmacia, Via Bonanno 33, 56126 Pisa, Italy*

**E-mail: phankiem@vast.ac.vn*

## ABSTRACT

Two new carbohydrate esters of cinnamic acid named gleditschiaside B and C were isolated from the methanolic extract of the leaves of *Gleditschia australis* Hemsl. (Caesalpiniaceae). Their structures were elucidated as *E*-cinnamic acid 1-*O*-[*E*-*p*-hydroxylcinnamoyl-(1→3)-α-L-rhamnopyranosyl-(1→6)-β-D-glucopyranosyl] ester (1) and *E*-cinnamic acid 1-*O*-{*E*-cinnamoyl-(1→3)-β-D-glucopyranosyl-[(1→6)-α-L-rhamnopyranosyl]-(1→3)-β-D-glucopyranosyl-[(1→6)-α-L-rhamnopyranosyl]} ester (2) by means of ESI-mass and HR-ESI-mass spectrometry, $^{1}$H-NMR, $^{13}$C-NMR (CPD and DEPT), HSQC and HMBC spectra in comparison with the literature.

***Keywords**: Caesalpiniaceae, Gleditschia australis, Gleditschiaside B, Gleditschiaside C.*

## 1.0 Introduction

*Gleditschia australis* Hemsl., belongs to family Caesalpiniaceae and is wildly distributed in Vietnam. The fruits are used to produce soaps, shampoo and medicinal drugs, and local people can sell them for income. It has been used in traditional medicine for various diseases such as inflammation, kidney stone, and diabetes mellitus (Chi, 1997; Bich, 2004). The fruits contain numbers of triterpenes and flavonoids (Bich, 2004; Hai, 1974). However, no studies on chemical constituents and bioactivity of the leaves have been carried out.

In previous chapter, we have reported the isolation and the structural elucidation of the new cinnamic acid derivative *E*-cinnamic acid 1-*O*-[*E*-cinnamoyl-(1→3)-α-L-rhamnopyranosyl-(1→6)-β-D-glucopyranosyl] ester (Kiem, 2007) from *Gleditschia australis* Hemsl. (Caesalpiniaceae). This paper deals with the isolation and structural determination of two new carbohydrate ester of cinnamic acid named gleditschiaside B and C from the same source. Their structures were elucidated as *E*-cinnamic acid 1-*O*-[*E*-*p*-hydroxylcinnamoyl-(1→3)-α-L-rhamnopyranosyl-(1→6)-β-D-glucopyranosyl] ester (1) and *E*-cinnamic acid 1-*O*-{*E*-cinnamoyl-(1→3)-β-D-glucopyranosyl-[(1→6)-α-L-rhamnopyranosyl]-(1→3)-β-D-glucopyranosyl-[(1→6)-α-L-rhamnopyranosyl]]} ester (2) by analysis of NMR spectral data including 2D techniques and ESI-mass and HR-ESI-mass spectrometry.

## 2.0 Experimental

### 2.1 Plant Material

The leaves of *G. australis* Hemsl. were collected in Tam Dao Mountain, Vinh Phuc province, Vietnam and was identified by Dr Tran Huy Thai, Institute of Ecology and Biological Resources, Vietnam Academy of Science and Technology.

A voucher of specimen was deposited at Institute of Natural Products Chemistry (INPC), Vietnam Academy of Science and Technology.

### 2.2 General Experimental Procedures

Melting points were determined using an Electro thermal IA-9200. The IR spectra were obtained on a Hitachi 270-30 type spectrometer with KBr discs. Optical rotations were determined on a Jasco DIP-1000 KUY polar meter. The electrospray ionization (ESI) mass spectra were obtained using an AGILENT 1100 LC-MSD Trap spectrometer. HRESIMS analyses: Q-TOF premier spectrometer equipped with a nanospray source. The $^{1}$H-NMR (500 MHz) and $^{13}$C-NMR (125 MHz) spectra were recorded on a Bruker AM500 FT-NMR spectrometer and TMS was used as an internal standard. Column chromatography (CC) was performed on silica gel (Kieselgel 60, 70-230 mesh and 230-400 mesh, Merck) and YMC RP-18 resins.

### 2.3 Extraction and Isolation

Dried leaves of *G. australis* were powdered and then extracted three times with MeOH. The MeOH extract (70 g) was suspended in water and partitioned in turn with *n*-hexane, chloroform, ethyl acetate, and *n*-BuOH to obtained *n*-hexane, chloroform, ethyl acetate, and *n*-BuOH fractions. The *n*-BuOH fraction (8.0 g) was chromatographed on a silica gel column using $CHCl_3$-MeOH-$H_2O$ (30:10:1, v/v/v) and on an YMC column using MeOH-$H_2O$ (3:1, v/v) to yield compounds 1 (13 mg) and 2 (18 mg) as amorphous powders.

*E*-Cinnamic acid 1-*O*-[*E*-*p*-hydroxylcinnamoyl-(1→3)-α-L-rhamnopyranosyl-(1→6)-β-D-glucopyranosyl] ester (gleditschiaside B, 1): Amorphous powder, mp. 188-189°C; $[\alpha]^{25}{}_{D}$–54°; IR (KBr) $\nu_{max}$ cm$^{-1}$: 3300-3450 (OH), 1710 (>C=O, ester), 1615 (C=C), 1032 (C-O-C); ESI-MS *m/z*: 625 [M+Na]$^+$; 601 [M-H]$^-$ HR-ESI-MS found *m/z* 603.2194 [M+H]+ (Calcd. 603.2078 for $C_{30}H_{35}O_{13}$), found *m/z* 625.2008 [M+Na]$^+$ (Calcd. 625.1897 for $C_{30}H_{34}O_{13}Na$); $^1$H-NMR (500 MHz, $CD_3OD$) and $^{13}$C-NMR (125 MHz, $CD_3OD$): see Table 15.1.

E-cinnamic acid 1-O-{E-cinnamoyl-(1→3)-β-D-glucopyranosyl-[(1→6)-α-L-rhamnopyranosyl]-(1→3)-β-D-glucopyranosyl-[(1→6)-α-L-rhamnopyranosyl]} ester (gleditschiaside C, 2): Amorphous powder., mp. 176-177°C; $[\alpha]^{25}{}_{D}$–57°; IR (KBr) $\nu_{max}$ cm$^{-1}$: 3300-3470 (OH), 1714 (>C=O, ester), 1610 (C=C), 1020 (C-O-C); ESI-MS *m/z*: 895 [M+H]$^+$; 893 [M-H]$^-$ HR-ESI-MS found *m/z* 895.3331 [M+H]$^+$ (Calcd. 895.3236 for $C_{42}H_{55}O_{21}$); $^1$H-NMR (500 MHz, $CD_3OD$) and $^{13}$C-NMR (125 MHz, $CD_3OD$): see Table 15.1.

Acid Hydrolysis of Compounds 1 and 2 (4 mg, each) in 10 per cent HCl-dioxane (1: 1, 1 ml) were heated at 80°C for 4 h in water bath. The reaction mixture was neutralized with $Ag_2CO_3$, filtered, and then extracted with $CHCl_3$ (1 ml). After concentration, the water layer was examined by TLC with $CHCl_3$-MeOH-$H_2O$ (55: 45: 10) and compared with authentic samples.

**Determination of Sugar Components**

The monosaccharide subunits were obtained by hydrochloric acid hydrolysis as described above. The sugar residue (of each compound) was then dissolved in 1 ml anhydrous pyridine, 2 mg L-leucine methyl ester hydrochloride was added, and the mixture was warmed at 60°C for 1 h. Then 2 mg $NaBH_4$ were added, and the mixture was stirred for 1 h at ambient temperature. Then 0.2 ml of trimethylsilylation reagent trimethylchlorosilane was added and warming at 60°C was continued for another 30 min. The leucine derivatives were subjected to GC analysis to identify the sugars. Column temperate 200°C; injection temperate 250°C; carrier gas $N_2$ at flow rate of 32.2 ml/min; derivatives of D-glucose and L-rhamnose 13.91 and 8.88 min, respectively.

## 3.0 Results and Discussion

Compound 1 was isolated from the methanolic extract of the leaves of *G. australis* Hemsl. The IR spectrum exhibited the presence of OH, >C=O, C=C and C-O-C groups at $\nu_{max}$ 3300-3470, 1714, 1610, 1020 cm$^{-1}$, respectively. The $^{13}$C/DEPT spectra (Table 15.1) revealed the presence of 30 carbon atoms, including 2 cinnamoyl units and 2 sugars, suggesting the presence of a derivative of the carbohydrate ester of cinnamic acid (Kiem, 2007). Analysis the NMR spectra, the presence of a disaccharide moiety in the up field range (12 resonances) and the downfield cinnamoyl groups was suggested. Comparing the NMR data of 1 with the corresponding data of 1-*O*-[*E*-cinnamoyl-(1→3)-[α-L-rhamnopyranosyl-(1→6)]-β-D-glucopyranosyl] ester (Kiem, 2007) noted that almost NMR data of these compound were found to match except for the other cinnamoyl group, suggesting that the *p*-hydroxyl group was attached to this cinnamoyl group. Protons resonance at δ 6.60 and 7.83 (1H, each, *J* = 16.0 Hz),

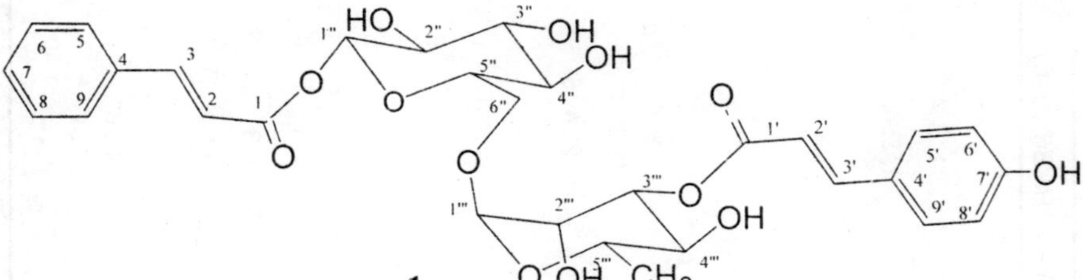


**1**

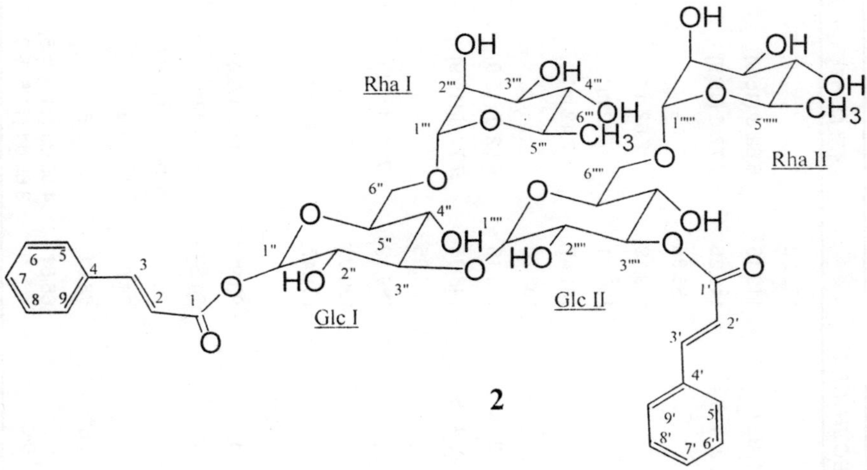


**2**

**Figure 15.1: Structures of 1 and 2**

and at $\delta$ 6.42 and 7.71 (1H, each, $J = 16.0$ Hz), were attributable to two *trans*-olefinic protons. A doublet at $\delta$ 5.61 (1H, $J = 7.5$ Hz) indicated a $\beta$-configuration anomeric proton (vicinal H-1''/2'' in *trans* position). A doublet at 4.78 ($J = 1.5$ Hz) indicated a $\alpha$-configuration anomeric proton (vicinal H-1'''/2''' in *cis* position).

All the NMR data of 1 were further deduced from the analysis of 2D-NMR spectra, including the heteronuclear single quantum coherence (HSQC), the $^1$H-$^1$H chemical shift correlation spectroscopy (COSY), and by the H-C long-range correlations in the heteronuclear multiple-bond correlation (HMBC) spectrum and summarized in Table 15.1.

In the HMBC spectrum, H-1'' ($\delta$ 5.61) correlated with C-1 ($\delta$ 167.04), H-1''' ($\delta$ 4.78) correlated with C-6'' ($\delta$ 67.83), and H-3''' ($\delta$ 5.10) correlated with C-1' ($\delta$ 168.90), H-3' ($\delta$ 7.71) correlated with C-1' and C-5' of the *p*-hydroxycinnamoyl. This evidence confirmed the linking of the two sugars and two cinnamoyl groups as shown in Figure 15.1. Acid hydrolysis of 1 afforded D-glucose and L-rhamnose. Furthermore, the HR-ESI-MS spectrum of 1 exhibited the quasi ion peaks at *m/z* 603.2194 [M+H]+ (Calcd. 603.2078 for $C_{30}H_{35}O_{13}$), and *m/z* 625.2008 $[M+Na]^+$ (Calcd. 625.1897 for $C_{30}H_{34}O_{13}Na$). From the above data, compound 1 was determined to be *E*-cinnamic

**Table 15.1: NMR Data of 1 and 1a**

| C | 1 | | | | 2 | | | |
|---|---|---|---|---|---|---|---|---|
| | $\delta_C^{a.c}$ | $\delta_H^{a.b}$ (J. Hz) | H-H COSY | HMBC (H–C) | $\delta_C^{a.c}$ | $\delta_H^{a.b}$ (J. Hz) | H-H COSY | HMBC (H–C) |
| 1 | 167.04 | - | | | 168.20 | - | | |
| 2 | 118.27 | 6.60 d (15.9) | 3 | 1, 3, 4 | 119.15 | 6.62 d (15.9) | 3 | 1, 3, 4 |
| 3 | 147.68 | 7.83 d (15.9) | 2 | 1, 2, 4, 5 | 146.35 | 7.77 d (15.9) | 2 | 1, 2, 4, 5 |
| 4 | 135.63 | - | | | 135.85 | - | | |
| 5, 9 | 129.39 | 7.64 m* | | | 129.19 | 7.62 m* | | |
| 6, 8 | 130.04 | 7.42 m* | | | 130.01 | 7.42 m* | | |
| 7 | 131.76 | 7.42 m* | | | 131.47 | 7.42 m* | | |
| 1' | 168.90 | - | | | 168.20 | - | | |
| 2' | 115.49 | 6.42 d (15.9) | 3' | 1', 3', 4' | 119.15 | 6.62 d (15.9) | 3' | 1', 3', 4' |
| 3' | 145.65 | 7.71 d (15.9) | 2' | 1', 2', 4', 5' | 146.35 | 7.77 d (15.9) | 2' | 1', 2', 4', 5' |
| 4' | 127.32 | - | | | 135.85 | - | | |
| 5', 9' | 131.62 | 7.47 d (8.5) | | | 129.19 | 7.62 d (8.5) | | |
| 6', 8' | 116.82 | 6.82 d (8.5) | | | 130.01 | 7.42 m* | | |
| 7' | 161.22 | - | | | 131.47 | 7.42 m* | | |
| | | | | **Glc I** | | | | |
| 1'' | 95.93 | 5.61 d (7.5) | 2'' | 1 | 93.95 | 5.11 d (7.5) | 2'' | 1 |
| 2'' | 74.01 | 3.50* | 1'', 3'' | 3'' | 74.87 | 3.42* | 1'', 3'' | 3'' |
| 3'' | 77.99 | 3.52* | 2'', 4'' | 1'', 2'' | 76.25 | 3.18 dd (9.0, 8.0) | 2'', 4'' | 1'', 2'' |
| 4'' | 71.12 | 3.49* | 3'', 5'' | | 71.85 | 4.00* | 3'', 5'' | |
| 5'' | 77.81 | 3.61 m | 4'', 6'' | 4'', 6'' | 78.01 | 3.88* | 4'', 6'' | 4'', 6'' |
| 6'' | 67.83 | 4.01 dd (11.5. 1.5) | 5'' | 1''' | 68.51 | 4.05 dd (11.5. 1.5) | 5'' | 1''' |
| | | 3.74 dd (11.5. 5.0) | 5'' | 1''' | | 3.65 dd (11.5. 5.0) | 5'' | 1''' |

*Contd...*

**Table 15.1–Contd...**

| C | 1 | | | | 2 | | | |
|---|---|---|---|---|---|---|---|---|
| | $\delta_C^{a.c}$ | $\delta_H^{a.b}$ (J. Hz) | H-H COSY | HMBC (H–C) | $\delta_C^{a.c}$ | $\delta_H^{a.b}$ (J. Hz) | H-H COSY | HMBC (H–C) |
| | | | | **Rham I** | | | | |
| 1''' | 102.21 | 4.78 (d. 1.5) | 2''' | 2''', 3''', 6'' | 102.12 | 4.78 d (1.0) | 2''' | 6'' |
| 2''' | 70.09 | 4.09 (dd. 3.5. 1.5) | 1''', 3''' | 1''' | 70.04 | 4.08* | 1''', 3''' | |
| 3''' | 75.53 | 5.10 (dd. 3.5. 1.0) | 2''', 4''' | 4''', 1' | 71.44 | 3.67* | 2''', 4''' | C-1'''' |
| 4''' | 71.48 | 3.66 (dd. 9.5. 1.0) | 3''', 5''' | 3''', 5''', 6''' | 72.03 | 3.34* | 3''', 5''' | |
| 5''' | 69.98 | 3.85 (dd. 9.5. 6.0) | 4''', 6''' | 4''', 6''' | 69.86 | 3.83 m | 4''', 6''' | |
| 6''' | 18.01 | 1.30 (3H, d. 6.0) | 5''' | 4''', 5''' | 18.04 | 1.32 d (6.5) | 5''' | 4''', 5''' |
| | | | | **Glc II** | | | | |
| 1'' | | | | | 98.20 | 4.51 d (7.5) | | C-3''' |
| 2'''' | | | | | 75.77 | 5.10* | | |
| 3'''' | | | | | 75.81 | 5.10* | | |
| 4'''' | | | | | 73.81 | 3.41* | | |
| 5'''' | | | | | 76.82 | 3.49 m | | |
| 6'''' | | | | | 68.45 | 4.05 dd (11.5. 1.5)<br>3.65 dd (11.5. 5.0) | | C-1'''''<br>C-1''''' |
| | | | | **Rham II** | | | | |
| 1''''' | | | | | 102.09 | 4.80 d (1.0) | | C-6'''' |
| 2''''' | | | | | 70.01 | 4.08* | | |
| 3''''' | | | | | 71.44 | 3.67* | | |
| 4''''' | | | | | 72.00 | 3.34* | | |
| 5''''' | | | | | 69.82 | 3.83 m | | |
| 6''''' | | | | | 17.98 | 1.32 d (6.5) | | C-5''''' |

[a]Measured in $CD_3OD$ [b]125 MHz, [c]500 MHz, Chemical shift ($\delta$) in ppm, *Overlapped signals.

acid 1-*O*-[*E*-*p*-hydroxylcinnamoyl-(1→3)-α-L-rhamnopyranosyl-(1→6)-β-D-glucopyranosyl] ester, and named as gleditschiaside B, a new natural product.

The NMR spectral data of 2 was similar to those of 1 except for the additional signals of two sugar units. Two *E*-cinnamoyl groups were confirmed at δ 7.62 (4H), 7.42 (6H), corresponding to two mono-substituted aromatic rings), and at δ 6.62 (2H, doublet, *J* = 15.9 Hz) and 7.77 (2H, doublet, *J* = 15.9 Hz), corresponding to two *trans*-olefinic protons. Four sugar units were suggested from the appearance of four anomeric carbon signals at δ 102.12, 102.09, 98.20 and 93.95 in the $^{13}$C-NMR spectrum. Of these sugars, two D-glucopyranose and two L-rhamnopyranose were confirmed by the H-C connections in the HSQC, H-H COSY, and by hydrolysis of 2 with the affording D-glucose and L-rhamnose. Typical signals of rhamnopyranosyl methyl groups were at $\delta_C$ 17.98/18.04 and at $\delta_H$ 1.32 (6H, *J* = 6.5 Hz). The higher chemical shifts ($\delta_C$ 68.51/68.45) of two oxymethylene carbons of glucopyranosyl groups suggested that these hydroxylmethylene groups were substituted. Detailed analysis of the 2D-NMR (HSQC, H-H COSY, HMBC) of 2 (Table 15.1) led to the connections of the partial structures as shown in Figure 15.1. In the HMBC spectrum, H-1"$_{glcI}$ (δ 5.11) and H-3""$_{glcII}$ (δ 5.10) correlated with two carbonyl at δ 168.20, the H-1"'$_{glcII}$ (δ 4.51) correlated with H-3" of glcI, as well as, two rhamnopyranosyl anomeric protons at δ 4.78 and 4.80 had long-range correlations with C-6"$_{glcI}$ (δ 68.51) and C-6"'$_{glcII}$ (δ 68.45), respectively. This evidence confirmed the sequences of each unit of 2 as shown in Figure 15.1. Furthermore, the HR-ESI-MS spectrum of 2 exhibited the quasi ion peaks at *m/z* 895.3331 $[M+H]^+$ (Calcd. 895.3236 for $C_{42}H_{55}O_{21}$). From the above data, compound 2 was determined to be *E*-cinnamic acid 1-*O*-{*E*-cinnamoyl-(1→3)-β-D-glucopyranosyl-[(1→6)-α-L-rhamnopyranosyl]-(1→3)-β-D-glucopyranosyl-[(1→6)-α-L-rhamnopyranosyl]} ester and named as gleditschiaside C, a new natural product.

## Acknowledgements

The authors would like to thank Dr Tran Huy Thai, Institute of Ecology and Biological Resources, VAST for the plant identification. Prof. Nunziatina De Tommasi and Prof. Fabrizio Dal Piaz, Dipartimento di Scienze Farmaceutiche, Università di Salerno for registering the HRESIMS spectra.

## References

Bich, D. H., Trung, D. Q., Chuong, B. X., Dong, N. T., Dam, D. T., Hien, P. V., Lo, V. N., Mai, P. D., Man, P. K., Nhu, D. T., Tap, N. and Toan, T., 2004. The medicinal plants and animals of Vietnam. Hanoi Science and Technology Publisher, 1st edition, Hanoi, Vol. 2. pp. 635-636.

Chi, V. V., 1997. Vietnam Medical Plant Dictionary. Medicinal Publishing House.

Hai, N. T. B., Glyzina, G. S., Libizov, N. 1. and Kogan, L. M., 1974. Flavonoids of the glumes of *Gleditschia australis*. Journal of Chemistry of Compounds, 8(5), pp. 617-619.

Kiem, P. V., Van, N. T. H., Tiep, P. K., Minh, C. V., Huong, L. M., Tomasi, N. D., Braca, A., 2007. A new E-cinnamic acid derivative from *Gledischia australis* Hemsl.. Vietnam Journal of Pharmacy, 372(4), pp. 33-36.

# Chapter 16

# A New Triterpene from *Baeckea frutescens* L. (Myrtaceae)

**Tran Hong Quang, Phan Van Kiem* and Chau Van Minh**
*Institute of Natural Products Chemistry, Vietnam Academy of Science and Technology,*
*18 Hoang Quoc Viet, Nghiado, Caugiay, Hanoi, Vietnam*
**E-mail: phankiem@vast.ac.vn*

## ABSTRACT

A new pentacylictriterpene 3β-hydroxylup-20(29)-ene-27,28-dioic acid 28-methyl ester (1) and six known compounds as ursolic acid (2), 11, 12-dehydroursolic acid lactone (3), uvaol (4), betulic acid (5), *p*-menthane-1β,2β,3α,4α-tetrol (6), *p*-menthane-1β,2β,4β-triol (7) were isolated from the methanolic extract of the aerial parts of *Baeckea frutescens*. Their chemical structures were determined by their spectroscopic data.

*Keywords*: *Baeckea frutescens, Myrtaceae, 3β-hydroxylup-20(29)-ene-27,28-dioic acid 28-methyl ester.*

## 1.0 Introduction

*Baeckea frutescens* L. (Myrtaceae) is a small herb, light-demanding, usually distributed on arid hills. *B. frutescens* L. distributed in Cambodia, Thailand, India, China and Vietnam. In Vietnam traditional medicine, it has been used to treat stomach ache, headache, fever and rheumatism (Bich, 2003). Previous studies on this plant have indicated the presence of chromones and chromanones (Tsui, 1996), chromone C-glycosides (Satake, 1999), phloroglucinols (BF-1, BF-2) (Fujimoto, 2003), flavanones (BF-4, BF-5, BF-6) (Makino, 1999). Our phytochemical investigation on the aerial parts of this plant resulted in the isolation and elucidation of a new pentacyclictriterpene 3β-hydroxylup-20(29)-ene-27,28-dioic acid 28-methyl ester (1), together with six known compounds as betulic acid (2), ursolic acid (3), uvaol (4), 11,

12-dehydroursolic acid lactone (5), *p*-menthane-1β,2β,3α,4α-tetrol (6), and *p*-menthane-1β,2β,4β-triol (7). Their structures were established by the means of MS, 1D–and 2D-NMR studies in comparison with the literature.

## 2.0 Materials and Methods

### 2.1 General Methods

Melting points were determined using an Electrothermal IA-9200. Optical rotations were determined on a Jasco DIP-1000 KUY polarimeter. The electrospray ionization (ESI) mass spectra were obtained using an AGILENT 1100 LC-MSD Trap spectrometer. The $^1$H-NMR (500 MHz) and $^{13}$C-NMR (125 MHz) spectra were recorded on a Bruker AM500 FT-NMR spectrometer and TMS was used as an internal standard. Column chromatography (CC) was performed on silica gel (Kieselgel 60, 70-230 mesh and 230-400 mesh, Merck) and YMC RP-18 resins.

### 2.2 Plant Material

The aerial parts of *B. frutescens* were collected in Tamdao, Vinh Phuc, Vietnam in February 2007 and identified by Dr. Tran Huy Thai, Institute of Ecology and Biological Resources, VAST. An authentic sample (No 20070217) was deposited at the Institute of Natural Products Chemistry, Vietnam Academy of Science and Technology

### 2.3 Extraction and Isolation

The dried aerial parts of *B. frutescens* (5.0 kg) were powdered and extracted with hot methanol three times to give the methanol extract (500.0 g), which was suspended in water and then partitioned with chloroform to give chloroform extract (80.0 g) and water layer. The chloroform extract (80.0 g) was then repeatedly subjected to chromatography on a silica gel column (Φ 100 x L 500 mm), eluted with *n*-hexane:ethyl acetate (gradient from 50:1 to 1:2 v/v) to give six fractions, F1 (19.5 g), F2 (12.5 g), F3 (6.0 g), F4 (18 g), F5 (12 g), and F6 (10.0 g). The fraction F3 was subjected to chromatography on a silica gel column (Φ 30 x L 500 mm) using chloroform–acetone (8:1) as eluent to give 6 (45 mg) as crystals. The fraction F4 was chromatographed on a silica gel column (Φ 60 x L 500 mm) using *n*-hexane–ethyl acetate (3:1) and then chloroform–ethyl acetate (15:1) as eluent to give 3 (40mg), 1 (30mg), 4 (20mg), and 5 (50mg). Compounds 2 (60mg) and 7 (25mg) were obtained from the fraction F5 after repeatedly chromatographing on a silica gel column (Φ 50 x L 500 mm), using chloroform–acetone (15:1 and 5:1) as eluent.

**3β-Hydroxylup-20(29)-ene-27,28-dioic acid 28-methyl ester (1)**

White crystals; positive ESI-MS *m/z*: 523.3 $[M+Na]^+$; negative ESI-MS *m/z*: 499.2 $[M-H]^-$. The $^1$H-NMR (500 MHz, $CDCl_3$) and $^{13}$C-NMR (125 MHz, $CDCl_3$): see Table 16.1.

**Ursolic Acid (2)**

White crystals, mp. 290-291 °C, $[\alpha]_D$ +66° (c 1,0, MeOH); ESI-MS *m/z*: 457 [M+H]+ ($C_{30}H_{48}O_3$); $^1$H-NMR (500MHz, $CDCl_3$) δ: 5.52 (1H, t, *J* = 3.5 Hz, H-12), 3.48 (1H, dd, *J* = 10.3, 4.1 Hz, H-3α), 2.66 (1H, d, *J* = 3.5 Hz, H-18), 1.27 (s, $CH_3$), 1.25 (s, $CH_3$),

1.03 (s, $CH_3$), 1.02 (3H, d, *J* = 6.5 Hz, H-30), 0,97 (3H, d, *J* = 6.3 Hz, H-29) and 0.91 (3H, s, H-25); $^{13}$C-NMR (125 MHz, $CDCl_3$): see Table 16.1.

**11,12-Dehydroursolic acid lactone (3)**

White crystals; mp 238°C; $[\alpha]_D^{10}$ + 44; ESI-MS *m/z*: 455.1 $[M+H]^+$ (positive mode), and 453.1 $[M-H]^-$(negative mode). $^1$H-NMR (500 MHz, $CDCl_3$) δ: 3.21 (1H, dd, *J* = 5.0, 10.0, H-3), 5.53 (1H, dd, *J* = 3.0 Hz, 10.0 Hz, H-11), 5.96 (1H, d, *J* = 10.0 Hz, H-12), 0.91 (3H, s, H-23), 1.05 (3H, s, H-24), 0.99 (3H, s, H-25), 1.16 (3H, s, H-26), 1.00 (3H, s, H-27), 0.93 (3H, s, H-29), and 0.78 (3H, s, H-30); $^{13}$C-NMR (125 MHz, $CDCl_3$): see Table 16.1.

**Uvaol (4)**

White crystals; mp 222-224°C; $[\alpha]_D^{24}$ +70 (c, 0.93 in $CHCl_3$); positive ESI-MS *m/z*: 443.1 $[M+H]^+$; negative ESI-MS *m/z*: 424.2 $[M-H_2O]^-$. $^1$H-NMR (500 MHz, $CDCl_3$) δ: 3.55 (1H, d, *J* = 11.0 Hz, H-3), 5.16 (1H, t, *J* = 3.5 Hz, H-12), 0.81 (3H, s, H-23), 0.95 (3H, s, H-24), 0.97 (3H, s, H-25), 1.02 (3H, s, H-26), 1.01 (3H, s, H-27), 3.23 (2H, t, *J* = 11.0 Hz, H-28), 0.90 (3H, d, *J* = 7.0 Hz, H-29), and 0.83 (3H, d, *J* = 6.0 Hz, H-30); $^{13}$C-NMR (125 MHz, $CDCl_3$): see Table 16.1.

**Betulic Acid (5)**

White crystals; mp 275-278°C, $[\alpha]_D^{23}$ +7.9 (c, 0.57 in Pyridine); positive ESI-MS *m/z*: 457.1 $[M+H]^+$; negative ESI-MS *m/z*: 455.1 $[M-H]^-$. $^1$H-NMR (500 MHz, $CDCl_3$) δ: 3.17 (1H, dd, *J* = 6.0 Hz, 11.5 Hz, H-3), 0.93 (3H, s, H-23), 0.75 (3H, s, H-24), 0.82 (3H, s, H-25), 0.95 (3H, s, H-26), 0.97 (3H, s, H-27), and 1.68 (3H, s, H-30). $^{13}$C-NMR (125 MHz, $CDCl_3$): see Table 16.1.

***p*-Menthane-1β,2β,3α,4α-tetrol (6)**

White crystals; $[\alpha]_D^{25}$ –1.6 (c 0.06, $CHCl_3$); positive ESI-MS *m/z*: 227.1 $[M+Na]^+$; negative ESI-MS *m/z*: 203.1 $[M-H]^-$, $^1$H-NMR (500 MHz, $CDCl_3$) δ: 3.77 (1H, ddd, *J* = 8.0, 5.5, 1.0, H-2), 3.57 (1H, ddd, *J* = 8.0 Hz, 5.5, 1.0, H-3), 2.00 (1H, m, $H_a$-5), 1.42 (1H, m, $H_b$-5), 2.00 (1H, m, $H_a$-6), 1.30 (1H, m, $H_b$-6), 2.01 (1H, m, H-8), 0.99 (3H, d, *J* = 7.0 Hz, H-9), 0.98 (3H, d, *J* = 7.0 Hz, H-10); $^{13}$C-NMR (125 MHz, $CDCl_3$) δ: 91.34 (C-1), 70.27 (C-2), 73.34 (C-3), and 84.67 (C-4), 29.16 (C-5), 25.02 (C-6), 20.08 (C-7), 32.75 (C-8), 17.63 (C-9), and 17.61 (C-10).

***p*-Menthane-1β,2β,4β-triol (7)**

White crystals; positive ESI-MS *m/z*: 210.7 $[M+Na]^+$; negative ESI-MS *m/z*: 186.7 $[M-H]^-$. $^1$H-NMR (500 MHz, $CDCl_3$) δ: 1.44 (2H, m, H-2), 1.61 (2H, m, H-3), 1.95 (2H, m, H-5), 3.52 (1H, d, *J* = 3.0 Hz, H-6), 1.25 (3H, s, H-7), 1.83 (1H, m, H-8), 0.94 (3H, d,, *J* = 7.0 Hz, H-9), and 0.92 (3H, d, *J* = 7.0 Hz, H-10); $^{13}$C-NMR (125 MHz, $CDCl_3$) δ: 75.70 (C-1), 30.28 (C-2), 30.39 (C-3), 72.04 (C-4), 34.84 (C-5), 75.74 (C-6), 27.09 (C-7), 39.00 (C-8), 17.12 (C-9), and 17.23 (C-10).

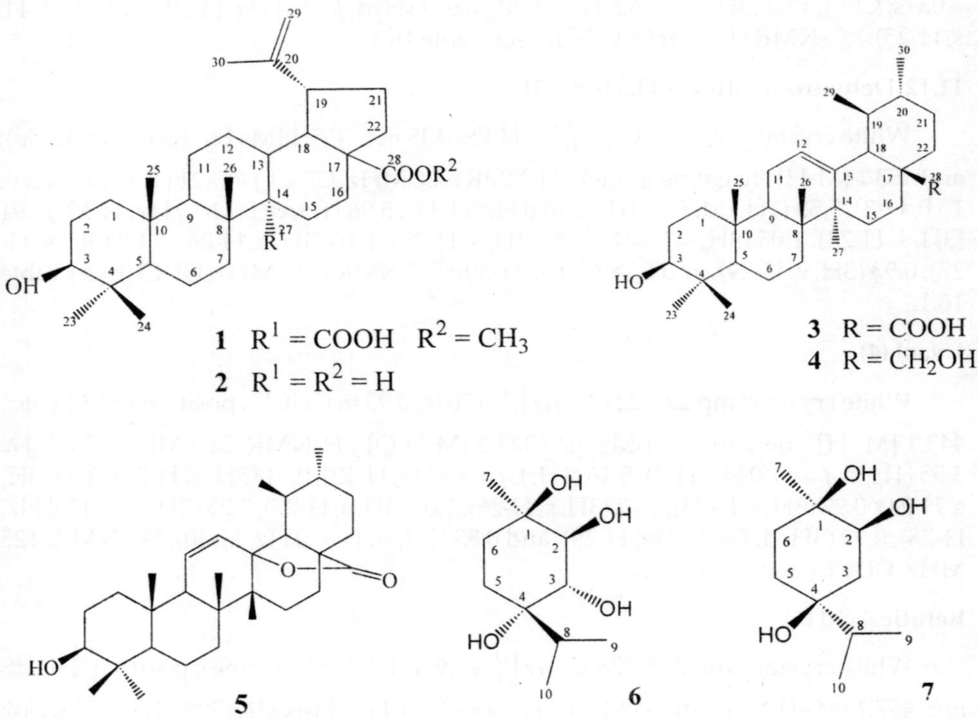

1 $R^1 = COOH$ $R^2 = CH_3$

2 $R^1 = R^2 = H$

3 R = COOH

4 $R = CH_2OH$

5

6

7

**Figure 16.1: Structures of Compounds 1-7**

## 3.0 Results and Discussion

Compound 1 was obtained as white crystals. The $^{13}$C-NMR and DEPT spectra revealed the presence of 31 carbons including five tertiary methyl groups, one methoxyl, 11 methylenes, 6 methines (one bearing oxygen atom), and 6 quaternary carbons and two carbonyl groups. The methyl signal at $\delta_C$ 19.04/$\delta_H$ 1.68 and at $\delta_C$ 110.18/$\delta_H$ 4.75/4.63 suggested a lupane skeleton with a double bond at C-20/C-29. The NMR spectra displayed the signal of a carboxyl group ($\delta_C$ 178.62), a carboxylate group ($\delta_C$ 176.72), a methylene double bond ($\delta_H$ 4.75 and $\delta_H$ 4.63/$\delta_C$ 110.18 and $\delta_C$ 149.88), a oxymethine group ($\delta_H$ 3.18/$\delta_C$ 79.04), a methyl ester ($\delta_H$ 3.67/$\delta_C$ 51.1), five tertiary methyl groups ($\delta_H$ 0.94, 0.75, 0.85, 1.02, 1.68/$\delta_C$ 28.07, 15.52, 16.69, 17.08, 19.04). The NMR data of 1 were resembled to that of melaleucic acid (Ahmad, 1994; Wenkert, 1978) except for the additional signal of a methoxyl group. The above data suggested that 1 was a lupane having a hydroxyl, one carboxyl, one methyl ester of the other carboxylic and a double bond at C-20/C-29, corresponding to the molecular formula of $C_{31}H_{48}O_5$, which was further confirmed by the exhibition of the quasi ion peaks at *m/z* 523.3 $[M+Na]^+$ (positive mode), and 499.2 $[M-H]^-$(negative mode) in the ESI-MS spectra. All the NMR data of 1 were carefully deduced from the heteronuclear single quantum coherence (HMQC) and the heteronuclear multiple-bond correlation (HMBC) experiments and summarized in Table 16.1. The methoxyl group was determined to attach to C-28 from the obviation of H-C long-range correlation of proton at $\delta$ 3.67 to carbon at δ 176.72 in the HMBC spectrum. Based on the above evidences and comparison with the published data, compound 1 was identified as 3β-hydroxylup-20(29)-ene-27,28-dioic acid 28-methyl ester, a new compound from nature.

**Table 16.1: The NMR Data of 1–5**

| C | $\delta_C$ of 5[a,b] | $\delta_C$ of 4[a,b] | $\delta_C$ of 3[a,b] | $\delta_C$ of 2[a,b] | 1[a,b] | | |
|---|---|---|---|---|---|---|---|
| | | | | | $\delta_C$ | $\delta_H$ mult. (J, Hz) | HMBC (H to C) |
| 1 | 38.31 | 38.80 | 38.50 | 38.89 | 38.80 | 1.70 m; 0.90 | |
| 2 | 22.82 | 27.28 | 23.41 | 27.19 | 27.71 | 2.03 m;1.24 m | |
| 3 | 78.83 | 79.05 | 77.07 | 78.98 | 79.04 | 3.18 dd (4.5, 11.5) | C–1, C–4, C–23, C–24 |
| 4 | 38.93 | 38.80 | 39.66 | 38.83 | 38.76 | – | |
| 5 | 54.78 | 55.20 | 52.54 | 55.45 | 55.53 | 0.64 d (11.5) | |
| 6 | 17.70 | 18.35 | 18.13 | 18.37 | 18.27 | 1.52*; 1.34* | |
| 7 | 30.85 | 32.85 | 32.85 | 34.42 | 37.59 | 1.62*; 1.38* | |
| 8 | 41.70 | 40.04 | 38.64 | 40.77 | 40.57 | – | |
| 9 | 53.04 | 47.69 | 47.17 | 50.64 | 51.34 | 1.35 m | |
| 10 | 36.37 | 38.03 | 36.46 | 37.21 | 37.49 | – | |
| 11 | 133.45 | 23.34 | 23.92 | 20.97 | 20.63 | 1.51 m; 1.24 m | |
| 12 | 128.83 | 125.07 | 124.70 | 25.63 | 27.30 | 2.02 m; 1.60 m | |
| 13 | 89.69 | 138.74 | 138.34 | 38.40 | 39.68 | 2.31 dd (3.5,12.5) | |
| 14 | 41.95 | 42.07 | 41.77 | 42.53 | 59.64 | | |
| 15 | 27.02 | 29.08 | 28.41 | 30.69 | 26.01 | 1.93 m; 1.71 m | |
| 16 | 25.55 | 22.50 | 23.54 | 32.35 | 34.14 | 2.34 m; 1.24* | |
| 17 | 45.10 | 36.90 | 47.17 | 56.31 | 56.29 | – | |
| 18 | 60.59 | 54.05 | 54.94 | 47.06 | 52.05 | 1.56 m | |
| 19 | 38.14 | 39.38 | 30.50 | 49.21 | 46.94 | 3.05 m | C–17, C–29, C–30 |
| 20 | 40.27 | 39.45 | 30.32 | 150.79 | 149.88 | – | |
| 21 | 31.25 | 30.64 | 27.01 | 37.26 | 30.41 | 1.91 m; 1.36 m | |
| 22 | 31.34 | 30.47 | 36.46 | 29.76 | 36.96 | 1.71 m; 1.29 m | |
| 23 | 27.77 | 28.14 | 23.40 | 27.99 | 28.07 | 0.94 s | C–3, C–4, C–5, C–24 |
| 24 | 14.92 | 15.62 | 16.20 | 15.41 | 15.52 | 0.75 s | C–3, C–4, C–5, C–23 |
| 25 | 16.12 | 15.70 | 16.90 | 15.99 | 16.69 | 0.85 s | C–1, C–5, C–9, C–10 |
| 26 | 18.90 | 17.35 | 15.31 | 16.16 | 17.08 | 1.02 s | C–7, C–8, C–9, C–14 |
| 27 | 17.90 | 23.40 | 25.72 | 14.73 | 178.62 | – | |
| 28 | 179.90 | 69.96 | 178.51 | 179.33 | 176.72 | – | |
| 29 | 17.82 | 16.79 | 21.23 | 109.55 | 110.18 | 4.75 d (2.0)<br>4.63 d (2.0) | C–19, C–20, C–30<br>C–19, C–20, C–30 |
| 30 | 19.16 | 21.33 | 23.51 | 19.38 | 19.04 | 1.68 s | C–19, C–20, C–29 |
| | | | | | 51.44 | 3.67 s | C–28 |

[a]125 MHz; [b]measured in $CDCl_3$; Chemical shift (δ) in ppm.

Compounds 2–7 were identified as ursolic acid (Poehland, 1987), 11,12-dehydroursolic acid lactone (Hao, 1996), uvaol (Siddiqui, 1986), betulic acid (Patra, 1988), *p*-menthane-1$\beta$,2$\beta$,3$\alpha$,4$\alpha$-tetrol (Ahmed, 2000), *p*-menthane-1$\beta$,2$\beta$,4$\beta$-triol (Mathur, 1967), respectively, by comparison with the literature.

## Acknowledgements

The authors would like to thank Dr Tran Huy Thai, Institute of Ecology and Biological Resources, Vietnam Academy of Science and Technology for the plant identification.

## References

Ahmad, V. U., and Rahman, A-U., 1994. Handbook of natural products data. Elsevier (2), pp. 1166.

Ahmed, A. A., 2000. Highly oxygenated monoterpenes from *Chenopodium ambrosioides*. J. Nat. Prod., 63: 989-991.

Bich, D. H., Chung, D.Q., Chuong, B.X., Dong, N.T., Dam, D.T., Hien, P.V., Lo, V.N., Mai, P.D., Man, P.K., Nhu, D.T., Tap, N. and Toan, T., 2004. Medicinal plants and animals of Vietnam. Vietnam publisher of science and technology (1), pp. 441-443.

Fujimoto, Y., Usui, S., Makino, M. and Sumatra, M., 2003. Phloroglucinols from *Baeckea frutescens*. J. Nat. Prod. 66, pp. 1144-1146.

Hao, H. Sun, H-D., and Zhao, S-X., 1996. Triterpenoids of *Isodon loxothyrsus*. Phytochemistry 42(6), pp. 1665-1666.

Makino, M., Fujimoto, Y., 1999. Flavanones from *Baeckea frutescens*. Phytochemistry 50, pp. 273-277.

Mathur, R. K., Ramaswamy, S. K., Rao A. S., and Bhattacharyya, S. C., 1967. Terpenoids–CVIII: Isolation of an oxidodiol from *Zanthoxylum rhetsa*. Tetrahedron 23(5), pp. 2495-2498.

Patra, A., Chaudhuri, S. K., and Panda, S. K., 1988. Betuli*n*-3-caffeate from *Quercus suber*, $^{13}$C-nmr spectra of some lupenes. J. Nat. Prod. 51(2), pp. 217–220.

Poehland, B.L., Carte, B.K., Francis, T.A., Hyland, L.J., Allaudeen, H.S., and Troupe, N., 1987. In vitro antiviral activity of Dammar resin triterpenoids. J. Nat. Prod. 50(4), pp. 706-713.

Satake, T., Kamiya, K., Saiki, Y., Hama, T., Fujimoto, Y., Endang, H., Umar, M., 1999. Chromone C-glycosides from *Baeckea frutescens*. Phytochemistry (50), pp. 303-306.

Siddiqui, S., Hafeez, F., Begum, S., Siddiqui B. S., 1986. Kaneric acid, a new triterpene from the leaves of *Nerium oleander*. J. Nat. Prod. 49(6), pp. 1086-1090.

Tsui, W-A., Brown, G. D., 1996. Chromones and chromanones from *Baeckea frutescens*. Phytochemistry 43(4), pp. 871-876.

Wenkert, E., Baddeley, G. V., Burfitt, 1. R., Moreno, L. N., 1978. Org. Magn. Resonance (1) pp. 337-343.

# Chapter 17

# Study on the Chemical Constituents of *Polygonum hydropiper* L.

**Tran Thi Quynh Hoa, Nguyen Xuan Nhiem, Hoang Thanh Huong, Ha Viet Hai, Phan Van Kiem and Chau Van Minh***

*Institute of Natural Products Chemistry, Vietnam Academy of Science and Technology, 18 Hoang Quoc Viet, Caugiay, Hanoi, Vietnam*

**E-mail: cvminh@fpt.vn*

## ABSTRACT

Vina-polygonum A, a new drimane derivative and six known flavonoids were isolated from the methanolic extract of the whole plant of *Polygonum hydropiper* L. The new natural product was elucidated as 3-*O*-$\beta$-D-glucopyranosyl-11$\alpha$-methoxy-11, 12-epoxydrim-7-ene (1), and the known compounds were identified as quercetin (2), 6,4'-dimethoxyquercetin (3), 3', 4'-dimethoxyquercetin (4), isoquercitrin (5), 3-*O*-galactopyranosyl-quercetin (6), and 3'-methoxyquercitrin (7) by spectroscopic evidences.

***Keywords***: *Polygonaceae, Polygonum hidropiper, Vina-polygonum A.*

## 1.0 Introduction

*Polygonum hydropiper* L., the folk medicinal plant, contains intense pungent substance in leaf and seed and is used against cancer. The young shoot is used as a spice with raw fish in Japan, and is toxic to fish, pigs and sheep, and that the water-soluble fraction shows haemolytic properties (Fukuyama, 1982). The major component of the lipophilic materials of the leaves is a pungent polygodial, adrimane-type sesquiterpene dialdehyde that shows intense antifeedant and plan growth inhibitory activities (Fukuyama, 1982). A previous investigation of the leaves of *P. hydropiper* L., have isolated polygodial polygonic acid and 11-ethoxycinnamolide, polygonal, isopolygonal and polygonone (Fukuyama, 1985), polygodial acetal (Ying, 1995), polygonolide possessing anti-inflammatory activity (Furuta, 1986). In addition, a number of flavonoids have been reported as antioxidative substances in leaves as 7,4'-dimethylquercetin, 3'-methylquercetin, quercetin, flavonoid glycoside (Haraguchi, 2001), and tamarixin 7-O-sulfate (Yagi, 1994), hydropiperoside with anticancer allelopathic effects (Takasaki, 2001). During the course of the investigation of the anticomplement and antitumor active substances of *P. hydropiper*, we report herein the isolation and the structural elucidation of the new drimane derivative named vina-polygonum A (1), and six known compounds as quercetin (2), 6,4'-dimethoxyquercetin (3), 3', 4'-dimethoxyquercetin (4), isoquercitrin (5), 3-O-galactopyranosyl-quercetin (6), and 3'-methoxyquercitrin (7). Their structures were established by the means of MS, 1D–and 2D-NMR studies.

## 2.0 Materials and Methods

### 2.1 General Experiment Procedures

The $^{1}H$-NMR (500MHz) and $^{13}C$-NMR (125MHz) spectra were recorded on a Bruker AM500 FT-NMR spectrometer. Chemical shifts are referenced to $\delta$ using tetramethylsilan (TMS) as an internal standard. The Electron Spray Ionization (ESI) mass spectrum was obtained using an AGILENT 1100 LC-MSD Trap spectrometer. Column chromatography (CC) was performed on silica gel 230-400 mesh (0.040-0.063 mm, Merck) or YMC RP-18 resins (30-50 µm, Fujisilisa Chemical Ltd.). Thin layer chromatography (TLC) was performed on DC-Alufolien 60 $F_{254}$ (Merck 1.05715) or $RP_{18}$ $F_{254s}$ (Merck) plates.

### 2.2 Plant Material

The stems of *Polygonum hydropiper* L., were collected in Tam Dao, Vinh Phuc province, Vietnam in January 2006 and identified by Dr. Tran Huy Thai, Institute of Ecology and Biological Resources, Vietnam Academy of Science and Technology (VAST). An authentic sample was deposited at the Institute of Natural Products Chemistry, VAST.

### 2.3 Extraction and Isolation

The dried stems of Polygonum hydropiper L. (5 kg) were extracted with MeOH three times, and then concentrated under low pressure to obtain 120 g MeOH extract. The MeOH extract was suspended in water and partitioned with hexane, $CHCl_3$ EtOAc and BuOH to obtain fractions hexane (15 g), $CHCl_3$ (25 g), EtOAc (30.0 g), and BuOH (11.0 g). The EtOAc (30.0 g), was then chromatographed on a silica gel column eluting with $CHCl_3$-MeOH gradient (from 30:1 to 1:1 v/v) to give five fractions F1 (3.5 g), F2 (5.8 g), F3 (6.0 g), F4 (4.0 g), F5 (8.0 g) and F6 (2 g). The F2 fraction was re-chromatographed on a silicagel column using $CHCl_3$-EtOAc (5:1) as eluent to give subfractions 1 (17.0 mg) as a colourless powder and 2 (10 mg) as yellow crystals. The F3 (6.0 g) fraction was chromatographed on an YMC RP-18 column using MeOH-$H_2O$ (7:2 v/v) system as eluent to give 3 (20 mg), 4 (10 mg) as yellow crystal. The F5 (8.0 g) fraction (6.0 g) was chromatographed on a silica gel column using a $CHCl_3$-MeOH (3:1 v/v) system as eluent yielded 5 (14 mg), 6 (14 mg) and 7 (15 mg) as yellow amorphous powders.

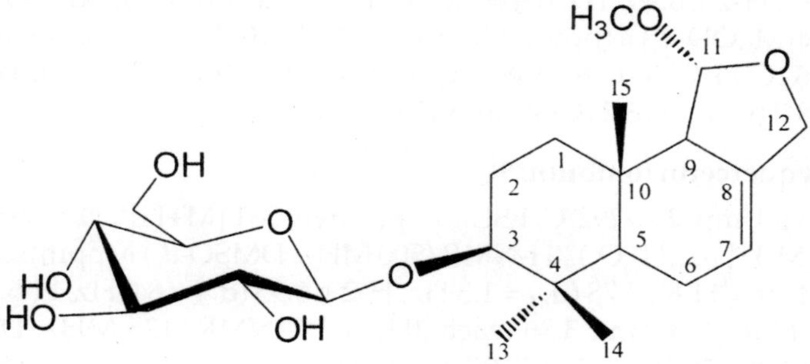

1

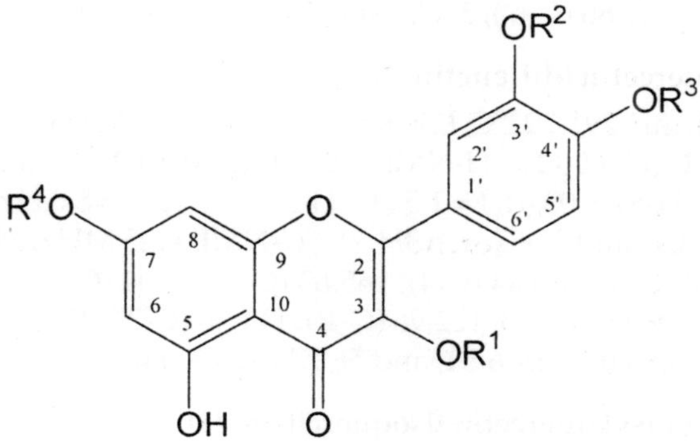

2

| | $R^1$ | $R^2$ | $R^3$ | $R^4$ |
|---|---|---|---|---|
| **2** | H | H | H | H |
| **3** | H | H | $CH_3$ | $CH_3$ |
| **4** | H | $CH_3$ | $CH_3$ | H |
| **5** | Glc | H | H | H |
| **6** | Gal | H | H | H |
| **7** | Glc | $CH_3$ | H | H |

**Figure 17.1: Structures of 1-7**

**3-*O*-β-D-glucopyranosyl-11α-methoxy-11, 12-epoxydrim-7-ene (vina-polygonum A, 1)**

Colourless amorphous powder; $[\alpha]_D^{25}$ -44.2° (*c* 0.5, EtOH); positive ESI-MS *m/z*: (positive) 429 $[M+H]^+$ and 451 $[M+Na]^+$, (negative) 427 $[M-H]^-$ ($C_{22}H_{36}O_8$); $^1$H-NMR (500 MHz, $CDCl_3$) and $^{13}$C-NMR (125 MHz, $CDCl_3$): see Table 17.1.

**Quercetin (2)**

Yellow crystal, mp 313-314°C; IR (KBr) $\nu_{max}$ (cm$^{-1}$): 3390, 3297 (br, OH), 2924, 2845 (CH), 1660 (C=O), 1616 (C=C), 1094 (C-O-C); ESI *m/z*: 303 $[M+H]^+$ ($C_{15}H_{10}O_7$); $^1$H-NMR (MeOD-$d_4$) δ (ppm): 6.20 (1H, d, $J$ = 2.1Hz, H-6), 6.41 (1H, d, $J$ = 2.1Hz, H-8), 7.75

(1H, d, *J* = 2.1 Hz, H-2'), 6.90 (1H, d, *J* = 8.2 Hz, H-5') and 7.65 (1H, dd, *J* = 8.2, 2.1 Hz, H-6'); $^{13}$C-NMR (MeOD-$d_4$) δ (ppm): 148.0 (C-2), 137.2 (C-3), 177.3 (C-4), 162.5 (C-5), 99.2 (C-6), 165.6 (C-7), 99.4 (C-8), 158.2 (C-9), 104.5 (C-10), 124.2 (C-1'), 116.0 (C-2'), 146.2 (C-3'), 148.7 (C-4'), 116.2 (C-5'), and 121.7 (C-6').

**7,4'-Dimethoxyquercetin (ombuin, 3)**

Yellow crystal, mp. 291-292°C, ESI *m/z*: (positive) 331 $[M+H]^+$; *m/z*: 353 $[M+Na]^+$, (negative) 329 $[M-H]^-$($C_{17}H_{14}O_7$). $^1$H-NMR (500 MHz, DMSO-$d_6$) δ (ppm): 6.34 (1H, br s, H-6), 6.76 (1H, br s, H-8), 7.78 (d, *J* = 1.5 Hz, H-2'), 6.93 (d, *J* = 8.0 Hz, H-5'), 7.73 (dd, *J* = 8.0, 1.5 Hz, H-6'), 3.33 and 3.36 (each 3H, s). $^{13}$C-NMR (125 MHz. DMSO-$d_6$) δ (ppm): 147.03 (C-2), 136.10 (C-3), 175.97 (C-4), 160.32 (C-5), 97.47 (C-6), 164.91 (C-7), 92.07 (C-8), 156.06 (C-9), 103.99 (C-10), 121.80 (C-1'), 111.76 (C-2'), 148.94 (C-3'), 147.39 (C-4'), 115.52 (C-5'), 121.86 (C-6'), 55.83, and 56.02 (2 x $OCH_3$).

**3', 4'-Dimethoxyquercetin (dillenetin, 4)**

Yellow crystal, mp. 291-292°C, ESI *m/z*: (positive) 331 $[M+H]^+$; *m/z*: 353 $[M+Na]^+$, (negative) 329 $[M-H]^-$($C_{17}H_{14}O_7$). $^1$H-NMR (500 MHz, MeOD-$d_4$) δ (ppm) 6.35 (1H. br s. H-6), 6.64 (1H, br s, H-8), 8.03 (d, *J* = 1.5 Hz, H-2'), 6.93 (d, *J* = 8.0 Hz, H-5'), 7.66 (dd, *J* = 8.0, 1.5 Hz, H-6'), 3.91 and 3.98 (each 3H, s). $^{13}$C-NMR (125 MHz, MeOD-$d_4$) δ (ppm): 147.44 (C-2), 133.70 (C-3), 180.44 (C-4), 165.63 (C-5), 99.04 (C-6), 167.31 (C-7), 93.16 (C-8), 158.23 (C-9), 106.69 (C-10), 122.96 (C-1'), 114.30 (C-2'), 151.10 (C-3'), 148.20 (C-4'), 116.08 (C-5'), 123.86 (C-6'), 56.51, and 56.73 (2 x $OCH_3$).

**3-*O*-β-D-glucopyranosyl quercetin (isoquercitrin) (5)**

Yellow amorphous powders, mp. 239-241°C, IR (KBr) $\nu_{max}$ (cm$^{-1}$): 3300, (br, OH), 2936 (CH), 1656 (C=O), 1601 (C=C), 1062 (C-O-C); ESI *m/z*: (positive) 465 $[M+H]^+$; *m/z*: 487 $[M+Na]^+$, (negative) 463,1 $[M-H]^-$($C_{21}H_{20}O_{12}$).$^1$H-NMR (500 MHz, MeOD-$d_4$) δ (ppm): 6.26 (1H, br s, H-6), 6.45 (1H, br s, H-8), 7.92 (1H, br s, H-2'), 6.94 (1H, d, *J* = 8.0 Hz, H-5'), 7.66 (1H, d, *J* = 8.0 Hz, H-6'), 5.29 (1H, d, *J* = 8.0 Hz, H-1''), 3.57 (1H, dd, *J* = 8.0, 8.0 Hz, H-2''), 3.29-3.38 (3H, overlapped, H-3'', H-5'', Ha-6), 3.65 (dd, *J* = 2.5, 2.5 Hz, H-4''), and 3.45 (1H. dd. *J* = 11.5, 5.0 Hz. $H_b$-6). $^{13}$C-NMR (125 MHz. MeOD-$d_4$) δ (ppm): 157.55 (C-2), 134.61 (C-3), 178.36 (C-4), 161.98 (C-5), 99.25 (C-6), 166.07 (C-7), 93.97 (C-8), 157.92 (C-9), 104.39 (C-10), 122.07 (C-1'), 116.55 (C-2'), 144.92 (C-3'), 148.90 (C-4'), 115.01 (C-5'), 122.18 (C-6'), 103.49 (C-1''), 74.73 (C-2''), 77.13 (C-3''), 70.22 (C-4''), 77.37 (C-5''), and 61.57 (C-6'').

**3-*O*-β-D-galactopyranosyl quercetin (hyperin) (6)**

Yellow amorphous powders, mp. 232-233°C, $^1$H-NMR (500 MHz, DMSO-$d_6$) δ (ppm): 6.20 (1H, br s, H-6), 6.40 (1H, br s, H-8), 7.53 (1H, d, *J* = 1.5 Hz, H-2'), 6.82 (1H,d, *J* = 8.0 Hz, H-5'), 7.67 (1H, dd, *J* = 8.0, 1.5 Hz, H-6'), 5.37 (1H. d. *J* = 7.5 Hz, H-1''), 3.57 (1H, d, *J* = 7.5 Hz, H-2''), 3.36 (1H, dd, *J* = 7.5, 2.5, H-3''), 3.65 (1H, dd, *J* = 2.5, 2.5, H-4''), 3.21 (1H, m, H-5''), 3.45 (1H, dd, *J* = 11.5. 5.0 Hz, $H_a$-6) and 3.31 (1H, overlapped, $H_b$-6). $^{13}$C-NMR (125 MHz. MeOD-$d_4$) δ (ppm): 156.29 (C-2), 133.47 (C-3), 177.45 (C-4), 161.20 (C-5), 98.68 (C-6), 164.23 (C-7), 93.49 (C-8), 156.20 (C-9), 103.86 (C-10), 121.96 (C-1'), 115.17 (C-2'), 144.81 (C-3'), 148.46 (C-4'), 115.93 (C-5'), 121.07 (C-6'), 101.81 (C-1''), 71.19 (C-2''), 73.18 (C-3''), 67.91 (C-4''), 75.82 (C-5''), and 60.11 (C-6'').

**3'-Methoxyquercitrin (3-glucosylisorhamnetin, 7)**

Yellow amorphous powders, mp. 215-217°C, ESI *m/z*: (positive) 479 $[M+H]^+$; *m/z*: 501 $[M+Na]^+$, (negative) 477. $[M-H]^-$($C_{22}H_{22}O_{12}$).$^1$H-NMR (500 MHz, MeOD-$d_4$) δ (ppm): 6.17 (1H, br s, H-6), 6.35 (1H, br s, H-8), 7.93 (1H, d, *J* = 1.5 Hz, H-2'), 6.91 (1H, d, *J* = 8.0 Hz, H-5'), 7.59 (1H, dd, *J* = 8.0, 1.5 Hz, H-6'), 5.35 (1H, d, *J* = 7.5 Hz, H-1''), 3.57 (1H, d, *J* = 7.5 Hz, H-2''), 3.36 (1H, dd, *J* = 7.5, 2.5, H-3''), 3.65 (1H, dd, *J* = 2.5, 2.5, H-4''), 3.21 (1H, m, H-5''), 3.45 (1H, dd, *J* = 11.5, 5.0 Hz, $H_a$-6) and 3.31 (1H, overlapped, $H_b$-6). $^{13}$C-NMR (125 MHz. MeOD-$d_4$) δ (ppm): 158.35 (C-2), 135.29 (C-3), 179.12 (C-4), 162.92 (C-5), 100.68 (C-6), 168.34 (C-7), 95.31 (C-8), 158.35 (C-9), 105.08 (C-10), 123.10 (C-1'), 114.34 (C-2'), 148.41 (C-3'), 150.89 (C-4'), 116.00 (C-5'), 123.83 (C-6'), 103.95 (C-1''), 75.90 (C-2''), 78.10 (C-3''), 71.48 (C-4''), 78.49 (C-5''), 62.56 (C-6''), and 56.77 ($OCH_3$).

## 3.0 Results and Discussion

Compound 1 was obtained as a colourless amorphous powder from the methanolic extract of the stems of *P. hydropiper*. The $^1$H-NMR spectrum of 1 showed a doublet signal of one anomeric proton at δ 4.36 (*J* = 7.5 Hz), a proton of the tri-substituted double bond at δ 5.57, an oxygenated methine proton at δ 4.81, an oxygenated methylene proton at δ 4.30 (broad-singlet, *J* = 11.0 Hz) and 4.15 (broad-singlet, *J* = 11.0 Hz), three tertiary methyl groups at 3.38 as a singlet. The $^{13}$C-NMR spectrum of 1 exhibited signal of 22 carbon atoms, including six signals of one D-glucopyranosyl (δ 106.67, 78.24, 77.65, 75.65, 71.67 and 62.80), a methoxyl (δ 55.68), and 15 signals were assigned for a drimane skeleton (Echeverro, 1997; Fukuyama, 1982 and 1985). In the HSQC experiment, proton signals at δ 3.31, 5.57, 4.81 correlated with carbon signals at δ 90.41, 118.19, 107.32, respectively, protons at δ 4.30 and 4.15 correlated with methylene carbon at δ 69.68, methyl protons at δ 0.96, 1.08 and 0.82 correlated with carbons at δ 16.70, 28.08 and 14.37, respectively, and other H-C correlations were analysis and gave in Table 17.1. Furthermore, signals were observed in the DEPT experiments were attributed to three quaternary carbons, ten methine carbons (five of them belongs to the glucopyranoside), five methylene carbons (one of them belongs to the glucopyranoside), and four methyl carbons (one is methoxyl carbon).

In addition, the partial structures of 1 were connected from the detailed analysis of the $^1$H-$^1$H chemical shift correlation spectroscopy (COSY). In the H-H COSY spectrum, H-2 correlated to H-1 and H-3, H-6 correlated to H-5 an H-7, H-9 correlated to H-11. All the NMR data of 1 were established from the above evidence in comparison with the reported literature (Echeverri, 1997), and confirmed by the heteronuclear multiple-bond correlation (HMBC) spectrum. The H-C long range correlations were observed between H-1' (δ 4.36) and C-3 (δ 90.41), between methoxyl protons (δ 3.38) and C-11 (δ 107.32), between H-11 (δ 4.81) and C-8 (δ 137.62), and between H-7 (δ 5.57) and C-9 (δ 61.60)/C-5 (δ 50.93) in the HMBC spectrum confirming the location of the methoxyl at C-11, the double bond at C-8/C-9, and the sugar linked to C-3 by ether linkage. The stereochemistry of the proton on C-3 must be α, and the methoxyl group at C-11 must be β by analogy with several drimanes isolated from Polygonum (Echeverri, 1997; Fukuyama, 1985; Ying, 1995). Finally, the structure of 1 was reconfirmed by the mass spectrum. The ESI-MS spectrum exhibited the quasi ion peaks at m/z 429 $[M+H]^+$ and 451 $[M+Na]^+$ (positive), 427 $[M-H]^-$(negative) corresponding to the molecular formula of $C_{22}H_{36}O_8$. Thus, compound 1 was determined to be 3-*O*-β-D-glucopyranosyl-11α-methoxy-11, 12-epoxydrim-7-ene, a new nature product and named as vina-polygonum A.

**Table 17.1: NMR Data of 1**

| *Position* | $\delta_C^{a,b\#}$ | $\delta_C^{a,b}$ | *DEPT* | $\delta_H^{a,c}$ *(J, Hz)* | *H–H COSY* | *HMBC (H to C)* |
|---|---|---|---|---|---|---|
| 1 | 37.61 | 38.72 | $CH_2$ | 1.73*/1.36* | H–2 | |
| 2 | 27.13 | 27.12 | $CH_2$ | 2.05*/1.73* | H–1, H–3 | |
| 3 | 79.00 | 90.41 | CH | 3.31* | H–2 | |
| 4 | 38.75 | 40.16 | – | – | H–5 | |
| 5 | 49.22 | 50.93 | CH | 1.37* | H–4, H–6 | |
| 6 | 23.45 | 24.38 | $CH_2$ | 2.10*/2.17* | H–5 | |
| 7 | 116.92 | 118.19 | CH | 5.57 br s | | 5, 8, 9, 12 |
| 8 | 136.31 | 137.62 | – | – | | |
| 9 | 61.40 | 61.60 | CH | 2.19* | H–11 | 7, 8, 10, 11 |
| 10 | 33.17 | 33.96 | – | – | H–9 | |
| 11 | 99.23 | 107.32 | CH | 4.81* | | |
| 12 | 68.83 | 69.68 | $CH_2$ | 4.30 br d (11.0)<br>4.15 br d (11.0) | | 7, 8, 9<br>7, 8, 9 |
| 13 | 14.86 | 16.70 | $CH_3$ | 0.96 s | | 3, 4, 5, 14 |
| 14 | 27.71 | 28.08 | $CH_3$ | 1.08 s | | 3, 4, 5, 13 |
| 15 | 14.07 | 14.37 | $CH_3$ | 0.82 s | | 1, 5, 9, 10 |
| 1' | | 106.67 | CH | 4.36 d (7.5) | H–2' | 3, 1', 2' |
| 2' | | 75.65 | CH | 3.25* | H–1', H–3' | |
| 3' | | 77.65 | CH | 3.32* | H–2', H–4' | |
| 4' | | 71.67 | CH | 3.31* | H–3', H–5' | |
| 5' | | 78.24 | CH | 3.36* | H–4', H–6' | |
| 6' | | 62.80 | $CH_2$ | 3.68 dd (5.5, 12.0)<br>3.87 dd (2.0, 12.0) | H–5'<br>H–5' | 4', 5'<br>4', 5' |
| $OCH_3$ | | 55.68 | $CH_3$ | 3.38 s | | 11 |

[a] Measured in $CDCl_3$; [b] 125 MHz, [c] 500 MHz, Chemical shift (δ) in ppm; # $\delta_C$ of danilol (Echeverri, 1997).

Compound 2-7 were identified as quercetin, 6,4'-dimethoxyquercetin, 3', 4'-dimethoxyquercetin, isoquercitrin, and 3-*O*-galactopyranosyl-quercetin, and 3'-methoxyquercitrin (Agrawal, 1989), respectively by comparison their NMR data with the literature.

## References

Agrawal, P. K., 1989. Carbon-13 NMR of flavonoids, Elsevier Science Publishers B. V., pp. 154-155, 334-335.

Bich, D. H., Chung, D. Q., Chuong, B. X., Dong, N. T., Dam, D. T., Hien, P. V., Lo, V. N., Mai, P. D., Man, P. K., Nhu, D. T., Tap, N., Toan, T., 2006. "Medicinal Animals and Plants in Vietnam". Hanoi Science and Technology Publishing House, Vol. 1.

Echeverri, F., Luis, J. G., Torres, F., Quinonens, W., Alzate, F., Cardona, G., Archbold, R., Roldan, J., Lanlou, E-H., 1997. Danilol, a new drimane sesquiterpene from *Polygonum punctatum* leaves. Natural Product Letters (10), pp. 295-301.

Fukuyama, Y., Sato, T., Asakawa, Y., and Takemoto, T., 1982. A potent cytotoxic warburganal and related drimane-type sesquiterpenoids from *Polygonum hydropiper*, Phytochemistry (21), pp. 2895-2898.

Fukuyama, Y., Sato, T., Miura, 1., and Asakawa, Y., 1985. Drimane-type sesqui–and norsesquiterpenoids from *Polygonum hydropiper*, Phytochemistry (24), 1521-1524.

Furuta, T., Fukuyama, Y., and Askawa, Y., 1986. Polygonolide, an isocoumarin from *Polygonum hydropiper* possessing anti-inflammatory activity. Phytochemistry (25), pp. 517-520.

Haraguchi, H., Hashimoto, K., Yagi, A., 1992. Antioxidative substances in leaves of *Polygonum hydropiper*. J-agric-food-chem (40(8)), pp. 1349-1351.

Takasaki, M. Kuroki, S., Kozuka, M., and Konoshima, T., 2001. New phenylpropanoid esters of sucrose from *Polygonum lapathifolium*, J. Nat. Prod. (64), pp. 1305-1308.

Yagi, A., Uemura, T., Okamura, N., Haraguchi, H., Imoto, T., and Hashimoto, K., 1994. Antioxidative sulphated flavonoids in leaves of *Polygonum hydropiper*. Phytochemistry (35), pp. 885-887.

Ying, B. P., Peiser, G., Ji, Y. Y., Mathias, K., Tutko, D., and Hwang, Y. S., 1995. Phytotoxic sesquiterpenoids from *Canella winterana*, Phytochemistry (38), pp. 909-915.

# Chapter 18

# Chemical Constituents from *Clerodendrum inerme* L.

*Tran Thi Minh*[1], *Nguyen Thi Hoang Anh*[2], *Vu Dao Thang*[1] and *Tran Van Sung*[2]

[1]*Ha Noi University of Technology, 1 Dai Co Viet Road, Hanoi, Vietnam*
[2]*Institute of Chemistry, Vietnamese Academy of Science and Technology, 18 Hoang Quoc Viet, Nghia Do, Cau Giay, Hanoi, Vietnam*

## ABSTRACT

Five compounds were isolated from the leaves of *Clerodendrum inerme* L., collected in Thai Binh province. Their structures were established from spectroscopic evidences as 20(29)-lupene-3-ol, 3β-form, hexacosanoyl; stigmast-5-ene-3-ol; apigenin; acacetin and andrographolide.

***Keywords:*** *Clerodendrum inerme, Spectroscopy.*

## 1.0 Introduction

*Clerodendrum inerme* L. (Verbenaceae) is widely distributed in coastal area and river mouth from the South to the North of Vietnam and the tropical countries. In the Vietnamese folk medicine, *C. inerme* has been used to cure several diseases such as ermatological diseases, marsh fever, hepatitis. Leaves in the form of poultice were used to resolve buboes. The obtained liniment by boiling of the roots in oil is useful for treatment of rheumatism..(Chi, 1997)

It has been reported that *C. inerme* was used in native medicine and some constituents were isolated. However, until now no reports on *Clerodendrum inerme* have been published in Vietnam. This paper deals with the isolation and structure elucidation of three compounds isolated from the leaves of this plant. They are stigmast-5-ene-3β-ol; 5,7,4′-trihydroxy flavone and 5,7-dihydroxy-4′-methoxy flavone.

# 2.0 Experimental

## 2.1 Instruments and Chemicals

Mps: Botius Engine (Germany). IR: IMPACT-410 Engine (Nicolet). NMR: Bruker AM500 FT-NMR using TMS as the internal standard. MS: HP5989B MS for EI-MS, AGILENT 1100 LC-MSD Trap for ESI-MS.

For analytical purposes: Merck TLC aluminium sheets silica gel 60 $F_{254}$ (layer thickness 0.2 mm) were used. Silica gel Merck 60 (0.040–0.063 mm) was used for column chromatography.

## 2.2 Plant Material

The leaves of *Clerodendrum inerme* was collected in Thai Binh province in February, 2006 and were identified by Dr Ngo Van Trai, Institute of Materia Medica, Hanoi.

## 2.3 Extraction and Isolation

The dried and powdered leaves of *C. inerme* (2 kg) were exhaustively extracted with methanol (80 per cent) at room temperature. The organic solvent was removed by distillation under reduced pressure. The obtained residue was added water and partitioned successively with n-hexane and then ethyl acetate. After evaporation of solvents, the n-hexane (29.9g) and ethyl acetate (27.7g) extracts were afforded. The amount of 10 g ethyl acetate extract was subjected over a silica gel column, washing with solvent system of $CH_2Cl_2$ and increasing amounts of MeOH to give 23 fractions.

Fraction 5 ($CH_2Cl_2$ 100 per cent) has a main constituent on TLC (n-hexane: ethyl acetate = 5: 1).

Crystallizing of this fraction in n-hexane gave 0.1g CE1 (1 per cent) with $R_f$ = 0.53 (n-hexane: ethyl acetate = 5: 1), white crystal, mp146–147°C; IR (KBr) $\nu_{max:}$ 3434, 2941, 2869, 1645, 1457, 1377, 1058; EI-MS *m/z* (per cent): 414 $[M]^+$ (1,6), typical fragments 271 (58), 255 (37), 213 (16), 159 (33), 119 (26), 109 (62), 81 (78), 67 (51), 55(100); $^1$H-NMR (500MHz, $CDCl_3$) δ(ppm): 5.34 (1H, s); 3.51 (1H, m); 2.27 (2H, m); 1.99 (2H, m); 1.83 (3H, m); 1.04 (6H, m); $^{13}$C-NMR (125MHz, $CDCl_3$) δ(ppm): 37.3 (C-1); 31.7 (C-2); 71.81 (C-3); 42.31 (C-4); 140.78 (C-5); 121.72 (C-6); 31.93 (C-7); 31.93 (C-8); 50.16 (C-9); 36.52 (C-10); 21.1 (C-11); 39.8 (C-12); 42.3 (C-13); 56.8 (C-14); 24.3 (C-15); 28.2 (C-16); 56.1 (C-17); 11.9 (C-18); 19.4 (C-19); 36.2 (C-20); 18.8 (C-21); 33.9 (C-22); 26.1 (C-23); 45.9 (C-24); 29.2 (C-25); 19.1 (C-26); 19.8 (C-27); 23.1 (C-28); 12.0 (C-29).

Fraction 16 ($CH_2Cl_2$: MeOH = 96: 4) was crystallized in $CHCl_3$: MeOH = 95: 5 to give 0,025g CE2 (0.25 per cent), yellow crystal, $R_f$ = 0.63 ($CH_2Cl_{2:}$ MeOH = 10: 1); mp 345–346°C; IR (KBr) $\nu^*_{max}$ (cm$^{-1}$): 3318, 1653 1609, 1556, 1496, 1445, 1353,1245, 1178, 831, 742; EI-MS (*m/z*): 270(100), typical fragments 242 (18.2); 213 (3.4); 153 (11.3); 124 (13.0); 118 (10.7); 96 (11.2); 89 (13.5); 78 (7.5); 69 (36.9); 55 (14.6); $^1$H–và $^{13}$C-NMR data were given in Table 18.1.

Fraction 11 ($CH_2Cl_{2:}$ MeOH = 98: 2) was crystallized in $CHCl_3$: MeOH = 95: 5 and washed with MeOH giving 0.017g CE3 (0.17 per cent), yellow crystal; mp 263–265°C; $R_f$ = 0.68 ($CH_2Cl_2$: MeOH = 15: 1); IR (KBr) $\nu_{max}$ (cm$^{-1}$): 3440; 3160; 2924; 2859; 1655;

1604; 1559; 1508; 1430; 1184; 1031; 830,48. ESI-MS (*m/z*): 285 $[M + H]^+$ ($C_{16}H_{12}O_5$). The $^1$H–and $^{13}$C-NMR data were given in Table 18.1.

**Table 18.1: $^1$H-, $^{13}$C–NMR Data for Compounds CE2 and CE3 (500, 125 MHz, DMSO-d6)**

| Position | CE2 (Apigenin) | | CE3 (Acacetin) | |
|---|---|---|---|---|
| | $\delta_H$, J in Hz | $\delta_C$ | $\delta_H$, J in Hz | $\delta_C$ |
| 2 | – | 163.7 s | | 163.3 s |
| 3 | 6.77 (1H, s) | 102.8 d | 6.86 (1H, s) | 103.5 d |
| 4 | – | 181.7 s | – | 181.7 s |
| 5 | – | 161.1 s | – | 161.4 s |
| 6 | 6.19(1H, d, J = 2.0) | 98.8 d | 6.20 (1H, d, J = 2.0) | 98.9 d |
| 7 | – | 164.1 s | – | 164.2 s |
| 8 | 6.48 (1H, d, J = 2.0) | 93.9 d | 6.51 (1H, d, J = 2.0) | 94.0 d |
| 9 | – | 157.3 s | – | 157.3 s |
| 10 | – | 103.7 s | – | 103.7 s |
| 1' | – | 121.1 s | – | 122.8 s |
| 2' | 7.92 (2H, dd, J = 6.9, 1.9) | 128.4 d | 8.03 (2H, d, J = 8.9) | 128.2 d |
| 3' | 6.93 (2H, dd, J = 6.9, 1.9) | 115.9 d | 7.11 (2H, d, J = 8.9) | 114.5 d |
| 4' | – | 161.4 s | – | 162.3 s |
| 5' | 6.93 (2H, dd, J = 6.9, 1.9) | 115.9 d | 7.11 (2H, d, J = 8.9) | 114.5 d |
| 6' | 7.92 (2H, dd, J = 6.9, 1.9) | 128.4 d | 8.03 (2H, d, J = 8.9) | 128.2 d |
| 5–OH | 12.95 (1H, s) | – | 12.91 (1H, s) | – |
| 7–OH | 10.82 (1H, s) | – | – | – |
| 4'–OH | 10.3 (1H, s) | – | – | – |
| 4'–$OCH_3$ | – | – | 3.86 (3H,s) | 55.5 q |

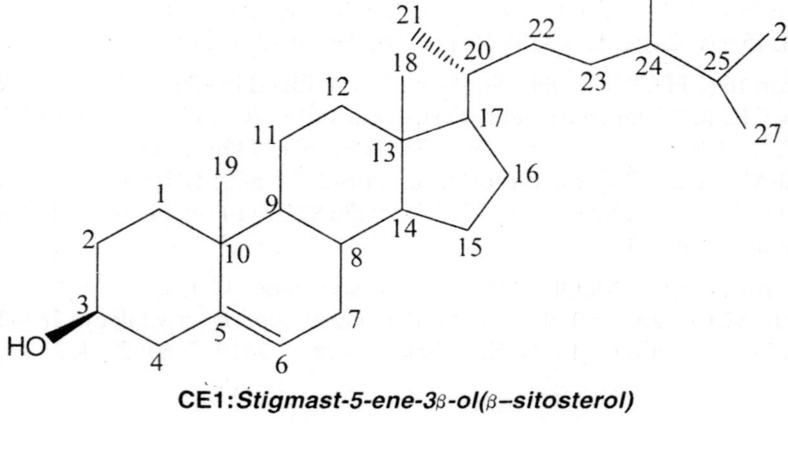


**CE1:*Stigmast-5-ene-3β-ol(β–sitosterol)***

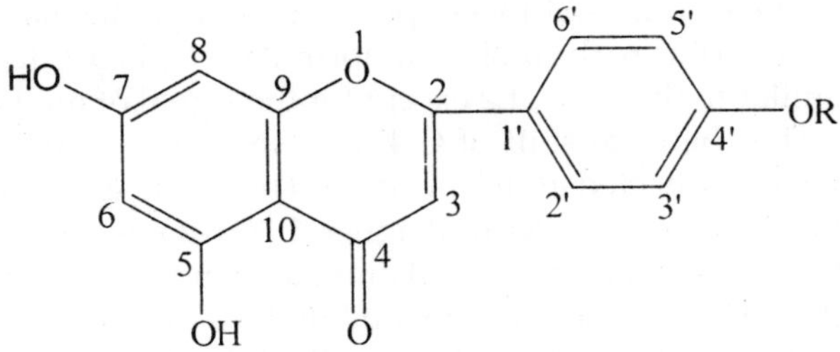

**CE2: R= H *5,7,4'–trihydroxyl flavone***

**CE3: R=$CH_3$ *5,7-dihidroxyl-4'-methoxy flavone***

## 3.0 Results and Discussion

The methanol extract (126.4g) of *C. inerme* leaves was partitioned successively with n-hexane and then ethyl acetate. The solvents were evaporated *in vacuo* to afford the *n*-hexane–(29.9g) and EtOAc–(27.7g) extracts. Column chromatography separation of 10g ethyl acetate extract over silica gel was carried out to yield three compounds.

Compound 1 (CE1) has the molecular formula of $C_{29}H_{50}O$ from positive ESI-MS (*m/z* 414 $[M]^+$) and $^{13}$C-NMR data. The molecule CE1 contains 29 carbons, including six methyl, 11 methylene, 9 methine groups and 3 quaternary carbons. The $^1$H-NMR spectrum indicated a multiplet signal at 3.25 ppm specific to proton of oxygenated methine group at C-3, a multiplet signal at $\delta_H$ 5.34 of double bond (-CH=C<). Its IR spectrum showed the presence of hydroxyl (3434cm-1) and double link (1645cm$^{-1}$). By detail comparison with the published spectral data (Gupta, 1994; Panday, 2003) the structure of 1 was determined as β–sitosterol or stigmast-5-en-3β-ol.

Compound 2 (CE2) was obtained as an yellow amorphous powder. IR spectrum showed the presence of hydroxyl group (3318 cm$^{-1}$), aromatic ring (1609 cm$^{-1}$ and 1556 cm$^{-1}$), carbonyl group (1653cm$^{-1}$). The molecular constitution of 2 was indicated to be $C_{15}H_{10}O_5$ from the molecular ion peak at *m/z* 270 $[M]^+$ in the EI-mass spectrum and $^{13}$C-NMR spectroscopic data. Its $^1$H–and $^{13}$C-NMR spectra indicated typical signals of flavone skeleton, containing a ketone signal at $\delta_C$181.7, the proton signal of 5-OH group shifted in the down field ($\delta_H$12.95) due to the intermolecular hydrogen-bridge with ketone group. Furthermore, a singlet signal at $\delta_H$ 6.77 was assigned to H-3 of flavone. In addition, $^1$H–and $^{13}$C-NMR spectra also showed the signals of two aromatic rings. Based on the proton multiplicities of two aromatic rings, the connecting positions of two hydroxyl groups at C-7 and C-4' were determined. Consequently, the structure of CE2 was established as 5,7,4'-trihydroxy flavone by comparison with the reported spectroscopic data of apigenin (Ersoz, 2002). This compound was isolated from different species. Apigenin is known to have antioxidant, anti-inflammatory and anti-tumor properties. This compound can also prevent the formation of uric acid, therefore probably use for treatment gout disease (Ersoz, 2002).

Compound 3 (CE3) was obtained as an yellow amorphous powder. Its IR spectrum showed the presence of 3440cm$^{-1}$ ($\nu_{OH}$); 1655cm$^{-1}$ ($\nu_{>C=O}$); 1604, 1559,

1508cm$^{-1}$ ($\nu_{C=C}$ benzene ring). ESI-mass spectrum gave molecular ion peak at *m/z* 285[M + H]$^+$, corresponding to the molecular formula of $C_{16}H_{12}O_5$. Its $^1$H–và $^{13}$C-NMR spectra is very similar to those of CE2 except for the signal of methoxyl group at $\delta_H$ 3.86 and $\delta_C$ 55.5. The chemical shift of C-4' was shifted at $\delta_C$ 162.3 indicating the methoxyl group was connected at this position. The NMR spectral data of CE3 are good agreement with those of acacetin (Wagner, 1976). It was reported that acacetin has antiperoxidant, antimutagenic, anti-inflammatory and antiplasmodial properties. Some recent studies showed that acacetin inhibited the proliferation of human lung and liver cancer cells (HepG2 and A549, respectively) (Martinez-Vazquez, 1998)

## References

Chi, V.V., 1997. Dictionary of Vietnamese Medicinal Plants, Publishing House Medicine, pp. 316

Ersoz, T., 2002, Phenolic compounds from *Scutellaria pontica*, Turk journal of chemistry, Vol. 26, p. 583.

Gupta, S. and Ali, M., 1994. Isolation and characterization of a dihidroxysterol from *Lawsonia inerme*, Natural Product Letters, Vol 4, pp 195-201.

Martinez-Vazquez M., Apan R.T.O., Lastra A.L. and Bye R., 1998, Planta Med., Vol 64, pp.134–137.

Pandey, R. and Verma, R. K., 2003. " 4α–Methyl–24β–ethyl–5α-cholesta-14,15-dien-3β-ol and 24β-ethylcholesta-5,9(11), 22-E-triene-3β-ol, sterol from *Clerodendrum inerme*", Phytochemistry, 63, pp 415-420.

Wagner, H. and Chari, V. M., 1976, Tetrahedron Letters, Vol 21, pp 1789-1802.

## *Chapter 19*

# Isolation and Characterization of Triterpenes and a Phenolic Glycoside from *Celastrus hindsii* Benth

***Trinh Thi Thuy*, Tran Van Sung, Nguyen Huy Cuong and Pham Thi Ninh***

*Institute of Chemistry, Vietnamese Academy of Science and Technology*
*18-Hoang Quoc Viet Road, Hanoi, Vietnam*
**E-mail: ttt@ich.vast.ac.vn*

## ABSTRACT

Clionasterol, 3-friedelanol, canophyllol, 3-friedelanone, friedelan-3, 21-dione, lup-20 (29)-ene-3β-ol, lup-12-ene-3β-ol, lup-20(29)-ene-3β,11β-diol, lup-20(29)-ene-3-one (lupenone) and lup-5,20(29)-diene-3-one as well as glucosyringic acid were isolated and structural determinated from the leaves and stems of *Celastrus hindsii* collected in Quang Binh, Vietnam. Their structures were determined on the basis of MS, NMR spectroscopic data and comparison with reported data.

***Keywords:*** *Celastrus hindsii, Celastraceae, Triterpenes, Friedelanol, Friedelanone, Canophyllol, Glucosyringic acid.*

## 1.0 Introduction

The Celastraceae constitutes approximately 88 genera and over 1300 species are widely distributed throughout South America, China and Vietnam. They have been chemically intensive studied due to many biological activities. Plant extracts of Celastraceae have been used for centuries as insect repellents and insecticides in traditional agriculture and also for the treatment of stomach disease and cancer

(Yao-Haur, 1997). *Celastrus hindsii* Benth is a small tree growing wild or cultivated in Son La, Hoa Binh, Quang Ninh, Nam Dinh, Ha Nam, Quang Binh provinces of Vietnam. The EtOH extract of its stems shows potent cytotoxicity against *hepatoma, cervix carcinoma, colon carcinoma* and *nasological carcinoma* cells as well as against HIV replication activity in H-9 lymphocytes *in vitro*. Phytochemical investigation of *C. hindsii* was reported to contain triterpenes, sesquiterpene pyridine alkaloids as its main components. The crude extract of C. under the local name "Xa den" is used successfully as antitumor, anticancer agents in the Army Hospital (QY108 Hospital) (Ly, 2006). In our search for biological active compounds from Celastrus species, we now report the isolation and structural determination of clionasterol (1), nine triterpenes 3-friedelanol (2), 3-friedelanone (3), D: A-friedo-oleanane (4), canophyllol (5), lup-20(29)-ene-3$\beta$-ol (6), lup-12-ene-3$\beta$-ol (7), lup-20(29)-ene-3$\beta$,11$\beta$-diol (8), lup-20(29)-ene-3-one (lupenone, 9), lup-5,20(29)-diene-3-one (10) as well as glucosyringic acid (11) from the leaves and stems of this plant collected in Quang Binh, Vietnam. These structures were determined on the basis of MS, NMR spectroscopic data and comparison with reported data.

## 2.0 Materials and Methods

### 2.1 General

NMR: BRUKER Avance 500 spectrometer at 499.8 MHz ($^1$H) and 125 MHz ($^{13}$C, $^{13}$C DEPT). Chemical shifts were referenced to internal TMS ($\delta$ = 0, $^1$H), $CDCl_3$ ($\delta$ = 77.0, $^{13}$C) and $CD_3OD$ ($\delta$ = 49.0, $^{13}$C). CC: Silica gel 60, 0.06-0.2 mm (Merck) for the first column, silica gel 60, 40-63 µm (Merck) for the following columns. TLC: Silica gel 60 F-254 (Merck).

### 2.2 Plant Material

The leaves of *C. hindsii* were collected in Quang Binh, Vietnam in October 2005. The species was identified by Mr. Nguyen Quoc Binh, Institute of Ecology and Natural Resources, VAST, Hanoi, Vietnam. A voucher specimen is deposited in the Herbarium of this Institute.

### 2.3 Extraction and Isolation

The dried and powdered leaves of *C. hindsii* were extracted with 90 per cent aq. EtOH at room temperature. EtOH was evaporated *in vacuo* at 45°C and the aq. solution was partitioned with *n*-hexane followed by EtOAc and *n*-BuOH. The organic solvents were evaporated *in vacuo* to afford 25.5; 2.5; 15 g of *n*-hexane, EtOAc and *n*-BuOH extracts, respectively. The extracts were chromatographed over silica gel or sephadex LH-20 and, recrystallized to give pure compounds.

## 3.0 Results and Discussion

Compound 1 was obtained as white needles from the EtOAc extract using column chromatography on silica gel. The ESI-MS spectrum gave a peak at *m/z* 414 $[M]^+$, corresponding to the molecular formula $C_{29}H_{50}O$. The $^1$H–and $^{13}$C-NMR spectral data of 1 contained six methyl, one hydroxyl groups. The $^{13}$C-NMR spectrum was similar to those of $\beta$-sitosterol, except for the significant changes in chemical shifts at C-24 and its neighbour, which could be explained the other configuration at C-24 is different.

Therefore, the structure of 1 was determined as clionasterol (γ-sitosterol), which was isolated for the first time from *Cliona celata* (Thuy, 2006b).

The ESI-MS of compound 2 gave a peak at *m/z* 411[M+H-$H_2O$]$^+$(100 per cent), corresponding to the molecular formula $C_{30}H_{52}O$. The IR spectrum indicated a hydroxyl (3478 $cm^{-1}$), a ketone (1703 $cm^{-1}$) group. The $^{13}$C-NMR and DEPT spectra showed the presence of signals for 30 carbons including $CH_3$ x 8, $CH_2$ x 11, CH x 5, Cq x 6, suggested that 2 have a friedelin triterpene skeleton. This was further confirmed by the signals of one secondary, 7 tertiary methyl groups in the $^1$H-NMR spectrum. The structure of 2 was identified as 3-friedelanol by comparison of the $^1$H–and $^{13}$C-NMR spectra with those of reported data.

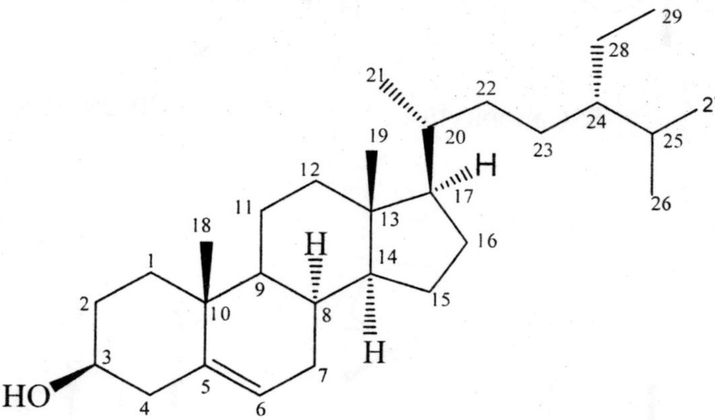

**1**: Clionasterol

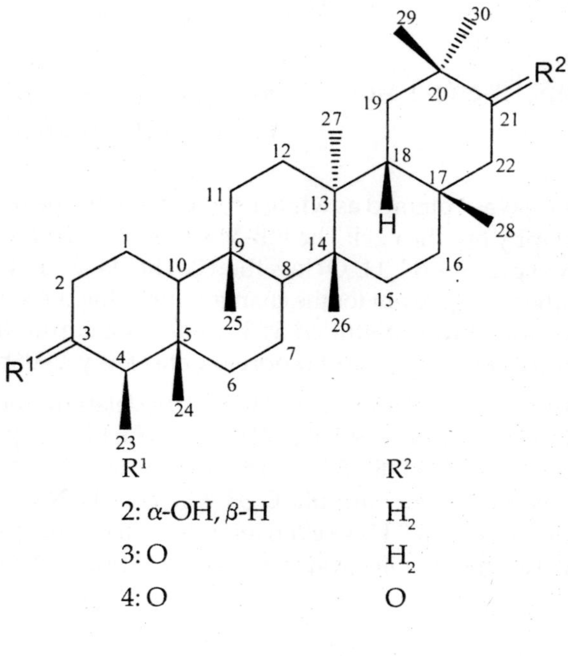

| | $R^1$ | $R^2$ |
|---|---|---|
| 2: | α-OH, β-H | $H_2$ |
| 3: | O | $H_2$ |
| 4: | O | O |

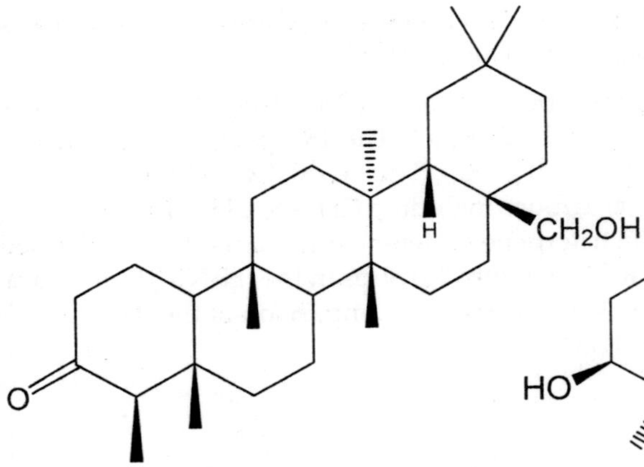


**5**: Canophyllol

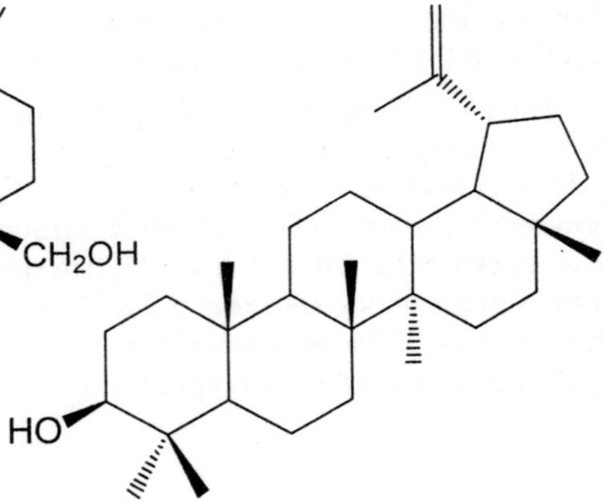


**6**: Lup-20(29)-ene-3β-ol

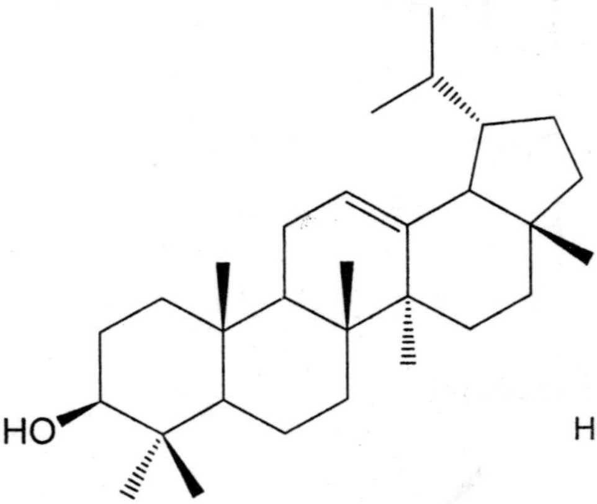


**7**: Lup-12-ene-3β-ol

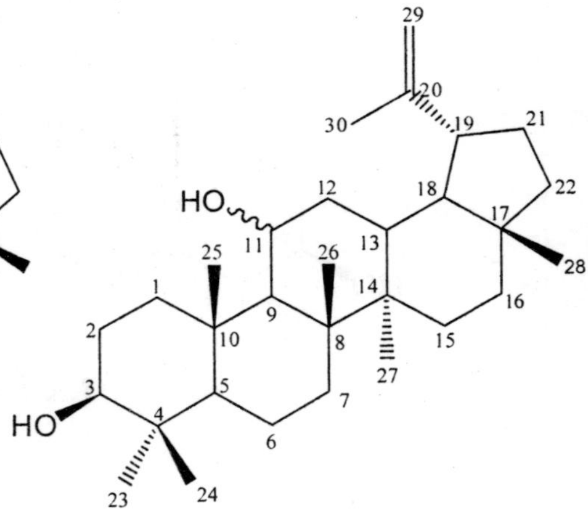


**8** : Lup-20,29-ene-3β,11β-diol
**8a**: Lup-20,29-ene-3β,11α-diol

3-Friedelanone (3) was obtained as white needles from the hexane extract using column chromatography on silica gel. The ESI-MS spectrum gave a peak at *m/z* 427 $[M+H]^+$ and have two protons ($C_{30}H_{50}O$) less than 2. The $^1$H–and $^{13}$C-NMR spectral data were similar to those of 2, except for the changes due to the presence of a carbonyl group ($\delta_C$ 213.2) therefore 3 was identified as 3-friedelanone from its identical $^1$H– and $^{13}$C-NMR spectral data with those of reported data (Thuy, 2006b).

Compound 4 is a pentacyclic triterpenoid with a friedelane dione skeleton. Its IR spectrum indicated a ketone group (>C=O, 1710 cm$^{-1}$). The EI-MS spectrum showed a molecular ion peak at *m/z* 440 (8) $[M]^+$, combination with $^{13}$C-NMR and DEPT spectra leading to the molecular formula $C_{30}H_{30}O_2$. The $^1$H-NMR displayed one secondary methyl (δ 0.89, d, J=6,5 Hz), seven tertiary methyl groups (δ 0.73, 1.05x2, 0.88, 1.08, 1.17, 1.16), two methylene groups, one of them [δ 2.60, 1.81 (each 1H, d, J=

**Table 19.1: $^{13}$C-NMR Spectral Data of 1–5, 8 and 9 [125 MHz, $CDCl_3$, δ (ppm)]**

| *C* | *1* | *2* | *3* | *4* | *5* | *8* | *8a** | *9* |
|---|---|---|---|---|---|---|---|---|
| 1 | 37.29 | 18.66 | 22.29 | 22.27 | 22.70 | 38.07 | 39.00 | 39.79 |
| 2 | 31.69 | 39.30 | 41.53 | 41.20 | 41.51 | 25.13 | 27.50 | 34.53 |
| 3 | 71.78 | 72.78 | 213.18 | 212.96 | 213.13 | 79.03 | 78.60 | 216.76 |
| 4 | 42.34 | 53.22 | 58.24 | 58.22 | 58.23 | 38.89 | 39.40 | 47.25 |
| 5 | 140.83 | 39.70 | 42.15 | 42.74 | 42.11 | 53.14 | 55.60 | 54.31 |
| 6 | 121.69 | 41.75 | 41.31 | 41.49 | 41.25 | 18.01 | 18.10 | 18.66 |
| 7 | 31.94 | 17.57 | 18.25 | 18.27 | 18.25 | 34.14 | 35.30 | 33.72 |
| 8 | 31.94 | 49.20 | 53.12 | 53.35 | 52.50 | 41.39 | 41.00 | 40.86 |
| 9 | 50.18 | 37.85 | 37.46 | 37.01 | 37.47 | 51.31 | 55.70 | 48.79 |
| 10 | 36.54 | 61.38 | 59.50 | 59.43 | 59.49 | 38.89 | 37.70 | 58.13 |
| 11 | 21.11 | 32.84 | 35.64 | 35.53 | 34.51 | 75.77 | 70.40 | 22.54 |
| 12 | 39.81 | 30.66 | 30.52 | 30.61 | 28.15 | 23.29 | 27.70 | 24.87 |
| 13 | 42.35 | 38.39 | 39.71 | 38.18 | 38.16 | 37.61 | 37.70 | 38.49 |
| 14 | 56.80 | 37.13 | 38.32 | 39.91 | 37.47 | 42.93 | 42.60 | 41.98 |
| 15 | 24.33 | 30.66 | 32.80 | 32.77 | 29.14 | 27.55 | 27.50 | 27.41 |
| 16 | 28.26 | 32.36 | 36.03 | 37.01 | 31.26 | 35.60 | 55.50 | 35.67 |
| 17 | 56.10 | 37.86 | 30.01 | 33.22 | 35.17 | 42.93 | 43.00 | 41.98 |
| 18 | 19.41 | 42.85 | 42.82 | 41.93 | 39.38 | 48.36 | 47.70 | 41.23 |
| 19 | 11.88 | 32.84 | 35.36 | 35.08 | 33.38 | 48.00 | 47.70 | 47.25 |
| 20 | 36.17 | 30.04 | 28.17 | 42.10 | 30.10 | 150.81 | 150.20 | 149.81 |
| 21 | 19.06 | 32.35 | 32.44 | 218.85 | 31.41 | 29.80 | 29.80 | 30.07 |
| 22 | 33.99 | 41.75 | 39.26 | 54.99 | 41.51 | 40.02 | 39.80 | 40.51 |
| 23 | 26.15 | 11.63 | 6.82 | 6.83 | 6.82 | 27.86 | 28.30 | 26.43 |
| 24 | 45.88 | 16.41 | 14.66 | 14.66 | 14.67 | 14.94 | 15.50 | 14.45 |
| 25 | 29.21 | 20.13 | 17.95 | 18.47 | 19.20 | 16.25 | 16.10 | 16.47 |
| 26 | 19.83 | 18.66 | 20.26 | 21.20 | 19.08 | 14.94 | 17.20 | 18.52 |
| 27 | 18.80 | 18.26 | 18.66 | 17.74 | 18.08 | 14.47 | 14.50 | 14.45 |
| 28 | 23.11 | 31.81 | 32.10 | 33.55 | 68.04 | 18.05 | 18.10 | 18.66 |
| 29 | 12.00 | 30.04 | 31.79 | 28.81 | 34.26 | 109.45 | 109.80 | 108.40 |
| 30 | | 32.10 | 35.03 | 26.62 | 32.85 | 19.24 | 19.40 | 18.66 |

* $\delta_C$ values in Lit. Ahmad, 1981.

13 Hz, $H_2$-22) was attached to a quaternary carbon atom and the other at δ 2.41 (ddd, J= 2, 5, 7 Hz, H-2A); 2.31 (dd, J= 13.7 Hz, H-2B). The EI-MS spectrum displayed four important fragment ions at *m/z* 219, 273, 233, 355, suggested that one of two carbonyl group attached at C-21 or C-22 in ring E (Scheme 1). The identity of 4 as D: A-friedelan-3,21-dione (21-oxofriedelan-3-one) was established by comparison of those spectral data with reported data (Anjaneyulu, 1993). This structure was confirmed by HMBC

and NOESY spectra. The HMBC showed a strong correlation of C-3 (δ 212.96)/Me-23 ($\delta_H$0.89), H-$2_{A,B}$ ($\delta_H$2.41; 2.31) and C-22 ($\delta_C$ 218.85)/Me-28 (δ1.08), Me-29 (δ1.17), H-18 (δ1.82), thus two carbonyl groups at C-3 and C-21. This is first time D:A-friedelan-3,21-dione was isolated from the plant, despite the fact that it was previously prepared by oxidation of D:A-friedelan-3α,21α-diol isolated from *Euphorbia tortilis* (Anjaneyulu, 1993).

**D:A-friedo-oleanan-3,21-dione (4)**

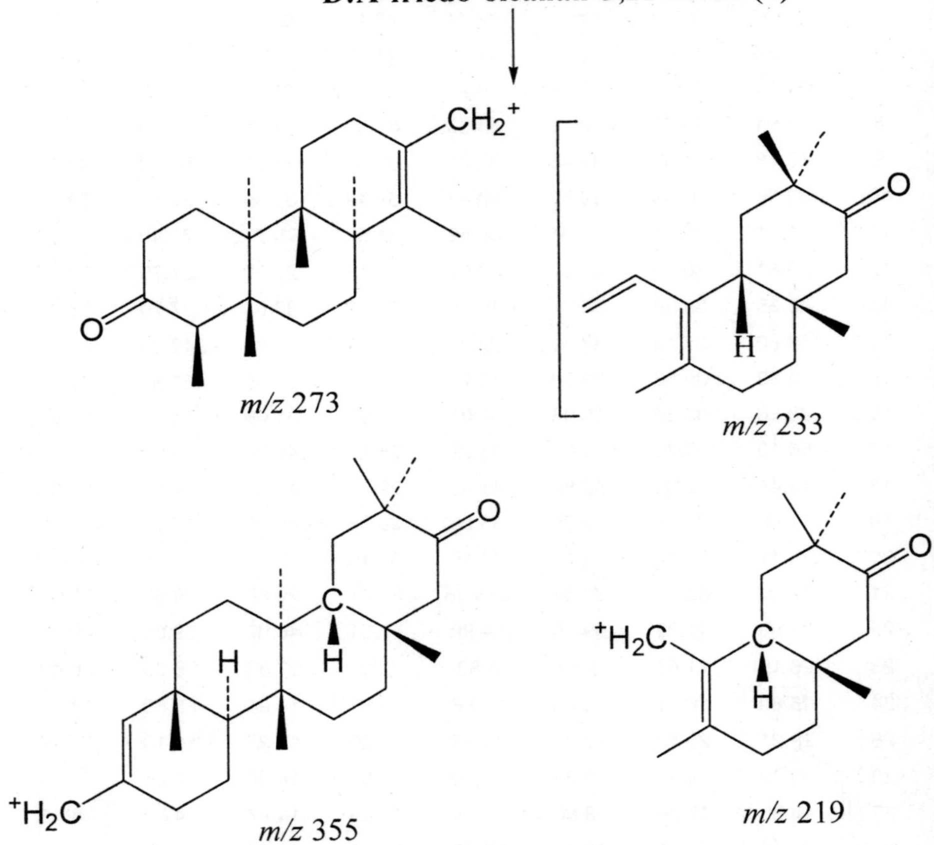


***Scheme 1:*** **EI-MS Spectral Fragmentation of 4**

Canophyllol (5) was obtained as white needles. Its IR spectrum showed bands for carbonyl (1705 $cm^{-1}$) and hydroxyl (3542 $cm^{-1}$) groups. The molecular formula was established as $C_{30}H_{50}O_2$ by combination of $^{13}$C-NMR spectral data and the peak at *m/z* 442 $[M+H]^+$(58), with one oxygen-atom more than 3. The $^1$H–and $^{13}$C-NMR spectral data were very similar to those of 3, except for the changes due to the presence of methylenoxy group ($\delta_H$ 3.64, $\delta_C$ 68.04). The $^{13}$C-NMR spectra indicated the presence of a carbonyl group ($\delta_C$213.13, C-3)) and hydroxyl group at C-28. Combination of $^1$H-$^{13}$C-NMR spectra, structure of 5 was determined as canophyllol (28-hydroxy-3-

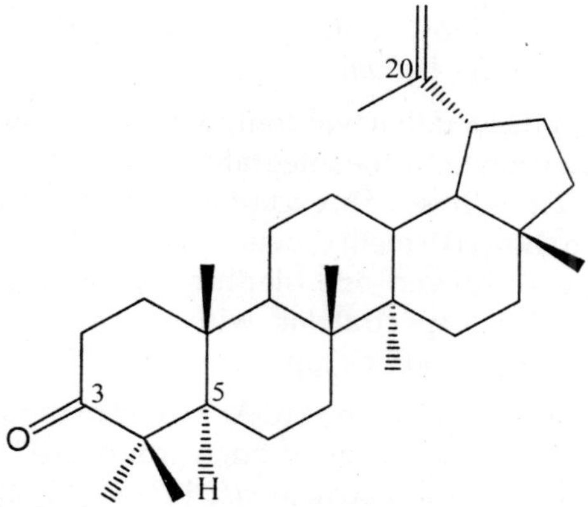

**9**: Lup-20(29)-ene-3-one

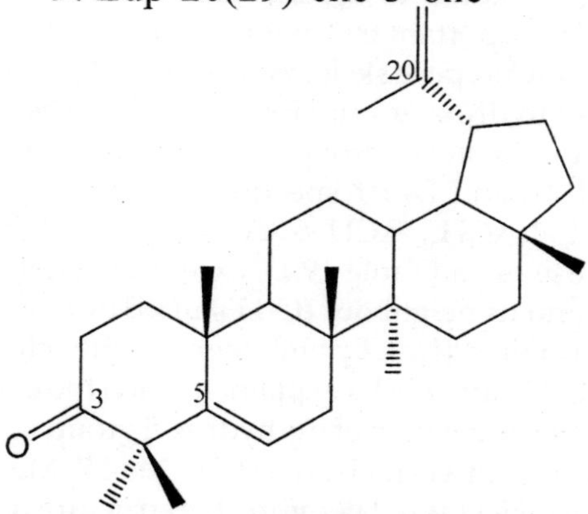

**10**: Lup-5,20(29)-diene-3-one

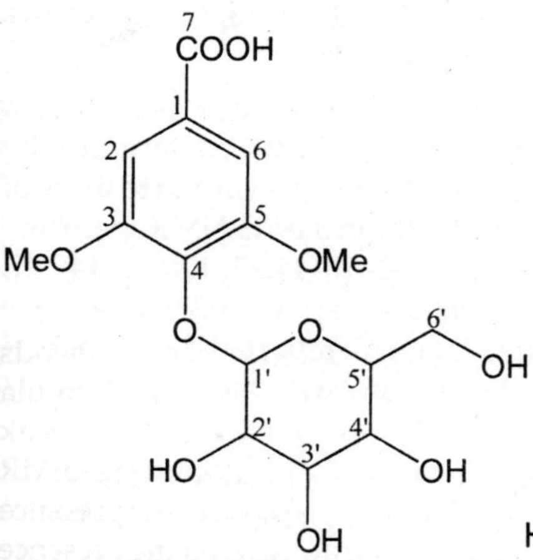

**11**: Glucosyringic acid

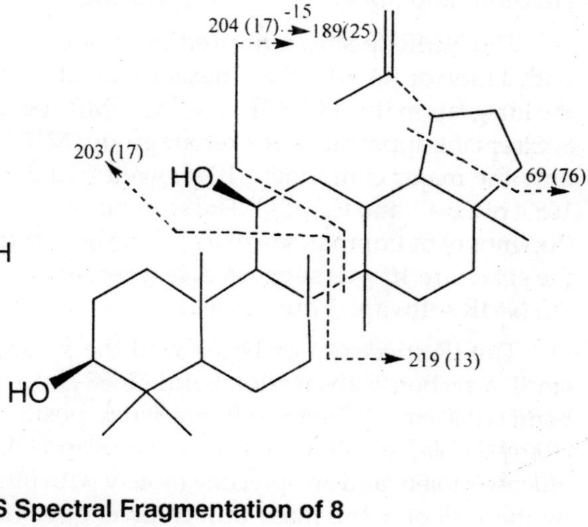


***Scheme 2:*** **EI-MS Spectral Fragmentation of 8**

friedelanone). Canophyllol shows antimicrobial activity and was isolated for the first time from *Calophyllum inophyllum*.

The NMR spectra indicated that two compounds 6+7 were isolated as a mixture with a ratio of 10:7, determined by the integrals in the $^1$H-NMR spectrum. Their $^{13}$C-NMR spectrum is similar to those of 8, except for the appearance of a double bond. The major component 6 showed a methylidene (>C=H$_2$) group ($\delta_H$ 4.56, 4.68; $\delta_C$ 109.33), while less component 7 showed one olephinic proton ($\delta_H$ 5.18; $\delta_C$ 121.75). By comparison of those $^{13}$C-NMR spectral data with reported data, 6 were identified as lup-20,29-ene-3*β*-ol (lupenol) and 7 as lup-12-ene-3*β*-ol (Thuy, 2006b).

Compound 8 was isolated from the EtOAc extract of the stems. The IR spectrum indicated a hydroxy (3363 cm$^{-1}$) and methyliden group (1641, 3070 cm$^{-1}$). The EI-MS spectrum showed a molecular ion peak at *m/z* 442 (2) [M]$^+$, combination with $^{13}$C-NMR and DEPT spectra leading to the molecular formula $C_{30}H_{50}O_2$. The EI-MS spectrum displayed three important fragment ions at *m/z* 219 (13), 203 (17), 189 (25), suggested that 8 is a lupan-triterpene skeleton. The peak at *m/z* 203 indicated fragment ion of ring A-B with C-3 hydroxy group; ion at *m/z* 219 was formed by the C-ring cleavage indicated that the second hydroxy was in the fragment of ring D-E as shown in *Scheme* 2. The $^{13}$C-NMR and DEPT spectra showed the presence of 30 carbon signals including 7xCH$_3$, 10xCH$_2$, 7xCH, 6xCq. The $^1$H–and $^{13}$C-NMR spectral data for 8 was similar to those of 8a (Table 19.1), except the significant changes in the chemical shifts at C-11 and its neighbour (C-11 shifted downfield (D$\delta$ 5.4 ppm), C-9 and C-12 were shifted up field (D$\delta$4.4 ppm). Significantly changes in the chemical shifts of C-11, C-9 and C-12 can only be explained when the configuration of C-11 is different to those of 8a. The orientation of the hydroxyl group was clarified by NOESY spectrum. The correlations between H-11$\alpha$/H-3$\alpha$, Me-27, Me-30 indicated that the relative configuration of OH-11 is *β*. Therefore, the structure of 8 was determined as lup-20,29-ene-3*β*,11*β*-diol. This compound was isolated for the first time from *Dodonaceae attennuata*. Its epimer, lup-20,29-ene-3*β*,11*a*-diol (nepeticin) shows antibiotic and blood cholesterol reducing activity (Thuy, 2006b).

The NMR spectra indicated that compounds 9+10 were isolated as a mixture with a ratio of 1:4 from the n-hexane extract of the leaves of *C. hindsii*, determined by the integrals in the $^1$H-NMR. The $^{13}$C-NMR spectrum of 9 and 10 is similar to those of 8, except the appearance of a ketone group ($\delta$216.76/216.71). In the $^{13}$C-NMR spectrum, only the major component 10 showed two double bonds ($\delta$144.25, 120.51, 149.81, 108.4 of $C_5$=$C_6$ and $C_{20}$=$C_{29}$). The structure of 9 was identified as lup-20(29)-ene-3-one (lupenone) by comparison of its $^{13}$C-NMR spectral data with reported data, whereas the structure 10 was suggested as lup-5,20(29)-diene-3-one with the help of ACD/$^{13}$C-NMR software (Thuy, 2006a).

The IR spectrum of 11 showed the presence of hydroxyl groups (3440-3524 cm$^{-1}$), a carbonyl absorption band (1668 cm$^{-1}$), aromatic ring (1600 cm$^{-1}$) and–C-O bond (1008 cm$^{-1}$). The ESI-MS spectrum (positive ions) gave the base peak at *m/z* 383 (100) [M+Na]$^+$ ($C_{15}H_{20}O_{10}$). The $^{13}$C-NMR and DEPT spectra showed the presence of a glucose moiety and an aglycone moiety with nine carbon atoms. This was supported by the loss of a 162 mass unit to give a peak at *m/z* 199 [M+H-162]$^+$ in the mass spectrum. The appearance of six signals in the $^{13}$C-NMR spectrum of the aglycone moiety corresponded to nine carbons, indicating that the molecule must be a degree of symmetry in its structure. This was confirmed by two singlets at δ7.39 (H-2 and H-6) and 3.92 (6H, 2x$OCH_3$), therefore two methoxyl groups were attached at C-3 and C-5. The $^1$H-NMR spectrum displayed one doublet at δ5.28 (d, J= 8.0 Hz, H-1') and the $^{13}$C-NMR signal at $\delta_C$104.29 (C-1'), suggesting that β-D-glucose moiety was attached to C-4. This was confirmed by the CH long-range correlation of $\delta_C$169.66 (C-4) / $\delta_H$5.09 (H-1'), whereas C-7 shows correlations to both H-2, H-6 ($\delta_C$169.66/$\delta_H$7.39) in the HMBC spectrum (Table 19.2). Therefore, structure of 11 was elucidated as glucosyringic acid, which was isolated for the first time from the roots of *Rododendron molle*. In a preliminary in *vitro* bioassay glucosyringic acid inhibited significantly the proliferation of murine B lymphocytes at a concentration of 1x $10^{-6}$ M (Thuy, 2006b).

**Table 19.2: $^{13}$C–and $^1$H-NMR Spectral Data of 11 [125 MHz, $CD_3OD$, δ (ppm)]**

| *C* | $\delta_C$ | $\delta_H$ *(J in Hz)* | *HMBC correlation* |
|---|---|---|---|
| 1 | 127.61 | | H-2, H-6 |
| 2,6 | 108.81 | 7.39, 2H | 5-OMe |
| 3,5 | 153.76 | | H-2, H-6, OMe, C-5/H-6, C-3/H-2 |
| 4 | 139.82 | | H-1', H-2, H-6 |
| 7 | 169.66 | | H-2, H-6 |
| 1' | 104.29 | 5.09 d (7.5) | H-2' |
| 2' | 75.28 | 3.56 m | H-1', H-3' |
| 3' | 77.34 | 3.52 m | H-2', H-4', H-5' |
| 4' | 70.86 | 5.52 m | H-3', H-5' |
| 5' | 77.91 | 3.33 m | H-4', H-6' |
| 6' | 62.05 | 3.72 dd (4.9; 11.5)<br>3.72 dd (4.9; 11.5) | H-5' |
| OMe | 57.33 | 3.92 s | H-6 |

This is the first time triterpenes 2-10 and glucosyringic acid was isolated from *Celastrus* sp. (Thuy, 2006 a,b). Some isolated compounds (1, 4, 6+7 and 8) were screened for antibacterial and antifungal activity. The micro organisms used are: *Escherichia coli (Ec); Pseudomonas aeruginosa (Pa); Bacillus subtillis (Bs); Staphylococcus aureus (Sa); Candida albicans (ca).* Lup-20,29-ene-3β,11β-diol (8) inhibited the growth of *Stahylococcus aureus* microorganisms.

## Acknowledgements

We thank Mr. Nguyen Quoc Binh, Institute of Ecology and Natural Resources, VAST, Hanoi, Vietnam for identification of plant materials.

## References

Ahmad, V. U., 1981. Nepeticin from *Nepeta hindostana*. Tetrahedron Letters 22, 1715.

Anjaneyulu, V., Suresh, B. J., Hari, B. K. B., Connolly, J. D., 1993. Two D: A-friedo-oleane derivatives from *Euphorbia tortilis*. Phytochemistry 33 (3), 647-649

Yao-Haur Kuo, Yang Kuo Li-Ming, 1997. Antitumor and anti-aids triterpenes from *Celastrus hinds2*. Phytochemisty 44 (7), 1275-1281

Ly, T. N., Makoto, S., Yamauchi, R., 2006. Isolation and characterization of rosmanic acid oligomers in *Celastrus hindsii* Benth leaves and their antioxidative activity. J. Agric. Food Chem. 54, 3786-3793.

Thuy, T. T., Cuong, N. H., Ninh, P. T., Nhung, L. T. H., Sung, T. V., 2008. Isolation and structural characterization of phenolic glycoside and triterpenes in *Celastrus hindsii*, Vietnamese J. of Chem. 46 (2), 224-228.

Thuy, T. T., Cuong, N. H., Sung, T. V., 2007. Triterpenes from *Celastrus hindsii*, Vietnamese J. of Chem. 45 (3), 373-376.

## Chapter 20

# Chemical Studies on Five Vietnamese *Fissistigma* Species (Annonaceae)

***Tran Van Sung*, Trinh Phuong Lien, Trinh Thi Thuy, Nguyen Thi Hoang Anh, Nguyen Hong Van and Tran Duc Quan***

*Institute of Chemistry, Vietnam Academy of Science and Technology, Cau Giay, Hanoi, Vietnam*

**E-mail: tvs@ich.vast.ac.vn*

## ABSTRACT

The genus *Fissistigma* has a large number of species, belonging to the Annonaceae family. Most of these plants have not yet been investigated pharmacologically and phytochemically. This paper reports our results on phytochemical investigation of five *Fissistigma* species growing in Vietnam. The structures of isolated compounds were characterized on the basis of MS, NMR spectroscopic data and comparison with reported data. Some isolated compounds were assayed *in vitro* for antibacterial activity.

***Keywords:*** *Annonaceae, Fissistigma, Fissistigmatin, Fissispallin, Aporphine, Pronuciferine, Nornuciferine, Roemerine.*

## 1.0 Introduction

The genus *Fissistigma* is a large tribe with ca.70 species in the Annonaceae family (Ban, 2000). The decoctions of some *Fissistigma* species have been used in Southeast Asia as traditional medicines for treatment of infections and enhancement of blood circulation and especially to stop wound bleeding (Perry, 1980). In continuation of our investigation on the constituents of *Fissistigma,* we now present the isolation and structural elucidation of five fissistigmatins from *Fissistigma species* (*F. bracteolatum, F.*

*pallens, F. chloroneurum, F. capitatum, F. acuminatissima).* MS, NMR techniques and comparison of those spectral data with reported data determined the structures of these compounds.

## 2.0 Materials and Methods

### 2.1 General

EI-MS (70 eV, DIS): ADM 402, Finnigan TSQ 700 and HR-ESI-MS (resolution ca. 5000): QStar Pulsar (Applied Biosystems). NMR: Bruker Avance 500, 499.84 MHz ($^1$H) and 125 MHz ($^{13}$C, $^{13}$C DEPT). TMS ($\delta$ = 0.0, $^1$H), $CDCl_3$ ($\delta$= 77.0, $^{13}$C), $CD_3OD$ ($\delta$= 49.0, $^{13}$C), $(CD_3)_2CO$ ($\delta$=21.6, $^{13}$C) were references. CC: Silica gel 60, 0.06-0.2 mm (Merck) for the first column, silica gel 60, 40-63 µm (Merck) for the following columns. TLC: silica gel 60 $F_{254}$ (Merck).

### 2.2 Plant Material

Leaves of *Fissistigma* species were collected provinces in Vietnam. The species were identified by Dr. Ngo Van Trai, Institute of Materia Medica, Hanoi and A voucher specimens were deposited at the same Institute.

### 2.3 Extraction and Isolation

The plant materials were dried, ground and extracted with MeOH at room temperature. MeOH was evaporated in *vacuo* and the aq. solution was extracted with hexane, followed by EtOAc and BuOH. The solvents were evaporated under reduced pressure. The extracts were separated on silica gel with gradient hexane-EtOAc, $CHCl_3$-MeOH or EtOAc-MeOH-$H_2O$ to afford fractions. The crude compounds were separated and further purified by chromatography on silica gel or sephadex and crystallization.

## 3.0 Results and Discussion

### 3.1 *Fissistigma bracteolatum* Chatt.

*F. bracteolatum* is a creeper growing in the north Vietnam. It is used with other ingredients to treat infections and also to enhance blood circulation (Ban, 2000; Perry, 1980). Our first phytochemical investigation on the leaves of *F. bracteolatum* yielded four novel fissistigmatins A-D (1-4) and five novel chalconoids (5-9) besides two known compounds (10-11).

Fissistigmatin A (1) was isolated as white needles in a yield of 0.0080 per cent to the dry material. The molecular formula of compound 1 ($C_{33}H_{42}O_5$) was deduced from combined analysis of HR-ESI-MS at *m/z* 541.2922 $[M+Na]^+$ (calc. 541.2930) and $^1$H– and $^{13}$C-APT NMR spectra (Tables 20.1 and 20.2). The EI-MS displayed a highly conjugated flavylium type (Porzel, 2000; Lien, 2000) ion at *m/z* 297 as base peak. The chemical shift of C-4 at 30.1 clearly indicated C-4 as $sp^3$ hybridized carbon. By combination of homo–and heteronuclear two-dimensional NMR experiment the remaining moiety was identified as a eudesmane. The relative stereochemistry was deduced from the NOESY and NOE difference experiment. The absolute configuration of 1 was confirmed by X-ray crystallographic analysis of its *p*-bromo-benzoate derivative (Porzel, 2000).

Fissistigmatin B (2) was isolated as colorless oil in a yield of 0.0012 per cent, exhibiting the same EI–and ESI-MS spectra as fissistigmatin A (1) and consequently the same molecular formula ($C_{33}H_{42}O_5$). $^1$H–and $^{13}$C-NMR spectra of 2 (Tables 20.1 and 20.2) were quite similar to those of 1. Noticeable differences in chemical shifts in comparison with 1 were observed for position C-2, 3, 4, 1'', 2'', 9'', 14'', suggesting that 2 is stereoisomer of 1 with S-configuration at C-4. This was confirmed by the CD spectrum, which showed a mirrored curve compared with that of 1 (Porzel, 2000).

Fissistigmatin C (3) was isolated as white needles in a yield of 0.0011 per cent. The molecular formula of 1 as $C_{33}H_{40}O_4$, established by ESI-MS (*m/z* 523, [M+Na]$^+$) as well as analysis of and $^{13}$C-APT and HSQC-NMR spectra (Tables 20.1 and 20.2) indicated the loss of one $H_2O$ molecule compared with 1 and 2. The $^1$H–and $^{13}$C-NMR spectral data of 3 were quite similar to those of 1, except for one methyl group replaced by a terminal methylene group ($\delta$c 105.9, $\delta_H$ 4.64 and 4.43).

Fissistigmatin D (4) was isolated as colourless amorphous solid in a yield of 0.0012 per cent. The EI-MS displayed a highly conjugated flavylium type (Porzel, 2000; Lien, 2000) ion at *m/z* 297 as base peak. The NMR spectra showed the presence of a flavonoid moiety with the same substitution pattern as for 1-3, however the sesquiterpene moiety was quite different to those of 1, 2 and 3. Based on comparison of the NMR data the sesquiterpene moiety was determined as globulol. The flavonoid and the sesquiterpene moiety connected *via* a C-4–C-11'' bond were confirmed by the HMBC correlations of H-4 with C-1''/C-11''/C-12'' and Me-12'' with C-4. The (4*S*)-configuration is determined by strong cross peak between H-3 and H-1$\beta$''/$H_3$-13'' and between H-4 and H-1$\beta$''/H-10$\beta$'' in the NOESY spectrum. Fissistigmatins A-D (1-4) belongs to a novel type of natural product bearing a flavonoid and a sesquiterpene unit connected *via* a C-C bond (Porzel, 2000).

The structures of five new chalconoids were elucidated as 2-hydroxy-3,4,6-trimethoxychalcone (5), 2-hydroxy-3,4,6-trimethoxychacone (6), 2'-hydroxy-3',4',6'-trimethoxydihydrochalcone (7), 2'-hydroxy-3',4',6'-trimethoxy-$\beta$'-methoxychalcane (8), 2-hydroxy-3',4',6'-trimethoxy-$\beta$'-ethoxychalcane (9) by combination of MS and 2D-NMR techniques (Lien, 2000).

## 3.2 *Fissistigma pallens* (Fin. and Gagn.) Merr.

*F. pallens* is growing in the North Vietnam, its chemical constituents have not yet been studied. From the leaves and branches of *F. pallens* a novel eudesmane glycoside named fissispallin (12) have been isolated besides afzelin (13).

The HR-ESI-MS of compound 12 gave the [M+Na]$^+$ peak at *m/z* 537.2835 (calc. 537.2823) leading to the molecular formula $C_{30}H_{42}O_7$. The sugar moiety was identified from its characteristic signals in the $^1$H–and $^{13}$C-NMR spectra as $\beta$-glucopyranose. The presence of the *trans*-cinnamate moiety is confirmed by the appearance of two doublets at $\delta$ 7.73 and 6.44 (each 1H, d, *J*=16.0 Hz) in the $^1$H-NMR spectrum.

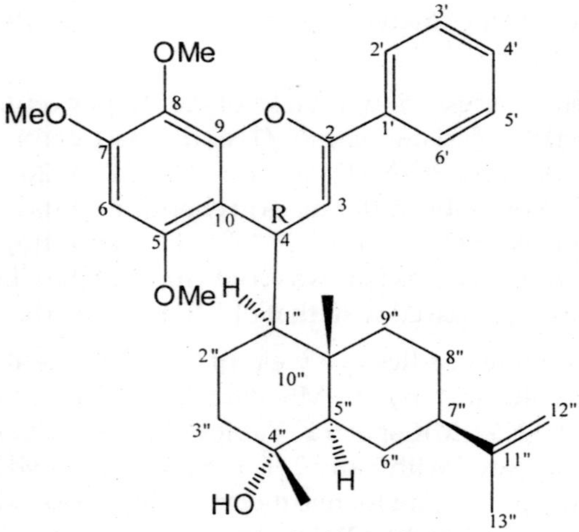

**1**: Fissistigmatin A

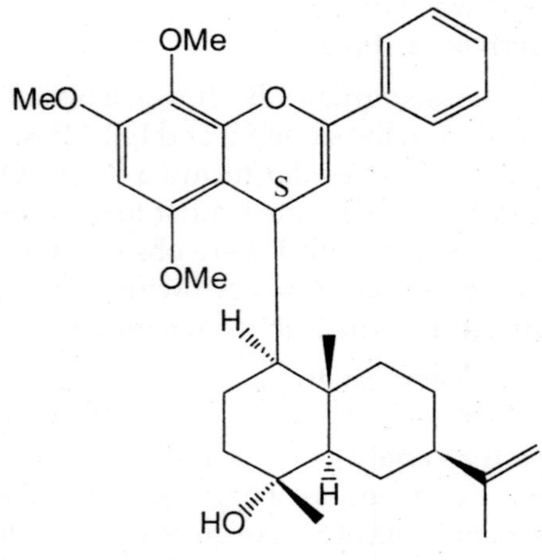

**2:** Fissistigmatin B

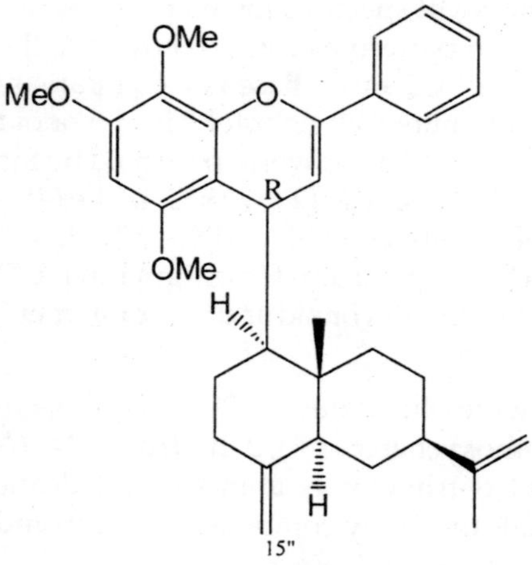

**3**: Fissistigmatin C

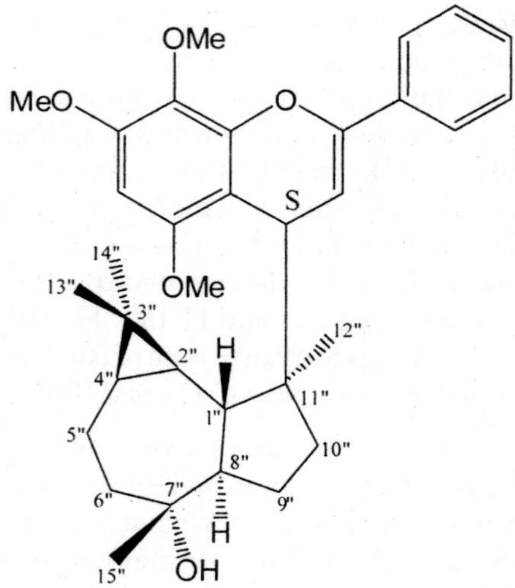

**4:** Fissistigmatin D

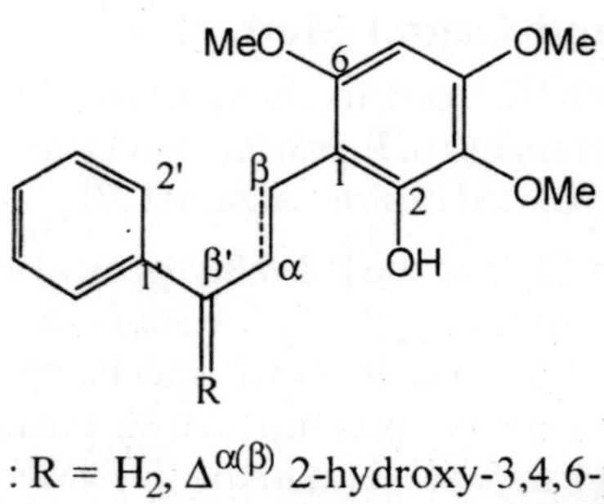

**5** : R = $H_2$, $\Delta^{\alpha(\beta)}$ 2-hydroxy-3,4,6-trimethoxychalcene

**6** : R = O 2-hydroxy-3,4,6-trimethoxydihydrochalcone

**10** : R = O, $\Delta^{\alpha(\beta)}$ 2-hydroxy-3,4,6-trimethoxychalcene

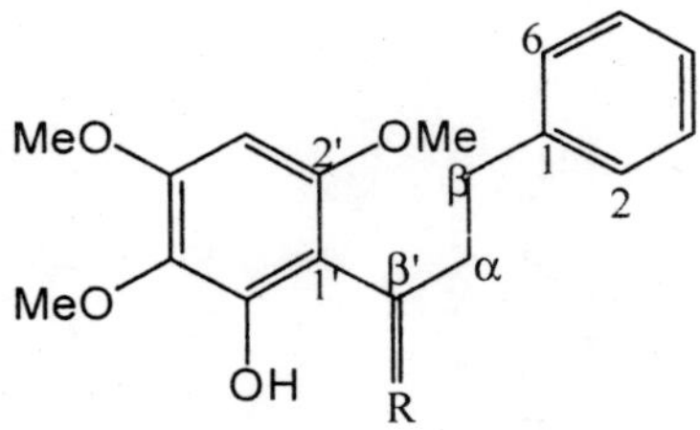

**7**: R = O : 2'-hydroxy-3',4',6'-trimethoxychalcone
**8**: R = OMe, H : 2'-hydroxy-3',4',6'-trimethoxy-β'-methoxychalcane
**9**: R = OEt, H : 2-hydroxy-3',4',6'-trimethoxy-β'-ethoxychalcanchalcane

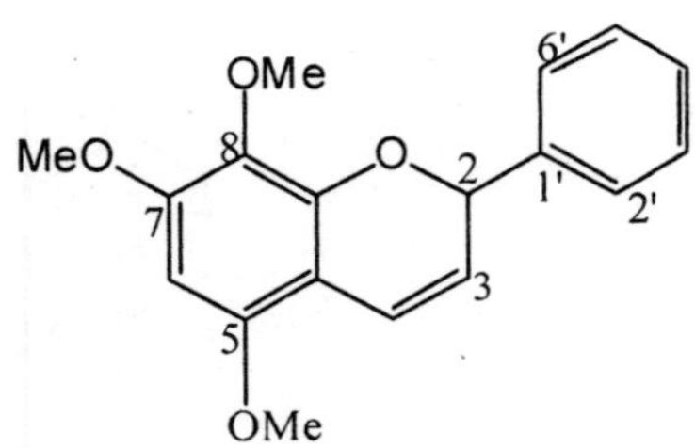

**11**: 5,7,8-trimethoxyflav-3-ene

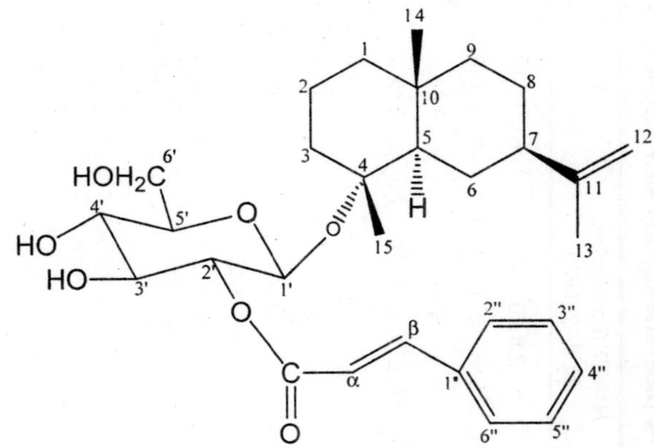

**12**: Fissispalin

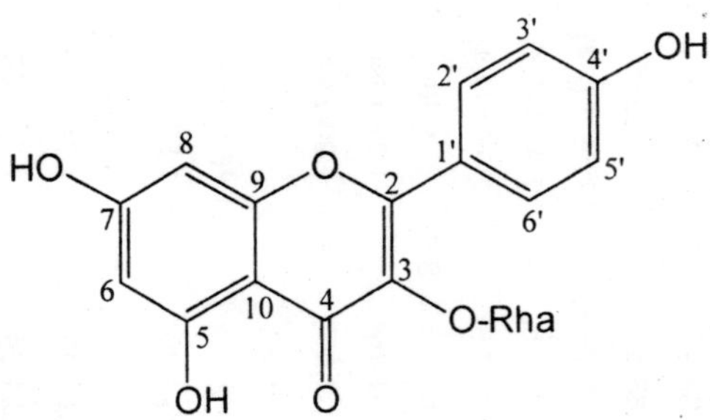

**13**:Afzelin

The linkage between cinnamic acid and glucose could be revealed by a broad triplet in the lower field at δ 4.79 (J=7.9 Hz, H-2´) in the $^{1}$H-NMR and confirmed by the HMBC correlations C=O/H-2´, H-α, H-β. The structure of 12 is elucidated as eudesm-11-ene-4-α-O-β-2-cinnamoyloxy glucopyranoside, named as fissispallin. Fissispallin is the first natural representative of ester of cinnamic acid and sesquiterpene glycoside. Compound 13 was identified as afzelin by comparison of its spectral data with reported values (Thuy, 2006a,b).

**Table 20.1: $^1$H-NMR Spectral Data of 1–4 [acetone-$d_6$, 500 MHz, $\delta$ppm ($J$ in Hz)]**

| *H* | *1* | *2* | *3* | *HMBC Correlations of 1–3 (H/C)* | *4* | *HMBC Correlations of 4 (H/C)* |
|---|---|---|---|---|---|---|
| 3 | 5.68 d (6.0) | 6.05 d (6.4) | 5.68 d (6.1) | 2,4,10, 1' | 6.00 d (6.8) | 2,4,10, 1' |
| 4 | 4.09 dd (6.0, 1.2) | 3.77 dd (6.4, 5.4) | 4.16 dd (6.1, 1.3) | 2, 3, 5, 9, 10, 1", 2", 10" | 3.69 d (6.8) | 2, 3, 5, 9, 10, 1", 10", 11", 12" |
| 5–OMe | 3.88 s | 3.86 s | 3.90 s | 5 | 3.84 s | 5 |
| 6 | 6.49 s | 6.49 s | 6.51 s | 4, 5, 7, 8, 9, 10 | 6.52 s | 4, 5, 7, 8, 9, 10 |
| 7–OMe | 3.88 s | 3.89 s | 3.89 s | 7 | 3.89 s | 7 |
| 8–OMe | 3.82 s | 3.83 s | 3.82 s | 8 | 3.82 s | 8 |
| 2'/6' | 7.78 d (7.4) | 7.81 d (7.5) | 7.76 d (7.4) | 2, 6'/2', 4' | 7.83 d (7.4) | 2, 6'/2', 4' |
| 3'/5' | 7.43 t (7.4) | 7.43 t (7.5) | 7.43 t (7.4) | 1', 2'/6', 5'/3' | 7.44 t (7.4) | 1', 5'/3' |
| 4' | 7.36 t (7.4) | 7.35 t (7.5) | 7.35 t (7.4) | 2'/6' | 7.34 t (7.4) | 2'/6' |
| 1" | 1.44 | 1.60 ddd (12.4, 5.4, 2.9) | 1.68 | | 1.45 | C–4, 2", 7", 8", 11" |
| 2" | 1.36/1.56[a] | 1.13/1.46[a] | 1.47/1.64[a] | | 0.59 | |
| 3" | 1.28/1.66[a] | 1.37/1.66[a] | 1.90/2.24[a] | | – | |
| 4" | – | – | – | | 0.58 | |
| 5" | 1.31 | 1.27 | 1.86 br d 11.5 | | 1.81 brd/1.10[a] | |
| 6" | 2.01/1.26[a] | 1.96/1.20[a] | 1.52/1.49[c] | | 1.53/1.73[a] | 4", 7", 15" |
| 7" | 1.94 | 1.86 | 2.02 | | – | |
| 8" | 1.67/1.51[a] | 1.53/1.39[a] | 1.71/1.49[a] | | 2.02 | 1", 2", 7", 9", 15" |
| 9" | 1.43/2.22[a] | 1.20/1.94[a] | 1.61/2.29[a] | | 1.62/1.78[a] | 1" |
| 10" | – | – | – | | 0.97/1.79[a] | 4, 1", 8", 9", 11", 12" |
| 12" | 4.75 br s/ 4.69 br s[b] | 4.70 br s/ 4.66 br s[b] | 4.77 br s/ 4.72 br s[b] | 7", 13" | 0.86s | 4, 1", 10", 11" |
| 13" | 1.76 dd 1.3/0.7 | 1.72 t 1.1 | 1.78 br s | 7", 11", 12" | 1.16 s | 2", 3", 4", 14" |
| 14" | 1.14 s | 1.08 s | 0.94 s | 1", 5", 9", 10" | 1.01 s | 2", 3", 4", 13" |
| 15" | 1.02 s | 1.02 s | 4.43 br s[b] | 3", 4", 5" | 1.20 s | 6", 7", 8" |

[a] H-$\alpha$/H-$\beta$; [b] H-$Z$/H-$E$.

### 3.3 *Fissistigma chloroneurum* (Hand-Mazz) Tsiang

*F. chloroneurum* (Hand-Mazz) Tsiang is a creeper growing in the North mountain of Vietnam, the chemical constituents of which have not yet been studied. We have isolated and determinated the structures of octadecanoic acid (14), geranylfarnesol (15), as well as *β*-sitsterol (stigmast-5-ene-3-ol, 16) from the leaves of this plant (Tam, 2005).

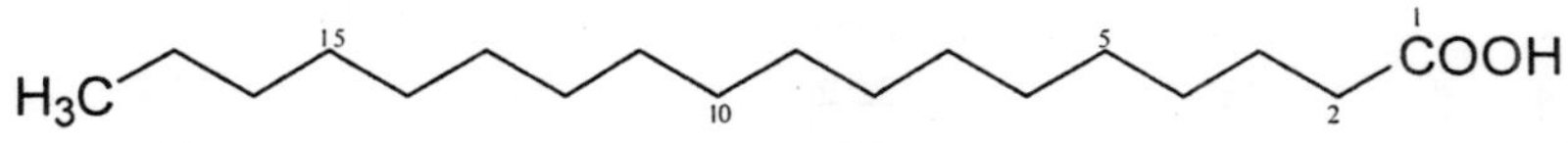

**14**: Octadecanoic acid

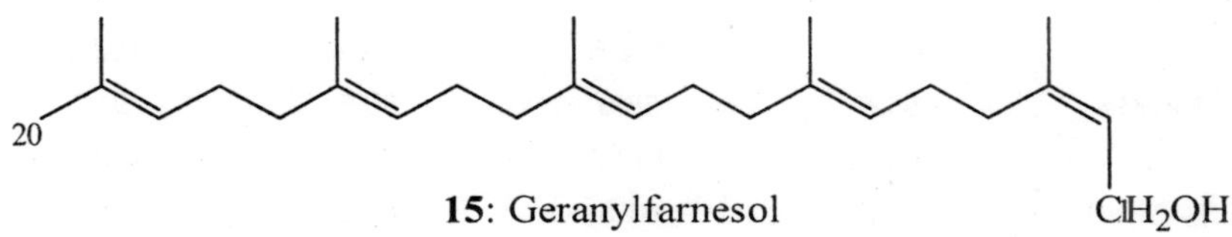

**15**: Geranylfarnesol

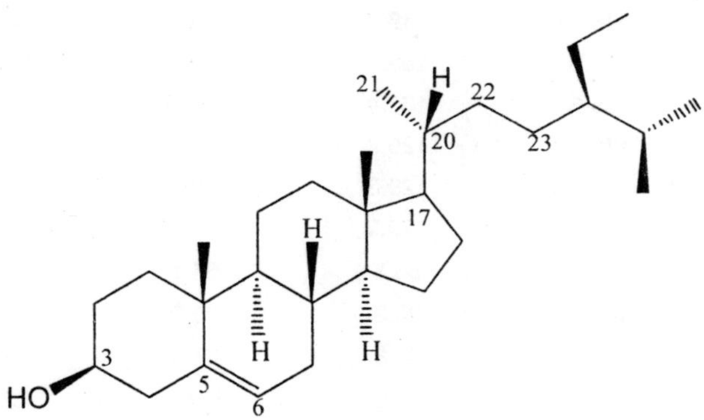

**16**: β-Sitosterol

### 3.4 *Fissistigma capitatum* Merr. Ex. Li.

From the n-hexane and ethyl acetate extract of the leaves and branches of *F. capitatum*, four compounds were isolated. Their structures were elucidated as taraxerol (17), 16-hentriacontanone (18), α-acetylamino-phenylpropyl-α-benzoylamino-phenylpropanoate (patricabratine, 19) and kaempferol-3,7-di-α-L-rhamnopyranoside (20) by using IR, MS and NMR spectroscopic methods.

The EI-MS spectrum of 17 gave a peak at *m/z* 426 $[M]^+$. The DEPT and $^{13}C$-NMR spectra showed the presence of 30 carbon signals ($CH_3$x8, $CH_2$x10, CHx5, Cqx7), suggested that 17 has a triterpene skeleton. This was further confirmed by the signals of 8 tertiary methyl signals, olefinic methin at $\delta_H$ 5.53 (*dd*) and methinoxy at $\delta_H$ 3.20 (*m*) in the $^1H$-NMR spectrum. One double bond was confirmed by signals at $\delta_C$ 158.1 (C-14), 116.9 (C-15) in the $^{13}C$-NMR spectrum. The structure of 17 was identified as 14-taraxeren-3*β*-ol (taraxerol). Taraxerol was isolated for the first time from *Taraxacum officinale* and then frequently found in other plants (*Rhododendron*, *Euphorbia* sp.).

Taraxerol possesses antiulcer activity and was used as cancer chemopreventive agent (Anh, 2005).

**Table 20.2: $^{13}$C–NMR Spectral Data of 1–4 [acetone–$d_6$, 76.5 MHz]**

| *C* | *1* | *2* | *3* | *4* |
|---|---|---|---|---|
| 2 | 150.3 | 149.1 | 150.4 | 151.9 |
| 3 | 101.9 | 106.7 | 101.7 | 103.9 |
| 4 | 30.1 | 32.2 | 30.5 | 39.2 |
| 5 | 152.9 | 153.6 | 152.9 | 153.6 |
| 5–OMe | 56.0 | 55.8 | 56.1 | 55.7 |
| 6 | 93.3 | 92.8 | 93.4 | 93.0 |
| 7 | 152.8 | 152.6 | 152.8 | 152.6 |
| 7–OMe | 56.6 | 56.6 | 56.6 | 56.7 |
| 8 | 132.1 | 132.7 | 132.2 | 132.7 |
| 8–OMe | 61.2 | 61.3 | 61.2 | 61.3 |
| 9 | 148.1 | 148.2 | 148.2 | 149.5 |
| 10 | 108.9 | 108.6 | 108.7 | 107.9 |
| 1' | 135.3 | 135.4 | 135.2 | 135.0 |
| 2'/6' | 125.2 | 125.2 | 125.2 | 125.3 |
| 3'/5' | 129.3 | 129.3 | 129.3 | 129.2 |
| 4' | 129.1 | 129.0 | 129.2 | 129.1 |
| 1" | 57.5 | 58.8 | 57.1 | 45.8 |
| 2" | 22.4 | 25.2 | 25.8 | 31.4 |
| 3" | 44.1 | 44.8 | 37.3 | 20.4 |
| 4" | 71.2 | 71.2 | 151.4 | 27.2 |
| 5" | 56.9 | 57.2 | 51.7 | 21.0 |
| 6" | 26.4 | 26.8 | 30.1 | 45.6 |
| 7" | 47.0 | 46.8 | 46.3 | 74.4 |
| 8" | 27.8 | 28.1 | 27.8 | 59.7 |
| 9" | 42.6 | 43.6 | 39.4 | 25.6 |
| 10" | 39.2 | 39.8 | 40.5 | 37.9 |
| 11" | 151.6 | 151.6 | 151.5 | 53.6 |
| 12" | 108.5 | 108.4 | 108.8 | 17.6 |
| 13" | 21.2 | 21.1 | 21.1 | 17.3 |
| 14" | 17.7 | 16.0 | 15.0 | 29.3 |
| 15" | 22.9 | 23.1 | 105.7 | 20.7 |

Compound 18 was isolated as colourless needles from the hexane extract by column chromatography. The IR band at 1699 cm$^{-1}$ revealed the presence of carbonyl group. The molecular formula ($C_{31}H_{62}O$) was established on the basis of EI-MS (*m/z*

450), combined with data from the DEPT and $^{13}$C-NMR spectra, which showed 16 signals including a keto carbonyl ($\delta_C$ 211.8) and 14 methylene groups (*ca.* $\delta_C$ 22.0-32.0 ppm). As indicated in the NMR spectra, compound 16 is consisting of two symmetrical moiety $C_{15}H_{31}$ *via* the C=O group. The structure of 18 is determined as 16-hentriacontanone (palmiton), which has been isolated from the leaves of *Annona diversifolia* and possess *anticonvulsive* activity (Anh, 2005; Van, 2005).

**Table 20.3: $^1$H–and $^{13}$C–NMR Spectral Data of 12 [$CDCl_3$, $\delta$ (J in Hz)]**

| C | *δC, 125 MHz* | *δH (J in Hz), 500 MHz* | *HMBC* |
|---|---|---|---|
| 1 | 40.85 | 1.25 m; 1.05 1H, m | $H_3$–14 |
| 2 | 19.61 | 2.0 m; 1.5 m | $H_2$–3 |
| 3 | 39.77 | 1.62 dt (13.8, 3.9); 1.68 [a] m | $H_3$–15 |
| 4 | 79.69 | – | H–1', $H_2$–2, $H_2$–3, $H_3$–15 |
| 5 | 47.49 | 1.43 br dt (13.7, 3.3) | $H_3$–14, $H_3$–15 |
| 6 | 22.54 | 1.97 dd (13.3; 2,0); 1.27 m | H–5 |
| 7 | 39.34 | 2.27 br s | $H_3$–13 |
| 8 | 23.27 | 1.60 m | $H_2$–6, $H_2$–9 |
| 9 | 40.56 | 1.35 m; 1.26 m | $H_3$–14 |
| 10 | 35.05 | – | $H_3$–14 |
| 11 | 146.80 | – | H–6b, H–7, $H_2$–12, $H_3$–13 |
| 12 | 110.81 | 4.87 br s; 4.85 br s | $H_3$–13 |
| 13 | 22.82 | 1.69 s | $H_2$–12 |
| 14 | 18.87 | 0.91 s | H–5 |
| 15 | 18.21 | 1.10 s | $H_2$–1, H–5 |
| 1' | 94.34 | 4.75 d (7.8) | H–2' |
| 2' | 74.37 | 4.79 t[b] (7.9) | H–1' |
| 3' | 75.20 | 3.39 m | H–4' |
| 4' | 75.60 | 3.61 br t (9.1) | H–1', H–2' |
| 5' | 70.77 | 3.69 t (9.1) | $H_2$–6' |
| 6' | 62.09 | 3.91 dd (11.8, 3.5) 3.79 dd (11.8, 5.5) | H–5' |
| C=O | 166.39 | – | H–2', H–α, H–β |
| α | 145.44 | 7.73 d (16.0) | H–2"/H–6" |
| β | 117.81 | 6.44 d (16.0) | H–α |
| 1" | 134.37 | – | H–α, H–β, H–2"/H–6" |
| 2", 6" | 128.16 | 7.54 d (7.4) | H–β, H–3"/H–5" |
| 3", 5" | 128.86 | 7.42 dd (7.4, 2.5) | H–2"/H–6", H–4" |
| 4" | 130.32 | 7.43 m | H–2"/H–6", H–3"/H–5" |

[a] hidden under δ1.69; [b] t like dd.

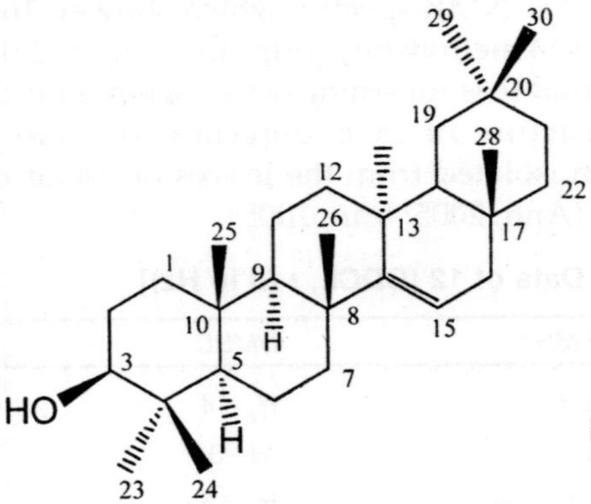

**17**: Taraxerol

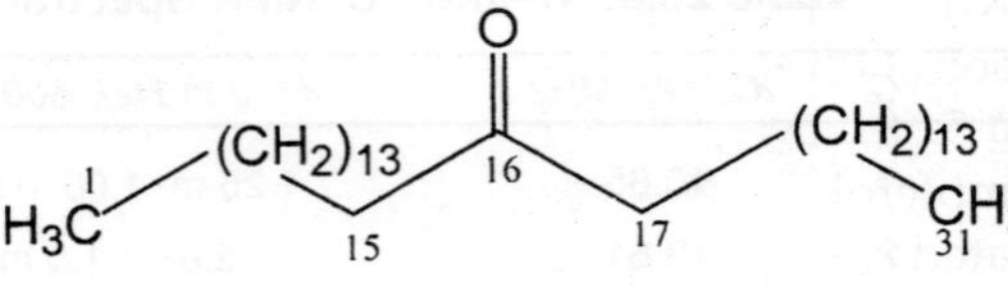

**18:** 16-Hentriacontanon

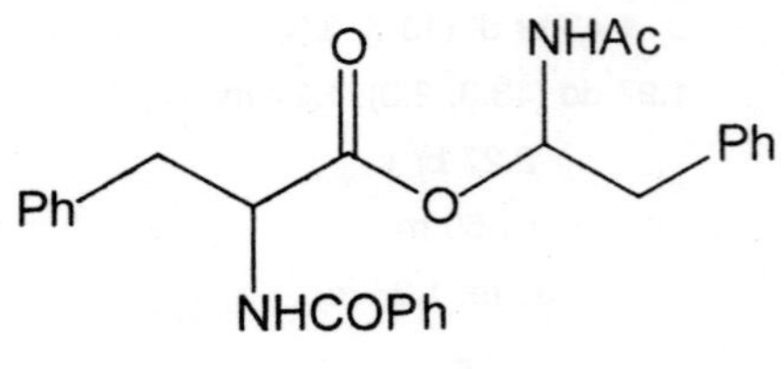

**19**: Patriscabratine

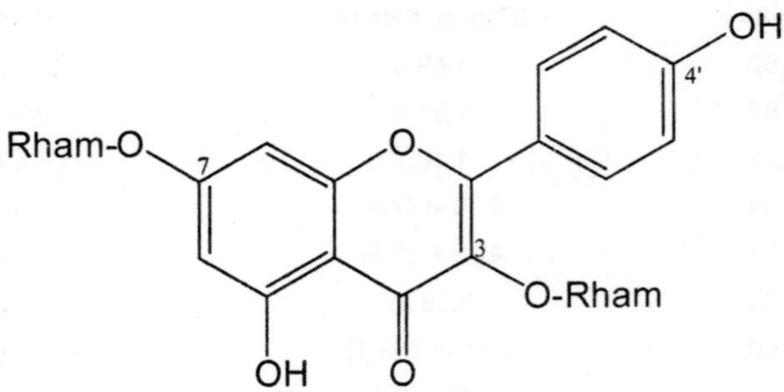

**20**: Kaempferol-3, 7-di-α-L-rhamnopyranoside

The ESI-MS spectrum of compound 19 gave the $[M+H]^+$ peak at $m/z$ 579 corresponding to the molecular formula $C_{27}H_{28}N_2O_4$. The $^1$H-NMR spectrum indicated the presence of 15 aromatic protons (δ 7.0-7.8), two N-H protons (δ 5.97, 6.76), three methylenes (δ 3.96 *dd*; 3.85 *dd*; 3.25 *dd*; 3.08 *dd*; 2.78 *m*), two methine groups (δ 4.78; 4.37) and one acetyl at δ 2.05 (3H, *s*). This was supported by three ester carbonyl at $\delta_C$ 167.1, 170.2 and 170.8; two methine; three methylene groups in the $^{13}$C-NMR and DEPT spectra. Combination of the MS and NMR spectral data led to the structure 2-acetylamino-3-phenylpropyl-2-benzoylamino-3-phenylpropanoat (patriscabratine) for 19. Patriscabratine was isolated for the first time from the tubers of *Gastrodia elata* Blume (Anh, 2005).

The ESI-MS spectrum (positive ions) of 20 gave the $[M+H]^+$ peak at *m/z* 579 and two important peaks at *m/z* 433 $[M+H\text{-rham}]^+$ and 289 $[M+H\text{-}2 \times \text{rham}]^+$. Combination with $^{13}C$-NMR and DEPT spectra leading to the molecular formula $C_{27}H_{30}O_{14}$. Two sugar moieties were identified as α-L-rhamnopyranose by two anomeric protons ($\delta_H$ 5.42, 5.58) and two anomeric carbons (δc 99.9, 103.5) in the NMR spectra. The aglycone moiety was identified as kaempferol by MS, $^1H$–and $^{13}C$-NMR spectra. The connection of two rhamnoses at C-3 and C-7 was deduced from CH long-range correlations of carbon with the anomeric protons: C-3 (δ136.5)/H-1"(δ 5.42) and C-7 (δ163.6)/H-1"'(δ 5.58). From the MS and NMR data the structure of 20 was determined as kaempferol 3,7-di-α-rhamnopyranoside (kaempferitrin, lespedin). Kaempferitrin was isolated from *Indigofera arecta*, *Lespedeza cyrtobotrya* etc. (Van, 2005).

### 3.5 *Fissistigma acuminatissima* Merr.

*F. acuminatissima* Merr. is a climbing shrub growing in north Vietnam (Ban, 2000).The chemical constituents of this plant have not yet been studied. From the leaves of *F. acuminatissima*, a new proaporphine alkaloid, pronuciferine N-oxide (21), three known aporphine alkaloids, nornuciferine (22), roemerine N-oxide (23), liriodenine (24) as well as catechin (25) and isorhamnetin-3-rutinoside (26) were isolated and determinated (Sung, 2007).

The molecular formula of 21 ($C_{19}H_{21}NO_4$) was deduced from combined analysis of HR-ESI-MS at *m/z* 328.15438 $[M+H]^+$ (calc. 328.15433), $^1H$–and $^{13}C$-DEPT-NMR spectra. The $^{13}C$-NMR spectral data of 21 were similar to those of stepharine, except for the downfield shifts of the signals of carbons attached to the nitrogen atom at δ 57.0 (N-Me), 67.0 (C-5) and δ 74.8 (C-6a). The $^1H$-NMR spectrum showed a *dd* at δ 5.15 (H-6a) and a singlet at δ 3.26 (N-Me) suggested the presence of an N-oxide group. This was confirmed by a peak at *m/z* 311 $[M\text{-}O]^+$ for a loss of one oxygen atom in the EI-MS spectrum. Interpretation of the NOESY correlation of H-3 (6.92, s) with 2-OMe (3.85, s) permitted the assignment of the methoxy substituents. From above spectral analysis, alkaloid 21 has been determined as pronuciferine N-oxide, which is a new natural product (Sung, 2007).

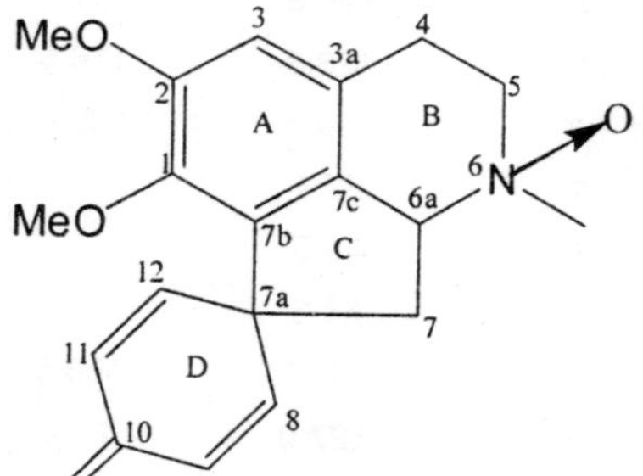


**21**: Pronuciferine N-oxide

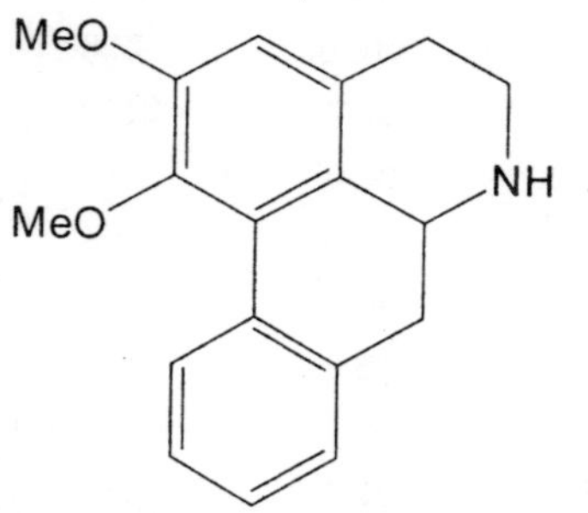


**22**: Nornuciferine

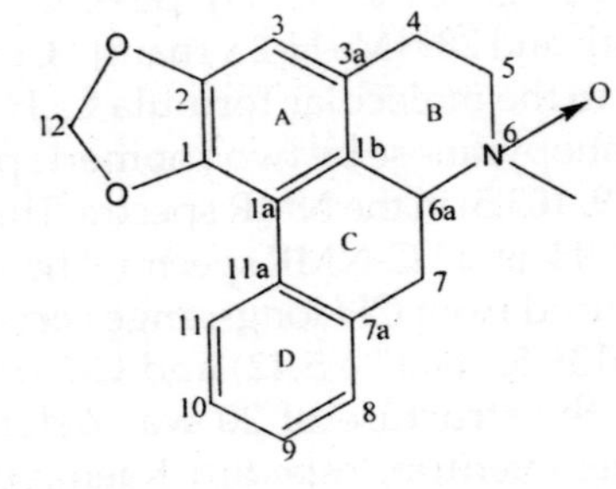

**23**: Roemerine N-oxide

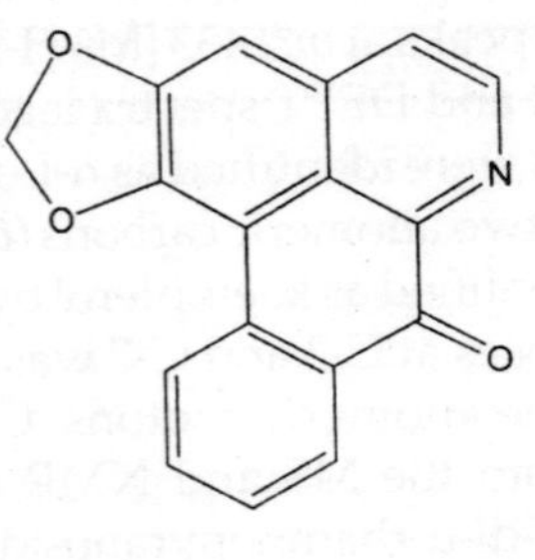

**24**: Liriodenine

**Table 20.4: $^{13}$C-NMR Spectral Data of Compounds 17, 18, 19 ($CDCl_3$) and 20 ($CD_3OD$) (δ ppm, 125 MHz)**

| *C* | *17* | *18* | *C* | *19* | *20* |
|---|---|---|---|---|---|
| 1 | 38.0 | 14.1 | 1 | 136.6 | – |
| 2 | 27.2 | 22.7 | 2 | 129.3 | 159.9 |
| 3 | 79.1 | 31.9 | 3 | 128.8 | 136.5 |
| 4 | 39.0 | 29.3* | 4 | 127.1 | 179.8 |
| 5 | 55.6 | 29.4* | 5 | 128.8 | 163.6 |
| 6 | 18.8 | 29.4* | 6 | 129.3 | 100.6 |
| 7 | 35.1 | 29.5* | 7 | 38.4 | 163.0 |
| 8 | 38.8 | 29.6* | 8 | 55.0 | 95.6 |
| 9 | 48.8 | 29.7* | 9 | 170.2 | 158.1 |
| 10 | 37.6 | 29.7* | 10 | – | 107.6 |
| 11 | 17.5 | 29.7* | 1' | 136.7 | 122.4 |
| 12 | 35.8 | 29.7* | 2' | 129.1 | 132.0 |
| 13 | 37.6 | 29.7* | 3' | 128.6 | 116.6 |
| 14 | 158.1 | 23.9 | 4' | 126.8 | 161.8 |
| 15 | 116.9 | 42.8 | 5' | 128.6 | 116.6 |
| 16 | 36.7 | 211.8 | 6' | 129.1 | 132.0 |
| 17 | 38.0 | – | 7' | 37.4 | – |
| 18 | 49.3 | – | 8' | 49.5 | – |
| 19 | 41.4 | – | 9' | 64.6 | – |
| 20 | 28.8 | – | 1" | 133.7 | 103.5 |
| 21 | 33.7 | – | 2" | 127.0 | 71.9 |
| 22 | 33.1 | – | 3" | 128.6 | 72.2 |
| 23 | 28.0 | – | 4" | 131.9 | 73.6 |
| 24 | 15.5 | – | 5" | 128.6 | 72.1 |
| 25 | 15.5 | – | 6" (Me) | 127.0 | 17.7 |

*Contd.*

**Table 20.4–Contd...**

| *C* | *17* | *18* | *C* | *19* | *20* |
|---|---|---|---|---|---|
| 26 | 29.9 | – | 7" | 167.1 | – |
| 27 | 25.9 | – | 1" | – | 99.9 |
| 28 | 29.9 | – | 2" | – | 71.7 |
| 29 | 33.4 | – | 3" | – | 72.1 |
| 30 | 21.3 | – | 4" | – | 71.3 |
| | | | 5" | – | 73.2 |
| | | | 6" (Me) | – | 18.1 |
| | | | $CH_3$–<u>CO</u> | 170.8 | – |
| | | | $CH_3$–CO | 20.1 | – |

* Exchangeable.

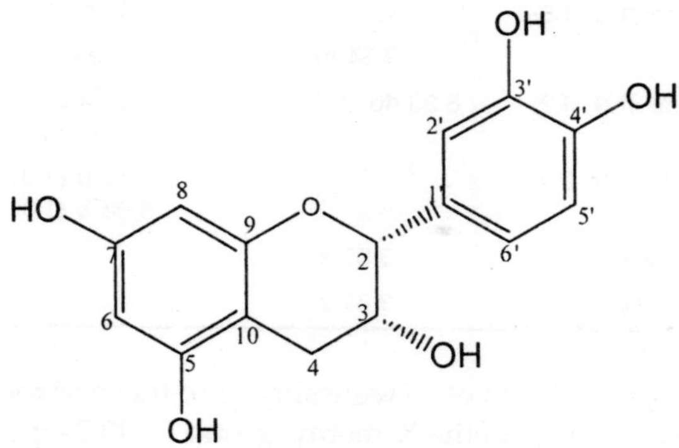

**25**: Epicatechin

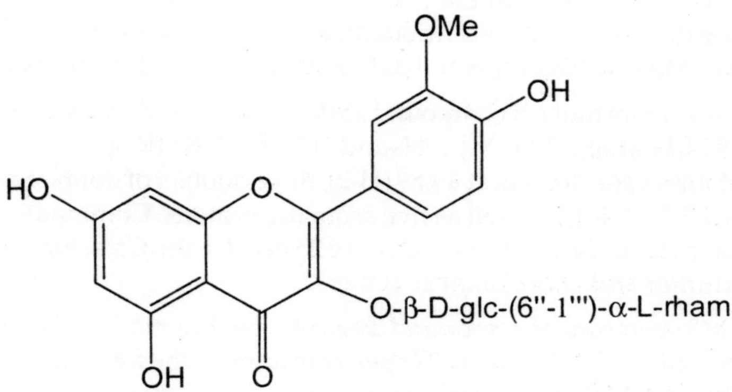

**26**: Isorhamnetin-3-rutinoside

**Table 20.5: $^1$H-NMR Spectral Data of Compounds 21–24 (500 MHz in $CD_3OD$, δ ppm, J in Hz)**

| *H* | *21* | *22* | *23* | *24* |
|---|---|---|---|---|
| 3 | 6.92 s | 6.88 s | 6.69 s | 7.30 s |
| 4 | 3.02 dd (5.3, 17.3) | 3.07 dd (4.5, 13.5)<br>2.91 t (13.8) | 3.65 m<br>3.27 m | 8.70 d (5.2) |
| 5 | 2.42 dd (6.5, 12.0)<br>2.96 ddd (1.6, 5.7, 10.3) | 3.00 d (14.4)<br>3.25 br d (*ca* 5.5) | 3.73 m<br>3.63 m | 7.93 d (5.2) |
| 6 (N–Me) | 3.26 s | – | 3.10 s | – |
| 6a | 5.15 dd (6.7, 9.8) | 4.18 dd (4.4, 14.0) | 4.43 dd (3.5; 14.5) | – |
| 7 | 3.69 dd (6.5, 8.2)<br>3.85 m | 3.65 m | 3.10 m | – |
| 8 | 7.12 dd (2.9, 9.9) | 7.26 m | 7.37 m | 8.63 d (8.1) |
| 9 | 6.42 dd (1.8, 9.6) | 7.34 m | 7.32 m | 7.78 dt (1.5, 8.1) |
| 10 | – | 7.34 m | 7.29 m | 7.60 dt (1.0, 8.1) |
| 11 | 6.29 dd (1.9, 9.9) | 8.33 dd (1.7, 7.6) | 8.04 dd (0.9, 7.7) | 8.42 dd (1.5, 8.1) |
| 12 | 7.14 dd (2.9, 9.9) | | 6.15 d (1.0)<br>5.98 d (1.0) | 6.43 s |
| 1–OMe | 3.64 s | 3.65 s | – | – |
| 2–OMe | 3.85 s | 3.89 s | – | – |

The $^{13}$C-NMR spectral data of 23 were similar to those of roemerine, except for the significant chemical shifts of the N-methyl group ($\delta_C$ 49.2) and its neighbours (C-6a: 75.7, C-5: 68.1). The molecular formula of 23 ($C_{18}H_{18}NO_3$) was determined by HR-ESI-MS spectrum at *m/z* 296.12829 $[M+H]^+$ (calc. 296.12812) and *m/z* 278 $[M\text{-}H\text{-}O]^+$, which also revealed the presence of an N-oxide group. Roemerine N-oxide was isolated for the first time from the plant *Papaver glaucum* [10]. Two other known alkaloids, nornuciferine (22) and liriodenine (24) were isolated and identified by comparison of MS and NMR spectral data with published data (Sung, 2007).

The molecular formula of compound 25 ($C_{15}H_{14}O_6$) was deduced from combined analysis of EI-MS at *m/z* 290 $[M]^+$, $^1$H–and $^{13}$C-DEPT NMR spectra. The $^1$H-NMR spectrum exhibited one doublet at δ 4.89 (H-2), three doublet of doublet at δ 3.99 (H-3), 2.53 (H-4*ax*), 2.87 (H-4*eq*), as well as five aromatic protons. Combination of MS and NMR spectral data confirmed the structure of 25 as catechin. Catechin and its analogs showed antitumor and antioxidant activities.

The EI-MS spectrum of compound 26 gave a peak at *m/z* 316 [M-sugar chain]$^+$, combination with $^{13}$C-NMR and DEPT spectra leading to the formula $C_{16}H_{12}O_7$ for the aglycone. The $^1$H-NMR spectrum showed one methoxy group ($\delta_H$3.53, $\delta_C$56.81) and five aromatic protons. The β-D-glucopyranose was identified by anomeric signals at $\delta_H$ 5.25 (d, J=7.4 Hz) and the rhamnopyranose was identified by methyl signal at $\delta_H$1.64 (d, J=6.2 Hz) in the $^1$H-NMR spectrum. The $^1$H–and $^{13}$C-NMR spectra of sugar moiety were identical with those of rutinoside and the aglycone moiety was identical with those of isorhamnetin (Van, 2007). Therefore the structure of 26 was determined as 3-*O*-α-rhamnopyranosyl-(1→6)-β-glucopyranyloxy-4',5,7-trihydroxy-3'-methoxyflavone (isorhamnetin-3-rutinoside), which was isolated for the first time from the flowers of *Narcissus tazetta* and then in *Lilium aurantum, Herniaria glabra* (Van, 2007).

**Table 20.6: $^{13}$C-NMR Spectral Data of Compounds 21–24 (125 MHz, δppm in $CD_3OD$)**

| *C* | *21* | *22* | *23* | *24* |
|---|---|---|---|---|
| 1 | 146.1 | 147.2 | 145.2 | 150.4 |
| 1a | – | 127.8 | 117.6 | 108.1 |
| 1b | – | 128.1 | 124.5 | 124.3 |
| 2 | 155.7 | 154.9 | 150.1 | 154.0 |
| 3 | 113.2 | 113.1 | 108.3 | 104.3 |
| 3a | 127.6 | 132.8 | 131.4 | 145.5 |
| 4 | 25.1 | 26.9 | 29.9 | 126.3 |
| 5 | 67.0 | 42.8 | 68.1 | 145.0 |
| 6(N–$\underline{C}H_3$) | 57.0 | – | 49.2 | – |
| 6a | 74.8 | 56.5 | 75.7 | 137.8 |
| 7 | 40.1 | 35.5 | 28.1 | 183.5 |
| 7a | 52.1 | 135.0 | 133.9 | 132.0 |
| 7b | 129.6 | – | – | – |
| 7c | 134.3 | – | – | – |
| 8 | 155.4 | 129.6 | 128.1 | 129.2 |
| 9 | 129.0 | 129.2 | 128.6 | 129.6 |
| 10 | 188.2 | 128.6 | 129.4 | 135.5 |
| 11 | 127.9 | 129.2 | 129.5 | 128.7 |
| 11a | – | a | 123.2 | 134.2 |
| 12 | 152.6 | – | 102.9 | 104.7 |
| 1–OMe | 56.8 | 54.4 | – | – |
| 2–OMe | 61.2 | 60.6 | – | – |

**Table 20.7: Antimicrobial Activity[a] of Compounds 12, 22, 23 and 24**

| *Compounds* | *Microorganisms* | | | | |
|---|---|---|---|---|---|
| | *Ec* | *Pa* | *Bs* | *Sa* | *Ca* |
| Fissispalin (12) | 12,5 | 50 | 12,5 | 12,5 | >128 |
| Nornuciferine (22) | >128 | >128 | >128 | >128 | >128 |
| Roemerine N–oxide (23) | >128 | >128 | >25.5 | 16.5 | >128 |
| Liriodenine (24) | >128 | >128 | 5.8 | 17.9 | >128 |

[a] $IC_{50}$ µg/ml.

Some of isolated compounds (12, 22, 23 and 24) were screened for antibacterial and antifungal activity. The *microorganisms* used are: *Escherichia coli (Ec); Pseudomonas aeruginosa (Pa); Bacillus subtillis (Bs); Staphylococcus aureus (Sa); Candida albicans (ca).* Fissispalin (12) inhibited the growth of three microorganisms *(Esherichia coli, Bacillus subtillis* and *Staphylococcus aureus),* while liriodenine (24) showed most effective with *Bacillus subtillis* (Table 20.7).

## Acknowledgements

This research was supported financially by the Vietnamese Ministry of Science and Technology (MOST) in form of a project in basic research (Code: 510506, 2006-2008), as well as the International Foundation for Science, Stockholm, Sweden (IFS) and the Organisation for the Prohibition of Chemical Weapons (OPCW), through a grant to Mr. Tran Duc Quan. We thank Dr. Ngo Van Trai, Institute of Materia Medica, Hanoi for identification of the plant materials.

## References

Anh, N. T. H., Van, N. T. H., Nhung, L. T. H., Sung, T. V., 2005. Chemical study of *Fissistigma capitatum* Merr. ex L1., Annonaceae. Tap chi Hoa hoc, 43 (4): pp. 475–478

Ban, N. T., 2000. Thuc vat chi Viet Nam (Flora of Vietnam), Hanoi Publishing House for Science and Technics: pp.209-210.

Lien, T. P., Porzel, A., Schmidt, J., Sung, T. V., Adam, G., 2000. Chalconoids from *F. brateolatum*. Phytochemistry (53): pp. 991-995

Perry, L. M., 1980. In Medicinal plants of East and Southeast Asia Cambridge: MIT press, pp. 19.

Porzel, A., Lien, T. P., Schmidt, J., Susane, D., Sung, T.V., Adam, G., 2000. Fissistigmatins A-D: Novel type natural products with flavonoid-sesquiterpene hybrid structure from *F. brateolatum*. Tetrahedron (56): pp. 865-872.

Sung, T. V., Thuy, T. T., Van, N. T. H., 2007. Proaporphine and Aporphine Alkaloids from *Fissistigma acuminatissima*, Asian Chemistry Letters, 11 (3 and 4): pp. 231-234.

Tam N. T., Thuy T. T., Anh N. T.H., Sung T.V., 2005. First results in chemical study of *Fissistigma chloroneurum* (Hanz-Mazz) Tisiang. Tap Chi Duoc lieu, 10 (2): pp. 49–51.

Thuy, T. T., Sung, T. V., Hao, N. T., 2006. An eudesmane glucoside from *Fissistigma pallens*. Pharmazie (61); pp. 570–571.

Thuy, T. T., Sung, T. V., Hao, N. T., 2006. Results on chemical study on the leaves of *Fissistigma pallens*. Vietnamese J. of Chem (44 (4)): pp. 412-417.

Van, N. T. H., Thuy, T. T., Sung, T. V., 2007. Flavonoids from *Fissistigma acuminatissima*, Vietnamese J. of Chem., 45 (5): pp. 648-651.

Van, N.T., Anh, N. T. H., Sung, T. V., 2005. Results on Phytochemical Study of *Fissistigma capitatum* Merr. ex L1. Tap chi Duoc lieu, 10 (3): pp. 86-88.

## Chapter 21

# The Synthesis of a Novel Bibenzopyran Relied on Electro-oxidation of Malloapelta B by Cyclic Voltammetry

*Phan Thi Binh[1]*, Bui Hai Ninh[1], Chau Van Minh[2], Nguyen Hoai Nam[2], Le Mai Huong[2] and Phan Van Kiem[2]*

*[1]Institute of Chemistry, [2]Institute of Natural Products Chemistry, Vietnam Academy of Science and Technology, Hanoi, Vietnam*

**E-mail: ptbinh@ich.vast.ac.vn, thao_binhvn@yahoo.com*

## ABSTRACT

A novel bibenzopyran named bimalloapelta (1) was synthesized relying on electro-oxidation of malloapelta B by cyclic voltammetry in acetonitrile adding $LiClO_4$ 0.1M as supporting electrolyte. Its structure determination based on extensive NMR studies and ESI mass spectral measurements. The new compound showed significant cytotoxicity against two cancer cell lines as human hepatocellular carcinoma (Hep-2; $IC_{50}$: 0.46 µg/m) and rhabdosarcoma (RD; $IC_{50}$: 0.33 µg/m). These results were the same as that of malloapelta B (Hep-2, $IC_{50}$: 0.49 µg/ml and KB, $IC_{50}$: 0.54 µg/ml).

***Keywords***: *Malloapelta B, Bimalloapelta, Cytotoxicity, Electro-organic synthesis.*

## 1.0 Introduction

As part of an ongoing program to discover new anti-cancer agents from nature resources, we have reported previously the isolation and the structural elucidation of malloapelta B, a new cytotoxic compound from *Mallotus apelta* (Minh *et al.*, 2005). To seek malloapelta B's derivatives, which have stronger cytotoxic activities than that of malloapelta B, we have synthesized a series of its derivatives based on organic synthesis and electro-organic reactions.

Currently, electro-organic synthetic method has been used often to synthesize organic compounds. The advantages of electro-organic reactions are that they react quickly and very selectively (Weinberg, 1974). Malloapelta B, a new cytotoxic component and new inhibitor against NF-kB activation from *Mallotus apelta* is an organic agent having some double bonds (Minh *et al.*, 2005). Therefore, it can be also used as an electro-organic active agent. That means malloapelta B can be oxidised or reduced by electro-organic methods. Among them is the cyclic voltammetric method, which is an efficient synthetic way. In our experiment we chose the voltage located in oxidation area. The voltammograms of base solvent as well as research solvent were taken by electro-organic workstation system IM6 from Zahner Elektrik (Germany) in the voltage range from 1V to 1.5V at a scan rate of 150mV/s. This report deals with the electro-organic synthesis of bimalloapelta (1), the structural determination and the evaluation of its cytotoxic activity by *in vitro* assay.

## 2.0 Materials and Methods

### 2.1 General Experimental Procedures

The IR spectra were obtained on a Hitachi 270-30 type spectrometer using KBr discs. The Electron Spray Ionization Mass (ESI) spectrum was obtained using a AGILENT 1100 LC-MSD trap spectrometer. The $^{1}$H-NMR (500 MHz) and $^{13}$C-NMR (125 MHz) spectra were recorded on a Bruker AM500 FT-NMR spectrometer using TMS as the internal standard. Column chromatography (CC) was performed on silica gel (Kieselgel 60, 70-230 mesh and 230-400 mesh, Merck). Thin layer chromatography (TLC) was performed on DC-Alufolien Kiesegel 60 F254 (Merck).

### 2.2 Synthesis

#### Electro-organic Cell

Using Electro-organic cell (100 ml) in three electrodes compartment with a platine net as counter electrode (CE), a platine plate of 1cm$^2$ as working electrode (WE), and a Ag/AgCl electrode as reference electrode (RE).

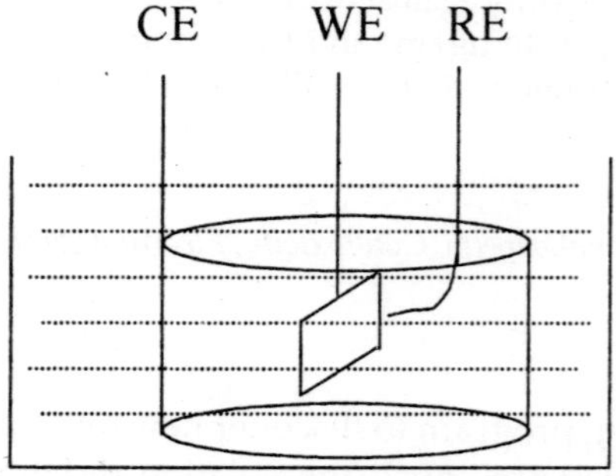


**Figure 21.1: Electrochemical Cell**

**Electrolyte**

Base electrolyte was acetonitrile with $LiClO_4$ 0.1M as supporting electrolyte. 200 mg Malloapelta B agent (12 g/l) was added to base electrolyte.

**Cyclic Voltammetry**

The current-potential curves (Figure 21.3) obtained by the application of a triangular impulse of potential was shown in Figure 21.2. Investigations of electrosynthesis by cyclic voltammetry are usually carried out by choosing the voltage

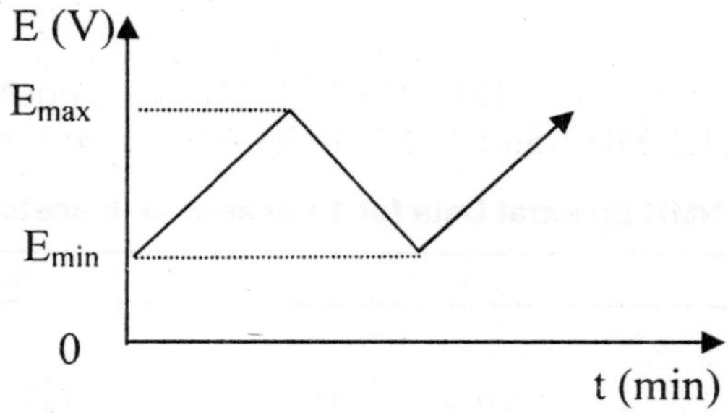


**Figure 21.2: Variation of Applied Potential with Time in Cyclic Voltammetry Shows the Maximum ($E_{max}$) and Minimum ($E_{min}$) Potentials. The Sweep Rate |dE/dt| = $\nu$**

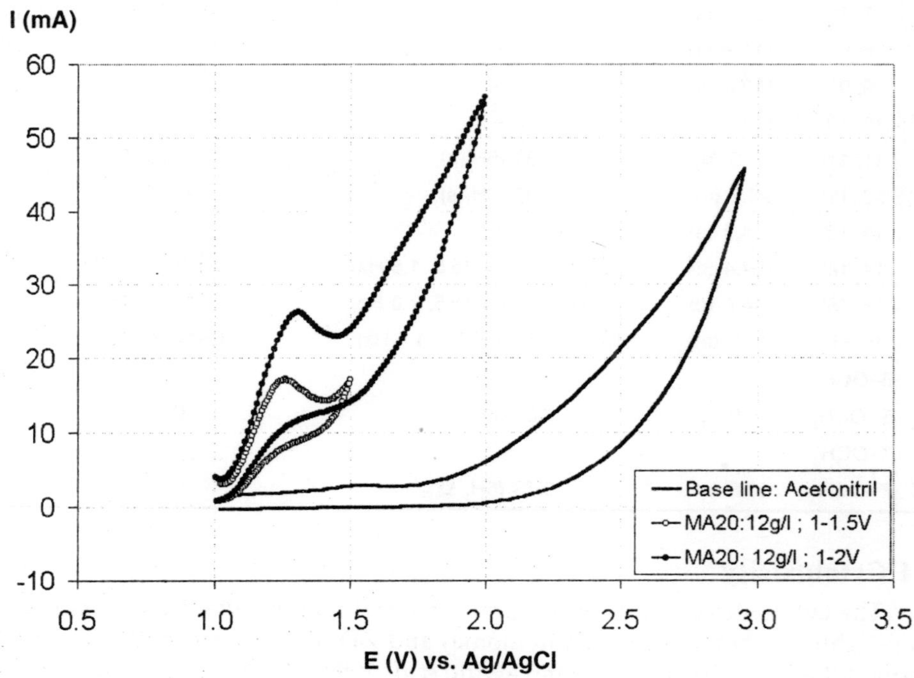


**Figure 21.3: Cyclic Voltammograms from Mallopelta B (MA20) in $LiClO_4$ 0.1M + $CH_3CN$ 0.1M**

spans and sweep rates ($v$). The voltammograms were taken using electrochemichal workstation system IM6 from Zahner Elektrik unit (Germany) in the voltage range from 1V to 1.5V at a scan rate of 150mV/s (2000 cycles).

## 2.3 Purification

After finishing reaction, the reactive solvent was evaporated in vaccum to get 250 mg extract, which was then chromatographed on a silica gel column (Φ 20 x L 500 mm) eluted with hexane-acetone (4: 1) as the eluent to give 1 (180 mg) as white powder.

**Bimalloapelta (1)**

White powder, IR $^{KBr}v_{max}$ $cm^{-1}$: 1745 (C=O), 1625 (C=C); positive ESI ($m/z$) 593 $[M+H]^+$; the $^{13}C$-NMR (125 MHz) and $^1H$-NMR (500 MHz): see Table 21.1.

**Table 21.1: NMR Spectral Data for 1 (measured in acetone-$d_6$)**

| *C* | *$\delta_C$ (ppm)* | *$\delta_H$ (ppm)* | *HMBC* |
|---|---|---|---|
| 2, 2' | 77.2 (s) | – | |
| 3, 3' | 47.8 (d) | 2.33 (2H, d, J = 6.5 Hz) | C–2, C–4, C–10, C–11, C–12 |
| 4, 4' | 68.2 (d) | 4.89 (2H, d, J = 6.5 Hz) | C–2, C–3, C–5, C–9, C–10, C–4' |
| 5, 5' | 160.8 (s) | – | |
| 6, 6' | 88.5 (d) | 6.09 (2H, s) | C–5, C–7, C–8, C–10, |
| 7, 7' | 158.3 (s) | – | |
| 8, 8' | 111.2 (s) | – | |
| 9, 9' | 153.0 (s) | – | |
| 10, 10' | 104.2 (s) | – | |
| 11, 11' | 27.3 (q) | 1.33 (6H, s) | C–2, C–3 |
| 12, 12' | 24.7 (q) | 1.33 (6H, s) | C–2, C–3 |
| 13, 13' | 194.5 (s) | – | |
| 14, 14' | 134.4 (d) | 6.30 (2H, dd, J = 15.5, 1.5 Hz) | C–8, C–13, C–16 |
| 15, 15' | 144.6 (d) | 6.55 (2H, dq, J = 15.5, 7.0 Hz) | C–13, C–16 |
| 16, 16' | 18.2 (q) | 1.87 (6H, dd, J = 7.0, 1.5 Hz) | C–14, C–15 |
| 5–$OCH_3$ | | | |
| 5'–$OCH_3$ | 56.9 (q) | 3.81 (6H, s) | C–5 |
| 7–$OCH_3$ | | | |
| 7'–$OCH_3$ | 56.8 (q) | 3.78 (6H, s) | C–7 |

## 2.4 Cytotoxicity

The cytotoxic activities of compounds 1 and malloapelta B were assayed on Hep-2 (human hepatocellular carcinoma) and RD (rhabdosarcoma) cells by SRB method (Lee *et al.*, 2003; Likhitwitayawuid *et al.*, 1993; Minh *et al.*, 2004). In brief, the cell lines were stored in the liquid $N_2$ then were cultured in Dulbeco's Modified Eagle Medium (DMEM) supplemented with 7–10 per cent Fecal Bovine Serum (FBS) for test.

Cells were typically grown to 60 per cent–70 per cent confluence, the medium was then changed and the cells were used for test procedures one day later. In each case, 96-well tissue culture plates were used. Test samples (4–10mg) were initially dissolved in 1ml of 100 per cent DMSO, then diluted 10 fold with $H_2O$. Serial dilutions were performed using 10 per cent aqueous DMSO as the solvent, and 10µl were added to each well. Control groups were also added in which 10µl of 10 per cent DMSO and 10µl of 0,01mM Elipticine in DMSO were added to each well as negative and positive control in turn. After the plates were prepared, cell were removed from the tissue culture flasks by treatment with trypsin 0.05 per cent, enumerated, and diluted with fresh media. The quantities of cells (in 190 µl of media) were added to the 96-well plates (KB: 3x $10^4$;Hep-G2 and FL: 4 x $10^4$), and incubation was performed for three days at 37°C in a $CO_2$ incubator with the plates capped in the normal fashion. After the incubation period, cells were fixed to the plastic substratum by the addition of 50µl of cold 50 per cent aqueous Trichloroacetic acid (TAC). The plate were incubated at 4°C for 1h, washed with tap water (4 x), and air-dried. Cells then were stained by the addition of 0.4 per cent Sulforhodamine B (w/v) dissolved in 1 per cent AcOH (30 min). Free sulforhodamine B solution were then removed by washing with 1 per cent aqueous AcOH (4x). The plates were air-dried, and the bound dye was solubilized by the addition of 10mM unbuffered Tris base, pH 10. The plates were placed on a shake for 5 min, and the absorption was determined at 515 nm using an ELISA plate reader.

## 3.0 Results and Discussion

As known about the electro-organic reactions that cation radicals, carbonium or uncharged radicals are formed at the anode, and anion radicals, carbanions, or uncharged radicals are formed at the cathode (Weinberg, 1974). Figure 21.3 showed the cyclic voltammograms of the solution with and without malloapelta B in acetonitrile plus $LiClO_4$ (0.1M) as supporting electrolyte. There was a clear appearance of the oxidation peak of malloapelta B when the potential ranged from 1 to 1.5V versus Ag/AgCl. Some derivatives of malloapelta B were formed during oxidation process. The main product among them was found. The electro-organic reaction could be:

$$\text{MALLOAPELTA B} \xrightarrow[\text{LiClO}_{4/}\text{CH}_3\text{CN}]{e^-} \text{BIMALLOAPELTA} \qquad (1)$$

An electro-organic oxidation mechanism of malloapelta B was proposed as shown in Scheme 1. Firstly, malloapelta B transferred one electron to convert into corresponding cation radical, which was further oxidised by $LiClO_4$, ($LiClO_4$ is much oxidative than $CH_3CN$) then converted into 1.

By chromatography on silica gel, compound 1 was obtained as white powder from the reactive solution. The $^1$H-NMR spectrum of 1 inhibited one singlet of two methyl groups at $\delta$ 1.33, one doublet of doublet of the other methyl group at $\delta$ 1.87 (J = 7.0, 1.5 Hz), one singlet at $\delta$ 6,09 was assigned to H-6, a doublet of doublet at $\delta$ 6.30 (J = 15.5, 1.5 Hz) and a doublet of quartet at 6.55 (J = 15.5, 7.0 Hz) were assigned to two proton H-14 and H-15, respectively at *trans* configuration. Two other singlets at 3.81

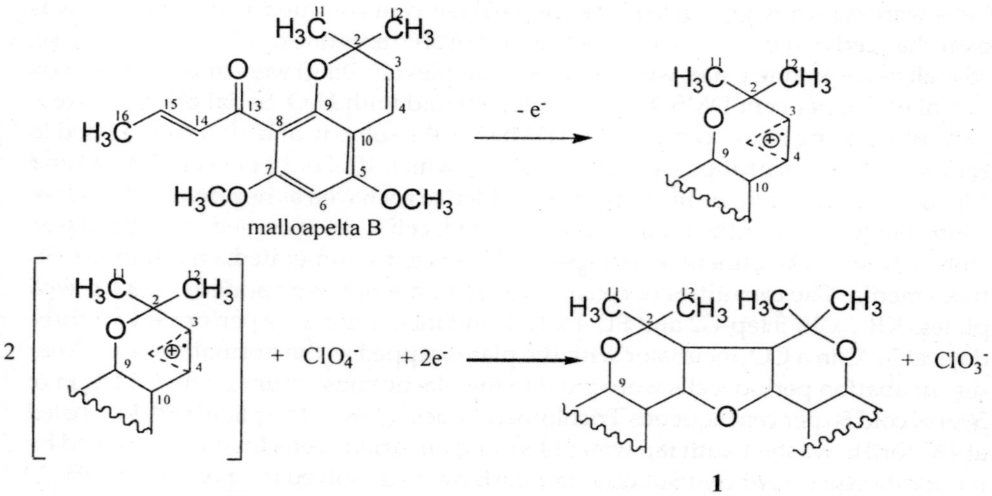

**Scheme 1: The Electro-organic Oxidation Mechanism of Malloapelta B**

and 3.78 were assigned to two methoxyl groups. A methine proton resonance at higher field (δ 2.33, d, J = 6.5 Hz) coupled with the other methine proton bearing to oxygen atom at δ 4.89 (d, J = 6.5 Hz). The $^{13}$C-NMR, DEPT 135° and DEPT 90° spectra of 1 confirmed the presence of 17 carbons, including 3 methyl, 2 methoxyl, 5 methine and 7 quaternary carbon groups. Comparing the NMR of 1 with that of malloapelta B suggested the quite difference between them at C-3 and C-4 of the benzopyran ring. The double bond at C-3/C-4 of malloapelta B ($\delta_H$ 5.45 and 6.58; $\delta_C$ 127.1 and 116.7) was oxidised and changed into single bond ($\delta_H$ 2.33 and 4.89; $\delta_C$ 47.8 and 68.2) in 1. All the other NMR signals of 1 were similar to that of malloapelta B. In addition, the positive electron spray ionization mass spectrum (ESI) of 1 inhibited a quasi-molecular ion peak with the highest intensity at *m/z* 593 [M+H]$^+$, correspond to the molecular formula of $C_{34}H_{40}O_9$. This evidence suggested the chemical structure of 1 as shown in Figure 21.4. To further confirm this structure, the heteronuclear multiple quantum coherence (HMQC) and heteronuclear multiple bonds correlation (HMBC) spectra were taken and analysed in detail as shown in Table 21.1. Cross peaks were observed between the methine proton at δ 2.33 and carbon C-4 (δ 68.2)/C-10 (δ 104.2)/C-11 (δ 27.3), between the oxymethine proton at δ 4.89 and carbon C-2 (δ 77.2)/C-5 (δ 160.8)/ C-9 (δ 153.0) in the HMBC spectrum indicating further that the double bond at C-3/ C-4 of malloapelta B was oxidised and changed into single bond in 1. The coupling constant between protons H-3 and H-4 ($J_{3\text{-}4}$ = 6.5 Hz) confirmed that they are all *axial* configuration (Silverstein *et al.*, 1998). Accordingly, the structure of 1 was determined as shown in Figure 21.4, which named bimalloapelta.

Compounds 1 and malloapelta B were assayed on Hep-2 (human hepatocellular carcinoma) and RD (rhabdosarcoma) cells by SRB method. As a result, 1 also inhibited strongly cytotoxic activity on both tested cancer cell lines Hep-2 and RD with the $IC_{50}$ values of 0.46 μg/ml and 0.33 μg/ml, respectively. Comparing these results with

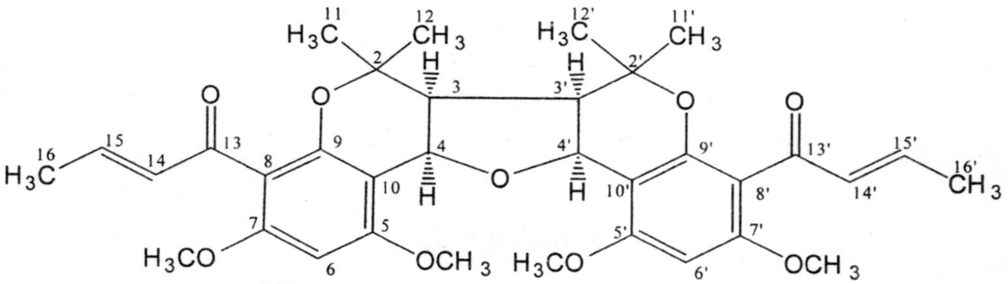


**Figure 21.4: Structure of Compound 1**

those of malloapelta B (Hep-2, $IC_{50}$: 0.49 µg/ml and KB, $IC_{50}$: 0.54 µg/ml) indicated that $IC_{50}$ values of both compounds were the same and that the oxidation of double bond at C-3/C-4 did not affect to its cytotoxic activity.

## Acknowledgements

The authors wish to thank the Humboldt-Fellowship for the support of the IM6 equipment. We are grateful to the colleagues of NMR and LC-MS Lab, Institute of Chemistry, VAST for the measurements of NMR and ESI spectra.

## References

Lee, H. J., Park, S. Y., Kim, J. S., Song, H. M., Suh, M. E. and Lee, C. O., 2003. Bioorg. Med. Chem.(11); pp. 4791-4796.

Likhitwitayawuid, K., Angerhofer, C. K., Cordell, G. A. and Pezzuto, J. M., 1993. J. Nat. Prod. (56); pp. 30-38.

Minh, C. V., Kiem, P. V., Huong, L. M and Kim, Y. H., 2004. Archives of Pharmacol Research (27); pp. 734-737.

Minh, C. V., Kiem, P. V., Huong, H. T., Nam, N. H., Lee, J. J. and Kim, Y. H., 2005. Chemical investigations and biological studies of Mallotus apelta, V1. Cytotoxic constituents from *Mallotus apelta*, Journal of Chemistry (43(1)); pp. 5-6.

Silverstein, R. M. and Webster, F. X., 1998. Spectrometric Identification of Organic Compounds, Six Edition, John Wiley and Sons, Inc. Press; pp. 212.

Weinberg, N. L., 1974. Technique of electro-organic synthesis. John Wiley and Sons Press (5(1)).

Chapter 22

# A New Dammarane-Type Triterpene Saponin from *Eriochloa ramosa* (Retz) Hack (Poaceae)

*Le Thi Kim Loan*[1], *Nguyen Xuan Nhiem*[2], *Chau Van Minh*[2] *and Phan Van Kiem*[2]*

[1]*National Institute of Medicinal Materials, Ministry of Health, Vietnam*

[2]*Institute of Natural Products Chemistry, Vietnam Academy of Science and Technology, Vietnam*

**E-mail: phankiem@vast.ac.vn*

## ABSTRACT

Combined chromatographic methods of the methanolic extract of the whole plant *Eriochloa ramosa* led to the isolation of a new compound named as vina-erioramoside A (1), together with 4 known compounds (2-5). The new natural product was elucidated as 3β, 6β, 20(*S*)-trihydroxydammar-24-ene-3-*O*-[β-D-glucopyranoside]-20-*O*-[β-D-glucopyranosyl-(1'3)-β-D-glucopyranosyl-(1'6)-β-D-glucopyranoside] and the known compounds were identified as ginsenoside-$Rg_1$ (2), quercitrin (3), (-) palmatine (4), and daucosterol (5) by spectroscopic methods including ESI-MS, 1D and 2D NMR and in comparison with the literature.

***Keywords***: *Eriochloa ramosa, Poaceae, Vina-erimoside A.*

## 1.0 Introduction

*Eriochloa* is small genus, mainly distributed in tropical areas, in which *Eriochloa ramosa* (Retz.) Kuntze is a popular species. In Vietnam, this species is widely found in plain and midland areas, rarely found in low mountainous areas. The plant, perennial herb is light and moisture demanding. In some local areas in Vietnam (Son Tay, Nam Dinh), whole plant of this species is used to treat influenza, fever and petechial fever (Bich *et al.*, 2004). To date, no studies on chemical constituents of this species are reported. In few preliminary pharmacological investigations, ethanol extract of this species at doses of 0.5g/kg and 1.0g/kg moderately reduced fever and decreased the effects of analgin at dose of 0.2g/kg (Bich *et al.*, 2004). As part of our investigation on chemical constituents of this plant, this paper deals with the isolation and elucidation of a new dammarane-type triterpene 3*β*, 6*β*, 20(*S*)-trihydroxydammar-24-ene-3-*O*-[*β*-D-glucopyranoside]-20-*O*-[*β*-D-glucopyranosyl-(1'3)-*β*-D-glucopyranosyl-(1'6)-*β*-D-glucopyranoside] named vina-erioramoside A (1), along with four known compounds as 3*β*,6*α*,12*β*,20*S*-tetrahydroxydammar-24-en 6-*O*-[*β*-D-lucopyranoside]-20-*O*-[*β*-D-lucopyranoside (ginsenoside $A_2$) (2), quercitrin (3), palmatine (4), and daucosterol (5) from the methanolic extract of this plant. Their structures were established by spectroscopic methods.

## 2.0 Materials and Methods

### 2.1 General Experiment Procedures

The $^1$H-NMR (500MHz) and $^{13}$C-NMR (125MHz) spectra were recorded on a Bruker AM500 FT-NMR spectrometer. Chemical shifts are referenced to $\delta$ using tetramethylsilan (TMS) as an internal standard. The Electron Spray Ionization (ESI) mass spectrum was obtained using an AGILENT 1100 LC-MSD Trap spectrometer. Column chromatography (CC) was performed on silicagel 230-400 mesh (0.040-0.063 mm, Merck) or YMC RP-18 resins (30-50 µm, Fujisilisa Chemical Ltd.). Thin layer chromatography (TLC) was performed on DC-Alufolien 60 $F_{254}$ (Merck 1.05715) or $RP_{18}$ $F_{254s}$ (Merck) plates.

### 2.2 Plant Material

The whole plant of *Eriochloa ramosa* were collected in Dong Anh District, Hanoi City, Vietnam in September 2006 and identified by graduate Ngo Van Trai. An authentic sample was deposited at the National Institute of Medicinal materials.

### 2.3 Extraction and Isolation

The dried stems of *E. ramosa* (0.8 kg) were extracted with MeOH three times, and then concentrated under low pressure to obtain 21 g MeOH extract. The MeOH extract was suspended in water and partitioned in turn with *n*-hexane, $CHCl_3$, EtOAc and *n*-BuOH to obtain fractions *n*-hexane (2.2 g), $CHCl_3$ (3.5 g), EtOAc (5.0 g), and *n*-BuOH (4.5 g). Compounds 3 (15 mg) were obtained as yellow amorphous powder from the EtOAc fraction (5.0 g) after combined chromatography on normal phase and reversed phase silica gel column. The $CHCl_3$ (3.5 g) was chromatographed on a silica gel column eluting with $CHCl_3$-MeOH (from 20:1 to 1:2 v/v) to give four fractions F1 (0.5 g), F2 (0.8 g), F3 (1.0 g), and F4 (1.2 g). The F4 fraction was then chromatographed on a silica gel column using $CHCl_3$-EtOAc (10:1) as eluent to give 4 (10.0 mg) as white crystals and 5 (20 mg) as a colourless solid. The water layer was chromatographed on a Dianion HP-20 column eluting with MeOH: $H_2O$ (gradient from 0 per cent MeOH to 100 per cent MeOH, v/v) to give five fractions FW1 (0 per cent MeOH), FW2 (25 per

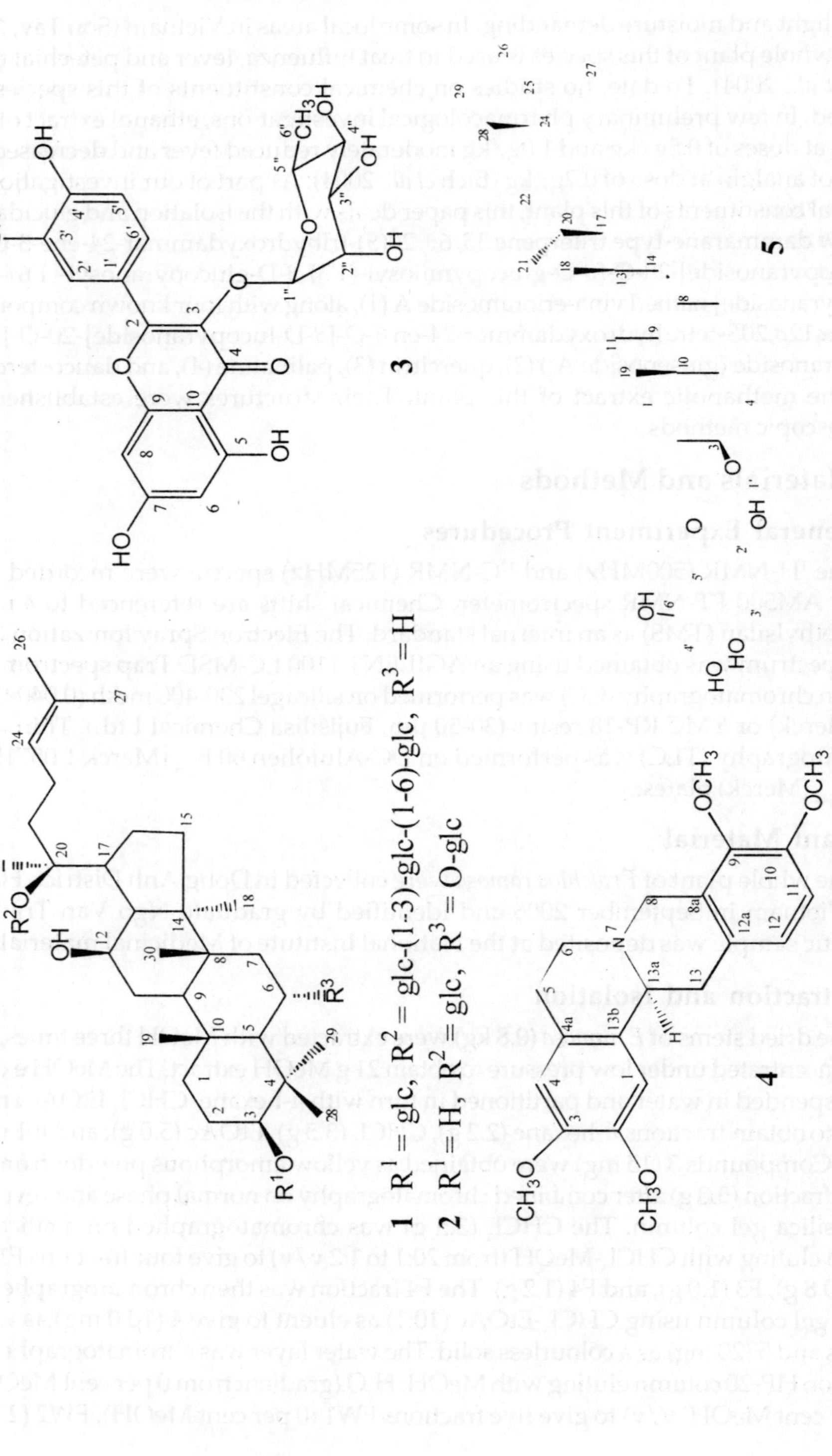


**Figure 221: The Structures of Compounds 1–5**

cent MeOH), FW3 (50 per cent MeOH), FW4 (75 per cent MeOH) and FW5 (100 per cent MeOH). Compound 1 (13 mg) was obtained from the FW2 fraction and compound 2 (9.0 mg) were obtained from the FW4 fraction as a colorless amorphous powder after combined chromatography on the normal phase and reversed phase silica gel column.

**3β,6β,20(*S*)-Trihydroxydammar-24-ene-3-*O*-[β-D-glucopyranoside]-20-*O*-[β-D-glucopyranosyl-(1'3)-β-D-glucopyranosyl-(1'6)-β-D-glucopyranoside](vinarioramoside A, 1)**

Colorless amorphous powder, mp. 183-184°C; ESI *m/z*: (positive) 1131 $[M+Na]^+$; (negative) 1107$[M-H]^-$($C_{54}H_{92}O_{23}$); $^1$H-NMR (500 MHz, $CD_3OD$) and $^{13}$C-NMR (125 MHz, $CD_3OD$): see Table 22.1.

**3β,6α,12β,20*S*-Tetrahydroxydammar-24-en 6-*O*-[β-D-glucopyranoside]-20-*O*-[β-D-glucopyranoside (ginsenoside $A_2$) (2)**

Colorless amorphous powder, mp. 194-196°C; ESI *m/z*: (positive) 823.3 $[M+Na]^+$; (negative) 799.2 $[M-H]^-$($C_{42}H_{72}O_{14}$); $^1$H-NMR (500 MHz, $CD_3OD$) δ (ppm): 1.09 and 1.77 (H-2), 1.62 and 1.68 (H-2), 3.36 (m, H-3), 1.15 (d, *J* = 3.0 Hz, H-5), 4.12 (dt, *J* = 3.0, 10.5 Hz, H-6), 1.65 and 2.06 (H-7), 1.52 (dd, *J* = 2.5, 13.0 Hz, H-9), 1.32 and 1.88 (H-11), 3.70 (m, H-12), 1.76 (overlapped, H-13), 1.16 and 1.63 (H-15), 1.42 and 1.95 (H-16), 2.29 (m, H-17), 1.03 (s, H-18), 1.12 (s, H-19), 1.36 (s, H-21), 1.64 and 1.84 (H-22), 2.12 (m, H-23), 5.13 (br t, *J* = 7.0 Hz, H-24), 1.70 (s, H-26), 1.64 (s, H-27), 1.35 (s, H-28), 1.03 9s, H-29), 0.97 (s, H-30), 20-O-Glc: 4.37 (d, *J* = 7.5 Hz, H-1'), 3.23 (H-2', H-3'), 3.35 (H-4'), 3.29 (H-5'), 3.65 (Ha-6'), 3.83 (dd, *J* = 2.0, 12.0 Hz, Hb-6'), 6-O-Glc: 4.62 (d, *J* = 7.5 Hz, H-1''), 3.10 (H-2''), 3.13 (H-3''), 3.35 (H-4''), 3.37 (H-5''), 3.67 (Ha-6''), and 3.80 (dd, *J* = 2.0, 12.0 Hz, Hb-6''); $^{13}$C-NMR (125 MHz, $CD_3OD$) δ (ppm): 40.38 (C-1), 27.66 (C-2), 78.26 (C-3), 40.49 (C-4), 61.80 (C-5), 80.92 (C-6), 45.31 (C-7), 41.89 (C-8), 50.61 (C-9), 40.19 (C-10), 30.97 (C-11), 71.74 (C-12), 49.84 (C-13), 53.13 (C-14), 31.54 (C-15), 27.24 (C-16), 53.13 (C-17), 17.65 (C-18), 17.80 (C-19), 84.94 (C-20), 22.82 (C-21), 36.65 (C-22), 24.23 (C-23), 125.86 (C-24), 132.29 (C-25), 25.84 (C-26), 17.93 (C-27), 31.38 (C-28), 16.10 (C-29), 17.11 (C-30), 20-O-Glc: 98.31 (C-1'), 75.41 (C-2'), 77.94 (C-3'), 71.24 (C-4'), 77.67 (C-5'), 62.94 (C-6'), 6-O-Glc: 105.57 (C-1''), 75.51 (C-2''), 79.88 (C-3''), 71.86 (C-4''), 79.09 (C-5''), and 62.57 (C-6'').

**Quercetin 3-*O*-α-L-rhamnopyranoside (quercitrin) (3)**

Yellow amorphous powders, mp. 182-185°C; ESI *m/z*: (positive) 449 $[M+H]^+$ ($C_{21}H_{20}O_{11}$); $^1$H-NMR (500 MHz, $CD_3OD$) δ (ppm): 6,21 (1H, d, *J* = 1.5 Hz, H-6), 6,38 (1H, d, *J* = 1.5 Hz, H-8), 7,35 (1H, d, *J* = 2,0 Hz, H-2'), 6,92 (1H, d, *J* = 8,5 Hz, H-5'), 7,32 (1H, dd, *J* = 8,5, 2,0 Hz, H-6'), 5,37(1H, d, *J* = 1,5 Hz, H-1''), 4,23 (1H, dd, *J* = 2,0, 3,0 Hz, H-2''), 3,76 (1H, dd, *J* = 3,0, 9,5 Hz, H-3''), 3,56 (1H, dd, *J* = 9,5, 9,5 Hz, H-4''), 3,43 (1H, m, H-5''), and 0,97 (3H, d, *J* = 6,0 Hz, H-6''). $^{13}$C-NMR (125 MHz, $CD_3OD$) δ (ppm) 159.29 (C-2), 136,21 (C-3), 179,61 (C-4), 163,53 (C-5), 99,81 (C-6), 165,81 (C-7), 94,73 (C-8), 158.18 (C-9), 105,89 (C-10), 122,97 (C-1'), 116,96 (C-2'), 146,35 (C-3'), 149,75 (C-4'), 116,37 (C-5'), 122,86 (C-6'), 103,51 (C-1''), 72,01 (C-2''), 72,12 (C-3''), 73,26 (C-4''), 71,88 (C-5''), and 17,62 (C-6'').

**Palmatine (4)**

Yellow needles, mp. 204-205°C; ESI *m/z*: (positive) 352 $[M]^+$ ($C_{21}H_{22}O_4N$); $^1$H-NMR (500 MHz, $CD_3OD$) δ (ppm): 7.58 (s, H-1), 7.01 (s, H-4), 3.28 (t, *J* = 6.0 Hz, H-5), 4.94 (t, *J* = 6.0 Hz, H-6), 9.73 (s, H-8), 8.00 (d, *J* = 9.5 Hz, H-11), 8.06 (d, *J* = 9.5 Hz, H-12), 8.75 (s, H-13), 3.92, 3.98, 4.06, and 4.20 (4 x $OCH_3$); $^{13}$C-NMR (125 MHz, $CD_3OD$) δ (ppm): 109.89 (C-1), 150.75 (C-2), 151.79 (C-3), 112.21 (C-4), 129.93 (C-4a), 27.77 (C-5), 57.31 (C-6), 146.22 (C-8), 123.13 (C-8a), 153.69 (C-9), 145.54 (C-10), 124.49 (C-11), 127.90 (C-12), 135.10 (C-12a), 121.20 (C-13), 139.56 (C-13a), 120.30 (C-13b), 57.09 (2-$OCH_3$), 57.59 (3-$OCH_3$), 62.55 (9-$OCH_3$), and 56.66 (10-$OCH_3$).

**Daucosterol (5)**

mp. 283-286°C; $[\alpha]^{25}_D$–41,5° (MeOH); $^1$H-NMR (500 MHz, $CD_3OD$) δ: 3.52 (1H, dd, *J* = 11.7, 5.1 Hz, H-3), 5.35 (1H, br d, *J* = 5.0 Hz, H-6), 0.68 (3H, s, H-18), 1,00 (3H, s, H-19), 0.92 (3H, d, *J* = 6.5 Hz, H-21), 0.84 (3H, t, *J* = 7.6 Hz, H-26), 0.81 (3H, d, *J* = 6.8 Hz, H-28), 0.83 (3H, d, *J* = 7.3 Hz, H-29), and 4,30 (1H, d, *J* = 7.8 Hz, H-1'). $^{13}$C-NMR (125 MHz, $CD_3OD$) δ: 36.78 (C-1), 31.32 (C-2), 76.89 (C-3), 39.75 (C-4), 140.41 (C-5), 121.12, 31,37 (C-7), (C-6), 31.32 (C-8), 49.56 (C-9), 36.16 (C-10), 20.54 (C-11), 38.27 (C-12), 41.80 (C-13), 55.39 (C-14), 25.43 (C-15), 29.21 (C-16), 56.13 (C-17), 11.61 (C-18), 19.04 (C-19), 35.42 (C-20), 18.56 (C-21), 33.31 (C-22), 27.72 (C-23), 45.11 (C-24), 28.67 (C-25), 19.64 (C-26), 18.89 (C-27), 22.56 (C-28), 11.73 (C-29), 100.76 (C-1'), 73.42 (C-2'), 76.73 (C-3'), 70.07 (C-4'), 76.69 (C-5'), and 61.06 (C-6').

## 3.0 Results and Discussion

Compound 1 was obtained as a colorless amorphous powder from the methanolic extract of whole plant of *E. ramosa*. The $^{13}$C-NMR spectrum exhibited signals of 54 carbon atoms including 30 carbons of the triterpene and 24 carbons belong to four sugar units, suggesting the presence of the triterpene saponin. A tri-substituted double bond was assigned at δ 126.03 (d)/132.24 (s), and a *gem* methyl group linked to the double bond were at δ 25.93 and 18.02. Two oxymethine carbons of the aglycon were at δ 91.32 and 71.69, and a tertiary carbon bearing oxygen atom was at δ 84.97. In addition, eight quaternary methyl groups were assigned at δ 16.32, 16.69, 16.73, 17.40, 18.02, 22.49, 25.93, and 28.42. Comparing the carbon chemical shifts of the aglycon of 1 with those of dammarane type saponins, which have a hydroxyl group at C-12, a double bond at C-24/C-25 and two sugars attached to C-3 and C-20 and found to match well (Yoshikawa *et al.*, 2003; Yahara *et al.*, 1979). Four anomeric carbons were at δ 98.10, 104.99, 104.52 and 105.39, together with four oxymethylene carbons at δ 62.28, 63.12, 62.83, and 70.26 suggested the presence of four D-glucopyranosyl groups, which were further confirmed by the appearance of four β-configuration anomeric protons (each, vicinal H-1/2 in *trans* position) as doublets at δ 4.46, 4.70, 4.38 and 4.61 (each, *J* = 7.5 Hz) in the $^1$H-NMR spectrum. From the above data, the suggested molecular formula of 1 was $C_{54}H_{92}O_{23}$, which was further confirmed by the ESI mass spectrum with the exhibition of the quasi molecular ion peaks at *m/z* 1131 $[M+Na]^+$ (positive ion mode) and *m/z* 1107 $[M-H]^-$(negative ion mode). All the NMR data of 1 were first established by comparison its NMR data with those of 3β,6β,20(*S*)-trihydroxydammar-24-ene-3-*O*-[β-D-glucopyranoside]-20-*O*-[β-D-xyllopyranosyl-(1'3)-β-D-xyllopyranosyl-(1'6)-β-D-glucopyranoside] (Yoshikawa,

2003) (Table 22.1), and further deduced by the heteronuclear single quantum coherence (HSQC) and the heteronuclear multiple-bond correlation (HMBC) experiments. All the chemical shifts of the protons were established by the analysis of the cross peaks observed in the HSQC spectrum. The partial structures, the linking of substitution groups and all the chemical structure of 1 were reconfirmed by the H-C long range correlations in the HMBC spectrum and summarized in Table 22.1.

**Table 22.1: NMR Data of 1 and Notoginsenoside O**

| *C* | $\delta_C^{\#}$ | *1* | | |
|---|---|---|---|---|
| | | $\delta_C^{a,b}$ | $\delta_H^{a,c}$ (J, Hz) | *HMBC (H to C)* |
| 1 | 39.3 | 40.27 | 1.04 m/1.75 m | |
| 2 | 26.7 | 27.25 | 1.75 m/2.03 m | |
| 3 | 88.7 | 91.32 | 3.22* | |
| 4 | 39.6 | 40.58 | – | |
| 5 | 56.4 | 57.56 | 0.80 d (11.5) | |
| 6 | 18.4 | 19.24 | 1.51 m/1.60 m | |
| 7 | 35.1 | 35.86 | 1.32 m/1.58 m | |
| 8 | 40.1 | 40.99 | – | |
| 9 | 50.2 | 51.10 | 1.47* | |
| 10 | 37.0 | 37.93 | – | |
| 11 | 30.7 | 31.50 | 1.06*/1.60* | |
| 12 | 70.1 | 71.69 | 3.28* | C–13, C–14, C–17 |
| 13 | 49.5 | 49.85 | 1.77 br d (11.5) | C–12, C–17 |
| 14 | 51.7 | 52.41 | – | |
| 15 | 30.7 | 30.84 | 1.28*/1.82 m | |
| 16 | 26.8 | 27.25 | 1.36*/1.92 m | |
| 17 | 51.7 | 52.90 | 2.32 m | |
| 18 | 16.1 | 16.32 | 1.30 s | C–8, C–13, C–14, C–15 |
| 19 | 16.3 | 16.69 | 0.94 s | C–1, C–5, C–9, C–10 |
| 20 | 83.4 | 84.97 | – | |
| 21 | 22.3 | 22.49 | 1.38 s | C–17, C–20, C–22 |
| 22 | 36.2 | 36.79 | 1.57*/1.82 m | |
| 23 | 23.2 | 23.88 | 2.16 m | |
| 24 | 125.9 | 126.03 | 5.16 br d (7.0) | |
| 25 | 130.8 | 132.24 | 1.71 s | |
| 26 | 25.8 | 25.93 | 1.65 s | C–24, C–25, C–27 |
| 27 | 18.0 | 18.02 | 1.65 s | C–24, C–25, C–26 |
| 28 | 28.1 | 28.42 | 1.95 s | C–3, C–4, C–5, C–29 |
| 29 | 16.8 | 16.73 | 0.88 s | C–3, C–4, C–5, C–28 |
| 30 | 17.5 | 17.40 | 0.94 s | C–7, C–8, C–9, C–14 |

*Contd...*

**Table 22.1–Contd...**

| *C* | $\delta_C^{\#}$ | *1* | | |
|---|---|---|---|---|
| | | $\delta_C^{a,b}$ | $\delta_H^{a,c}$ (J, Hz) | *HMBC (H to C)* |
| GlcI | *GlcI* | | | |
| 1' | 106.7 | 105.39 | 4.46 d (7.5) | C–3 |
| 2' | 75.7 | 75.29 | 3.14* | |
| 3' | 78.6 | 77.93 | 3.58 dd (8.0, 8.0) | |
| 4' | 71.9 | 71.60 | 3.23* | |
| 5' | 78.1 | 77.93 | 3.46* | |
| 6' | 63.1 | 63.12 | 3.66*/3.78* | |
| GlcII | *GlcII* | | | |
| 1' | 97.9 | 98.10 | 4.61 d (7.5) | C–20 |
| 2' | 75.3 | 75.14 | 3.24* | |
| 3' | 79.2 | 78.54 | 3.38* | |
| 4' | 71.4 | 71.55 | 3.30* | |
| 5' | 76.8 | 77.70 | 3.27* | |
| 6' | 70.1 | 70.26 | 4.09 dd (2.0, 11.5)<br>3.80 dd (5.0, 11.5) | |
| XylI | *GlcIII* | | | |
| 1''' | 105.2 | 104.99 | 4.38 d (7.5) | C–6'' |
| 2''' | 73.4 | 76.79 | 3.46* | |
| 3''' | 86.2 | 81.14 | 3.60* | |
| 4''' | 70.8 | 71.93 | 3.75* | |
| 5''' | 66.1 | 78.54 | 3.68* | |
| 6''' | | 62.83 | 3.66*/3.78* | |
| XylII | *GlcIV* | | | |
| 1'''' | 105.9 | 104.52 | 4.70 d (7.5) | C–3''' |
| 2'''' | 74.7 | 76.32 | 3.38* | |
| 3'''' | 77.9 | 78.31 | 3.27* | |
| 4'''' | 71.0 | 71.69 | 3.38* | |
| 5'''' | 67.2 | 78.50 | 3.78* | |
| 6'''' | | 62.83 | 3.66*/3.78* | |

[a]Measured in $CD_3OD$, [b]125 MHz, [c]500 MHz, Chemical shift (d) in ppm, [#]$d_C$ of notoginsenoside O in Py–$d_5$ (Yoshikawa *et al.*, 2003).

In the HMBC spectrum, H-1'''' (δ 4.70) correlated with C-3''' (δ 81.14), H-1''' (δ 4.38) correlated with C-6'' (δ 77.70), H-1'' (δ 4.61) correlated with C-20 (δ 84.97), and H-1' (δ 4.46) correlated with C-3 (δ 91.32) confirming that the C-1' of GlcI attached to C-3, C-1'''' of GlcIV linked to C-3''' of the GlcIII, C-1''' of GlcIII linked to C-6'' of GlcII,

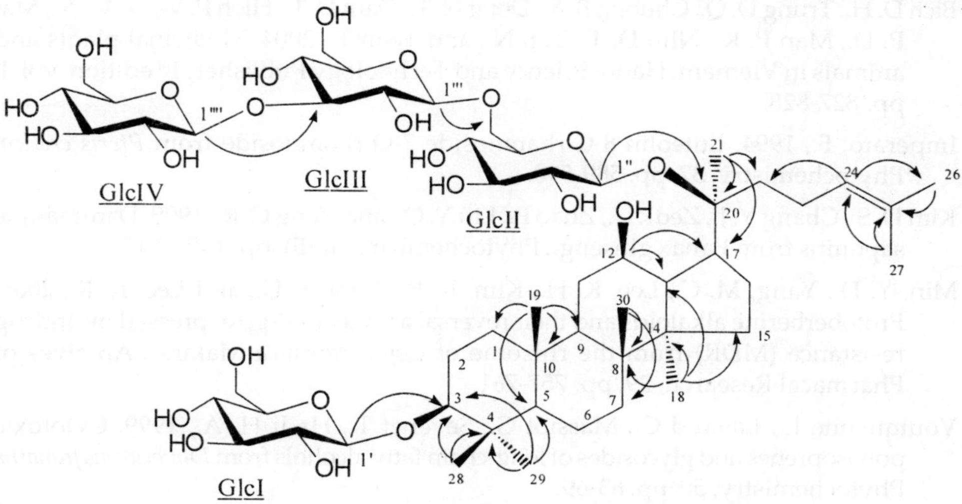


**Figure 22.2: Selected HMBC Correlations of 1**

and C-1'' of GlcII attached to C-20 of the aglycon. Furthermore, cross peaks were observed between H-21 (δ 1.38) and C-20 (84.97)/C-17 (δ 52.90)/C-22 (δ 36.79), between H-24 (δ 5.16) and C-22 (δ 36.79)/C-23 (δ 23.88)/C-25 (δ 132.24)/C-26 (25.93)/C-27 (δ 18.02), between H-28 (δ 1.95)/H-29 (δ 0.88) and C-3 (δ 91.32), and between H-17 (δ 2.32) and C-12 (δ 71.69)/C-13 (δ 49.85) in the HMBC spectrum. This evidence confirmed the location of carbons bearing oxygen atom at C-3, C-12 and C-20, as well as, the *gem* dimethyl attached to the double bond. The absolute configuration of C-3, C-12 and C-20 were determined as shown in Figure 22.1 from the good agreement of the NMR data (the chemical shifts and the coupling constants) of 1 with those of relative dammarane-type saponins (Yoshikawa *et al.*, 2003; Yahara *et al.*, 1979; Min *et al.*, 1999), the stereochemistry frequently appeared in the nature. Consequently, the structure of saponin 1 was established as 3β,6β,20(*S*)-trihydroxydammar-24-ene-3-*O*-[β-D-glucopyranoside]-20-*O*-[β-D-glucopyranosyl-(1'3)-β-D-glucopyranosyl-(1'6)-β-D-glucopyranoside], a new nature product and named as vina-erimosa A.

Compounds 2-5 were identified as 3β,6α,12β,20*S*-tetrahydroxydammar-24-en 6-*O*-[β-D-glucopyranoside]-20-*O*-[β-D-glucopyranoside (ginsenoside $A_2$) (Yahara *et al.*, 1979). quercitrin (Agrawal, 1989), (-) tetrahydropalmatine (Min *et al.*, 2006), and daucosterol (Voutquenne *et al.*, 1999), respectively, by comparison their NMR data with the literature. All their NMR data were established by the detail analysis of 1D-NMR ($^1$H-, $^{13}$C-NMR, DEPT 90°, DEPT 135°) and 2D-NMR (HSQC, HMBC) spectra. This is the first report of these compounds from *Eriochloa ramosa*.

## References

Agrawal, P. K., carbon-13 NMR of flavonoids, Elsevier Science Publishers B. V. 1989, pp. 154-155, 334-335.

Bich D. H., Trung D. Q., Chuong B. X., Dong N. T., Dam D. T., Hien P. V., Lo V., N., Mai P. D., Man P. K., Nhu D. T., Tap N., and Toan T., 2004. Medicinal plants and animals in Vietnam, Hanoi Science and Technology Publisher, 1st edition, vol. I, pp. 827-828.

Imperato, F., 1994. Luteolin 8-C-rhamnoside-7-O-rhamnoside from *Pteris cretica*. Phytochemistry, 37, pp. 589-590.

Kim D. S., Chang Y. J., Zedk U., Zhao P., Liu Y. Q., and Yang C. R., 1995. Dammarane saponins from Panax ginseng., Phytochemistry, 40(5), pp. 1493-1497.

Min, Y. D., Yang, M. C., Lee, K. H., Kim, K. R., Choi, S. U., and Lee, K. R., 2006. Protoberberine alkaloids and their reversal activity of P-gp expressed multidrug resistance (MDR) from the rhizome of *Coptis japonica* Makino. Archives of Pharmacal Research, 29, pp. 757-761.

Voutquenne L., Lavaud C., Massiot G., Sevenet T., Hadi H. A., 1999. Cytotoxic polyisoprenes and glycosides of long-chain fatty alcohols from *Dimocarpus fumatus* Phytochemistry, 50, pp. 63-69.

Yahara, S., Kaji, K., and Tanaka, O., 1979. Further study on dammarane-type saponins of roots, leaves, flower-buds, ang fruits of Panax ginseng C.A. Meyer. Chem. Pharm. Bull., 27, pp. 88-92.

Yoshikawa M., Morikawa T., Kashima Y., Ninomiya K., and Matsuda H., 2003. Structures of new dammarane-type triterpene saponins from the flower buds of Panax notoginseng and hepatoprotective effects of principal ginseng saponins., Journal of Natural Products, 66, pp. 922-927.

# Chapter 23

# Indole Alkaloids from *Kopsia pitardii* Merr. (Apocynaceae)

***Do Thi Thu Huong[1]*, Nguyen Ngoc Hanh[2], Nguyen Quyet Chien[1] and Nguyen Van Hung[1]***

[1] *Institute of Chemistry, Vietnamese Academy of Science and Technology, Hanoi, Vietnam*

[2] *Institute of Chemical Technology, Vietnamese Academy of Science and Technology, Ho Chi Minh City, Vientam*

**E-mail: dothuhuong58@hotmail.com, dothuhuong58@gmail.com*

## ABSTRACT

Four indole alkaloids: methyl 11, 12-methylenedioxy-$N_1$-decarbomethoxy-$\Delta^{14,15}$-chanofruticosinate (1), methyl $N_1$-decarbomethoxy chanofruticosinate (2), methyl 11,12-methylenedioxychanofruticosinate (3) and methyl 12-methoxychanofruticosinate (4) were isolated from the Vietnamese medicinal plant Trang Nam (*Kopsia pitardii* Merr., Apocynaceae) with 0.12, 0.038, 0.005 and 0.01 per cent yield, respectively. MS and NMR analysis determined their structures.

***Keywords:** Indole alkaloids, Vietnamese medicinal plant Trang Nam, Kopsia pitardii Merr., Apocynaceae.*

## 1.0 Introduction

The plant *Kopsia pitardii* Merr. (Vietnamese name: Trang Nam) grows in the South of Vietnam. Its leaves were described to possess anti-inflammatory activity and are used to treat throat inflammation and arthritis (Chi, 1996). On international level, many Kopsia species have been investigated chemically and are known to contain indole alkaloids of various structure types (Kan, 1984; Sevenet, 1994; Kam,

2004; Lim, 2006; Sevenet, 1991; Mok, 1998; Rho, 1999). In the present paper we report the isolation and structure elucidation of the alkaloids: methyl 11, 12-methylenedioxy-$N_1$-decarbomethoxy-$\Delta^{14,15}$-chanofruticosinate (1), methyl $N_1$-decarbomethoxy chanofruticosinate (2), methyl 11,12-methylenedioxychanofruticosinate (3), and methyl 12-methoxychanofruticosinate (4) from the leaves of this plant.

## 2.0 Experimental

### 2.1 General Experimental Procedures

FTIR spectra were measured on a Nicolet Impact 410 spectrometer. EIMS spectra were measured on an HP 599B mass spectrometer at 70 eV. ESIMS was measured on an Agilent LC-MSD-Trap-SL at the Institute of Chemistry (Vietnamese Academy of Science and Technology, Hanoi). NMR spectra were acquired on a Bruker Advance 500 spectrometer. TLC was performed on Merck 60-$F_{254}$ silica gel plates, detected with Dragendoffs reagent. Column chromatography was accomplished with silica gel (230-400 mesh or 70-230 mesh).

### 2.2 Plant Material

Leaves and branches of *Kopsia pitardii* Merr., Apocynaceae (Synonym: *K. cochinchinensis* auct. Non Kuntze) were collected in Nui Dinh, Dong Nai province in June 1998 and identified by Mr. Nguyen Van Dau (Ho Chi Minh Plant Park).

### 2.3 Extraction and Isolation

The dried and powdered leaves and branches of *K. pitardii* (100g) were alkalized with $NH_4OH$ 10 per cent and extracted with $CH_2Cl_2$. The extract was concentrated under reduced pressure and dissolved in ether. The ether solution was extracted with HCl 5 per cent in water. This acid solution was washed with ether, alkalized with $NH_4OH$ and extracted with $CH_2Cl_2$. After evaporation 0.85 g of total alkaloids was obtained. Column chromatography of the total alkaloids on silica gel (230-400 mesh) was performed using solvent mixtures of increasing polarity (n-hexane/ethyl

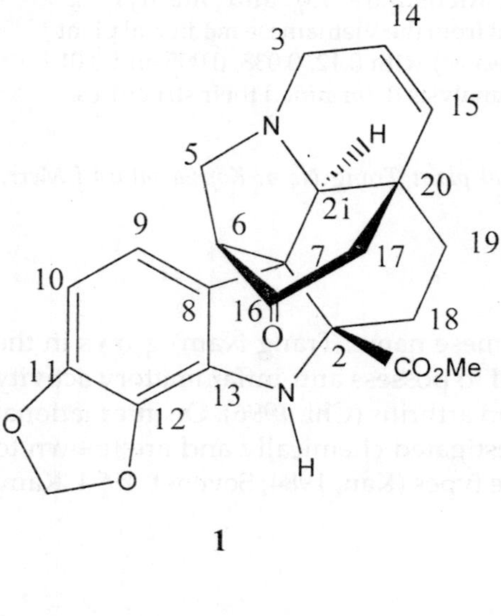


**1**

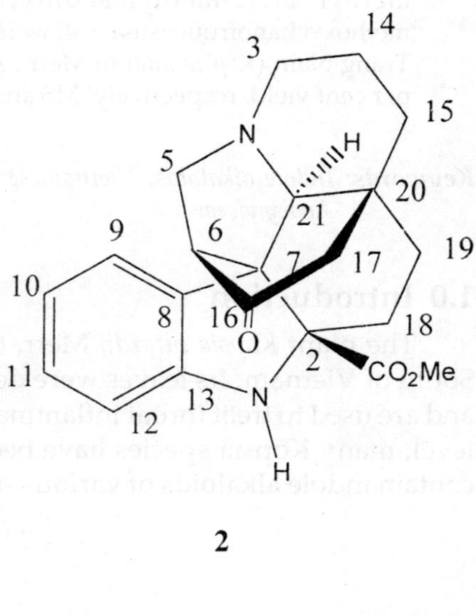


**2**

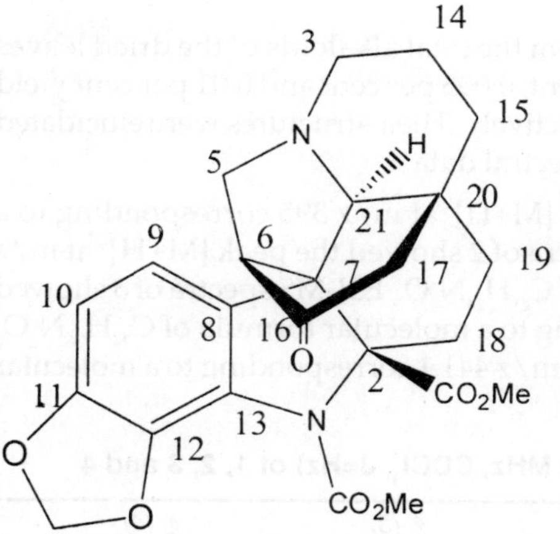

3

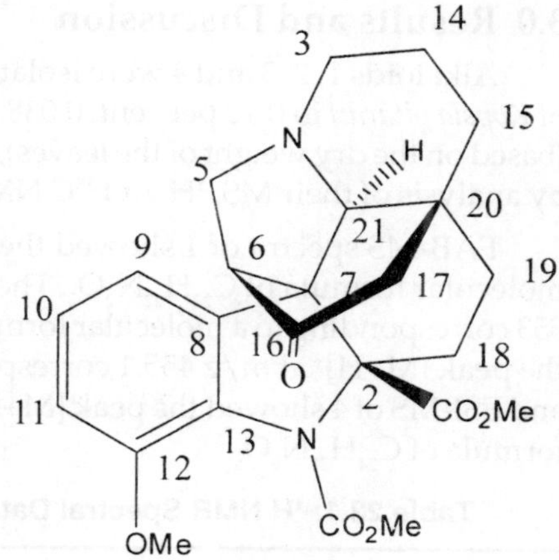

4

acetate and $CH_2Cl_2$/ethyl acetate) to give alkaloid 1 (120 mg, 0.12 per cent), alkaloid 2 (38 mg, 0.038 per cent), alkaloid 3 (5 mg, 0.005 per cent) and alkaloid 4 (10 mg, 0.01 per cent).

**Methyl 11,12-methylenedioxy-N$_1$-decarbomethoxy-$\Delta^{14,15}$-chanofruticosinate (1)**

mp = 175-178 °C, TLC (n-hexane/EtOAc 1:1) $R_f$: 0.48, IR (KBr) $\nu_{max}$ ($cm^{-1}$): 3340, 2931, 2888, 2852, 1728, 1731, 1609, 1458, 1241, 1157, 1001, 742; EI-MS m/z (per cent): 394 $[M]^+$ ($C_{22}H_{22}N_2O_5$, 3.8), 335 (19.8), 294 (23.0), 293 (100), 220 (1,7), 180 (1.5), 129 (1.7), 115 (1.8), 83 (10.4), 58 (16.8), 55 (17.5).

**Methyl N$_1$–decarbomethoxychanofruticosinate (2)**

mp = 197-198 °C, TLC (n-hexane/EtOAc 1:1) $R_f$: 0.51, IR (KBr), $\nu_{max}$ ($cm^{-1}$): 3347, 2931, 2888, 2852, 1726, 1714, 1610, 1459, 1240, 1163, 1000, 742; EI-MS m/z (per cent): 352 $[M]^+$ ($C_{21}H_{24}N_2O_5$, 17.3), 294 (23.6), 293 (100), 223 (3.0), 179 (3.6), 115 (4.5), 83 (15.3), 58 (30.7), 55 (30.4).

**Methyl 11,12-methylendioxychanofruticosinate (3)**

Yellow paste, TLC (n–hexane/EtOAc 1:1) $R_f$: 0,49, IR (KBr), $\nu_{max}$ ($cm^{-1}$): 3448 (broad), 3347, 2924, 2867, 1775, 1722, 1674, 1460, 1376, 1245, 1057, 985; EI-MS m/z (per cent): 454 $[M]^+$ ($C_{24}H_{26}N_2O_7$, 4.7), 395 ((34.8), 365 (6.3), 323 (9.5), 294 (6.2), 293 (24.7), 173 (3.4), 115 (11.1), 107 (60.3), 83 (23.4), 58 (30.7), 57 (31.3), 55 (100).

**Methyl 12-methoxychanofruticosinate (4)**

Colourless crystal, IR (KBr) $\nu_{max}$ ($cm^{-1}$): 3428 (broad), 2934, 2869, 1740, 1714, 1605, 1492, 1460, 1359, 1258, 1110, 1053, 804, 740, 572, 446; EI-MS (m/z), (per cent): 440 $[M]^+$ ($C_{25}H_{32}N_2O_5$, 22.3), 409 (4.6), 381 (100), 349 (9.1), 321 (27.3), 83 (10.1), 59 (56.3), 55(28.8).

## 3.0 Results and Discussion

Alkaloids 1, 2, 3 and 4 were isolated from the total alkaloids of the dried leaves of *Kopsia pitardii* in 0.12 per cent, 0.038 per cent, 0.005 per cent and 0.01 per cent yield (based on the dry weight of the leaves), respectively. Their structures were elucidated by analysis of their MS, $^1$H and $^{13}$C NMR spectral data.

FAB-MS spectra of 1 showed the peak $[M+H]^+$ at m/z 395 corresponding to a molecular formula of $C_{22}H_{22}N_2O_5$. The spectra of 2 showed the peak $[M+H]^+$ at m/z 353 corresponding to a molecular formula of $C_{21}H_{24}N_2O_3$. ESI-MS spectra of 3 showed the peak $[M+H]^+$ at m/z 455.1 corresponding to a molecular formula of $C_{24}H_{26}N_2O_7$ and ESI-MS of 4 showed the peak $[M+H]^+$ at m/z 441.1 corresponding to a molecular formula of $C_{24}H_{28}N_2O_6$.

**Table 23.1: $^1$H NMR Spectral Data (500 MHz, $CDCl_3$, J=Hz) of 1, 2, 3 and 4**

| *Position* | $\delta_H$ *(1)* | $\delta_H$ *(2)* | $\delta_H$ *(3)* | $\delta_H$ *(4)* |
|---|---|---|---|---|
| 3 | 2.96–3.08 m<br>2.96–3.08 m | 3.38 dt (19.5; 2.6)<br>3.84 ddd (19.5; 2.4; 1.5) | 2.80–3.04 m | 2.95–3.05 m |
| 5 | 2.87 d (11.2)<br>3.76 d (11.2) | 2.83 dd (11.0)<br>4.10 d (11.0; 6.0) | 2.84–3.04 m | 3.78 dd (10.8, 6.1)<br>2.96 d (10.8) |
| 6 | 2.96 d (6.2) | 3.25 d (6.0) | 3.31 d (6.2) | 3.20 brd (6.1) |
| 9 | 6.74 d (8.0) | 6.70 d (7.9) | 7.09 br d (7.5) | 6.88 dd (7.6, 0.8) |
| 10 | 6.52 d (8.0) | 6.33 d (7.9) | 6.78 br t (7.4) | 7.02 dd (8.1, 7.7) |
| 11 | – | – | 7.06 dt (0.9; 7.7) | 6.83 dd (8.2, 0.8) |
| 12 | – | – | 6.73 br d (7.7) | – |
| 14 | 1.20–1.50 m<br>1.80–2.00 m | 5.60 dt (9.8; 2.4) | 1.23–1.39 m<br>1.68–1.96 m | 1.30–1.45 m |
| 15 | 1.20–1.50 m<br>1.20–1.50 m | 5.96 ddd<br>(9.8; 2.4; 1.5) | 1.23–1.39 m<br>1.68–1.96 m | 1.85–2.00 m<br>1.30–1.40 m |
| 17 | 2.10 d (18.3)<br>2.83 d (18.3) | 2.31 d (18.2)<br>2.47 d (18.2) | 2.04 d (18.8)<br>2.83 d (18.8) | 2.90 d (18.7)<br>2.07 d (19.0) |
| 18 | 2.23 dd (16.2; 7.7) | 1.81 m–1.98 m<br>1.81 m–1.98 m | 1.68–1.96 m<br>1.68–1.96 m | 2.95–3.10 m<br>3.28 m |
| 19 | 1.20–1.50 m<br>1.58 | 1.55 dt (10.1; 2.1)<br>1.78–1.99 m | 1.23–1.39 m<br>1.52 brd (13) | 1.56 brd (13.0)<br>1.28–1.35 m |
| 21 | 2.48 s | 2.61 s | 2.48 s | 2.52 s |
| NH | | 4.49 s | 4.50 s | |
| $OCH_2O$ | 5.95 s (2H) | 5.87 d (1.5) | | |
| 5.93 d (1.5) | – | | | |
| O<u>Me</u> | 3.61 s | 3.65 s | 3.60 s | 3.82 s |
| $NCO_2$<u>Me</u> | 3.84 s | – | – | 3.85 s |
| 2–$CO_2$<u>Me</u> | – | – | – | 3.68 s |

s: Singlet, d: Doublet, t: Triplet, q: Quartet, br: Broad.

The molecular structures of these alkaloids were elucidated by the analysis of their EI-MS, ESI-MS, FAB-MS, $^{1}H$, $^{13}C$ NMR and DEPT, COSY, HMQC and HMBC spectral data. Their $^{1}H$, $^{13}C$ NMR spectral data are shown in Tables 23.1 and 23.2. By comparing these spectral data with published ones, the isolated compounds were identified as the indole alkaloids:

- 1 is methyl 11, 12-methylenedioxy-$N_1$-decarbomethoxy-$\Delta^{14,15}$-chanofruticosinate (Kam, 1993; Husain, 2001; Huong, 2007).
- 2 is methyl $N_1$–decarbomethoxychanofruticosinate (Kam, 1993; Huong, 2007).
- 3 is methyl 11, 12-methylendioxychanofruticosinate (Husain, 2001; Huong, 2007).
- 4 is methyl 12-methoxychanofruticosinate (Husain, 2001).

**Table 23.2: $^{13}C$–NMR Spectra Data (125 MHz, $CDCl_3$) of 1, 2, 3 and 4**

| *Position* | $\delta_C$ *(1)* | $\delta_C$ *(2)* | $\delta_C$ *(3)* | $\delta_C$ *(4)* |
|---|---|---|---|---|
| 2 | 75.0 | 73.8 | 76.1 | 77.8 |
| 3 | 50.3 | 46.6 | 46.5 | 46.9 |
| 5 | 59.5 | 52.7 | 52.4 | 53.3 |
| 6 | 54.5 | 55.3 | 55.5 | 54.8 |
| 7 | 57.8 | 57.7 | 58.4 | 60.4 |
| 8 | 130.2 | 133.2 | 129.2. | 138.4 |
| 9 | 116.2 | 124.0 | 116.9 | 116.5 |
| 10 | 100.9 | 119.8 | 103.4 | 125.3 |
| 11 | 148.1 | 128.1 | 149.1 | 112.8 |
| 12 | 128.1 | 110.2 | 124.1 | 149.1 |
| 13 | 131.7 | 147.8 | 133.8 | 130.5 |
| 14 | 126.1 | 17.5 | 17.5 | 17.9 |
| 15 | 136.0 | 35.0 | 35.2 | 36.1 |
| 16 | 207.6 | 209.3 | 208.1 | 209.1 |
| 17 | 46.9 | 42.6 | 42.4 | 43.6 |
| 18 | 27.2 | 27.5 | 23.5 | 23.8 |
| 19 | 31.9 | 34.7 | 34.9 | 34.9 |
| 20 | 37.1 | 36.2 | 38.0 | 37.1 |
| 21 | 65.7 | 68.4 | 68.5 | 69.2 |
| O<u>CH₂</u>O → $O\underline{CH_2}O$ | 100.9 | – | 100.7 | – |
| $C_2$–$\underline{C=O}$ | 174.6 | 175.0 | 174.7 | 171.8 |
| N–$\underline{C=O}$ | – | – | 153.1 | 153.8 |
| O$\underline{Me}$ | 52.3 | 52.2 | 52.6 | 56.6 |
| $NCO_2\underline{Me}$ | – | – | 53.0 | 53.4 |
| 2–$CO_2\underline{Me}$ | – | – | – | 52.9 |

## Acknowledgements

We thank Mr. Nguyen Van Dau, Ho Chi Minh Plant Park for the identification of the plant. We wish to thank Dr. Mary Pais and Dr. Thierry Sevenet, Institute of Natural Products ICSN-CNRS, France for the FAB-MS.

## References

Huong, D.T.T., Hanh, N.N. and Chien, N.Q., 2007. Three indole alkaloids from *Kopsia pitardii* Merr., *Journal of Chemistry* (Vietnamese), 45 (II), 152-155.

Husain, K., Jantan, I., Kamarudin, Said, I.M, Aiami, N. and Takayama, H.I., 2001. Methyl chanofruticosinates from leaves of *Kopsia flavida* Blume, *Phytochem.*, 57, 603-606.

Kan, C.,Husson, H.P., Potier, P. and Kosoffine, C., 1984.A new dimeric indole alkaloid of pleiomutine type from *Kopsia officinalis*, *J. Nat. Prod.*, 47, 117-122.

Kam, T. and Choo, Y., 2004. Venalstonine and dioxokopsan derivatives from *Kopsia fruticosa*, *Phytochem.*, 65, 2119-2122.

Kam, T., Tan, P., Hoong, P. and Chu, C., 1993. Methyl chanofruticosinates from leaves of *Kopsia arborea*, *Phytochem.*, 3, 489-491.

Lim, K.H. and Kam, T.S., 2006. Arboflorine, an unusual pentacyclic monoterpenoid indole alkaloid incorporating a third nitrogen atom, *Org. Lett.*, 8(8), 1733-5.

Mok, S.L., Yoganathan, K., Lim, T.M. and Kam, T.S., 1998. Cardiovascular effects of aspidofractinine-type alkaloids from Kopsia, *J. Nat. Prod.*, 61(3), 328-32.

Rho, M.C., Toyoshima, M., Hayashi, M., Koyano, T., Subramaniam, G., Kam, T.S. and Komiyama, K., 1999. Reversal of multidrug resistance by kopsiflorine isolated from *Kopsia dasyrachis*, *Planta Med.*, 65(4), 307-10.

Sevenet, T., Allorge, L., David, B., Awang, K., Hamid, A., Hadi, A., Kan-Fan, C., Quirion, J.C., Remy, F., Schaller, H. and Teo, L.E., 1994. A preliminary chemotaxonomic review of *Kopsia* (Apocynaceae), *Journal of Ethnopharmacology*, 41, 147-183.

Sevenet, T., 1991. Looking for new drugs: what criteria?, *J. Ethnopharmacol.*, 32(1-3), 83-90.

Vo Van Chi, 1996. Dictionary of Vietnamese Medicinal Plants, Medical Publishing House, pp. 1250.

# Chapter 24

# Review of Lupane Triterpenoids from *Acanthopanax* Species and their Pharmacological Activities

***Nguyen Xuan Nhiem*[1,2], *Nguyen Huu Tung*[1,2], *Eun Mi Choi*[2] and *Young Ho Kim*[2]***

[1]*Institue of Natural Products Chemistry, Vietnamese Academy of Science and Technology, Hanoi, Vietnam*

[2]*College of Pharmacy, Chungnam National University, Daejeon 305-764, Korea*

**E-mail: yhk@cnu.ac.kr*

## ABSTRACT

*Acanthopanax* species (Araliaceae) are widely distributed in Korea, China, Vietnam, Malaysia, Polynesia, Europe, North Africa and America. The barks and leaves of *Acanthopanax* species have traditionally been used as a tonic and a sedative as well as in the treatment of rheumatism and diabetes. Chemical components of *Acanthopanax* species and their pharmacological activities were studied by several groups worldwide. Lignans, phenylpropanoids, coumarins, flavonoids, terpenoids and polyacetylenes have been isolated from *Acanthopanax* species and have been shown to have various levels of activities such as anti-bacterial, anti-cancer, anti-gout, anti-hepatitis, anti-hyperglycemic, anti-inflammatory, antioxidant, anti-pyretic, anti-xanthine oxidase, choleretic, hemostatic, hypocholesterolemic, immunostimulatory and radioprotectant effects, etc. Herein, we review the recent chemical components of lupane triterpenoides from *Acanthopanx* species and their pharmacological activities. Additionally, we describe the effect of chiisanoside on the function of osteoblasts using pre-osteoblastic target cell line, MC3T3-E1, which has been a well-characterized as an *in vitro* model for osteoblast differentiation.

***Keywords**: Acanthopanax, Lupane triterpenoid, Pharmacological activity, Chiisanoside.*

## 1.0 Introduction

*Acanthopanax* species (Araliaceae) are widely distributed in Asia, Malaysia, Polynesia, Europe, North Africa and the America. *Acanthopanax* species have traditionally been used as a tonic and a sedative as well as in the treatment of rheumatism and diabetes. The ingredients of *Acanthopanax* species were reported to have various pharmacological activities such as anti-bacterial, anti-cancer, anti-gout, anti-hepatitis, anti-hyperglycemic, anti-inflammatory, antioxidant, anti-pyretic, anti-xanthine oxidase, choleretic, hemostatic, hypocholesterolemic, immunostimulatory, radioprotectant effects, etc.

Chemical components of *Acanthopanax* species were studied by many researchers worldwide. Several types of compounds have been isolated from *Acanthopanax* species. Major active constituents are reported as lignans (eleutheroside E, sesamin, liriodendrin, etc), phenylpropanoids (syringin, coniferin, chlorogenic acid, etc.), cuomarins (isofraxidin, scoparone, etc.), flavonoids (hyperin, kaempferitrin, etc), diterpenoids (acanthoic acid, sumogaside, etc.), polyacetylenes (falcarinol, falcarindiol, etc.) and others. Various types of triterpene saponins were reported form the leaves from *Acanthopanax* species. On the basis of the type of aglycone, these saponis can be classified into the oleanane, lupane, taraxane, ursane, and 3,4-secolupane classes. Of these saponins, lupane triterpenes were reported as major components of *Acanthopanax* leaves and showed significant biological effects on several bioassay systems.

Herein, we have reviewed the recently reported lupane triterpenoides from *Acanthopanx* species and their pharmacological activities. Additionally, we described the effect of chiisanoside on the function of osteoblasts using pre-osteoblastic target cell line, MC3T3-E1, which has been a well-characterized as an *in vitro* model for osteoblast differentiation.

### Lupane Triterpenoids

Firstly, lupane triterpenoids containing carboxylic acid at C-28 were mainly isolated from the leaves of *Acanthopanx* species.

Impressic acid [3α,11α-dihydroxy lup-20(29)-en-28-oic acid] [1] was isolated from the leaves of *A. trifoliatus* (Ty *et al.*, 1984) and from the root of *A. koreanum* (Cai *et al.*, 2004).

3α, 11α, 23-Trihydroxy lup-20(29)-en-28-oic acid [2] (Ty *et al.*, 1984) and 3α, 11α-dihydroxy-23-oxo–lup-20(29)-en-28-oic acid [3] (Ty *et al.*, 1985) were isolated from the leaves of *A. trifoliatus* (Ty *et al.*, 1985).

Acantrifoside A [4] was isolated from the leaves of *A. koreanum* (Chung and Hahn, 1991; Yook *et al.*, 1998) and *A. trifoliatus* (Yook *et al.*, 1998) and from the leaves of *Acanthopanax gracilistylus* (Yook *et al.*, 2002). B cell proliferation to lipopolysaccharide was significantly increased by acantrifoside A (Kim *et al.*, 1999).

Acanthodilol [5] was isolated from the leaves of *A. koreanum* (Chung *et al.*, 1991).

Methyl betulin [6] was isolated from the leaves of *Acanthopanax* fruits (Shin *et al.*, 1992)

Acankoreoside A [7] was isolated from the leaves of *A. koreanum* (Chang *et al.*, 1998) and from the leaves of *A. gracilistylus* (Liu *et al.*, 2002). T cell proliferation to concanavalin A and B cell proliferation to lipopolysaccharide were significantly increased by acankoreoside A (Kim *et al.*, 1999).

Acankoreoside B [8] and D [10] were isolated from the leaves of *A. koreanum* (Chang *et al.*, 1998; 1999).

Acankoreoside C [9] was isolated from the leaves of *A. koreanum* (Chang *et al.*, 1999) and from the leaves of *Acanthopanax gracilistylus.* (Yook *et al.*, 2002).

Acanthodiol glycoside [11] was isolated from the leaves of *A. trifoliatus* (Yook *et al.*, 1999).

Wujiapioside B [12] was isolated from the leaves of *A. gracilistylus.* (Yook *et al.*, 2002).

3-Epibetulinic acid 28-O-α-L-rhamnopyranosyl-(1→4)-β-D-glucopyranosyl-(1→6)-β-D-glucopyranosyl ester [13] was isolated from the leaves of *A. gracilistylus.* (Yook *et al.*, 2002).

Wujiapioside A[14] was isolated from the leaves of *A. gracilistylus* (Liu, *et al.*, 2002).

Protochiisanoside [15]was isolated from the leaves of *A. divaricatus* (Shirasuna *et al.*, 1997).

Acantrifoside B [16] was isolated from the leaves of *A. trifoliatus* (Kiem *et al.*, 2003b).

24-nor-3α,11α-Dihydroxy-lup-20(29)-en-28-oic acid [17] and 24-nor-11α-hydroxy-3-oxo-lup-20(29)-en-28-oic acid [18] were isolated from the leaves of *A. trifoliatus* (Lischewski *et al.*, 1985).

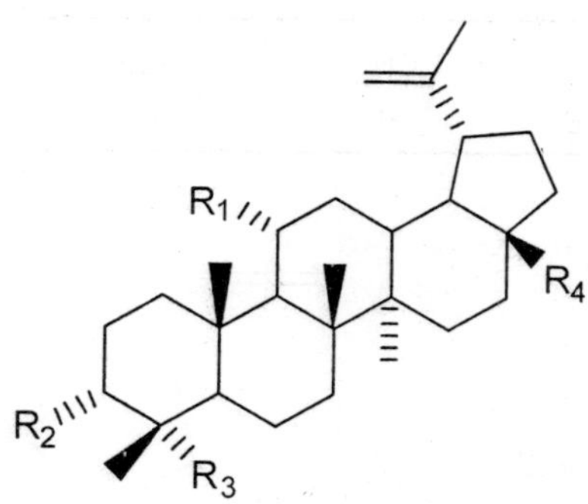


| | | $R^1$ | $R^2$ | $R^3$ | $R^4$ | Reference |
|---|---|---|---|---|---|---|
| 1 | Impressic acid | OH | OH | $CH_3$ | COOH | Ty, 1984 |
| 2 | 3α,11α,23-Trihydroxylup-20(29)-en-28-oic acid | OH | OH | $CH_2OH$ | COOH | Ty, 1984 |
| 3 | 3α,11α-Dihydroxy-23-oxo-lup-20(29)-en-28-oic acid | OH | OH | CHO | COOH | Ty, 1985 |

| | | $R^1$ | $R^2$ | $R^3$ | $R^4$ | Reference |
|---|---|---|---|---|---|---|
| 4 | Acantrifoside A | OH | OH | $CH_3$ | COOGlc-Glc-Rha | Chung, 1991; Yook, 1998 |
| 5 | Acanthodiol | OH | β–OH | $CH_3$ | COOH | Chung, 1991 |
| 6 | Methyl betulin | H | β-$OCH_3$ | $CH_3$ | $CH_2OH$ | Shin, 1992 |
| 7 | Acankoreoside A | H | OH | COOH | COOGlc-Glc-Rha | Chang, 1998 |
| 9 | Acankoreoside B | OH | OH | $CH_2OH$ | COOGlc-Glc-Rha | Chang, 1998 |
| 9 | Acankoreoside C | OH | OGlc | $CH_3$ | COOGlc-Glc-Rha | Chang, 1999 |
| 10 | Acankoreoside D | OH | OH | CHO | COOGlc-Glc-Rha | Chang, 1999 |
| 11 | Acanthodiol glycoside | OH | β–OH | $CH_3$ | COOGlc-Glc-Rha | Yook, 1999 |
| 12 | Wujiapioside B | H | OH | $CH_2OH$ | COOGlc-Glc-Rha | Yook, 2002 |
| 13 | 3-Epibetulinic acid 28-O-glc-glc-rha | H | OH | $CH_3$ | COOGlc-Glc-Rha | Yook, 2002 |
| 14 | Wujiapioside A | H | OH | CHO | COOGlc-Glc-Rha | Liu, 2002 |

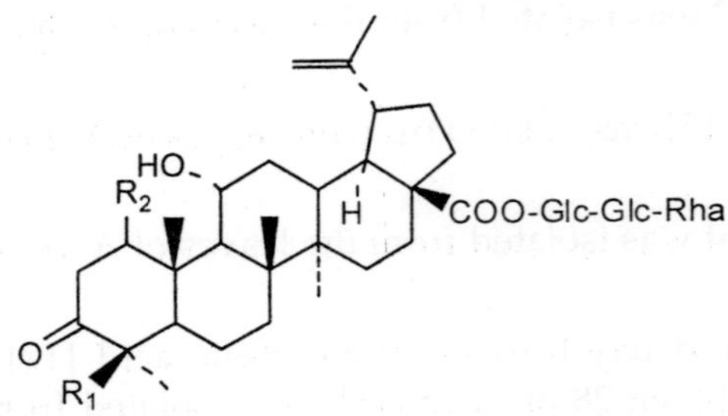


| | | $R^1$ | $R^2$ | Reference |
|---|---|---|---|---|
| 15 | Protochiisanoside | $CH_3$ | β-OH | (Shirasuna, 1997) |
| 16 | Acantrifoside B | H | H | (Kiem, 2003b) |

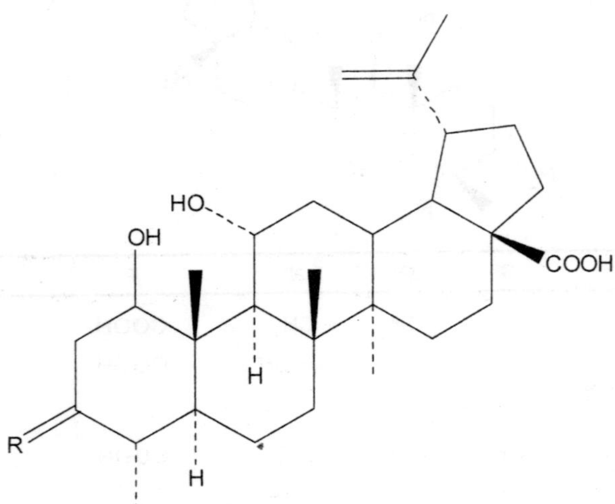

| | | *R* | *Reference* |
|---|---|---|---|
| 17 | 24-nor-3α,11α-Dihydroxylup-20(29)-en-28-oic acid | α-OH, β–H | Lischewski, 1985; Kutschabsky, 1985 |
| 18 | 24-nor-11α-Hydroxy-3-oxo-lup-20(29)-en-28-oic acid | O | Lischewski, 1985 |

Acantrifoic acid A [19] was isolated from the leaves of A. trifoliatus (Kiem *et al.*, 2003a). Acantrifoic acid A had strong inhibitory effects against monoamine oxidase.

Acantrifoside C [20] was isolated from the leaves of *A. trifoliatus* (Kiem *et al.*, 2003a).

Acankoreoside E [21] were isolated from the leaves of *A. koreanum* (Park *et al.*, 2005)

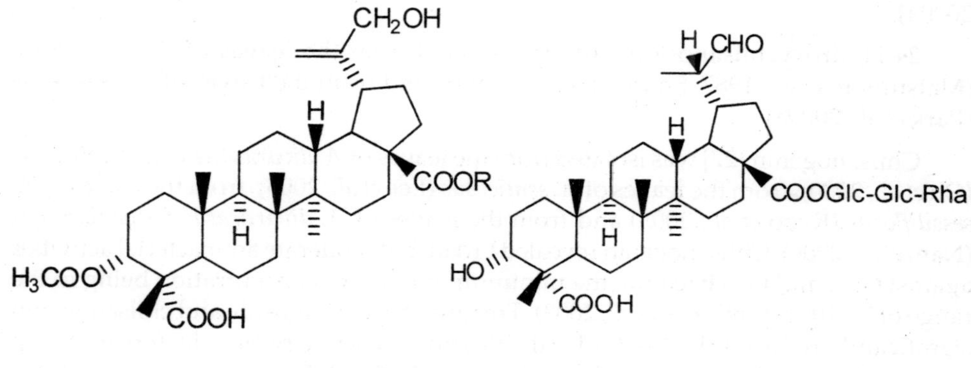


| | | | |
|---|---|---|---|
| 19 | Acantrifoic acid A | R = H | Kiem, 2003a |
| 20 | Acantrifoside C | R = Glc-Glc-Rha | Kiem, 2003a |
| 21 | Acankoreoside E | | Park *et al.*, 2005 |

## Seco-lupane Triterpenoid

Divaroside [22] (3,4-seco-lupane-type triterpene glycosyl esters) was isolated from the leaves of *A. senticosus* forma *inermis* (Park *et al.*, 2000).

Chiisanoside [23] was isolated from leaves and stem-bark from *A. chiisanensis*. (Han *et al.*, 1984), from the leaves of *A. divaricatus* var. *albeofructus* (Oh *et al.*, 2000), from the leaves of *A. senticosus* forma *inermis* (Park *et al.*, 2000, Lee *et al.*, 2003; Jiang *et al.*, 2006), from the leaves of *A. sessiliflorus* (Ryoo *et al.*, 2003), from the leaves of *A. sessiliflorus* (Ryoo *et al.*, 2003; Yoshizumi *et al.*, 2006) and from the leaves of *A. divarticatus forma flavi-flos* (Nam *et al.*, 2006). Chiisanoside exhibited non-toxic effects and significant anti-histaminic activities; the anti-diabetic activities against epinephrine and alloxan induced diabetes, decreased the toxicities by ephedrine hydrochloride and promoted the elimination of chloramphenicol from blood. It also increased the survival rate in rats intoxicated by carbon tetrachloride and led to the re-establishment of normal enzymatic function. An anti-cancer effect of chiisanoside was much lower than that of cisplatin (Yook *et al.*, 1996). Chiisanoside decreased the clearance rate of carbon (Lee *et al.*, 1987).

T cell proliferation to concanavalin A was significantly increased by chiisanoside (Kim *et al.*, 1999). Chiisanoside inhibited NO and $PGE_2$ production and reduced the release of inflammatory cytokines like TNF–$\alpha$ and IL-1$\beta$. The protein and mRNA expression levels of iNOS and COX-2 enzyme and NF-kB activation were also inhibited (Won *et al.*, 2005). Chiisanoside inhibited pancreatic lipase activity in vitro ((Jiang *et al.*, 2006).

22$\alpha$-Hydroxychiisanoside [24] was isolated from the leaves of *A. divaricatus* (Shirasuna *et al.*, 1997), from the leaves of *A. senticosus* forma *inermis* (Park *et al.*, 2000) and from the leaves of *A. sessiliflorus* (Ryoo *et al.*, 2003).

1-Deoxychiisanoide [25] was isolated from the leaves of *A. senticosus* (Park *et al.*, 2000a).

24-Hydroxychiisanoside [26] was isolated from the leaves of *A. divaricatus.* (Matsumoto *et al.*, 1987; Shirasuna *et al.*, 1998) and from the leaves of *A. senticosus* (Park *et al.*, 2000a)

Chiisanogenin [27] was isolated from the leaves of *A. divaricatus* var. *albeofructus* (Oh *et al.*, 2000), from the leaves of *A. senticosus* (Lee *et al.*, 2003), from the leaves of *A. sessiliflorus* (Ryoo *et al.*, 2003) and from the leaves of *A. divarticatus forma flavi-flos* (Nam *et al.*, 2006). Chiisanogenin revealed broad, but moderate antibacterial activities against G(+) and G(-) bacteria, the minimum inhibitory concentration being in the range of 50-100 µg/ml (Lee *et al.*, 2003). Treatment of chiisanoside and chiisanogenin significantly reduced rheumatoid arthritis and C-reactive protein factors in the rat induced by Freund's complete adjuvant reagent. Both compounds inhibited xanthine oxidase activity and increased superoxide dismutase, glutathione peroxidase and catalase (Jung *et al.*, 2005).

Sachunoside [28] was isolated from the leaves of *A. divaricatus* (Park *et al.*, 2001).

*iso*-Chiisanoside [29] was isolated from the leaves of *A. chiisanensis* (Kasai *et al.*, 1986), from the leaves of *A. senticosus* forma *inermis* (Park *et al.*, 2000).

11-Deoxyisochiisanoside [30] was isolated from the leaves of *A. senticosus* (Park *et al.*, 2000a), from the leaves of *A. sessiliflorus* (Yoshizumi *et al.*, 2006) and from the leaves of *A. divarticatus* forma *flavi-flos* (Nam *et al.*, 2006).

iso-Chiisanoside methyl ester [31] was isolated from the leaves of *A. chiisanensis* (Kasai *et al.*, 1986), from the leaves of *A. senticosus* forma *inermis* (Park *et al.*, 2000), from the leaves of *A. sessiliflorus* (Yoshizumi *et al.*, 2006) and from the leaves of *A. divarticatus forma flavi-flos* (Nam *et al.*, 2006).

Inermoside [32] was isolated from the leaves of *A. senticosus* forma *inermis* (Park *et al.*2000).

Sessiloside [33] was isolated from the leaves of *A. sessiliflorus* (Yoshizumi *et al.*, 2006). Sessiloside inhibited pancreatic lipase activity *in vitro* (Jiang *et al.*, 2006).

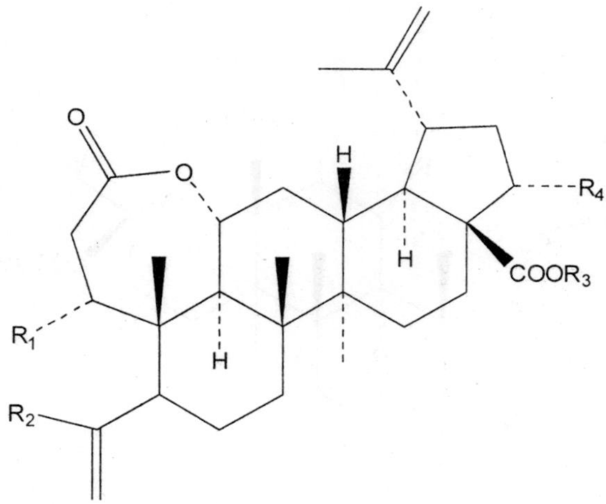


| | | $R^1$ | $R^2$ | $R^3$ | $R^4$ | *Reference* |
|---|---|---|---|---|---|---|
| 22 | Divaroside | OH | $CH_3$ | glc-glc | H | Matsutomo, 1987, Shirasuna, 1997, Park, 2000 |
| 23 | Chiisanoside | OH | $CH_3$ | glc-glc-rha | H | Yook, 1991 etc. |
| 24 | 22α-Hydroxychiisanoside | OH | $CH_3$ | glc-glc-rha | OH | Shirasuna, 1997, Park, 2000b |
| 25 | 1-Deoxychiisanoside | H | $CH_3$ | glc-glc-rha | H | Park, 2000a |
| 26 | 24-hydroxychiisanoside | OH | $CH_2OH$ | glc-glc-rha | H | Park, 2000a |
| 27 | Chiisanogenin | OH | $CH_3$ | H | H | Oh, 2000 |

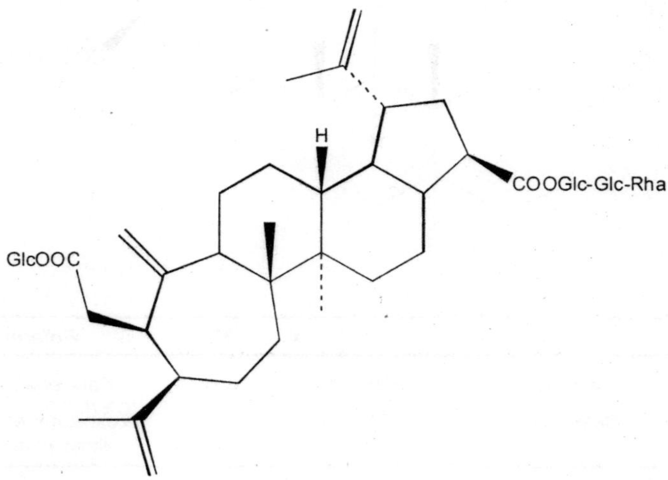


28 Sachunoside, Park *et al.*, 2001

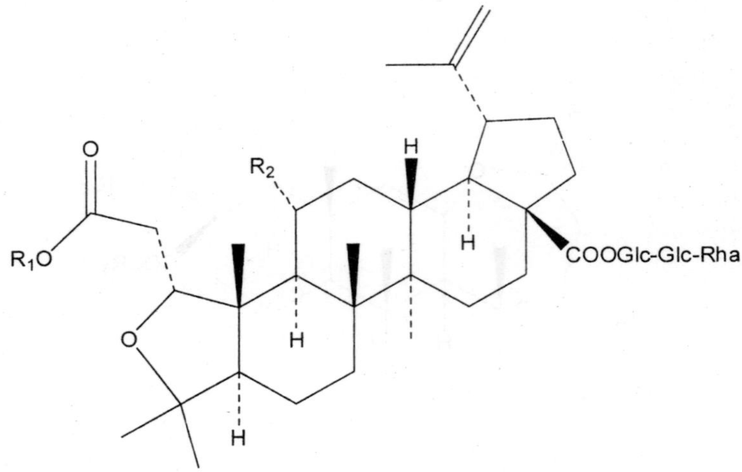


| | | $R^1$ | $R^2$ | Reference |
|---|---|---|---|---|
| 29 | *iso*-Chiisanoside | H | OH | Kasai, 1986, Park, 2000a |
| 30 | 11-Deoxyisochiisanoside | H | H | Park, 2000a |
| 31 | *iso*-Chiisanoside methyl esters | $CH_3$ | OH | Park, 2000b |

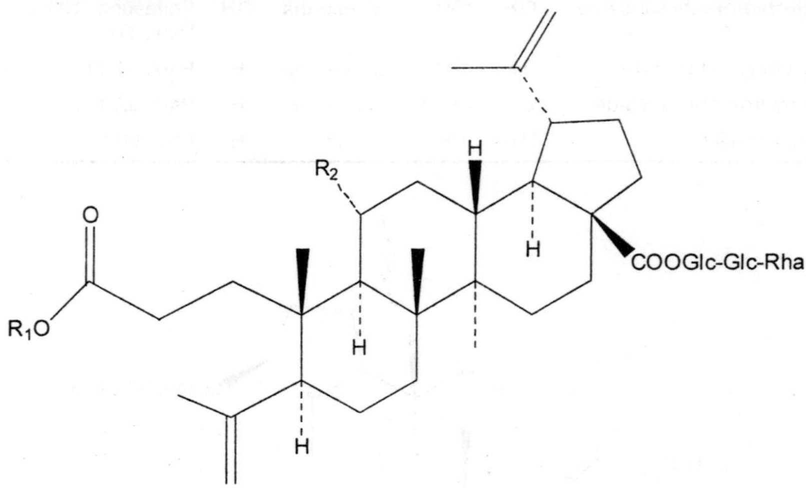


| | | $R^1$ | $R^2$ | Reference |
|---|---|---|---|---|
| 32 | Inermoside | $CH_3$ | OH | Park *et al.*, 2000a |
| 33 | Sessiloside | H | H | Yoshizumi *et a.*, 2006<br>Jiang *et al.*, 2006, |

## Biological Effects of Osteoblastic MC3T3-E1 Cells

Osteoporosis is a major health concern for aging communities. The progressive decrease in bone mass leads to an increased susceptibility to fractures, which results in substantial morbidity and mortality (Riggs and Melton, 1992). Bone tissue is constantly resorbed and rebuilt in a coupled process, referred to as remodelling. The process of bone remodelling is controlled by a balance of bone formation and bone resorption (Roodman, 1996). Excessive bone resorption exceeding that of bone formation results in bone abnormalities, such as osteoporosis. Many osteoporotic patients have already lost a substantial amount of bone; therefore, a method of increasing bone mass by stimulating new bone formation is required (Mohan *et al.*, 2000). We investigated the effect of chiisanoside on the function of osteoblasts using pre-osteoblastic target cell line, MC3T3-E1, which has been well-characterized as an *in vitro* model for osteoblast differentiation (Sudo *et al.*, 1983). MC3T3-E1 cells were incubated with chiisanoside and cell growth was measured (Figure 24.1). MC3T3-E1 cell growth was elevated significantly by the presence of chiisanoside (0.02~20 μM). Based on this preliminary observation, we evaluated the differentiation-inducing activities of chiisanoside on MC3T3-E1 cells by assessing for intracellular ALP activity, collagen content, and calcium deposition. The effect of chiisanoside on osteoblast differentiation was first assessed by measuring the ALP activity, one of the major osteoblast differentiation markers. Chiisanoside significantly increased the ALP activity at concentrations of 0.2~20 μM (Figure 24.2). At the concentration of 2 μM, chiisanoside increased ALP activity up to 131 per cent compared to that of control. Since chiisanoside significantly increased ALP activity in osteoblastic MC3T3-E1 cells, we further investigated the effect of chiisanoside on collagen synthesis using Sirius Red-based colorimetric assay. As shown in Figure 24.3, chiisanoside significantly increased collagen synthesis at concentrations of 0.02-20 μM. Next, we examined the effects of chiisanoside on mineralization, another important process in

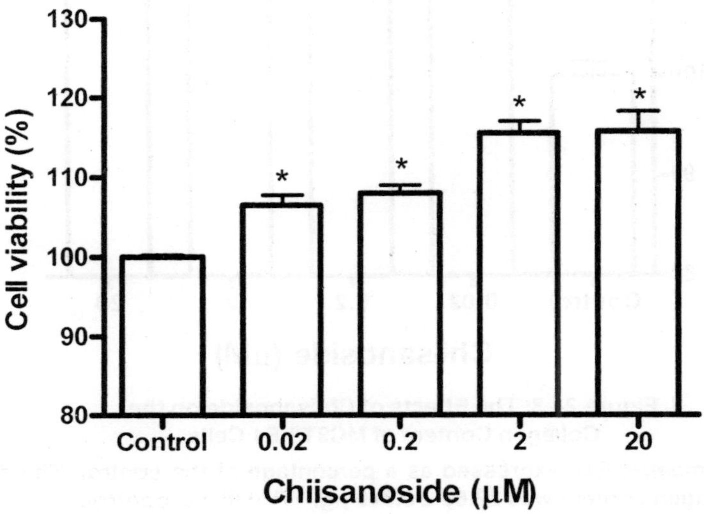


**Figure 24.1: The Effects of Chiisanoside on the Viability of MC3T3-E1 Cells**

**Data are the mean±SEM, expressed as a percentage of the control. The control value for MTT assay was 0.408 ± 0.005 OD. * *P*<0.05 vs. control.**

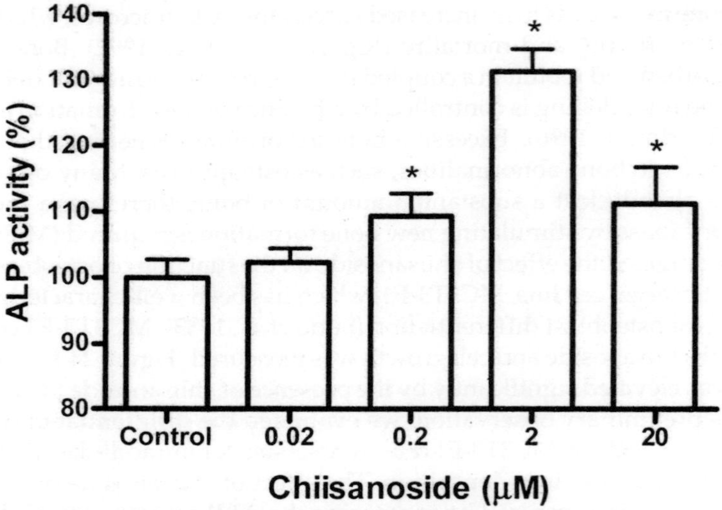


**Figure 24.2: The Effects of Chiisanoside on the Alkaline Phosphatase Activity of MC3T3-E1 Cells**

**Data are the mean±SEM, expressed as a percentage of the control. The control ALP activity was 0.510±0.015 Unit/$10^6$cells. * *P*<0.05 vs. control.**

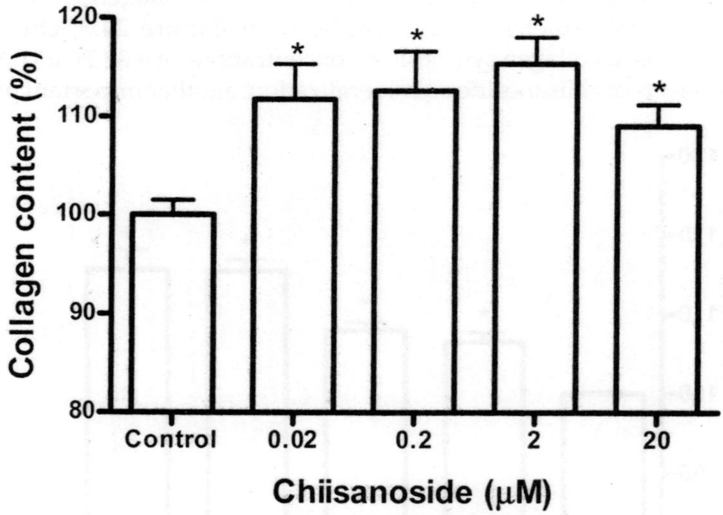


**Figure 24.3: The Effects of Chiisanoside on the Collagen Content of MC3T3-E1 Cells**

**Data are the mean±SEM, expressed as a percentage of the control. The control value for collagen content was 22.69 ± 0.349 μg. * *P*<0.05 vs. control.**

differentiation, by measuring the calcium deposition by Alizarin Red staining. The results were consistent with the effects on ALP activity and collagen synthesis, chiisanoside showed significant stimulatory effect on mineralization (Figure 24.4).

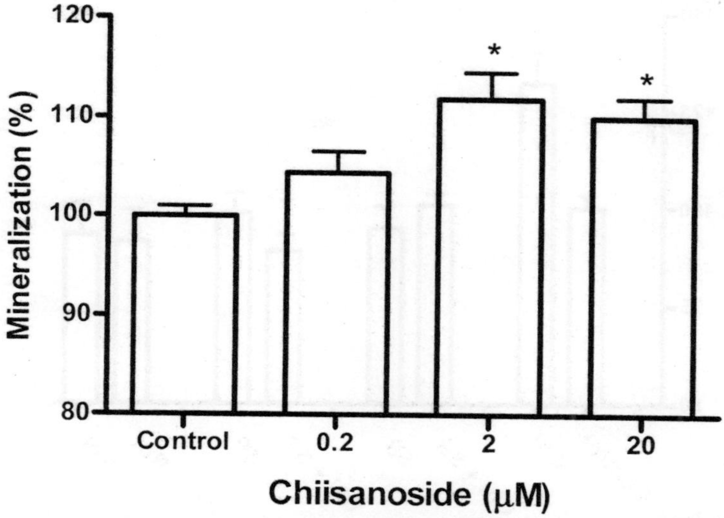


**Figure 24.4: The Effects of Chiisanoside on the Mineralization of MC3T3-E1 Cells**
**Data are the mean±SEM, expressed as a percentage of the control. The control mineralization value was 0.640±0.006 OD. * *P*<0.05 vs. control.**

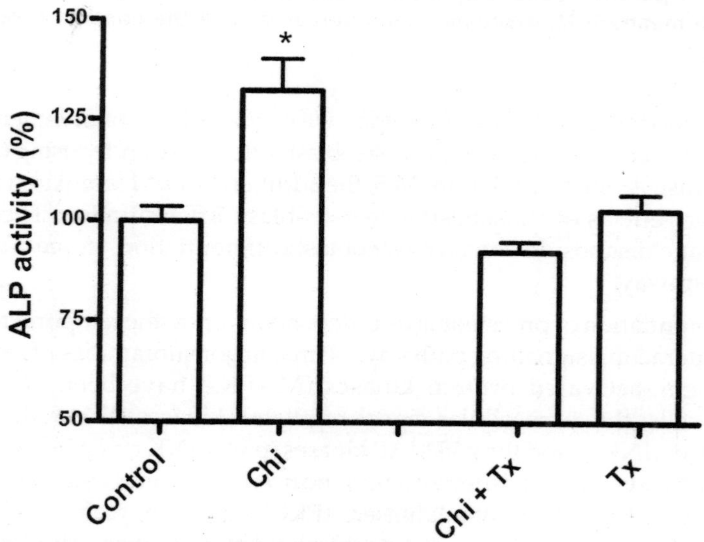


**Figure 24.5: Effect of Tamoxifen on ALP Activity Increased by Chiisanoside**
**One hour before the treatment with 2 μM chiisanoside (Chi), cultures were pre-treated with 1 μM tamoxifen (Tx). Data are the mean±SEM, expressed as a percentage of the control. * *P*<0.05 vs. control.**

At the concentration of 2 μM, about 112 per cent increase in mineralization was observed by the treatment with chiisanoside, as compared to control. Phytoestrogens are known to exert stimulatory effects on osteoblast differentiation, in part, *via* estrogen

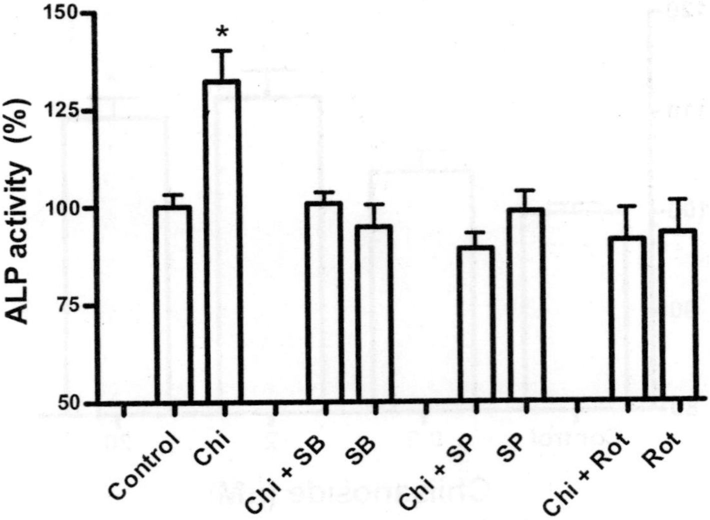


**Figure 24.6: Effect of p38, JNK, and PKC Inhibitors on ALP Activity Increased by Chiisanoside**

**One hour before the treatment with 2 μM chiisanoside (Chi), cultures were pre-treated with 1 μM SB203580 (SB), 3 μM SP600125 (SP), and 1 μM Rottlerin (Rot). Data are the mean±SEM, expressed as a percentage of the control. * *P*<0.05 vs. control.**

receptor (ER)-mediated pathway. Therefore, we examined the involvement of ER in the stimulatory effects of chiisanoside on osteoblast differentiation, by using tamoxifen, an ER antagonist. As shown in Figure 24.5, the addition of 1 μM tamoxifen abolished the stimulatory effects of chiisanoside on osteoblast differentiation. These results suggested that chiisanoside enhance osteoblast differentiation, in part, *via* an ER-dependent pathway.

The differentiation of preosteoblasts is dependent upon the temporal regulation of multiple interacting signalling pathways. Three major subfamilies of structurally related mitogen-activated protein kinases (MAPKs) have been identified in mammalian cells: the extracellular signal-regulated kinases (Erks); the c-Jun N-terminal kinases (JNKs); and the p38 MAP kinases (p38s). JNK and p38 are important signalling pathways for cell differentiation induced by several osteotropic factors (Guicheux *et al.*, 2003). The protein kinase C (PKC) signalling pathways have been also implicated in the regulation of osteoblastic differentiation. PKC-dependent mechanisms mediate the differentiation of osteoblastic cells and gene expression in response to parathyroid hormone (Yang *et al.*, 2006). Evaluation of the role of MAP kinases in chiisanoside-induced MC3T3-E1 osteoblastic differentiation was performed using selective inhibitors of p38 and JNK pathways. As presented in Fig. 6, the p38 inhibitor SB203080 and JNK inhibitor SP600125 significantly reduced the stimulation of ALP by chiisanoside. These observations strongly suggested that p38 and JNK are involved in mediating the stimulation of ALP by chiisanoside. To determine whether activation of ALP by chiisanoside is PKC-dependent or-independent, we investigated the influence of the PKC inhibitor Rottlerin on chiisanoside-induced activation of ALP. As depicted in Fig. 6, the stimulation of ALP by chiisanoside was also decreased by Rottlerin, an inhibitor of PKC, further supporting a role of the PKC pathway in the stimulation of ALP by chiisanoside. In the present study, we show that chiisanoside can stimulate ALP activity in early differentiating osteoblastic cells, probably by a p38-, JNK-, and PKC-dependent mechanism and that activation of p38, JNK, and PKC by chiisanoside may be important for the stimulation of ALP and matrix calcification induced by chiisanoside.

## References

Cai, X. F., Lee, J. S., Shen, G., Dat, N. T., Lee, J. J., Kim, Y. H., 2004. Triterpenoids from *Acanthopanax koreanum* root and their inhibitory activities on NFAT transcription. Arch. Pharm. Res. 27, 825-828.

Chang, S. Y., Yook, C. S. and Nohara, T., 1998. Tow new lupane triterpene glycosidies from leaves of *Acanthopanax koreanum.* Chem. Pharm. Bull, 46, 163-165.

Chang, S. Y., Yook, C.S. and Nohara, T., 1999. Lupane-triterpene glycosidies from leaves of *Acanthopanax koreanum.* Phytochemistry, 50, 1369-1374.

Chung, B. S. and Kim, Y. H., 1986. Studies on the constituents of *Acanthopanax Koreanum* leaves. Yakhak Hoji 17, 62-66.

Chung, J. Y. and Hahn, D. R., 1991. Constituents of *Acanthopanax koreanum* leaves. Yakhak Hoeji, 35, 240-244.

Guicheux, J., Lemonnier, J., Ghayor, C., Suzuki, A., Palmer, G. and Caverzasio J., 2003. Activation of p38 mitogen-activated protein kinase and c-Jun-$NH_2$-terminal kinase by BMP-2 and their implication in the stimulation of osteoblastic cell differentiation, J. Bone Miner. Res. 18, 2060–2068.

Hahn, D.-R., Kim, J.-H., Taniyasu, S., Tanaka, O., 1985. A new glycosyl esterof a 3,4-seco-triterpene from Korean medicinal plant, *Acanthopanax chiisanensis* (Araliaceae). Chem. Pharm. Bull. 32, 1244-1247.

Jiang, w., Li, W., Han, L., Liu, L., Zhang, Q., Zhang, S., Nikaido, T., and Koike K., 2006. Biologically active triterpenoid saponins from *Acanthopanax senticosus.* J. Nat. Prod. 69, 1577-1581.

Jung, H. J., Nam, J. H., Choi, J., Lee, K. T, and Park, H. J., 2005. Antiinflammatory effects of chiisanoside and chiisanogenin obtained from the leaves of *Acanthopanax chiisanensis* in the carrageenan–and Freund's complete adjuvant-induced rats. J. Ethopharmacol. 97, 359-367.

Kiem, P. V., Cai, X. F., Minh, C. V., Lee, J.J., Kim, Y. H. 2003a. Lupane-triterpene carboxylic acids from the leaves of *Acanthopanax trifoliatus.* Chem. Pharm. Bull. 51, 1432-1435.

Kiem, P. V., Minh, C. V., Cai, X. F., Lee, J. J., and Kim, Y. H. 2003b A new-nor-lupane-glycoside of *Acanthopanax trifoliatus.* Arch. Pharm. Res. 26, 706-708.

Kim, Y. H., Chung, B. S. Ko, Y.S., and Han, H.J. 1988. Kaurane derivatives from *Acanthopanax Koreanum*. Arch Pharm Res 11, 159-162.

Kim, Y. O., Cho, D. H., Chung, H. J., Kim, J. H., Chang, S. Y., Yook, C. S., Yang, K. S., and Oh, O. J. 1999. Effects of lupane-triterpenoids on mitogen-induced proliferation of lymphocytes. Yakhak Hoeji 43, 208-213.

Kutschabsky.L., Pfeifer, D., Lischewski, M., Ty, P.D. and Adam, G. 1985. Molecula and crystal structure of a new 24-nor triterpenoid carboxylic acid from *Acanthopanax trifoliatus*. Croatia Chemica Acta 58, 427-434.

Lee, M. W., Chung, J. Y., Kim, Y. C. and Hahn, D. R., 1987. Chung Ang J. Pharm. Sc1. 1, 1-3.

Lee, S., Shin D. S., Oh, K. B., Shin K. H., 2003. Antibacterial compounds from the leaves of *Acanthopanax senticosus*. Arch. Pharm. Res. 26, 40-42.

Liu, X. Q., Chang, S. Y., Park, S. Y., Nohara, T. and Yook, C. S. 2002. A new lupine-triterpene glycosidie from the leaves of *Acanthopanax gracilistylus*. Arch. Pharm. Res., 25, 831-836.

Lischewski, M., Ty, P. D., Kutschabsky, L., Pfeiffer, D., Phiet, H. V., Preiss, A., Sung, T. V. and Adam, G., 1985, Two 24-nor triterpenoid carboxylic acids from *Acanthopanax trifoliatus*. Phytochemistry. 24, 2355-2357.

Matsumoto, K., Kasai, R., Kanamaru, F., Kohda, H. and Takana, O., 1987. 3,4-Seco-lupane-type triterpene glycosyl esters from leaves of *Acathopanax divaricatus*. Chem. Pharm. Bull. 35, 413-415.

Mohan, S., Kutilek, S., Zhang, C., Shen, H. G., Kodama, Y., Srivastava, A. K., Wergedal, J. E., Bermer, W. G., and Baylink, D. J., 2000. Comparison of bone formation responses to parathyroid hormone (1-34), (1-31), and (2-34) in mice. *Bone*, 27, 471-478.

Nam, S. G., Yook, C. S., Kim, 1. S., Choi, H. S., and Park S. Y., 2006. Studies on the constituents of the leaves of *Acanthopanax divaricatus* forma *flavi-flos*. Nat. Prod. Sc1. 12, 119-121.

Oh, O. J., Chang, S. Y., Kim, T. H., Yang, K. S., Yook, C. S., Park, S. Y. and Nohara, T., 2000. Constituents of *Acanthopanax divaricatus* var. *albeofructus*. Nat. Med. 54, 29-32.

Park, S. Y., Chang, S. Y., Yook, C. S. and Nohara, T., 2000a. New 3,4-Seco-lupane-type triterpene glycosides from *Acanthopanax senticosus* forma *inermis*. J. Nat. Prod. 63, 1630-1633.

Park, S. Y., Chang, S. Y., Yook, C. S. and Nohara, T., 2000b. Triterpene glycosides from leaves of *Acanthopanax senticosus* forma *inermis*. Nat. Med. 54, 43.

Park, S. Y., Yook, C. S., and Nohara, T., 2001. A novel 3,4-seco-migrated-lupane glycoside with a seven-membered B-ring from Acanthopanax divaricatus var. sachunensis. Tetrahed. Letts. 42, 2825-2828.

Park, S. Y., Choi H. Y., Yook, C. S. and Nohara, T., 2005. A new lupane glycoside from the leaves of *Acanthopanax koreanum*. Chem. Pharm. Bull. 53, 97-99.

Riggs, B. L. and Melton III, L. J., 1992. The prevention and treatment of osteoporosis. *N. Engl. J. Med.* 327, 620-627.

Ryoo, H. S., Park, S. Y., Chang, S. Y. and Yook, C. S., 2003. Triterpene components from the leaves of *Acanthopanax sessiliflorus* Seem. Kor. J. Pharmacogn. 34, 269-273.

Sang, Y. P., Hyun,S. C., Chang, S. Y. and Nohara, T., 2005. A New Lupane Glycoside from the Leaves of *Acanthopanax koreanum*. Chem. Pharm. Bull. 53(1) 97-99.

Shin, A. T., Kim, C.J. and Yook, C. S. 1992. Study on chemical constituents of *Acanthopanax* fruits. Bull. K. H. Pharma. Sc1. 20, 63-73.

Shirasuna, K., Miyakoshi, M., Mimoto, S., Isoda, S., Satoh, Y., Hirai, Y., Ida, Y. and Soji, J. 1997. Lupane triterpenoid glycosyl esters from leaves of *Acanthopanax divaricatus*. Phytochemistry. 45, 579-584.

Sudo, H., Kodama, H., Amagi, Y., Yamamoto, S., and Kasai, S., 1983. In vitro differentiation and calcification in a new clonal osteogenic cell line derived from newborn mouse calvaria. *J. Cell. Biol.*, 96, 191-198.

Ty, P. D., Lischewski, M., Phiet, H. V., Preiss, A., Nguyen, P. V. and Adam, G., 1985, 3$\alpha$, 11$\alpha$-Dihydroxy-23-oxo-lup-20(29)-en-28-oic acid from *Acanthopanax trifoliatus*. Phytochemistry 24, 867-869.

Ty, P. D., Lischewski, M., Phiet, H. V., Preiss, A., Sung, T. V., Schmidt, J. and Adam, G., 1984, Two triterpenoid carboxylic acids from *Acanthopanax trifoliatus*. Phytochemistry 23, 2889-2891.

Won, J. H., Pa, S. Y., Nam, S. K., Park, H. J., Choi, J. and Lee, K. T., 2005. Inhibition of lipopolysacchride-induced expression of inducile nitric oxide and cyclooxygenase-2 by chiisanoside via suppression of nuclear factor-kB activation in RAW 264.7 macrophage cells. Biol. Pharm. Bull. 28, 1919-1924.

Yang, D., Guo, J., Divieti, P., and Bringhurst, F. R., 2006. Parathyroid hormone activates PKC-delta and regulates osteoblastic differentiation via a PLC-independent pathway. Bone 38, 485-496.

Yook, C. S., Rho, Y. S., Seo, S. H., Leem, J. H. and Han, D. R., 1996, Chemical components of *Acanthopanax divaricatus* and anti cancer effect in leaves. Yakhak Hoeji 40, 251-261.

Yook, C. S, Kim, S. C., Kim, C. J. and Hahn, D. R., 1991, Phytochemical studies on the barks of *Acanthopanax* senticosus forma inermis. Yakhak Hoeji 35 Phytochemistry 22, 629-632.

Yook, C. S, Kim, Y. H., Hahn, D. R., Nohara, T. and Chang, S. Y., 1998, A lupane-triterpene glycoside from leaves of two *Acanthopanax*. Phytochemistry 49, 839-843.

Yook, C. S, Chang, S. Y., Lai, J. H., Ko, S. K., Jeong, J. H. and Nohara, T., 1999, Lupane-glycoside of *Acanthopanax trifoliatus* forma tristigmatis leaves. Arch. Pharm. Res. 22, 629-632.

Yook, C. S., Liu, X. Q., Chang, S. Y., Park, S. Y. and Nohara, T., 2002. Lupane-triterpene glycosides from the leaves of *Acanthopanax gracilistylus*. Chem. Pharm. Bull. 50, 1383-1385.

Yoshizumi, K., Hirano, K., Ando, H., Hirai, Y., Ida, Y., Tsuji, T., Tanaka, T., Satouchi, K., and Terao, J., 2006. Lupane-type saponins from leaves of *Acanthopanax sessiliflorus* and their inhibitory activity on pancreatic lipase. J. Food. Chem. 54, 335-341.

# *Part III*
# Clinical and Bioactivity Studies

# Chapter 25

# Traditional and Modern Applications of *Aegle marmelos* (L.) Corr. and *Azadirachta indica* A Juss–Vital Trees of South India

**C. Rajasekaran*, E. Meignanam, N. Premkumar, T. Kalaivani, R. Siva and V. Vijayakumar[1]**

*School of Biotechnology, Chemical and Biomedical Engineering*

*[1]School of Humanities and Social Sciences*

*VIT University, Vellore – 632 014, Tamil Nadu, India*

**E-mail: drcrs70@gmail.com*

## ABSTRACT

There is an increasing awareness among people towards nature and natural products. Because it is pollution free and less toxic without side effects, natural medicine is attracting more attention than allopathic system. Even though 6000 plants are mentioned in the traditional systems of medicine, only 350 species are under use and most of them are herbs. Although several trees possess medicinal properties, it has been ignored by indigenous and modern systems of medicine. Nevertheless, trees attract major attention from traditional communities of southern parts of India due to their multiple medicinal properties. Among them, *Aegle marmelos* (L.) Corr. and *Azadirachta indica* A Juss species play a vital role in day to day usage of different indigenous communities, due to their sacred and medicinal value.

In the present investigation, major focus is on the traditional uses, antimicrobial and hepatoprotective activities of these two species. Leaves were dried under shade and extracted with different solvent systems, namely, petroleum ether, benzene, dichloromethane, chloroform, ethanol, and water. These isolates were subjected to antimicrobial activity tests against various gram positive and gram negative bacteria, which revealed that chloroform, ethanolic and aqueous extracts of *A. marmelos* showed potent inhibitory activity. In case of *A. indica*, dichloromethane, ethanolic and aqueous extracts had maximum inhibition. Hepatoprotective activities of the ethanolic and aqueous extracts of both the plants were studied against carbon tetrachloride induced liver damage in mice using silymarin as the internal control. Enzyme activities of Serum Glutamate Oxaloacetate Transaminase (SGOT), Serum Glutamate Pyruvate Transaminase (SGPT) and Alkaline phosphatase (ALP) showed that both plant extracts had moderate activity over carbon tetrachloride treatment as compared to the control. Similar trend was observed in the histopathological analysis. The results of the present investigation revealed various traditional uses, potent antimicrobial and hepatoprotecive activity of these plants.

***Keywords***: *Ethnobotany, Antimicrobial, Sacred value, Hepatoprotective, Photomicrograph, Aegle marmelos, Azadirachta indica.*

## 1.0 Introduction

India has a very rich biodiversity and it is not only, one of the world's twelve megadiversity countries but also one of the eight major centres of origin and diversification of domesticated taxa. It has approximately 490,000 plant species of which, about 17,500 are angiosperms; more than 400 are domesticated crop species and almost an equal number are their wild relatives (NBPGR, 2000). Since ages plants have been playing a vital role in life supporting systems of contemporary civilization by serving the purpose of maintaining good health and well being of mankind (Jain, 1979; Maikhuri, 2005). Medicinal plants are a major source of raw material for the traditional systems like Ayurveda, Siddha and Unani. Even the modern system of medicine has more than 25 per cent of drugs in use, which are either plant based or plant derived.

India and China are the two great producers of medicinal plants having more than 40 per cent of global biodiversity. China is at present exporting herbal medicines worth of US$ 5 billion. India has a potential of achieving export of US$ 250 crores by 2010. Although 6000 plants are mentioned in the traditional systems of medicine, 350 species are considered to be most important (Ahmedullah, 1999). Although several trees possess various medicinal properties, it has been ignored by indigenous and modern systems of medicine. Nevertheless, trees attract major attention from traditional communities of southern parts of India due to their multiple medicinal properties. Among them, *Aegle marmelos* (AM) and *Azadirachta indica* (AI) species play a vital role in day-to-day usage of different indigenous communities, due its sacred and medicinal value. AM is a moderate-sized, slender, aromatic, tropical deciduous tree commonly known as "Wood Apple" belonging to the family *Rutaceae* and possesses sacred value in India. The fruits have numerous seeds, which are densely covered with fibrous hairs and are embedded in a thick, glüey, aromatic pulp. AI commonly known as "Neem" is a tropical evergreen tree belonging to the family *Meliaceae*. Emerging young terminal leaves are reddish to purplish in colour.

AM is used to treat traditionally various aliments such as diarrhea, dysentery, intestinal parasites, dryness of the eyes, and the common cold (Bakhru, 1997). In

India, neem is known as "Divine Tree", "Heal All", "the village pharmacy", because of its healing versatility, and it has been used by various traditional means of medicine due to its multiple medicinal properties (Agrawal, 2003; Puri, 1999).

Keeping the above in view, the present investigation was focused on the traditional uses, antimicrobial and hepatoprotective activities of these two species.

## 2.0 Materials and Methods

### 2.1 Plant Materials

*Aegle marmelos* belonging to the family *Rutaceae* and *Azadirachta indica* belonging to the family *Meliaceae* were chosen for the present investigations.

### 2.2 Ethnobotanical Documentation

The ethnobotanical data were collected from the local villagers, tribal communities and traditional vaidhyas of Vellore District (Tamil Nadu) and adjacent areas.

### 2.3 Preparation of Plant Extracts

The leaves of (AM) and (AI) were freshly collected during the month of December 2006 from Ranipet and forests near Sholingar respectively at Vellore district, Tamil Nadu India. The leaves were dried under shade and coarsely powdered. The powder was successively extracted using soxhlet apparatus with various solvents such as petroleum ether, benzene, chloroform, dichloromethane, ethanol and water. These extracts were condensed using rotary vacuum evaporator followed by vacuum evaporator and stored in desiccator at 8°C. The powder of all the extracts was suspended in appropriate solvent systems and was subjected to further analysis.

### 2.4 Anti-Microbial Assay

The following microorganisms were selected for the present study:

**Gram Positive**

*Micrococcus luteus, Staphylococcus aureus, Staphylococcus pyogenes, Streptococcus faecalis, Bacillus stearothermophilus, Micrococcus glutamics, Lactobacillus bulgaris.*

**Gram Negative**

*Escherichia coli, Pseudomonas denitrificans.*

The Mueller Hinton Agar (MHA) plates were prepared and well diffusion method was used to screen the antimicrobial activity (Bauer, 1966). The different extracts at 500 ppm concentration were loaded on 9 mm well. The zone of inhibition was measured after 24hrs with transparent ruler in millimetre. These studies were performed in triplicate.

### 2.5 Hepatoprotective Study

#### 2.5.1 Experimental Animals

The cross breed albino mice weighing 20-25g were housed in clean propylene cages and maintained at 30±2°C under natural light/dark conditions. They were fed with standard pellet diet and water was given *ad libitum*. The animals were acclimatized to laboratory conditions for 2 weeks. Animals were divided into eleven groups of six mice each. The body weight of each of the animals was recorded initially. The period of experimentation was 5 days.

### 2.5.2 Carbon Tetrachloride induced Hepatotoxicity

Group I animals received 1 per cent CMC in distilled water (2ml/kg body weight) for five days with olive oil (2ml/kg body weight i.p) on second and third day. Group II animals received 1 per cent CMC (2ml/kg body weight) for 5 days with 1: 1 mixture of olive oil and $CCl_4$ (2ml/kg body weight i.p.) on 2nd and 3rd day. Group III animals served as positive control and were given silymarin (200mg/kg) for five days.

Group IV and Group V animals were given ethanolic extract of AM (500mg/kg) and (600mg/kg) body weight respectively. Group VI and Group VII animals received respectively 500mg/kg and 600mg/kg body aqueous extract of AM weight. Group VIII and Group IX animals were given 500mg/kg and 600mg/kg body weight ethanolic extract of AI. Group X and Group XI animals received respectively 500mg/kg and 600mg/kg body weight aqueous extract of AI. In addition to ethanolic and aqueous extracts, 1: 1 mixture of olive oil and $CCl_4$ (2ml/kg body weight i.p.) were given to Group IV to Group XI animals on 2nd and 3rd day.

### 2.5.3 Enzyme Assay

On the fifth day, blood was collected from the retro orbital plexus of the animals and serum was allowed to coagulate at 37°C for 30 mins, and subjected to centrifugation at 2500 rpm. Serum samples were stored at 2-8°C until further use. The enzyme assay was determined for Serum Glutamate Oxaloacetate Transaminase (SGOT), Serum Glutamate Pyruvate Transaminase (SGPT) (Reitman, 1957), and Alkaline Phosphatase (ALP) (Modified method of Kind, 1954) using commercially available enzyme kit (Crest Biosystems, Goa, India).

### 2.5.4 Histopathological Analysis

Two animals from each group were sacrificed by decapitation, liver dissected out, blotted off blood, washed in saline and stored in 10 per cent formalin before sectioning for histopathological studies. The specimen was embedded in paraffin, cut into 5 μm sections, stained with haematoxylin-eosin dye and then observed under a microscope and photomicrographs taken.

## 2.6 Statistical Analysis

The results were expressed as mean S.E.M. for each parameter. The data obtained were subjected to one way ANOVA. P value of $<0.01$ were considered to be statistically significant. Sigma stat software was used for statistical analysis.

# 3.0 Results

## 3.1 Ethnobotanical Uses in South India

Table 25.1 indicates the ethnobotanical use of AM and AI, which were collected from the local tribes/villagers from study area. It is also shows their traditional practices currently followed.

**Table 25.1: Ethnobotanical Information obtained from the Local Tribes/Villagers from Vellore District of Tamil Nadu and their Traditional Practices**

| *Uses* | *Description* | |
|---|---|---|
| | *Aegle marmelos* | *Azadirachta indica* |
| Sacred Value | In Hindu mythology leaves and wood are essential for worshipping Lord Shiva. The villagers belonging to Garhwal and Kolli malai regions offer leaves in the month of July/August, to god to overcome sterility problem and subsequent year the couples are blessed with the child. It is considered as an emblem of fertility. | The tree is sacred to the God worshipped by women in seasons when epidemics prevail. Since neem leaves repel snakes, the tree is also connected with their worship, and upright snake stones are frequently erected round its trunk. The tree is still regarded as *'Village dispensary'* in India. It is also believed to considered to drive the *"evil sprit"*. |
| General Uses | Beverage is prepared with fruit pulp and tamarind, used for body heating problems. Cologne is obtained by distillation from flowers. The wood is used for carving, small-scale turnery, tool and knife handles, pestles and combs, taking a fine polish.<br><br>The ripen fruit, tamarind and sugar is mixture is used as laxative to overcome constipation and body heating problems.<br><br>Mature but still unripe fruits are made into jam. A firm jelly is made from the pulp alone or better still, combined with guava to modify the astringent flavour. The pulp is also pickled. | Effective in treating eczema, ringworm and acne. Traditionally, leaf paste is applying directly to wounds or skin diseases. Intake of neem leaves acts as immunizer to prevent various diseases–immunity development, blood, digestive, nervous disorders, sexually transmitted diseases (STD). During "Ugadi festival" mixture of tamarind, jaggery, mango and neem Buds/Flowers are taken in the empty stomach. The emerging tender leaves are given to the kids to overcome the *Ascoris lumbricoids* infection. |
| External Uses | The shell of hard fruits has been fashioned into pill–and snuff boxes, sometimes decorated with gold and silver. The ornaments placed in this shell looks like the new one for ever. The gum from seeds is used as household glue and as an adhesive by jewellers.<br><br>The fruit pulp used as detergent for washing clothes in olden days. It has been eliminated in recent days. It is still used to wash the silver ornamentals and shields.<br><br>The fruit pulp used for head wash. The dried pulp is also used in local based hair cosmetics along with mehandi and amla. | The leaves are used to treat viral based infectious diseases such as small pox, chicken pox, measles and flu The sprinkle fresh neem leaf near the beds or used as a hand fan and hang a cluster of leaves on the door curtains. This acts as disinfectant and prevent the spread of disease. The leaves were soaked with water (100g/L) in metallic vessel (Bronze metal) kept in the sun light for 10 hours during the day time. The neem leaves treated water is used for bathing purpose for 10 days or till get the recovery.<br><br>The decoction of neem leaves used to soak feet for treating various foot fungi. |

*Contd...*

**Table 25.1–Contd...**

| *Uses* | *Description* | |
|---|---|---|
| | *Aegle marmelos* | *Azadirachta indica* |
| Pesti/ Insecticide | — | Neem seed oil is used as pest/insecticide. The oil is mixed with the dried leguminous seeds to preserve for long time usage. Fresh neem seeds were soaked in water and it acts as soil born pest and insecticide. It also act as Nemeticide. |
| Dye | Yellow colour dye is obtained from unriped fruit, which is used for painting and printing work. | — |
| Medicinal uses | "Sherbet" acts as mild laxative, tonic and digestive effects. A decoction of the unripe fruit, with fennel and ginger, is prescribed for haemorrhoids. It has been surmised that the psoralen in the pulp increases tolerance of sunlight and aids in the maintaining of normal skin colour. It is employed in the treatment of leucoderma. The leaf decoction is also said to alleviate asthma. | Neem bark is commonly used as antipyretic agent to clean the teeth. The traditional method is to snap off a twig of the tree and chew on it. The astringent qualities of the bark prevented bleeding gums, tooth decay and foul smell long before the advent of toothpaste. |
| | The bitter, pungent leaf juice, mixed with honey, is given to allay catarrh and fever. With black pepper to alleviate jaundice and constipation accompanied by oedema. | Neem oil have been found to be spermicidal, Irrulars and Malaiyali tribal communities belonging to Tamil Nadu region use this neem oil as contraceptive. |
| | A hot poultice of the leaves is considered as an effective treatment for ophthahmia and various inflammations, also febrile delirium and acute bronchitis. | Neem bark and roots also have medicinal properties. Bark and roots in powdered form are also used to control fleas and ticks on pets. |
| | An infusion of Bael leaf water is regarded as an effective remedy for peptic ulcer. | |
| | The pulp of the fresh fruit is mixed with sugar and curd/ buttermilk is given to patient with severe fever. | |

## 3.2 Antimicrobial Activity

The antimicrobial activity of AM and AI in different solvent extracts against various organisms are given in the Table 25.2.

In case of AM, ethanolic and chloroform extracts showed maximum inhibition against Gram-positive and Gram-negative bacteria. In aqueous extract, moderate activity was observed followed by dichloromethane extract. Petroleum ether extract was not effective against any of the organisms tested. Among the different microorganisms tested, maximum inhibition was found in *Micrococcus glutamicus* and *E. coli*. In case of *Bacillus cereus* and *Lactobacillus bulgaris* growth was not inhibited by any of these extracts.

In case of AI, dichloromethane extract showed maximum inhibitory activity followed by ethanolic and aqueous extracts against various organisms tested. Chloroform extract showed inhibition against only *Bacillus cereus*. Petroleum ether extract was not effective against any of the organism tested. Among the different microorganisms tested maximum inhibition was found in *Micrococcus glutamicus* followed by *Staphylococcus aureus, Bacillus stearothermophilus, B. cereus* and *Streptococcus faecalis*.

## 3.3 Hepatoprotective Activity

### 3.3.1 Enzyme Assays

Table 25.3 reveals the analysis of SGOT, SGPT and ALP levels in $CCl_4$ induced hepatotoxicity in mice using aqueous and ethanolic extracts of AM and AI.

As compared to the normal control group, the animals treated with $CCl_4$ showed significant increase in serum levels of hepatic marker enzymes such as SGOT, SGPT and ALP. Aqueous extract of AI (600mg/kg) was found to have maximum hepatoprotecive activity and there reduced levels of SGOT, SGPT and ALP were measured. This effect was as equivalent as the effect of silymarin, positive control (Group II). In case of AM ethanolic extract (500mg/kg) was found to have moderate activity as compared to silymarin.

### 3.3.2 Histopathological Observations

Figure 25.1 shows the effect of various concentration of ethanolic and aqueous extract from AM and AI on liver sections.

Histopathological results reveal that Group I Section of the liver tissue from mice used as control showed normal level architecture with neither inflammation nor necrosis. Group II $CCl_4$ treated Sections showed extensive liver cell damage, congested veins, and scattered inflammatory infiltrates. Group III section of the liver tissue of mice treated with a dose of 200mg/kg silymarin showed minimal congestion and patchy scattered areas of necrosis. Group IV Section showed mild to moderate damage with focal necrotic hepatocytes of mice treated with a dose of 500mg/kg of ethanolic AM. Group V Section of the liver tissue of mice treated with a dose of 600mg/kg of ethanolic AM showed marked damage centrilobular necrosis, patchy loss of hepatocytes, and dilated veins with congestion. Group VI Section showed marked damage with area of necrosis at aqueous AM (500 mg/kg). Group VII section of the

**Table 25.2: Anti–microbial Sensitivity Test for Various Extracts of *Aegle marmelos* and *Azadirachta indica* by using Gram Positive and Gram Negative Bacteria**

| Sl.No. | Strains Used | Zone of Inhibition (mm) | | | | | | | | | | |
|---|---|---|---|---|---|---|---|---|---|---|---|---|
| | | | *Aegle marmelos* | | | | | *Azadirachta indica* | | | | |
| | | *Cont.* | *P* | *D* | *C* | *E* | *A* | *P* | *D* | *C* | *E* | *A* |
| 1. | *Escherichia coli* | – | – | – | 18 | 19 | 9 | – | 15 | – | 13 | 10 |
| 2. | *Micrococcus glutamicus* | – | – | 9 | 20 | 12 | – | – | 18 | – | 15 | – |
| 3. | *Lactobacillus bulgaris* | – | – | – | – | – | – | – | 15 | – | – | – |
| 4. | *Streptococcus faecalis* | – | – | 14 | 13 | 12 | 13 | – | 15 | – | 13 | 15 |
| 5. | *Staphylococcus aureus* | – | – | – | 14 | 11 | 10 | – | 16 | – | 12 | 12 |
| 6. | *Bacillus stearothermophilus* | – | – | 11 | 14 | 18 | 12 | – | 16 | – | 14 | 10 |
| 7. | *Staphylococcus pyogenes* | – | – | 11 | 15 | 13 | 11 | – | 15 | – | 12 | – |
| 8. | *Pseudomonas denitrificans* | – | – | – | 15 | 12 | 12 | – | 15 | – | 14 | 11 |
| 9. | *Micrococcus luteus* | – | – | 12 | 15 | 10 | 12 | – | 15 | – | 13 | 9 |
| 10. | *Bacillus cereus* | – | – | – | – | – | – | – | 16 | 11 | 15 | 10 |

Cont.: Control; P: Petroleum ether extract; D: Dichloromethane extract; C: Chloroform extract; E: Ethanolic extract; A: Aqueous extract.

**Figure 25.1: Effect of Various Concentration of Ethanolic and Aqueous Extract from *Aegle marmelos* and *Azadirachta indica* on Mice Liver–Photo Micrographic Sections**

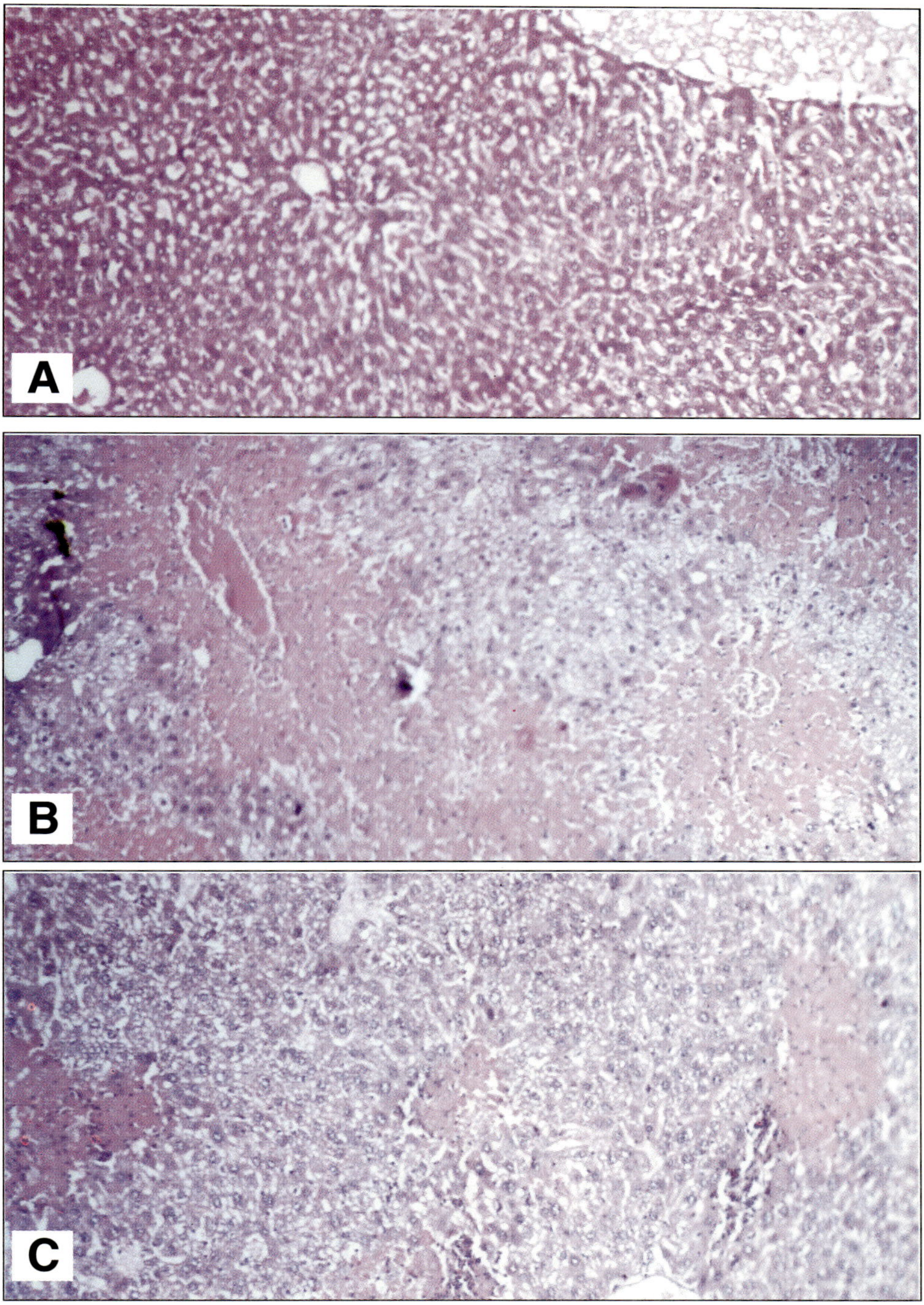


*Contd...*

**Figure 25.1–Contd...**

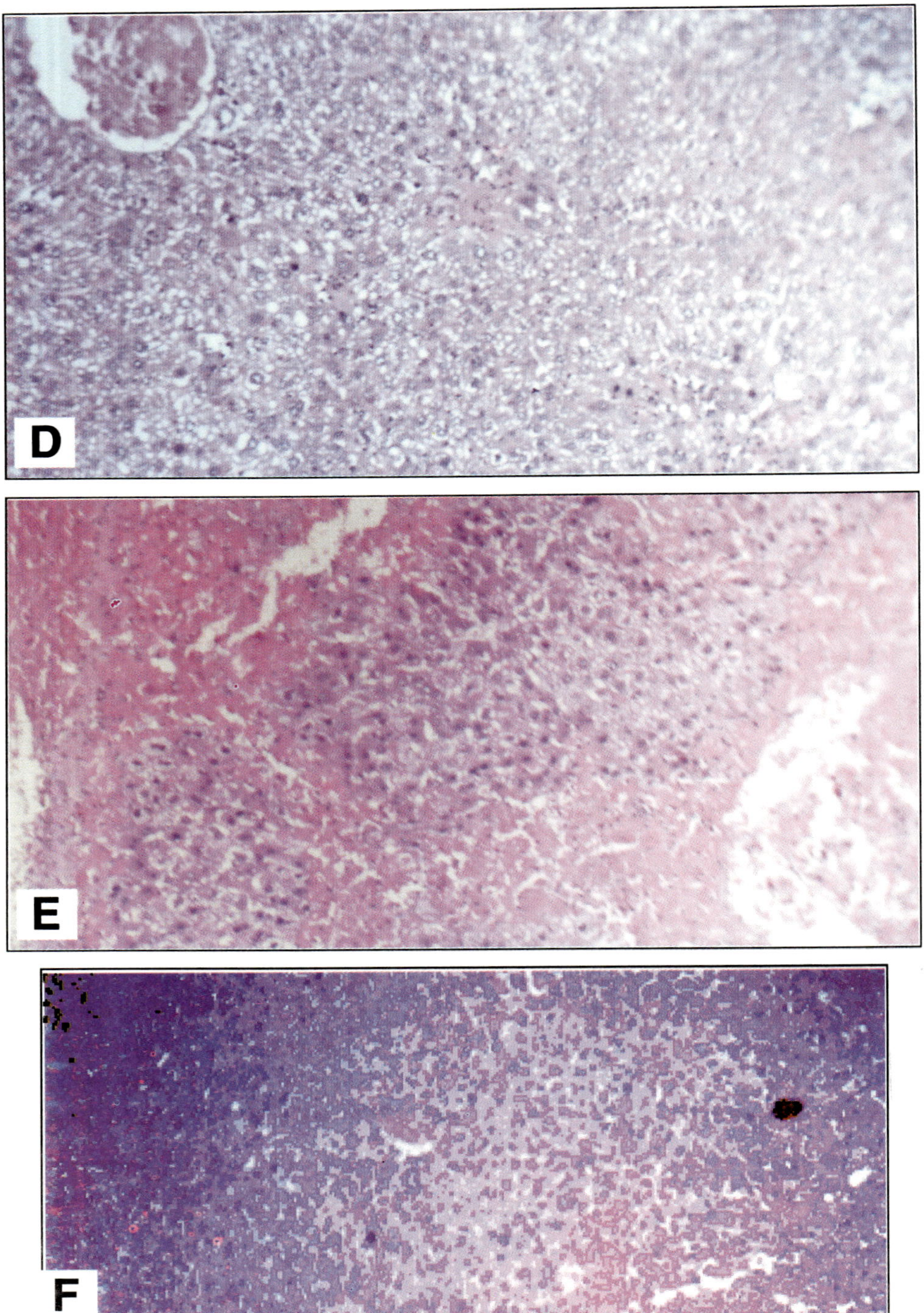


Contd...

**Figure 25.1–Contd...**

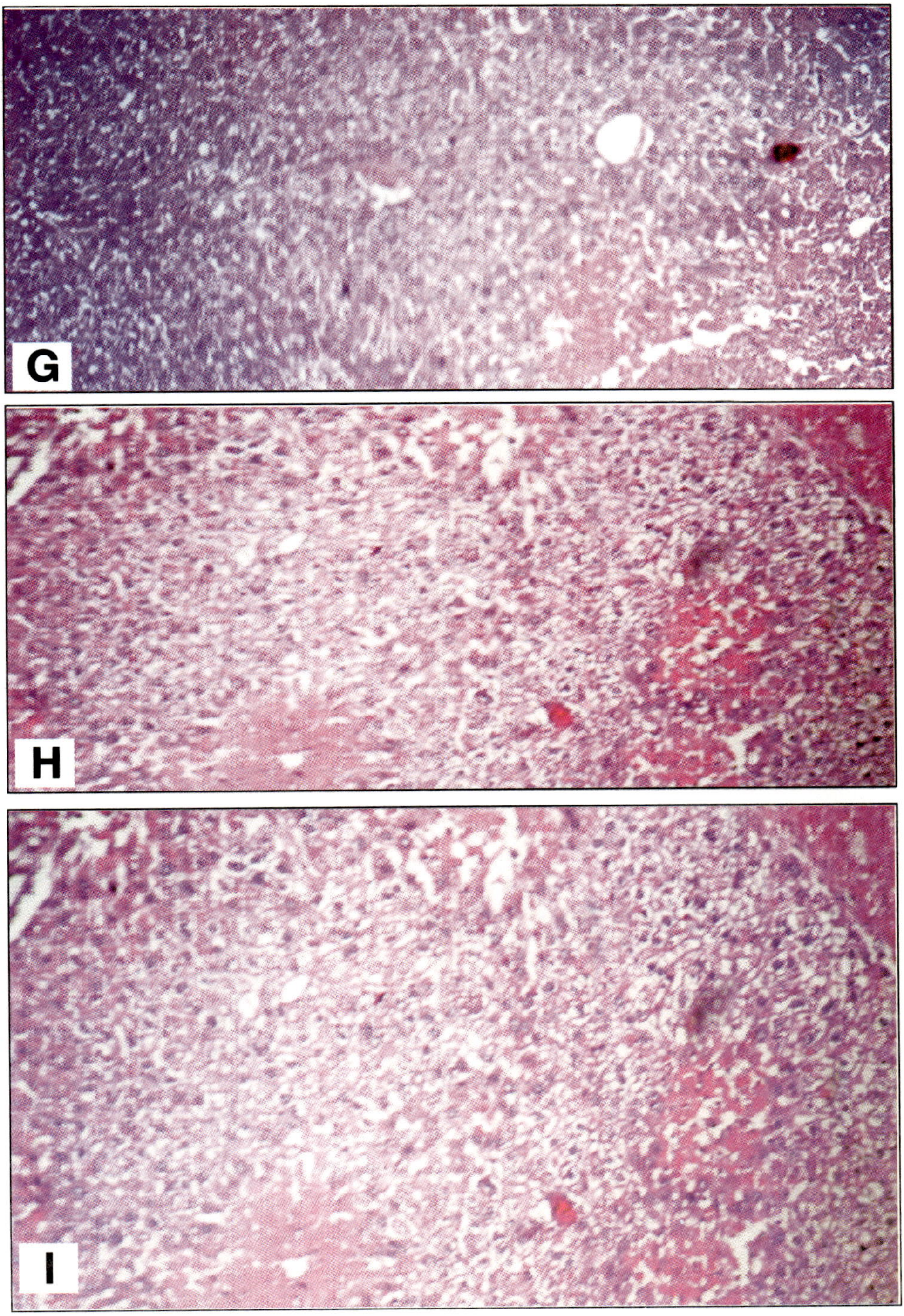


*Contd...*

**Figure 25.1–Contd...**

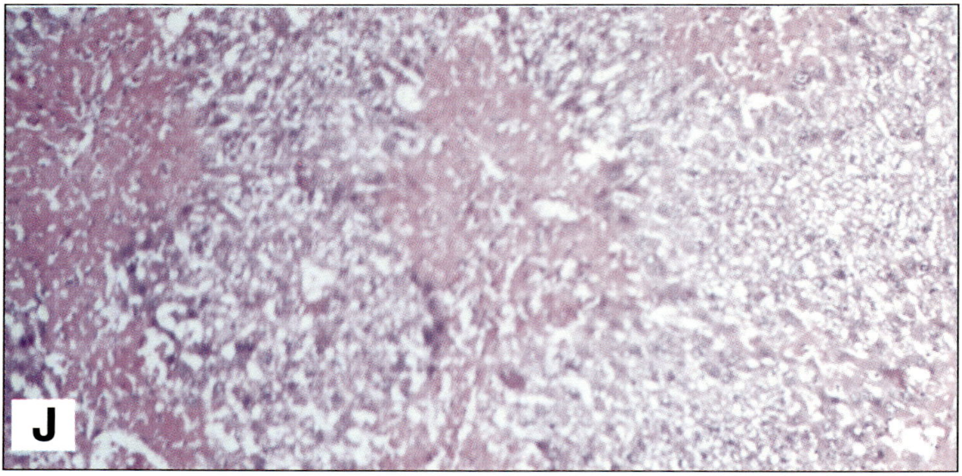

J

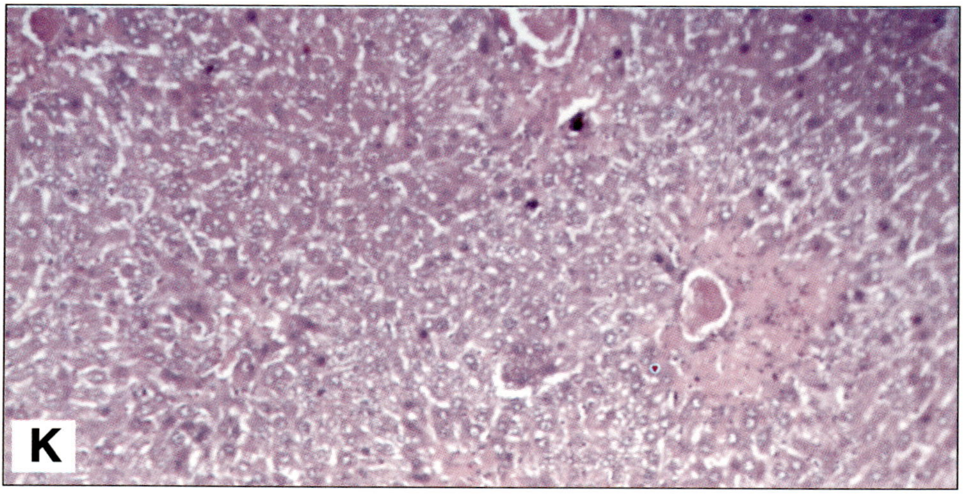

K

liver tissue of mice treated with a dose of 600mg/kg of aqueous AM showed extensive damage with large areas of necrosis, Hyperemia and congestion. Group VIII ethanolic extract (500 mg/kg) treated animals, the liver showed centrilobular necrosis and prominent dilated central veins. Group IX animals treated with ethanolic (600 mg/kg) showed marked centrilobular necrosis and dilated veins. Group X pretreatment with aqueous extract (500 mg/kg) showed moderate degree of damage with centrilobular necrosis and dilated veins. In group XI animals treated with aqueous extract (600 mg/kg) liver showed minimal congestion and patchy scattered areas of necrosis.

**Table 25.3: Analysis of SGOT, SGPT and ALP Levels in Carbontetrachloride Induced Hepatotoxicity in Mice against Aqueous and Ethanolic Extracts of *Aegle marmelos* and *Azadirachta indica***

| *Group* | *Treatment* | *SGOT (U/ml)* | *SGPT (U/ml)* | *ALP (K.A units)* |
|---|---|---|---|---|
| I | Control (1 per cent CMC) | 61.3 ± 5.2 | 41.3 ± 2.9 | 5.7 ± 0.4 |
| II | $CCl_4$ treated | 142 ± 11.5* | 100 ± 8.7* | 12.0 ± 0.2* |
| III | Silymarin(200 mg/kg) + $CCl_4$ | 54 ± 5.7* | 35.3 ± 1.7* | 4.4 ± 0.3* |
| IV | AM EtOH. (500 mg/kg) + $CCl_4$ | 99.3 ± 7.8** | 53.3 ± 2.9** | 6.0 ± 0.3* |
| V | AM EtOH (600 mg/kg) + $CCl_4$ | 115.3 ± 8.5*** | 80 ± 4.1*** | 9.8 ± 0.2*** |
| VI | AM Aqueous (500 mg/kg) + $CCl_4$ | 120.2 ± 6.1*** | 85.6 ± 4.7*** | 9.6 ± 0.4** |
| VII | AM Aqueous (600 mg/kg) + $CCl_4$ | 111.3 ± 6.3*** | 82 ± 5.2*** | 9.0 ± 0.3** |
| VIII | AI EtOH. (500 mg/kg) + $CCl_4$ | 91.3± 5.8*** | 64± 2.3*** | 8.9 ± 0.5*** |
| IX | AI EtOH (600 mg/kg) + $CCl_4$ | 90. 6 ± 5.4*** | 62.3 ± 1.9*** | 8.7 ± 0.4*** |
| X | AI Aqueous (500 mg/kg) + $CCl_4$ | 70 ± 3.0*** | 56 ± 1.1*** | 7.3 ± 0.1** |
| XI | AI Aqueous (600 mg/kg) + $CCl_4$ | 56.6± 6.5*** | 53.3±2.9*** | 5.5 ± 0.3** |

Values are expressed in Mean ± S.E.M for three animals in each group.

* $P < 0.001$; ** $P < 0.01$; *** $P < 0.1$

1a: Liver histophathology of control mice (Group I, H and Ex100); 1b: Liver histophathology of $CCl_4$ treated mice (Group II, H and Ex100); 1c: Liver histophathology of Silymarin (200 mg/kg) treated mice (Group III, H and Ex100); 1d: Liver histophathology of AM ethnolic extracted (500 mg/kg) treated mice (Group IV, H and Ex100); 1e: Liver histophathology of AM ethnolic extracted (600 mg/kg) treated mice (Group V, H and Ex100); 1f: Liver histophathology of AM aqueous extracted (500 mg/kg) treated mice (Group VI, H and Ex100); 1g: Liver histophathology of AM aqueous extracted (600 mg/kg) treated mice (Group VII, H and Ex100); 1h: Liver histophathology of AI ethnolic extracted (500 mg/kg) treated mice (Group VII, H and Ex100); 1i: Liver histophathology of AI ethnolic extracted (600 mg/kg) treated mice (Group IX, H and Ex100); 1j: Liver histophathology of AI aqueous extracted (500 mg/kg) treated mice (Group X, H and Ex100); 1k: Liver histophathology of AI aqueous extracted (600 mg/kg) treated mice (Group XI, H and Ex100).

## 4.0 Discussion

Since time immemorial AM and AI is used for treating various aliments traditionally in Southern India and utilized in day today life (Ross, 2005). Both the species have its own importance in the regions rituals, in case of AM, *in* Hinduism, Lord Shiva is believed to live under the Bael tree whereas, AI is important for performing Goddess pooja. The neem tree is still regarded as 'village dispensary' in various parts of India. The exposure of our body parts to the leaves may enhance the diffusion of the active ingredients, which is the major reason to overcome various ailments. Recent scientific studies have proved this concept (Karunanayake, 1984; Kamalakannan, 2005; Suresh Kumar, 2005).

Traditionally AM leaves are used in the religious poojas and fruits are consumed during the month of August–November. Fruit jam and juice are used in the summer. In the case of AI, leaves are offered in the religious "poojas" and flowers are consumed along with sweet and sour additives (*"Ugadi pachidi"*) during the month of March to

July to overcome the seasonal epidemics such as fever, bacterial, viral infections. These two plants are used on a day to day basis throughout the year except during winter months. It may be the reason why our forefathers have identified the season specific usage of these plants. During the winter season infectious epidemics are not common in Southern India thereby explaining why it is not utilized in the winter season. Both the plants possess antimicrobial, antifungal and other activities are scientifically proved by various scientific workers (Saisidharan, 1998; Sudharameshwari, 2007; Rojanapo, 1985; Siddique, 2002; Parida, 2002).

The bitter pungent leaf juice of AM, mixed with honey, is given to allay catarrh and fever. With black pepper added, it is taken to relieve jaundice and constipation accompanied by oedema. In the foot hills of Shevaroys hill region the tribal communities use this leaf and pulp juices along with neem and phyllanthus leaves to treat jaundice. The leaf decoction is also said to alleviate asthma in this region. The jaundice and asthmatic treatment against animal systems are successfully proved (Alam, 1990; Mishra, 1990). The yellow dye obtained from the fruits is traditionally used in the textile painting and printing works (Siva, 2007).

The emerging tender neem leaves are given to the children to overcome the *Ascoris lumbricoids* infection. Costa, (2006) reported the anthelmintic activity in sheep against gastrointestinal nematodes. In Tamil Nadu, Andra Pradesh and Karnataka farmers and local tribes are using dried neem leaves as a pesticide, nematicide and insecticide. Recently, entomologist found that neem can affect more than 200 insect species as well as mites, fungi, bacterial and even virus (Agrawal, 2003; Mahesh Kumar, 2005). Neem oil have been found to be spermicidal, Irrulars and Malaiyali tribal communities belonging to Tamil Nadu region using this neem oil as contraceptive. This contraceptive property was reported in the rats treated with neem seed extracts (Garg, 1998).

Various organic solvent extract from AM (Bael) showed anti-microbial activity against both Gram positive and Gram negative bacteria except in the case of petroleum ether extract, which did not show inhibitory zone against various strains studied. In the case of AI (Neem) anti bacterial effect was observed from various extracts. Anti-microbial activity against different solvent extracts of both the species is mentioned in Table. Our results confirmed the earlier report indicating the antimicrobial activity of leaf and bark of Bael tree against Gram positive and Gram negative bacteria (Saisidharan, 1998; Sudha Rameshwari, 2007). Previous workers reported that various such as leaves, seeds and barks have the antibacterial activity (Sairam, 2000; Thakurta, 2007). In this present investigation, a higher number of organisms was studied. The present results support the view that these plants can be used for the treatment of diseases in humans and animals thereby showing the importance of ethnobotanical approaches as potential sources of bioactive substances.

Analysis of SGOT, SGPT and ALP levels in Carbontetrachloride induced hepatotoxicity in mice against aqueous and ethanolic extracts of AM and AI are shown in the Table 25.3. Among AM extracts, ethanolic extract was found to be effective as compared to aqueous extracts. In ethanolic extract 500 mg/kg was found to be effective (Table 25.3). This is the first attempt to study the hepatoprotective activity of AM. AI aqueous extract 600mg/Kg was found as effective as compared to silymarin treatment. In both cases P < 0.01 values were significant. In Neem, the present results also follow the previous trend *i.e.* aqueous extracts having the hepatoprotective activity. However, in the present investigation 600mg/Kg. showed maximum effect in mice (Group XI). The enzymes assay was cross examined with histopatholoical studies and photo micrographic examination (Figure 25.1). The histopathological analysis also followed the similar trend as found in the enzymes Assays. The overall results of the present investigation revealed various ethnobotanical uses, potent antimicrobial and hepatoprotective activity of these plants.

## 5.0 Conclusion

India is one among the 12 mega biodiversity country in the world, possessing enormous biological resources. Suitable usage of the biological resources is essential for the improvement of the socio-economic status of the region, state and nation. Various medicinal plants, trees are very important and possess multiple medicinal properties. The plant species chosen in the present investigation possess multiple usages in routine life. The *Aegle marmelos* and *Azadirachta indica* plant has very good sacred value due to its multiple medicinal properties and ancient people of India have insisted to use them regularly to get rid of various ailments. Since these plants are used as food as well as medicine, they do not have any side effects. The antimicrobial studies in AM revealed that ethanolic and chloroform extracts exhibit maximum antibacterial activity as compared to dichloromethane, aqueous and petroleum ether extracts. Where as, AI, dichloromethane, ethanolic extracts had maximum inhibition as compared to aqueous, chloroform and petroleum ether extracts.

Hepatoprotective activity of the ethanolic and aqueous extracts of both the plants were studied against carbon tetrachloride induced liver damage in mice using silymarin as the internal control. The enzyme activities of Serum Glutamate Oxaloacetate Transaminase (SGOT), Serum Glutamic Pyruvic Transaminase (SGPT) and Alkaline phosphatase (ALP) were studied. In AM ethanolic extract 500 mg/kg was found to be effective whereas AI aqueous extract (600mg/Kg) was found to be as effective when compared to ethanolic extracts. Similar trend was observed in the histopathological analysis. The results of the present investigation revealed various traditional uses, potent antimicrobial and hepatoprotecive activity of these plants.

## Acknowledgements

The authors are thankful to VIT Management for their constant support and encouragements. Thanks are due to Prof. Lazar Mathew for his valuable comments and suggestions to carry out this research successfully.

## References

Agrawal, D.P., 2003. Medicinal properties of Neem: New Findings. ttp://www.infinityfoundation.com/mandala/t_es/t_es_agraw_neem_frameset.htm

Ahmedullah, M. and Nayar, M.P., 1999. *Red data book of Indian plants*, vol. 4 (Peninsular India), Calcutta: *Botanical Survey of India*.

Alam, M.M., Siddiqui, M.B., Hussain, W., 1990. Treatment of diabetes through herbal drug in rural India. Fitoterapia, 61, pp. 240-242.

Bakhru, H.K., 1997. *Foods that Heal. The Natural Way to Good Health*. Orient Paperbacks. ISBN 81-222-0033-8.

Bauer, R.W., Kirby, M.D.K., Sherris, J.C., Turck, M., 1966. Antibiotic susceptibility testing by standard single disc diffusion method. Am J. Clinical Pathol., 45, pp. 493-496.

Costa, C.T.C., Bevilaqua, C.M.L., Maciel, M.V., Camurc, A.L.F., Vasconcelos Morais, S.M., Monteiro, M.V.B., Farias.V.M., Da Silva.M.V. and Souza, M.M.C., 2006. Anthelmintic activity of *Azadirachta indica* A. Juss against sheep gastrointestinal nematodes. Veterinary parasitology, 137, pp. 306–310

Garg, S., Talwar, G.P. and Upadhyay, S.N., 1998. Immunocontraceptive activity guided fractionation and characterization of active constituents of neem (*Azadirachta indica*) seed extracts. J. Ethnopharmacol, 60, pp. 235–246

Jain, S.K. and Sastry, A.R.K. (1979). *Threatened Plants in India*. Botanical Survey of India.

Kamalakkannan, N., Prince, P.S., 2005. The effect of Aegle marmelos fruit extract in streptozotocin diabetes: a histopathological study, J Herb Pharmacother, 5, pp. 87-96.

Karunanayake, E.H., Welihinda, J., Sirimanne, S.R. and Sinnadorai, G., 1984. Oral hypoglycaemic activity of some medicinal plants of Sri Lanka, J. Ethnopharmacol, 11, pp. 223–231.

Kind, P.R. and King's, E.J., 1954. Estimation of plasma phosphatase by determination of hydrolysed phenol with antipyrin, J. Clin. Pathol., 7, pp. 322–326.

Mahesh Kumar, K. Krisshnaiah, N.V. Lingaiah, T. Pasalu, C. and Krishnaiah, K., 2005. Effect of some commercial neem based insecticides against *Nilaparvata lugens* (BPH), *Sogatella furcifera* (WBPH) and *Nephotettix virescens* (GLH)–Part 1. Practical Oriented Results on Use and Production of Neem–Ingredients and Pheromones. Trifolio-M Sonnenstr.22 D-35633 Lahnau, Germany. ISBN: 3-925614-28-1.

Maikhuri, R.K., Rao, K.S., Kusum Chauhan, Laxman Kandari, Prasad, P., Negi, G.S., Nautiyal, S., Purohit Aditya, Rajasekaran, C. and Saxena, K.G., 2005. Cultivation and conservation of higher Himalayan medicinal plants through participatory and action research: A case study from the Central Himalaya (Uttaranchal), India. *Himalayan Medicinal Plants, Balancing Use and Conservation*, pp: 281-301.

National Bureau of Plant Genetic Resources, 2000. Manual on exploration and collection of Plant Genetic Resources and related Indigenous Knowledge, New Delhi.

Mishra, A.K. and Dubey, N.K., 1990. Fungitoxicity of essential oil of amomum subulatum *Aspergillus flavus*. Economic Botany, 44, pp. 530-533.

Parida, M.M., Upadhyay, C., Pandya, G. and Jana, A.M., 2002. Inhibitory potential of neem (*Azadirachta indica* Juss) leaves on Dengue virus type-2 replication. J. Ethnopharmacol, 79, pp. 273–278.

Puri, H.S., 1999. Neem the Devine Tree, *Azadirachta indica*. Harwood Academic Publishers, The Netherlands. pp 182.

Rojanapo, W., Suwanno, S., Somaree, R., Glinsukon, T. and Thebtaranonth, Y., 1985. Mutagenic and Antibacterial Activity Testing of Nimbolide and Nimbic acid. J. Sci. Thailand, 11, pp. 177–181.

Reitman, S. and Frankel S., 1957. A colorimetric method for the determination of serum glutamic oxalacetic and glutamic pyruvic transaminases. Am. J. Clin. Pathol., 28, pp. 56-63.

Ross, I.A., 2005. Medicinal Plants of the World Vol.2.: Chemical Constituents, Traditional and Modern Uses. Humana Press Inc. Totowa, NJ

Sai Ram, M. Ilavazhagan, G., Sharma,S.K., Dhanraj, S.A., Suresh, B., Parida, M.M., Jana, A.M., Kumar Devendra and Selvamurthy, W., 2000. Anti-microbial activity of a new vaginal contraceptive NIM-76 from neem oil (*Azadirachta indica*). J. Ethnopharmacol., 71, pp. 377-382.

Sasidharan, V. K., Krishnakumar, T., Manjula, C. B., 1998. Antimicrobial Activity of Nine Common Plants in Kerala, India. *PJS*, 127(1)

Siddiqui, B. S., Afshan, F. and Faizi, S., 2002. Two New Triterpenoids from *Azadirachta indica* and Their Insecticidal Activity. J. Nat. Prod, 65, pp. 1216-1218.

Siva, R., 2007. Status of natural dyes and dye-yielding plants in India. Curr. Sci., 92, pp. 916-925.

Sudharameshwari,K. and Radhika, J., 2007. Antibacterial screening *of Aegle marmelos, Lawsonia inermis and Albizzia libbeck.* Afr J. Traditional, Complementary and Alternative Medicines, 4, pp. 205–210.

Suresh Kumar, Suresh, P.K., Vijayababu, M.R., Arunkumar, A. and Arunakaran, J., 2005. Anticancer effects of ethanolic neem leaf extract on prostate cancer cell line (PC-3). J. Ethnopharmacol, 105, pp. 246-250.

Thakurta, P., Bhowmika, P., Mukherjee, S., Hajra, T.K., Patra, A. and Bag, P.K., 2007. Antibacterial, antisecretory and antihemorrhagic activity of *Azadirachta indica* used to treat cholera and diarrhoea in India. J. Ethnopharmacol, 111, pp. 607–612

## Abbreviations

CMC: Carboxy methyl cellulose; AM: *Aegle marmelos;* AI: *Azadirachta indica;* $CCl_4$: Carbon tetrachloride.

## Chapter 26

# Antifungal Constituents from the Stems of *Dracaena cambodiana*

***Nguyen Hai Dang[1], Phan Van Kiem[1], Chau Van Minh[1]* and Tran Thu Huong[2]***

*[1]Institute of Natural Products Chemistry, Vietnam Academy of Science and Technology, Hanoi, Vietnam*

*[2]Faculty of Chemical Technology, Hanoi University of Technology, Hanoi, Vietnam*

**E-mail: cvminh@fpt.vn*

## ABSTRACT

The stems of *Dracaena cambodiana* have been investigated for antifungal constituents, resulting in the isolation of a new steroidal saponin dracagenin A (1) together with two known components 25*S*-namogenin B (2) and spriroconazole A (3). Their structures were elucidated on the basis of extensive spectroscopic analysis including 1D, 2D NMR and ESI MS. The isolated compounds were evaluated for their antifungal activities. 1 and 3 exhibited inhibitory activity against *Aspergilus niger* at the MICs of 50 μg/ml. No inhibition effects on *F. oxysporum*, *S. cerevisiae* and *C. albicans* have been found for the tested compounds. Interestingly, toxicity of 3 towards several cancer cell lines has been demonstrated. The $IC_{50}$ of 3 against Hep-G2, Lu, and RD are 2.00, 4.72, and 4.02 μg/ml, respectively.

***Keywords:*** *Dracaenaceae, Dracaena cambodiana, Steroidal saponin, Dracagenin A, 25S-namogenin B, Spriroconazole A.*

## 1.0 Introduction

*Dracaena cambodiana* (Dracaenaceae) is mostly distributed in the North of Vietnam. The plant has been found in ethnomedicine to treat menoschesis, ostealgia amongst others (Bich, 2006; Chi, 1997; Loi, 2001). Investigations on the chemical constituents of the genus revealed that the spirosterol and steroidal saponins are among the major components (Gonzalez, 2004; Mimaki, 1998). Interestingly, there has been no report so far on the phytochemicals of *D. cambodiana*. In our continuing studies for antifungal agents, we have isolated a new steroidal saponin namely dracagenin A (1), one sprirosterol 25*S*-namogenin B (2) and one known steroidal saponin spriroconazole A (3). The antifungal activities of these compounds were also described.

## 2.0 Materials and Methods

### 2.1 General Experiment Procedures

The $^1$H-NMR (500MHz) and $^{13}$C-NMR (125MHz) spectra were recorded on a Bruker AM500 FT-NMR spectrometer. Chemical shifts are referenced to $\delta$ using tetramethylsilan (TMS) as an internal standard. The Electron Spray Ionization (ESI) mass spectrum was obtained using an AGILENT 1100 LC-MSD Trap spectrometer. Column chromatography (CC) was performed on silica gel 230-400 mesh (0.040-0.063 mm, Merck) or YMC RP-18 resins (30-50 µm, Fujisilisa Chemical Ltd.). Thin layer chromatography (TLC) was performed on DC-Alufolien 60 $F_{254}$ (Merck 1.05715) or $RP_{18}$ $F_{254s}$ (Merck) plates.

### 2.2 Plant Material

The roots of *D. cambodiana* were collected in Hoa binh province, Vietnam in January 2006 and identified by Dr. Tran Huy Thai, Institute of Ecology and Biological Resources, VAST, Vietnam. An authentic sample was deposited at the Institute of Natural Products Chemistry, VAST, Vietnam.

### 2.3 Extraction and Isolation

The dried roots of *D. cambodiana* (4 kg) were extracted with MeOH three times (7 days each time) and then concentrated under low pressure to obtain 150 g MeOH extract. The MeOH extract was suspended in water and partitioned with hexane, $CHCl_3$ and BuOH to obtain hexane (60 g), $CHCl_3$ (35 g), and BuOH (65 g) fractions. The $CHCl_3$ fraction was then chromatographed on a silica gel column eluting with $CHCl_3$-MeOH gradient (from 10:1 to 1:1 v/v) to give fractions C1 (16 g), C2 (11 g), and C3 (7 g). The C1 fraction was chromatographed on a silica gel column using $CHCl_3$-EtOAc (3:1) as eluent to give subfractions C3A (6.5 g), C3B (3.4 g), C3C (6.0 g). The C3C sub-fraction (6.0 g) was chromatographed on a silica gel column using a $CHCl_3$-MeOH (3:1 v/v) system as eluent and yielded 2 (25 mg) as white powder. The BuOH fraction was chromatographed on a silica gel column eluting with $CHCl_3$-MeOH gradient (from 10:1 to 1:1 v/v) to obtain fractions B1 (25 g), B2 (20 g), and B3 (12 g). The B2 fraction showed the highest activity with regard to antifungal property. It was selected for further isolation of bioactive compounds. The B2 fraction (20 g) was chromatographed on an YMC RP-18 column using a MeOH-$H_2O$ (2:1 v/v) system as eluent and yielded 1 (18.5 mg) and 3 (9 mg) as white amorphous powders.

**25*S*-Namogenin B (2)**

White powder, positive ESI-MS *m/z*: 447 $[M+H]^+$, 429 $[M+H-H_2O]^+$, 411 $[M+H-2H_2O]^+$; negative ESI-MS *m/z*: 445 $[M-H]^-$; $^1$H-NMR (500 MHz, $CDCl_3$) $\delta$: 3.46 (dd, $J$ = 4.0, 11.5 Hz, H-1), 1.57/2.06 (m, H-2), 3.53 (m, H-3), 1.89/2.24 (m, H-4), 5.57 (d, $J$ = 5.5

Hz, H-6), 1.94/2.08 (m, H-7), 1.97 (m, H-8), 1.59 (m, H-9), 1.60/2.11 (m, H-11), 1.42/1.75 (m, H-12), 1.61/1.95 (m, H-15), 4.60 (m, H-16), 2.29 (m, H-17), 0.94 (s, H-18), 1.07 (s, H-19), 2.10/2.28 (m, H-20), 1.01 (d, *J* = 7.0 Hz, H-21), 1.94/2.02 (m, H-23), 1.40/2.11 (m, H-24), 1.72 (m, H-25), 3.29 (d, *J* =2.5 Hz, H-26a), 3.93 (d, *J* = 11.0 Hz, H-26b), and 16.1 (d, *J* = 7.0 Hz, H-27); $^{13}$C-NMR (125 MHz, $CDCl_3$) δ: 77.7 (C-1), 42.0 (C-2), 67.9 (C-3), 42.6 (C-4), 137.6 (C-5), 125.5 (C-6), 26.2 (C-7), 35.7 (C-8), 43.7 (C-9), 43.2 (C-10), 22.6 (C-11), 32.0 (C-12), 44.0 (C-13), 87.6 (C-14), 39.4 (C-15), 81.9 (C-16), 58.8 (C-17), 20.0 (C-

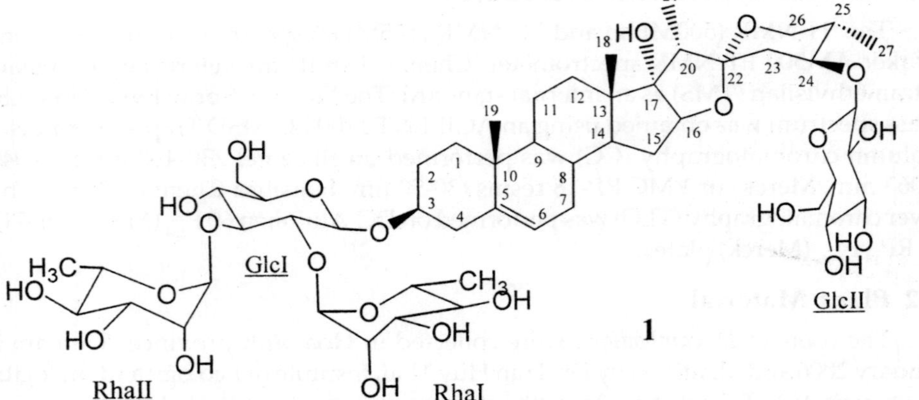

1

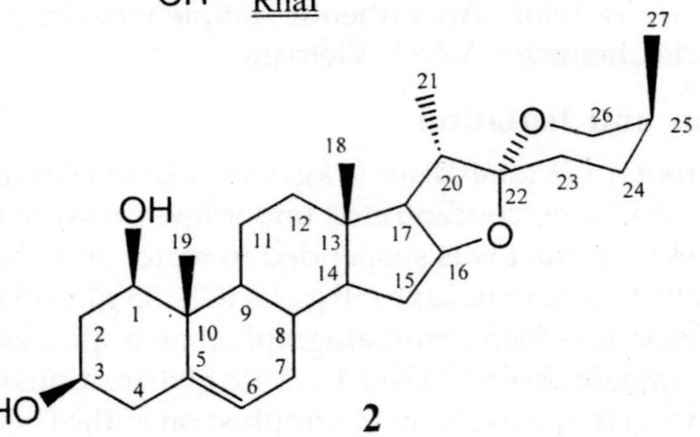

2

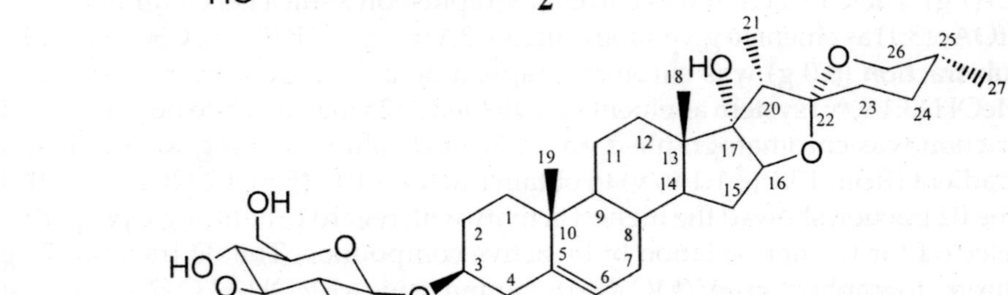

3

**Figure 26.1: Structures of 1-3**

18), 13.0 (C-19), 42.2 (C-20), 14.5 (C-21), 110.0 (C-22), 26.1 (C-23), 25.8 (C-24), 27.1 (C-25), 65.1 (C-26), and 16.1 (C-27).

**Spriroconazole A (3)**

White powder, positive ESI-MS *m/z*: 907 $[M+Na]^+$; negative ESI-MS *m/z*: 883 $[M-H]^-$; $^1$H-NMR (500 MHz, $CDCl_3$) δ: 1.11/1.90 (m, H-1), 1.31/1.91 (m, H-2), 3.66 (m, H-3), 2.29/2.47 (m, H-4), 5.40 (d, *J* = 5.0 Hz, H-6), 1.37/1.59 (m, H-7), 1.65 (m, H-8), 0.98 (m, H-9), 1.54/1.63 (m, H-11), 1.65/2.03 (m, H-12), 1.73 (m, H-14), 1.25/1.71 (m, H-15), 4.01 (dd, *J* = 7.0, 8.0 Hz, H-16), 0.85 (s, H-18), 1.07 (s, H-19), 2.11 (m, H-20), 0.94 (d, *J* = 7.0 Hz, H-21), 1.70/2.03 (m, H-23), 1.45/1.62 (m, H-24), 1.62 (m, H-25), 3.36/3.47 (m, H-26), 0.81 (d, *J* = 6.5 Hz, H-27), 4.53 (d, *J* = 7.0 Hz, H-1Glc), 3.58 (t, *J* = 9.0 Hz, H-3 Glc), 4.99 (d, *J* = 1.5 Hz, H-1 Rha), 1.26 (d, *J* = 6.5 Hz, H-6 Rha), 4.92 (d, *J* = 1.5 Hz, H-1 Rha'), and 1.28 (d, *J* = 6.5 Hz, H-6 Rha'); $^{13}$C-NMR (125 MHz, $CDCl_3$) δ: 38.6 (C-1), 30.8 (C-2), 79.1 (C-3), 39.3 (C-4), 141.9 (C-5), 122.9 (C-6), 32.8 (C-7), 33.3 (C-8), 51.5 (C-9), 38.0 (C-10), 21.7 (C-11), 33.2 (C-12), 45.8 (C-13), 53.1 (C-14), 32.1 (C-15), 90.6 (C-16), 91.3 (C-17), 17.5 (C-18), 19.8 (C-19), 45.5 (C-20), 9.1 (C-21), 111.0 (C-22), 32.5 (C-23), 29.4 (C-24), 31.3 (C-25), 67.7 (C-26), 17.5 (C-27), Glc (1) 100.2, (2) 97.4, (3) 88.4, (4) 70.5, (5) 77.5, (6) 62.6, RhaI (1) 102.8, (2) 72.3, (3) 72.5, (4) 73.6, (5) 70.1, (6) 17.8, RhaII (1) 103.9, (2) 72.2, (3) 72.4, (4) 73.8, (5) 70.9, and (6) 18.1.

## 3.0 Results and Discussion

Bioassay guided fractionation led to the isolation of three bioactive components. Compound 1 was obtained as white amorphous powder, The ESI MS (positive mode) showed the pseudomolecular $[M+Na]^+$ ion peak at *m/z* 1085 (corresponding to the molecular formula $C_{51}H_{82}O_{23}$). The $^{13}$C-NMR spectrum of 1 showed 51 signals, among which 27 were assigned to the aglycone, the remaining 24 signals were indicative of the presence of four hexoses (two D-glucose and two L-rhamnoses). The structure of the aglycone moiety was recognized to be penogenin (3b, 17a-dihydroxyspirost-5en) by $^1$H–and $^{13}$C-NMR spectral analysis using connectivities observed in the COSY, HSQC, and HMBC. The $^1$H-NMR spectrum of 1 showed two three-proton singlet signals at δ 0.83 and 1.07 and two three-proton doublet signals at δ 0.91 (*J* = 7.5 Hz) and 1.00 (*J* = 6.5 Hz), which were characteristic of the spirostanol skeleton, as well as signals for four anomeric protons at δ 4.54 (d, *J* =7.5 Hz), 4.37 (d, *J* = 7.5 Hz), 5.00 (d, *J* = 1.5 Hz), 1.92 (d, *J* = 1.5 Hz). The salient features of this aglycone were at δ 141.9 (C-5) and 122.6 (C-6), characteristic of $\Delta^5$-spirostene-type sapogenin. The proton coupling constant between H-25 and H-26$_{ax}$ (*J* = 11.5 Hz), and the $^{13}$C-NMR shifts of the F-ring part (C-25/δ 38.5) evident for the C-25*R* configuration.

The linkage of the sugar moiety to C-3 of the aglycone was confirmed by the correlation of an anomeric proton ($\delta_H$ 4.54) and C-3 position ($\delta_C$ 79.1) in the HMBC spectrum. This carbohydrate consisted of one disubstituted glucose and two terminal rhamnose moieties. The linkage positions of the sugars were determined by HMBC spectrum. Accordingly, the anomeric proton signal observed in $^1$H-NMR spectrum at $\delta_H$ 5.00 correlated with C-2 ($\delta_C$ 79.4) of glucose, the anomeric proton signal observed in $^{1}$H-NMR spectrum at $\delta_H$ 4.92 correlated with C-3 ($\delta$ 88.3) of glucose. Furthermore, the presence of two upfield signals of methyl protons at $\delta$ 1.26 (d, $J$ = 1.5 Hz), and 1.28 (d, $J$ = 1.5 Hz) in its $^{1}$H-NMR spectrum confirmed that the two-deoxyhexopyranose units were rhamnose moieties. The rhamnopyranosyl residues were shown to be terminal units as suggested by the absence of any glysosydation shift for their carbon resonances. The 2,3 distribution of the glucopyranosyl moiety was shown by downfield chemical shifts at $\delta$ 79.4 (C-2 Glc) and 88.3 (C-3 Glc) in the $^{13}$C-NMR spectrum. The NMR data were in good agreement with literature data (Tepono, 2001; Yokosuka, 2002).

**Table 26.1: NMR Data of 1**

| *C* | $\delta_C^{a,b}$ | $\delta_H^{a,c}$ *mult. (J, Hz)* | *HMBC (H to C)* |
|---|---|---|---|
| 1 | 38.6 | 1.13 m; 1.90 m | C–5 |
| 2 | 30.7 | 1.62 m; 1.91 m | |
| 3 | 79.1 | 3.65 m | C–1 Glc |
| 4 | 39.3 | 2.30 m; 2.47 m | C–2, C–5, C–6, C–10 |
| 5 | 141.9 | | |
| 6 | 122.6 | 5.40 d (5.5) | C–8, C–10 |
| 7 | 32.8 | 1.37 m; 1.68 m | |
| 8 | 33.3 | 1.65 m | |
| 9 | 51.5 | 0.97 m | |
| 10 | 38.0 | | |
| 11 | 21.7 | 1.49 m; 1.63 m | |
| 12 | 33.2 | 1.59 m; 2.03 m | |
| 13 | 45.7 | | |
| 14 | 53.9 | 1.74 m | |
| 15 | 32.0 | 1.31 m; 2.05 m | C–15, C–17 |
| 16 | 90.9 | 3.99 t (6.5) | |
| 17 | 91.8 | | |
| 18 | 17.5 | 0.83 s | C–12, C–13, C–14, C–17 |
| 19 | 19.8 | 1.07 s | C–4, C–9 |
| 20 | 45.9 | 2.16 m | C–14, C–17, C–21, C–23 |
| 21 | 9.0 | 0.91 d (7.5) | C–17, C–20, C–22 |
| 22 | 113.8 | | |
| 23 | | | |
| | 41.0 | 1.69 m; 2.22 m | C–24, C–25 |
| 24 | 82.0 | 3.62 m | |
| 25 | 38.5 | 1.67 m | |
| 26 | 65.8 | 3.38 m; 3.53 m | C–24, C–27 |
| 27 | 13.5 | 1.00 d (6.5) | C–24, C–26 |

*Contd...*

**Table 26.1–Contd...**

| C | $\delta_C^{a,b}$ | $\delta_H^{a,c}$ mult. (J, Hz) | HMBC (H to C) |
|---|---|---|---|
| **Glc (1 → C3)** | | | |
| 1 | 100.2 | 4.54 d (7.5) | C–3 |
| 2 | 79.4 | 3.47 m | |
| 3 | 88.4 | 3.60 m | C–2 Glc, C–4, Glc |
| 4 | 70.6 | 3.40 m | |
| 5 | 77.5 | 3.29 m | |
| 6 | 62.6 | 3.70 m; 3.88 m | |
| **Rha (1 → 2Glc)** | | | |
| 1 | 102.8 | 5.00 d (1.5) | C–2 Glc, C–3 Rha, C–5 Rha |
| 2 | 72.3 | 3.64 m | |
| 3 | 72.5 | 3.88 m | |
| 4 | 73.6 | 3.43 m | |
| 5 | 70.1 | 4.10 m | |
| 6 | 17.8 | 1.26 d (6.0) | |
| **Rha' (1 → 3Glc)** | | | |
| 1 | 103.9 | 4.92 d (1.5) | C–3 Glc, C–3 Rha', C–5 Rha' |
| 2 | 72.2 | 3.86 m | |
| 3 | 72.4 | 3.66 m | |
| 4 | 73.8 | 3.43 m | |
| 5 | 70.9 | 3.95 m | |
| 6 | 18.1 | 1.28 d (6.0) | |
| **Glc' (1 → C24)** | | | |
| 1 | 106.0 | 4.37 d (7.5) | C–24 |
| 2 | 75.5 | 3.17 m | |
| 3 | 78.1 | 3.39 m | |
| 4 | 71.7 | 3.33 m | C–5 Glc' |
| 5 | 77.7 | 3.31 m | |
| 6 | 62.8 | 3.70 m; 3.88 m | |

: Measured in $CD_3OD$; b: 125 MHz; c: 500 MHz. Chemical shift (δ) in ppm.

The remaining sugar moiety was also determined by extensive spectroscopic tudies. The strong downfield shift signal at C-24 (δ 82.0) in $^{13}$C-NMR spectrum was ndicative of the presence of one sugar moiety at this position. The correlation observed 1 HMBC spectrum between the anomeric proton ($\delta_H$ 4.37 (d, $J = 7.5$ Hz)) and C-24 ($\delta_C$ 2.0) confirmed that one glucose was unit connected to C-24 of the F-ring. From the bove evidence and comparison with published data (Mimaki, 2001), 1 was identified s 24-*O*-β-*D*-glucopyranosyl-3-*O*-α-L-rhamnopyranosyl-(1→2)-[α-L-rhamnopysano-yl-(1→3)]-β-D-glucopyranosylpennogenin which were named as dracagenin A. This the first report of this compound in nature.

Compound 2 was obtained as white powder. Inspecting the NMR data of 2 revealed that 2 were a spirostane-type sterol. The NMR data of 2 were similar to those of the aglycone of 1 except for the appearance of two-hydroxyl group at C-1 ($\delta_H$ 3.46 (dd, $J$ = 4.0, 11.5 Hz)/$\delta_C$ 77.7) and C-14 ($\delta_C$ 87.6) and the upfield shifts of the signals of F-ring from C-23 to C-27. This evidence led to suggesting a 25*S* configuration of 2. The 13C-NMR spectrum of 2 showed the upfield shift of the oxygenated signal ($\delta$ 58.8) assigned to C-17 in 1. Therefore, C-17 was considered as a methine group. The spectroscopic data of 2 were compared with those of 25*S*-namogenin B and found to match (Tran, 2001). Using the same methods of structure elucidation spectroscopy, compound 3 was determined to be spriroconazole A, which were isolated from *D. manii*, *D. arborea*, and *Dioscorea bulbifera* L.var *sativa* (Tepono, 2001).

The isolated compounds were evaluated for their antifungal activities. 1 and 3 exhibited inhibitory activity against *Aspergilus niger* at the MICs of 50 µg/ml. No inhibition effects on *F. oxysporum*, *S. cerevisiae* and *C. albicans* were found for the tested compounds. 2 were inactive against all tested fungi. Interestingly, toxicity of 3 towards several cancer cell lines was demonstrated. The $IC_{50}$ of 3 against Hep-G2, Lu, and RD are 2.00, 4.72, and 4.02 µg/ml, respectively. Thus, 1 and 3 should be considered to be promising antifungal agents from *D. cambodiana*.

## References

Bich, D. H., Chung, D. Q., Chuong, B. X., Dong, N. T., Dam, D. T., Hien, P. V., Lo, V. N., Mai, P. D., Man, P. K., Nhu, D. T., Tap, N., Toan, T., 2006. "Medicinal Animals and Plants in Vietnam". Hanoi Science and Technology Publishing House, vol. 1.

Chi, V. V. (ed.), 1997. "Vietnam Medical Plant Dictionary". Hanoi Medicinal Publishing House.

Gonzalez, A. G., Leon, F., Hernandez, J. C., Padron, J. 1., Pinto, L. S., Barrera, J. B., 2004. Flavan of dragon's blood from *Dracaena draco* and *Dracaena tamaranae*. Biochem. Syst. Ecol. (32), pp. 179-184.

Loi, D. T. (ed.), 2006. "Glossary of Vietnam Medicinal Plants". Hanoi Science and Technology Publishing House.

Mimaki, Y., Koruda, M., Takaashi, Y., Sashida, Y., 1998. Steroidal saponins from the stem of *Dracaena concinna*. Phytochem (47), pp. 1351-1356.

Mimaki, Y., Watanabe, K., Sakagami, H., Sashida, Y., 2001. Steroidal glycosides from the leaves of *Cestrum nocturnum*. J. Nat. Prod. (64), pp. 1127-1132.

Tepono, R.B., Tapondjou, A. L., Djoukeng, J. D., Abou-Mansour, E., Tabacci, R., Tane, P., Lontsi, D., Park, H. J., 2006. Isoaltion and NMR assignment of a pennogenin glycoside from *Dioscorea bulbifera* L. var *sativa*. Nat. Prod. Sc1. (12), pp. 62-66.

Tran, Q. L., Tezuka, Y., Banskota, A. H., Tran, Q. K., Saiki, 1., Kadota, S., 2001. New spirostanol steroids and steroidal saponins from roots and rhizomes of *Dracaena angustifolia* and their antiproliferative activity. J. Nat. Prod. (64), pp. 1127-1132

Yokosuka, A., Mimaki, Y., Sashida, Y., 2002. Spirostanol saponin from the rhizomes of *Tacca chantrieri* and their cytotoxic activity. Phytochem (61), pp. 73-78.

## Chapter 27

# Cytotoxic Activity Assessment of Traditional Anticancer Plants Belong to Some Species of *Selaginella* of Vietnam

**Le Minh Ha* and Le Mai Huong**

*Institute of Natural Products Chemistry,*

*Vietnamese Academy of Science and Technology,*

*18-Hoang Quoc Viet, Hanoi, Vietnam*

**E-mail: halm2vn@gmail.com*

### ABSTRACT

In traditional and folk medicine, some of *Selaginellaceae* family have been used in a decoction for treating symptoms of hepatitis, tuberculosis of lung, malign tumour and diabetic. In this report, seven species of this family have been collected, extracted, and then tested in cytotoxic assay with some Human cancer cell lines. Among them, the ethyl acetate extracts of four species: *S. uncinata*, *S. involvens*, *S. frondosa* Warb and *S. tamariscina* exhibited the cytotoxic activity with three human cancer cell lines: Hep-G2 (Heptonema carcinoma), RD (Rhabdosarcoma) and LU (Lung carcinoma). Especially, the extract of *S. frondosa* showed the strongest inhibitory effect against all three tested cell lines with the $IC_{50}$ values of 2.98μg/ml; 7.40μg/ml; and 19.27μg/ml against Hep-G2; RD, and LU cell lines, respectively. The chemical bioguided fractionation of bioactive extracts is continuing.

***Keywords:*** *Selaginella species, Cytotoxic activity, Selaginella frondosa.*

## 1.0 Introduction

In Vietnam, the only one *Selaginella* branch with about 40 different species has been found belong to Selaginellaceae family. These species are widely distributed in high and wet mountainous areas of the North and South of Vietnam. In the traditional and folk medicine, some of them have been used in a decoction for treating the symptoms of hepatitis, tuberculosis of the lung, malign tumour and diabetic (Chi V. V., 1991). In China, the whole herbs of *Selaginella tamariscina* have been used as a precious drug to cure cancer (Jiangsu., 1998). The biochemical works showed that biflavonoids were major components in the *Selaginella* species (Lin R.C., 1994), which exhibited the cytotoxic, antioxidant, antimicrobial, antivirus activities (Ohmoto *et al.*, 1983).

In this report, seven medicinal plants of Selaginellaceae family: *S. uncinata*, *S. monospora* Spring, *S. picta* A.Br.ex Baker, *S. doderleinii* Hieron, *S. involvens* Spring, *S. frondosa* Warb and *S. tamariscina* (Beauv.) Spring were collected, identificated their name, chemical extracted and bioassay evaluated in cytotoxic activity against three cell lines: Hep-G2 (*heptonema carcinoma*), RD (*rhabdosarcoma*) and LU (*lung cancer*).

## 2.0 Materials and Methods

### 2.1 Plant Materials and Preparation

#### Plant Materials

The whole herb of seven species of *S. uncinata*, *S. monospora* Spring, *S. picta* A.Br.ex Baker, *S. doderleinii* Hieron, *S. involvens* Spring, *S. frondosa* Warb and S. *tamariscina* (Beauv.) Springs were collected from different mountainous provinces in the North of Vietnam as Tam Dao, Lai Chau, and Gia Lai from the South of Vietnam in the cool season from September to December, 2006.

The names of collected plants were identified by biologist Ngo Van Trai. The voucher specimens are deposited at the Herbarium of Institute of Natural Products Chemistry, Vietnamese Academy of Science and Technology.

#### Plant Chemical Extraction

The powdered dried whole herbs (200g) of each of seven species were soaked successively in ethanol three times at 50°C. The ethanol solutions was filtered and evaporated under reduced pressure to give ethanol extracts. The ethanol concentrated solution were diluted with $H_2O$ and extracted successively with *n*-hexane and ethyl acetate, after removal the solvent *in vacuum* to give *n*-hexane and ethyl acetate extracts. The ethanol, *n*-hexane and ethyl acetate extracts used for cytotoxic activity test.

### 2.2 Cytotoxic Assay

Methodology of the cytotoxic test is adopted from the National Cancer Institute (Swanson 1988; Skehan 1990; Likhitwitayawuid 1993), and it is utilized as a routine test in the Bioassay laboratory of the Department of Medicinal Chemistry and Pharmacognosy, College of Pharmacy, UIC, USA.

The method is based on staining with sulforhodamine B (SRB), and measures the cellular protein content of adherent and suspension cultures in 96-well microtiter plates. Cultures fixed with tricloroacetic acid (TCA) were stained for 30 minutes with 0.4 per cent SRB dissolved in 1 per cent acetic acid. Then unbounded dye was removed by washing with 1 per cent acetic acid and protein-bound dye was extracted with 10mM unbuffered Tris base (Trishydroxymethyl aminomethane) for the determination of optical density (OD-515nm) with a 96 well microtiter plate reader.

The absorption values generated by each treatment procedures are averaged, and the average value obtained with the zero day control was subtracted.

The per cent of cell survival is caculated as below:

$$\frac{\text{OD (cells + sample)–OD (0 day)}}{\text{OD (cells +10\% DMSO)–OD (0 day)}} = \text{CS\% (\% cell survival)}$$

These resulting values are then expressed as a percentage relative to the solvent–treated control incubation.

*The $IC_{50}$ value* is the concentration required to inhibit cell growth by 50 per cent.

$IC_{50}$ values were calculated using non-linear regression analysis of plots of per cent survival versus for at least 5-10 folds of concentrations of each tested extract, then by the Table Curve logarithm program.

Plant extracts demonstrating $ED_{50}$ values of less than 20μg/ml, are considered to be active.

**Cell lines**

In our experiments, three cell lines have been used: Hep-G2 (heptonema carcinoma), RD (rhabdosarcoma) from National Institute of Hygienic and Epidemology and LU (human lung carcinoma) from UIC, USA.

## 3.0 Results and Discussion

The seven medicinal plants of Selaginellaceae family were collected at different provinces in Vietnam. List of collected plants display in Table 27.1.

**Table 27.1: List of *Selaginella* Species Collected in Vietnam**

| *Sl.No.* | *Name of Plant* | *Place of Collection* | *Time of Collection* | *Traditional Use* |
|---|---|---|---|---|
| 1. | *S. uncinata* | Gia Lai | 9/2006 | Antitumour, hepatitis |
| 2. | *S. monospora* Spring | Tam Dao | 9/2006 | Antimicrobial, inflammation |
| 3. | *S. picta* A.Br.ex Baker | Tam Dao | 10/2006 | Antijaundice, hacking cough |
| 4. | *S. doderleinii* Hieron | Lai Chau | 10/2006 | Antitumour, hepatitis |
| 5. | *S. involvens* Spring | Lai Chau | 11/2006 | Anticancer, yellow eye, burning |
| 6. | *S. frondosa* Warb | Lai Chau | 11/2006 | Anticancer, hepatitis |
| 7. | *S. tamariscina* (Beauv.) Spring | Gia Lai | 12/2006 | Anticancer, tuberculosis of the lung, diabetic |

The cytotoxic assay was used to screen extracts of some Vietnamese traditional medicinal plants of Selaginellaceae family. The ethanol extract of the seven *Selaginella* species were fractionated with *n*-hexane, ethyl acetate and all extracts tested for cytotoxic activity with three cell lines: Hep-G2 RD, and LU. The results of bioassay screening on cytotoxic activity of seven *Selaginella* species showed the ethanol and *n*-hexane extracts of them did not exhibit cytotoxic activity (the results displayed in Table 27.2), the only ethyl acetate extracts of four species: *S. uncinata, S. involvens, S. frondosa* and *S. tamariscina* exhibited the active against three cell lines (the results displayed in Tables 27.2 and 27.3).

**Table 27.2: Data of the % Cell Survival of Tested Ethanol and Ethyl Acetate Extracts of *Selaginella* Species**

| *Name of Plant* | *%CS of Ethanol Extracts* | | | *%CS of Ethyl Acetate Extracts* | | |
|---|---|---|---|---|---|---|
| | *HepG-2* | *RD* | *LU* | *HepG-2* | *RD* | *LU* |
| DMSO | 100,0 ± 0,0 | 100,0 ± 0,0 | 100,0 ± 0,0 | 100,0 ± 0,0 | 100,0 ± 0,0 | 100,0 ± 0,0 |
| Control (+) | 2,1± 0,0 | 1,5 ± 0,0 | 2,5 ± 0,0 | 2,1± 0,0 | 1,5 ± 0,0 | 2,35 ± 0,1 |
| *S. uncinata* | 93,3 ± 0,5 | 92,3 ± 0,5 | 96,0 ± 1,0 | 43,3 ± 0,3 | 35,4 ± 0,2 | 47,0 ± 1,2 |
| *S. monospora* | 98,2 ± 1,0 | 87,2 ± 0,7 | 97,0 ± 0,0 | 95,2 ± 1,1 | 59,5 ± 1,5 | 74,2± 0,5 |
| *S. picta* | 98,5 ± 0,5 | 95,5 ± 1,0 | 96,3 ± 0,7 | 98,5 ± 0,5 | 95,5 ± 1,0 | 96,29 ± 0,7 |
| *S. doderleinii* | 94,0± 0,5 | 94,6 ± 0,9 | 100,0 ± 3,1 | 74,1± 0,3 | 69,6 ± 0,2 | 82,7 ± 0,4 |
| *S. involvens* | 95,2 ± 1,0 | 99,1 ± 0,9 | 102,0 ± 2,4 | 45,2 ± 0,3 | 39,1 ± 0,1 | 48,0 ± 2,7 |
| *S. frondosa* | 80,9 ± 3,1 | 84,3 ± 2,5 | 94,9 ± 1,9 | 8,1± 2,1 | 12,8 ± 1,5 | 34,7 ± 0,2 |
| *S. tamariscina* | 82,9 ± 0,2 | 64,5 ± 2,3 | 67,8 ± 0,7 | 36,3 ± 0,4 | 38,9±0,3 | 46,7±0,1 |

**Table 27.3: The Cytotoxic Activity and the $IC_{50}$ Values of *Selaginella* Species**

| *Sl.No.* | *Sample* | *Cell Lines $IC_{50}$ (μg/ml)* | | |
|---|---|---|---|---|
| | | *Hep-G2* | *RD* | *LU* |
| | Control (+) | 0,32 | 0,25 | 0,35 |
| 1. | *S. uncinata* | 16,24 | 14,35 | 17,15 |
| 2. | *S. involvens* | 17,75 | 15,08 | 18,28 |
| 3. | *S. frondosa* | 2,98 | 7,4 | 19,27 |
| 4. | *S. tamariscina* | 14,74 | 16,11 | 17,92 |

The result from Table 27.2 and 27.3 showed that the ethyl acetate extract of *Selaginella frondosa* exhibited interesting cytotoxic activity with the $IC_{50}$ values of 2.98μg/ml (against Hep-G2); 7.40μg/ml (against RD); and 19.27μg/ml (against LU).

This is the first report of cytotoxic activity of *Selaginella* species. The chemical bioguided fractionation of bioactive extracts has been continuing.

## Acknowledgements

This work was supported by the Program of Basic Study in Natural Science, Vietnamese Ministry of Science and Technology (2005-2008).

## References

Loi, D. T., 1991. Vietnamese Traditional Medicine Plants, Hanoi Scientific and Technology Publisher, Hanoi, pp. 263.

Jiangsu, 1998. A dictionary of Traditional Chinese Drugs. Shanghai People's Ed., Shanghai, pp. 120.

Lin C. R., *et al.*, 1994. Planta Med, 60, pp.168-170.

Ohmoto T., Yoshoda O., 1983. Chem. Pharm. Bull, 31, pp. 919.

## Chapter 28

# Chemical and Biological Studies of Seed of Vietnamese Citrus Plant

*Doan Lan Phuong*[1], *Pham Quoc Long*[1]* *and B. Matthaus*[2]

[1]*Institute of Natural Products, VAST-18 Hoang Quoc Viet, Hanoi, Vietnam*

[2]*Institute for Lipid Research, Piusallee 68/76; 48147 Muenster, Germany*

**E-mail: mar.biochem@fpt.vn*

## ABSTRACT

Composition and content of lipid, fatty acid, tocopherol, total sterol, phenol of ten species of Vietnamese Citrus plant were investigated: *Citrus nobilis var. microcarpa* Hassk; *Citrus nobinis var. chryoscarpa* Lamk; *Citrus japonica* Thunb; *Citrus grandis* (L.) *Osb.var.gradis; Citrus grandis* (L.) Osbeck; *Citrus grandis; Citrus nobilis* Lour. *var. nobinis; Citrus sinensis* (L.) Osb.; *Citrus aurantifolia* (Christm and Panz) Sw.; *Citrus limonia* Osb. The antioxidant activity of MeOH extraction was *in vitro* tested by DPPH method on the Elisa at 515nm and discussed also.

***Keywords:*** *DPPH: 1, 1-diphenyl-2-picrylhydrazyl, SC%: Scavenging capacity, Lipid, Fatty acid composition, Seed oild (seed oil).*

## 1.0 Introduction

The Rutaceae are widely distributed in tropical, subtropical and temperate areas, especially in South Africa and Australia (Takhtajan, 1997). Nearly 30 genera with 110 species are in Vietnam at home and of these; the Citrus genus alone includes over 20 species (Anh, 2005).

All Citrus plants contain essential oils in the peel of their fruits, in leaves and flowers. As known these essential oils find large use in food processing, in perfumery and cosmetics. That is why they were thoroughly investigated, their main constituents being monoterpenic compounds (85-95 per cent) and not few are oxygenated (2–10 per cent) (Chavalit, 1991).

That and the fact alone let, Citrus fruits because of their scent, their taste and their vitamin are considered since old time as highly nourishing, other aerial plant parts are yet source of a lot of interesting bio-active compounds. Thus coumarine have been found in the bark (Davies and Goldberg, 1987) and insect deterrents in the husk of the seeds (Matthau, 1997). Lipids, tocopherols, sterols, phenolics have been isolated from the oils of the seeds (Badami and Patil, 1991).

However until now very little attention has been paid in Vietnam to the seed oils of the Citrus. The matter locks us. We will report in the present article of first and preliminary results, which we have lastly hid, by the seed oils of ten selected among the most common Vietnamese Citrus species.

## 2.0 Materials and Procedures

### 2.1 Plant Material

The ten selected species are indeed: *Citrus nobilis var. microcarpa* Hassk (M1), *Citrus nobinis var. chryoscarpa* Lamk (M2), *Citrus japonica* Thunb (M3), *Citrus grandis* (L.) *Osb var. gradis* (M4), *Citrus grandis* (L.) Osbeck (M5), *Citrus grandis* (M6), *Citrus nobinis* Lour, *var. nobinis* (M7), *Citrus sinensis* (L.) osb (M8), *Citrus aurantifolia* (Christm and Pang) Sw. (M9), *Citrus limonia* Osb (M10).

Sampling took place at sites in the North, the mid and the South of Vietnam during the 2005–2006 harvest. Seeds were colleted solely from ripe standard fruits. They were the well fan-dried and carefully preserved at room temperature and in contact with moisture.

### 2.2 Experimental Procedures

All experiments were performed in laboratories of the lipid Research Institute in Muenster, Germany (BAGKF, BRD). It was aimed to obtain.

#### The Total Lipid Content

By an extraction of the oil into n-hexane and following gravimetric determination, as prescribed as standard method in ISO/DIS. 659:1998 Germany.

#### The Fatty Acid Composition

By a methylation of the acids and following qualitative and quantitative analysis be capillary GC of the so obtained methyl esters, as prescribed as standard method in ISO/DIS 5590:1998 Germany.

#### The Total Composition

Be dilution of a oil drip in n-hexane and following qualitative and quantitative analysis by capillary GC of the so obtained methyl ethers, as prescribed as standard method in ISO 12228:1999.

**The Total Phenolic Content**

By a complevation of the phenolics with the help of the Tolin-liocaltean reagent and following spectrophotometric absorbency measurement, as prescribed by the method of Taga M.S (Pham, 2000).

**The Scavenging Capacity In Vitro**

Jrusthy the antioxidant capacity, by spectrophotometric absorbency measurement of a total methanolic extract of the oil at various concentrations and in a DPPH (1,1–cliphenyl–2–Picrylthydrazyl) system, method of Shela Goldstein (Shela *et al.*, 2003).

## 3.0 Results and Discussion

### 3.1 The Total Lipid Content

The results are listed in Table 28.1.

**Table 28.1: Lipid Contents of the Citrus Seeds**

| *Sl.No.* | *Common Name* | *Scientific Name* | *Symbol* | *Sampling Date and Site* | *Lipid Content (%)* | |
|---|---|---|---|---|---|---|
| | | | | | *With Shell* | *Without Shell* |
| 1 | Saigon mandarine | *Citrus nobilis var. microcarpa* Hassk | M1 | 10-12/2005, Sai Gon | 37.82 | 51.27 |
| 2 | Hanoi mandarine | *Citrus nobinis var. chryoscarpa* Lamk | M2 | 2-3/20006, Ha Noi | 33.43 | 45.11 |
| 3 | Hungyen Kumquat | *Citrus japonica* Thunb. | M3 | 1-3/2006, Ha Noi | 40.20 | 56.03 |
| 4 | Hanoi Shaddock | *Citrus grandis* (L.) *Osb.var.gradis* | M4 | 8-10/2005, Ha Noi | 41.68 | 58.96 |
| 5 | Saigon green ochinopeel | *Citrus grandis* (L.) Osbeck | M5 | 1-3/2006, Sai Gon | 46.91 | 49.15 |
| 6 | Dien shaddock | *Citrus grandis* | M6 | 10-12/2005, Ha Noi | 27.93 | 33.24 |
| 7 | Saigon orange | *Citrus nobilis* Lour. *var. nobinis* | M7 | 1-3/2006, Sai Gon | 41.74 | 54.49 |
| 8 | Vinh orange | *Citrus sinensis* (L.) *Osb.* | M8 | 3-5/2006, Vinh | 44.91 | 51.96 |
| 9 | Saigon lemon | *Citrus aurantifolia* (Christm and Panz) Sw. | M9 | 1-3/2006, Sai Gon | 30.4 | 38.01 |
| 10 | Vinh lemon | *Citrus limonia* Osb. | M10 | 5-7/2006, Vinh | 32.82 | 42.01 |

They show that the total lipid content, which reflects the economic value of the seed, with an average by 45 per cent is high enough. The lowest and value if found by

M6 (33, 24 per cent) of Dien shaddock (without shell) and the highest by M4 (58, 96 per cent) of Hanoi Shaddock (without shell).

## 3.2 The Fatty Acid Composition

The results are listed in Table 28.2. They show that the common acids exist in very sample. Thus with the saturated: palmitic C16:0 (20, 07-29, 91 per cent), stearic C18:0 (2, 31–5, 46 per cent) and with the unsaturated: oleic C18:1n-9 (17, 10–26, 26 per cent) linoleic C18:2n-6 (33.90–45, 22 per cent) values are relatively uniform and the linoleic content high enough. The unsaturated (70 per cent) make more than the double of the saturated (30 per cent). The polyunsaturated linolenic C18:3Δ9,12,15 in present in every sample and its average exceeds forums emerge in every sample. Usually these two forums are solely by the malvaceae, sapindaceae, Bombacaceae, Taliaceae, Thymalaceae, Anacardiaceae to b found (Taga *et al.*, 1984). Might this then be achaxacderistic peculiar to the Citrus genus inside the Rutaceae.

**Table 28.2: Fatty Acids Composition of the Citrus Seed Oils**

| *Fatty Acids* | *M1* | | *M2* | | *M3* | | *M4* | | *M5* | |
|---|---|---|---|---|---|---|---|---|---|---|
| | *a* | *b* | *a* | *b* | *a* | *b* | *a* | *b* | *a* | *b* |
| 14:0 | 0.06 | 0 | 0.06 | 0.07 | 0.04 | 0.05 | 0.11 | 0.08 | 0.10 | 0.10 |
| 14:1 | 0.02 | 0 | 0.04 | 0 | 0.02 | 0 | 0.02 | 0.02 | 0.02 | 0.02 |
| 16:0 | 22.56 | 20.96 | 21.04 | 23.71 | 20.07 | 20.75 | 27.69 | 26.90 | 29.03 | 29.03 |
| 16:1 n-9 | 0.02 | 0 | 0.02 | 0 | 0 | 0 | 0.30 | 0.02 | 0.03 | 0.03 |
| 16:1 n-7 | 0.67 | 0.63 | 0.70 | 0.63 | 3.25 | 3.06 | 0.40 | 0.37 | 0.37 | 0.37 |
| 17: 0 | 0.11 | 0.14 | 0.13 | 0.11 | 0.09 | 0.10 | 0.10 | 0.10 | 0.10 | 0.10 |
| 7.8-cpa-17:0 | 0.10 | 0 | 0.12 | 0 | 0.05 | 0 | 0.07 | 0 | 0.08 | 0.08 |
| 18:0 | 4.79 | 5.46 | 5.12 | 4.68 | 4.46 | 4.56 | 3.62 | 3.66 | 3.62 | 3.62 |
| 18:1 n-9 | 22.11 | 19.59 | 19.19 | 21.10 | 18.90 | 18.32 | 26.26 | 25.76 | 21.41 | 21.41 |
| 18:1 n-7 | 1.67 | 2.35 | 2.20 | 1.75 | 9.34 | 9.46 | 0.0 | 1.24 | 1.20 | 1.20 |
| 9,10-cpe-19:1 | 0.07 | 0 | 0.10 | 0 | 0.05 | 0 | 0.06 | 0.06 | 0.07 | 0.07 |
| 18:2n-6 | 42.50 | 45.22 | 44.95 | 43.15 | 33.90 | 34.80 | 36.72 | 36.85 | 38.18 | 38.18 |
| 20: 0 | 0.44 | 0.56 | 0.50 | 0.43 | 0.50 | 0.53 | 0.32 | 0.32 | 0.34 | 0.34 |
| 20:1n-9 | 0 | 0 | 0 | 0 | 0.03 | 0 | 0.02 | 0 | 0.02 | 0.02 |
| 18: 3 D9,12,15 | 4.37 | 5.10 | 5.33 | 4.36 | 8.60 | 8.26 | 4.21 | 4.59 | 4.88 | 4.88 |
| C20:1n-7 | 0 | 0 | 0 | 0 | 0.03 | 0 | 0 | 0 | 0 | 0 |
| C22: 0 | 0.12 | 0 | 0,14 | 0 | 0.15 | 0 | 0.06 | 0 | 0.06 | 0.06 |
| 24: 0 | 0.25 | 0 | 0.25 | 0 | 0.20 | 0 | 0.21 | 0 | 0.22 | 0.22 |
| **Total UFA** | **71.53** | **72.88** | **72.65** | **70.99** | **74.17** | **73.90** | **67.79** | **68.85** | **66.27** | **71.96** |
| **Total SFA** | **28.33** | **27.12** | **27.24** | **28.86** | **25.52** | **25.99** | **32.11** | **31.08** | **33.47** | **28.03** |
| **Sum** | **99.86** | **100** | **99.89** | **99.85** | **99.69** | **99.89** | **99.90** | **99.93** | **99.74** | **99.99** |

*Contd...*

**Table 28.2–Contd...**

| *Fatty Acids* | *M6* | | *M7* | | *M8* | | *M9* | | *M10* | |
|---|---|---|---|---|---|---|---|---|---|---|
| | *a* | *b* | *a* | *b* | *a* | *b* | *a* | *b* | *a* | *b* |
| 14:0 | 0.11 | 0.10 | 0.08 | 0.08 | 0.10 | 0.12 | 0.08 | 0.08 | 0.1 | 0.12 |
| 14:1 | 0.02 | 0 | 0.03 | 0 | 0.02 | 0 | 0.03 | 0 | 0.03 | 0 |
| 16:0 | 29.91 | 29.31 | 27.19 | 27.14 | 26.31 | 26.27 | 22.45 | 22.51 | 23.01 | 23.36 |
| 16:1 n-9 | 0.04 | 0 | 0.01 | 0 | 0.02 | 0 | 0.02 | 0 | 0 | 0 |
| 16:1 n-7 | 0.45 | 0.35 | 0.54 | 0.40 | 0.83 | 0.57 | 0.82 | 0.80 | 0.81 | 0.71 |
| 17: 0 | 0.10 | 0.10 | 0.12 | 0.13 | 0.11 | 0.11 | 0.10 | 0.10 | 0.10 | 0.11 |
| 7.8-cpa-17:0 | 0.08 | 0 | 0.11 | 0 | 0.11 | 0.11 | 0.31 | 0.30 | 0.24 | 0.25 |
| 18:0 | 2.31 | 3.57 | 4.81 | 4.90 | 4.82 | 4.80 | 3.74 | 3.92 | 4.08 | 4.13 |
| 18:1 n-9 | 22.33 | 20.75 | 19.72 | 19.72 | 21.61 | 22.09 | 17.62 | 17.10 | 19.51 | 19.64 |
| 18:1 n-7 | 1.31 | 1.40 | 1.17 | 1.23 | 1.05 | 1.31 | 1.46 | 1.70 | 1.60 | 1.57 |
| 9,10-cpe-19:1 | 0.05 | 0 | 0.06 | 0 | 0.07 | 0 | 0.11 | 0 | 0.14 | 0.14 |
| 18:2n-6 | 37.58 | 39.75 | 41.55 | 42.00 | 39.77 | 40.16 | 43.60 | 44.53 | 43.41 | 43.86 |
| 20: 0 | 0.27 | 0.34 | 0.45 | 0.44 | 0.40 | 0.39 | 0.41 | 0.42 | 0.39 | 0.39 |
| 20:1n-9 | 0.02 | 0 | 0.02 | 0.02 | 0.02 | 0 | 0.03 | 0 | 0.03 | 0 |
| 18: 3 D9,12,15 | 5.07 | 4.34 | 3.70 | 3.96 | 4.43 | 4.02 | 8.61 | 8.41 | 6.05 | 5.57 |
| C20:1n-7 | 0 | 0 | 0 | 0 | 0 | 0 | 0 | 0 | 0 | 0 |
| C22: 0 | 0.06 | 0 | 0.12 | 0 | 0,08 | 0 | 0.10 | 0 | 0.09 | 0 |
| 24: 0 | 0.23 | 0 | 0.25 | 0 | 0.25 | 0 | 0.20 | 0 | 0.19 | 0 |
| **Total UFA** | **66.95** | **66.59** | **67.91** | **67.31** | **67.63** | **66.95** | **72.62** | **66.95** | **71.82** | **71.7** |
| **Total SFA** | **32.99** | **33.41** | **32.02** | **32.69** | **32.06** | **31.70** | **27.09** | **27.04** | **27.96** | **28.10** |
| **Sum** | **99.94** | **100** | **99.93** | **100** | **99.69** | **98.65** | **99.71** | **99.88** | **99.78** | **99.8** |

a: With shell; b: Without shell.

## 3.3 The Tocopherol Composition

The results are listed in Table 28.3.

Tocopherols $\alpha$-T, $\beta$-T, $\delta$-T, P-8 (Plasmochromanol-8) and tocotrienols $\alpha$-T3, $\beta$-T3, $\gamma$-T3, $\delta$-T3 belongs to the class of the tocols. As natural anti-oxidizing agents they are usually to be found in every seed oil. Table 28.3 shows that in fact $\alpha$-T, $\gamma$-T, $\gamma$-T3 are present in every sample even though the contents are low the $\alpha$-T contents in M2 (Hanoi mandarine) M6 (Dien shaddock) M5 (Saigon shaddock), M7 (Saigon Orange), M9 (Saigon Lemon) vary from 11,56 to 18,72mg/100g. Besides that, it is to notify that: $\alpha$-T3 is present is every sample except in M6 (Dien-Shaddock); $\delta$-T appears only in M1 (Saigon mandarine) and M8 (Vinh orange); $\delta$-T3 is maisfert only in M1 (Saigon mandarine); P-8 emerges only in M9 (Saigon lemon) and M10 (Vinh lemon).

**Table 28.3: Tocopherol Composition of the Citrus Seed Oils without (with) Shell**

| Sample/10ml | | α-T | α-T3 | β-T | γ-T | p8 | γ-T3 | δ-T | δ-T3 | Sume |
|---|---|---|---|---|---|---|---|---|---|---|
| M1 0.908g | Area | 0.000 (1461) | 1834 (36) | 0.000 (28) | 0.000 (133) | 195 (0.00) | 0.000 (122) | 0.000 (2108) | 0.000 (26) | 2029 (3914) |
| | Content | 0.000 (11.66) | 13.96 (0.287) | 0.000 (0.153) | 0.000 (0.660) | 0.923 (0.00) | 0.000 (0.606) | 0.000 (9.416) | 0.000 (0.116) | 14.88 (22.90) |
| | Per cent | 0.000 (50.92) | 93.80 (1.25) | 0.000 (0.67) | 0.000 (2.88) | 6.20 (0.00) | 0.000 (2.65) | 0.000 (41.12) | 0.000 (0.51) | 100 (100) |
| M2 0.905g | Area | 3217 (1714) | 44 (93) | 0.000 (17) | 0.000 (52) | 195 (0.00) | 0.000 (84) | 390.000 | 0.000 (0.00) | 3300 (1960) |
| | Content | 24.569 (13.105) | 0.33 (0.711) | 0.000 (0.089) | 0.000 (0.247) | 0.920 (0.00) | 0.000 (0.400) | 0.1670.0 | 0.000 (0.00) | 25.07 (14.55) |
| | Per cent | 97.99 (90.06) | 1.34 (4.89) | 0.000 (0.61) | 0.000 (1.70) | 6.20 (0.00) | 0.000 (2.75) | 0.660.000 | 0.00 (0.00) | 100 (100) |
| M3 0.824g | Area | 1067 (779) | 16 (36) | 0.000 (14) | 352 (446) | 0.000 (0.000) | 0.000 (94) | 35 (0.00) | 0 (0.00) | 1470 (1369) |
| | Content | 8.950 (5.949) | 0.134 (0.275) | 0.000 (0.073) | 1.837 (2.119) | 0.000 (0.00) | 0.000 (0.447) | 0.164 (0.0) | 0.000 (0.00) | 11.09 (8.86) |
| | Per cent | 80.74 (67.12) | 1.21 (3.10) | 0.000 (0.82) | 16.57 (23.91) | 0.000 (0.00) | 0.000 (5.04) | 1.48 (0.00) | 0.00 (0.00) | 100 (100) |
| M4 0.929g | Area | 1934 (2035) | 27 (52) | 0.000 (11) | 108 (496) | 0.000 (42) | 0.000 (126) | 79 (0.0) | 0.000 (0.00) | 2148 (2762) |
| | Content | 14.389 (14.575) | 0.201 (0.372) | 0.000 (0.054) | 0.500 (2.210) | 0.000 (0.187) | 0.000 (0.561) | 0.329 (0.0) | 0.000 (0.00) | 15.42 (17.96) |
| | Per cent | 93.32 (81.15) | 1.30 (2.07) | 0.00 (0.30) | 3.24 (12.31) | 0.00 (1.04) | 0.00 (3.13) | 2.13 (0.00) | 0.00 (0.00) | 100 (100) |

Contd...

**Table 28.3–Contd...**

| Sample/10ml | | α-T | α-T3 | β-T | γ-T | p8 | γ-T3 | δ-T | δ-T3 | Sume |
|---|---|---|---|---|---|---|---|---|---|---|
| M5 0.932g | Area | 3207 (1114) | 32 (59) | 0.000 (0.000) | 279 (146) | 0.000 (0.00) | 0.000 (93) | 72 (0.00) | 0.000 (0.00) | 3590 (1412) |
| | Content | 23.783 (11.561) | 2.37 (0.612) | 0.000 (0.000) | 1.287 (0.943) | 0.000 (0.00) | 0.000 (0.600) | 0.299 (0.00) | 0.000 (0.00) | 25.61 (13.72) |
| | Per cent | 92.88 (84.29) | 0.93 (4.46) | 0.00 (0.000) | 5.03 (6.87) | 0.00 (0.00) | 0.00 (4.38) | 1.17 (0.0) | 0.00 (0.00) | 100 (100) |
| M6 0.784g | Area | 1113 (1113) | 0.000 (0.000) | 0.000 (0.000) | 150 (150) | 0.000 (0.000) | 79 (79) | 0.000 (0.00) | 0.00 (0.00) | 1342 (1342) |
| | Content | 9.812 (9.812) | 0.000 (0) | 0.000 (0.000) | 0.823 (0.823) | 0.000 (0.00) | 0.433 (0.433) | 0.000 (0.00) | 0.000 (0.00) | 11.07 (11.07) |
| | Per cent | 88.65 (88.65) | 0.00 (0.00) | 0.00 (0.000) | 7.43 (7.43) | 0.00 (0.00) | 3.91 (3.91) | 0.00 (0.00) | 0.00 (0.00) | 100 (100) |
| M7 0.975g | Area | 3787 (1083) | 47 (26) | 0.000 (27) | 124 (535) | 0.000 (0.00) | 0. 000 (60) | 85 (0.0) | 0.00 (0.00) | 4043 (1731) |
| | Content | 26.845 (8.997) | 0.333 (0.216) | 0.0000 (0.153) | 0.547 (2.765) | 0.000 (0.00) | 0.000 (0.310) | 0.337 (0.0) | 0.000 (0.00) | 28.06 (12.44) |
| | Per cent | 95.66 (72.31) | 1.19 (1.74) | 0.000 (1.23) | 1.95 (22.23) | 0.000 (0.00) | 0.00 (2.49) | 1.20 (0.00) | 0.00 (0.00) | 100 (100) |
| M8 0.957g | Area | 1418 (1083) | 21 (26) | 29 (27) | 759 (535) | 0.000 (0.00) | 0.000 (60) | 69 (0.00) | 0.000 (0.00) | 2296 (1731) |
| | Content | 10.241 (8.997) | 0.152 (0.216) | 0.143 (0.153) | 3.410 (2.765) | 0.000 (0.00) | 0.000 (0.310) | 0.279 (0.0) | 0.000 (0.00) | 14.23 (12.44) |
| | Per cent | 71.99 (72.31) | 1.07 (1.74) | 1.01 (1.23) | 23.97 (22.23) | 0.00 (0.00) | 0.00 (2.49) | 1.96 (0.0) | 0.00 (0.00) | 100 (100) |

Contd...

**Table 28.3–Contd...**

| Sample/10ml | | α-T | α-T3 | β-T | γ-T | p8 | γ-T3 | δ-T | δ-T3 | Sume |
|---|---|---|---|---|---|---|---|---|---|---|
| M9 0.959g | Area | 2855 (1581) | 82 (50) | 0.000 (17) | 529 (479) | 0.000 (84) | 0.000 (211) | 349 (0.0) | 0.000 (0.00) | 3815 (2422) |
| | Content | 20.576 (17.263) | 0.591 (0.546) | 0.000 (0.127) | 2.372 (3.254) | 0.000 (0.571) | 0.000 (1.433) | 1.408 (0.0) | 0.000 (0.00) | 24.95 (23.19) |
| | Per cent | 82.48 (74.43) | 2.37 (2.35) | 0.00 (0.55) | 9.51 (14.03) | 0.00 (2.46) | 0.00 (6.18) | 5.64 (0.0) | 0.00 (0.00) | 100 (100) |
| M10 0.942g | Area | 2002 (570) | 39 (17) | 0.000 (0.000) | 24 (31) | 0.000 (1.02) | 0.000 (69) | 124 (0.00) | 0.000 (0.00) | 2189 (789) |
| | Content | 14.689 (5.588) | 0.286 (0.167) | 0.000 (0.000) | 0.110 (0.189) | 0.000 (0.622) | 0.000 (0.421) | 0.509 (0.00) | 0.000 (0.00) | 15.59 (6.99) |
| | Per cent | 94.20 (79. 98) | 1.84 (2.39) | 0.000 (0.000) | 0.70 (2.71) | 0.000 (8.90) | 0.000 (6.02) | 3.27 (0.00) | 0.00 (0.00) | 100 (100) |

Generally said, the tocopherol and tocotriend contents in Citrus seed oil are low (11,07–28,06mg/100g). The total tocopherol contents set apart; differences rise here into view between samples with husk and sample without shell.

### 3.4 The Sterol Composition

The results are listed in Table 28.4.

**Table 28.4: Sterol Composition of the Citrus Seed Oil**

| *Content* | *Content% (Compared to the Total Sterol)* | | | | | | | | | |
|---|---|---|---|---|---|---|---|---|---|---|
| | *M1* | *M2* | *M3* | *M4* | *M5* | *M6* | *M7* | *M8* | *M9* | *M10* |
| Cholesterol | 1,03 | 0,99 | 4,82 | 1,28 | 1,19 | 1,90 | 7,34 | 1,73 | 1,88 | 2,87 |
| Brassicasterol | 0,1 | 0,0 | 0,70 | 0,0 | 0,0 | 0,0 | 0,0 | 0,26 | 0,0 | 0,0 |
| 24-methylene Cholesterol | 0,0 | 0,0 | 0,84 | 0,0 | 0,0 | 0,19 | 0,0 | 0,12 | 0,0 | 0,0 |
| Campesterol | 10,07 | 9,33 | 6,71 | 6,99 | 9,18 | 8,79 | 40,45 | 8,00 | 14,64 | 10,22 |
| Stigmasterol | 3,89 | 5,51 | 26,32 | 2,81 | 2,99 | 3,44 | 0,0 | 3,22 | 0,0 | 5,83 |
| Clerosterol | 1,29 | 1,02 | 5,45 | 1,38 | 1,24 | 1,36 | 3,53 | 1,30 | 0,77 | 0,0 |
| $\beta$ Sitosterol | 79,86 | 81,52 | 35,44 | 83,97 | 82,35 | 81,0 | 35,00 | 79,20 | 80,38 | 81,08 |
| Sitostanol | 0,51 | 0,0 | 0,00 | 0,00 | 0,0 | 0,0 | 0,0 | 0,65 | 0,0 | 0,0 |
| Δ5–Avenasterin | 1,83 | 1,17 | 12,40 | 3,05 | 1,17 | 1,76 | 10,58 | 3,69 | 2,33 | 0,0 |
| Δ5,24–Stigmastadienol | 0,89 | 0,0 | 4,97 | 0,0 | 1,06 | 0,94 | 3,09 | 0,95 | 0,0 | 0,0 |
| Δ7-Stigmastenol | 0,32 | 0,45 | 2,36 | 0,52 | 0,81 | 0,62 | 0,0 | 0,64 | 0,0 | 0,0 |
| Δ7-Avenasterol | 0,21 | 0,0 | 0,0 | 0,0 | 0,0 | 0,0 | 0,0 | 0,23 | 0,0 | 0,0 |
| **Total** | **100** | **99.99** | **100** | **100** | **99.99** | **100** | **99.99** | **99.99** | **100** | **100** |

Nearly every common sterol cholesterol, compestereol, stigonasterol, $\beta$–sitosterol is present as mixture in every oil. Yet with an average of 80 per cent sterol contents in the oils are all but uniform. Solely in M3 (Hungyen kumquat 35, 44 per cent) and in M7 (Saigon orange 35,00 per cent) emerge scarcely deviations. Quite high (10 per cent) is but there in these two oils the Δ5-avenasterol content while this is all the time lower than 5 per cent. Likewise is the compesterol content surprisingly high in M7 (40, 45 per cent Saigon orange) while this is all the time lower than 10 per cent.

### 3.5 The Total Phenolics Content

The results are listed in Table 28.5.

Beside the tocopherols phenolics too are considered as natural antioxidant agents. It is known that the total phenolic content often varies with the plant material and with the extracting solvent. It is found, it will reach its highest value when the material is extracted into MeOH and $H_2O$ (Shela *et al.*, 2003). The result shows that phenolics exits with a high content (>1000µg/g) in every sample, except in M9 (Saigon lemon, 79,53µg/g without husk and 517,55µg/g with husk). The highest total phenolic content is found by M3 (Hungyen kumquat, 2448.27 µg/g).

**Table 28.5: Phenolic Content of the Citrus Seeds**

| *Sl.No.* | *Sample* | *Total MeOH Extract µg/g (Without shell)* | *Total Phenolic µg/g (Without Shell)* | *Total MeOH Extract µg/g (With Shell)* | *Total Phenolic µg/g (With Shell)* |
|---|---|---|---|---|---|
| 1. | M1 | 948.8 | 318.71 | 839.6 | 1782.61 |
| 2. | M2 | 1226.1 | 1851.77 | 1192.8 | 1860.41 |
| 3. | M3 | 1315.8 | 2448.27 | 1049 | 1491.56 |
| 4. | M4 | 684.5 | 1217.80 | 532.1 | 872.00 |
| 5. | M5 | 614.0 | 2016.02 | 527.3 | 1939.75 |
| 6. | M6 | 557.6 | 1338.83 | 506.0 | 1557.84 |
| 7. | M7 | 810.4 | 1491.56 | 589.0 | 1719.21 |
| 8. | M8 | 881.2 | 1376.29 | 461.4 | 972.85 |
| 9. | M9 | 625.2 | 79.53 | 334.5 | 517.55 |
| 10. | M10 | 564.5 | 500.26 | 564.7 | 1592.42 |

## 3.6 Scavenging Capacity *in Vitro*

The results are listed in Table 28.6.

**Table 28.6: In *Vitro* Scavenging Capacity of the Citrus Seed Oils in DPPH System**

| *Minimale Inhibiting Concen-tration (mg/l)* | *SC (per cent) Value* | | | | | | | | | |
|---|---|---|---|---|---|---|---|---|---|---|
| | *Sample M1* | *Sample M2* | *Sample M3* | *Sample M4* | *Sample M5* | *Sample M6* | *Sample M7* | *Sample M8* | *Sample M9* | *Sample M10* |
| 100 | 58.89 | 56.91 | 87.03 | 45.78 | 60.81 | 46.21 | 44.58 | 33.66 | 24.59 | 43.02 |
| 75 | 49.68 | 46.85 | 74.42 | 40.04 | 55.78 | 39.48 | 35.93 | 26.51 | 22.47 | 36.00 |
| 50 | 34.94 | 34.02 | 61.87 | 34.66 | 45.50 | 33.38 | 28.92 | 20.69 | 22.82 | 22.96 |
| 25 | 28.07 | 17.65 | 53.01 | 27.92 | 33.03 | 20.69 | 21.40 | 13.89 | 21.55 | 20.84 |
| 10 | 22.89 | 6.09 | 48.76 | 24.95 | 24.03 | 18.14 | 18.43 | 14.32 | 20.55 | 16.23 |
| **Result** | + | + | + | + | + | + | + | + | – | + |

The capacity expressed in per cent (SC per cent) is evaluated as said by spectrophotometric absorbency measurements. Once obtained these measured values are computer-treated with the help of a special. Excel window to give the mean value. When SC per cent> 30 per cent IS considered as criterion of positively then the result is positive for every sample except M9 (Saigon lemon). The SC per cent value of M9 is lower than 30 per cent. Another exception but in the opposite direction, we could say, is M3 (Hung yen kimquat). The SC per cent value of M3 is in fact the highest observed.

## 4.0 Conclusion

Of the ten selected Vietnamese Citrus oils the total lipid content and total phenolic content have been determined. The fatty acid composition, tocopherol composition a sterol composition have been analyzed quality and qualitative. Their scavenging have been *in vitro* has been evaluated.

Noteworthy is it that in every oil the UFA(Unsaturated fatty acid) makes more than the double of the SFA (Saturated fatty acid), that the highly bioactive HUFA(Hight Unsaturated fatty acid) linoleic is all the time present with a content exceeding 4 per cent and, surprisingly that even acid of the two Cpa. and Cpe. forms everywhere emerge.

Noteworthy is yet, that irregularities are put up in some species, regarding the presence or absence or the fluctuations in content of ascertained bioactive compounds, chiefly of the tocols and the phenolics, which from near or from far are in touch with the scavenging capacity of the oils. All that deserves further investigation for a better understand.

## Acknowledgements

The experimental work has been performed at the Muenster Lipid Research Institute BAGKF, taking advantage of a three-month study stay in the cooperation frame between the Muenster LRI and the INPC in Hanoi. The Authors thank the Colleagues at Muenster LRI for their helpful advices. The Authors thank the taxonomists of the Centre for plant Ecology and Resources in Hanoi too, for the botanical identification of the collected seed oil of plant material.

## References

Anh, B. K., 2005. Study on chemistry and insect anti-feedant activity of seed oils in Citrus, and leaf in tetradium trichotomum lour–family Rutaceae.

Badami, R.C. and K. B. Paltil, 1991. Structure and occurrence of unusual fatty acids in minor seed oils. Prog. Lipid Res (19), pp 119-153.

Chavalit N., 1991. Citrus maxima (Burm) Merr. Plants resources of South–East asia–2, Edible funt and nuts, Pudoc wageningen, pp 128.

Davies, K. J. A., and Goldberg, A. L., 1987. 1,1-Diphenyl-2-pyerylhydrazyl radical (DPPH) scavenging. J. Biol. Chem, (17), pp 262-271.

Matthau, B., 1997. Antimutritive Compounds in Different Oilseeds. Fett/Lipid, pp170–174.

Pham Hoang Ho, 2000. Viet Nam vegetation, Vol. II, pp. 430-434.

Shela, G., Olga, M. B., Elena, K., Antonin, L., Milan, C., Nuria, G. M.,. Ratiporn, H., Yong–Seo, P., Soon–Teck, J., Simon, T., 2003. Comparison of the contents of the main biochemical compounds and the antioxidant activity of some spanish olive oils as determined by four different radical scavenging test, J. Biol. Chem (14), pp 154–159.

Taga, M. S., Miller, E. E.; Pratt, D. E., 1984. China seeds as a source of natural lipid antioxidants. J. Am. Oil Chem. Soc. (61), pp 928–931.

Takhtajan, A., 1997. Diversity and classification of flowering plants. Columbia University press, New York, pp 307-308.

# Chapter 29

# Study on Antipolyarthritic Activity of *Rhizoma cibotii*

***Dien Vu Van*, Tram Nguyen Thi and Duong Nguyen Thuy***

*Hanoi University of Pharmacy, Vietnam*

**E-mail: vandien1951@vnn.vn*

## ABSTRACT

Antipolyarthritic activity of *Rhizoma cibotii* was tested on S. pyogenes induced polyarthritis model. Result was showed that liquid extract 2:1 of *Rhizoma cibotii* inhibited polyarthritis in 3[th] stage (after inflammatory from 16 to 21 days) with $p<0.05$ at dose 20g dry material/kg body weight in comparison with inflamed control group. These results contributed explaining use this pharmacognosy to treat rheumatic disease being having scientific base and guiding rational, efficiently, safely use in therapy.

*Keywords: Rhizoma cibotii, Antipolyarthritis.*

## 1. Introduction

*Rhizoma cibotii* was a pharmacognosy having very many in Vietnam, utilized to treat kidney disease, chronic rheumatitis in traditional medicine since ancient (Loi D,T,1999) but was researched very little. Therefore, we researched antipolyarthritic activity on Steptococcus pyogenes induced polyarthritic model to contribute gradually demonstrating its pharmacoglogy action, basing on that guiding user safely, rationally and efficiently use.

## 2. Materials and Methods

### 2.1 Materials

*Rhizoma cibotii* were purchased from shop of pharmacognosy at Lan ong street, Hoan kiem Hanoi Vietnam and then processed by traditional method to reach standards of 3rd Vietnam pharmacopoeia and decocted with water and concentrated into liquid extract 2:1 for next experimental study

Referential drug: Prednisolon

Agent to cause polyarthritis: Steptococcus pyogenes A hemolysin $\beta$ was supplied by microbiological department of Hanoi university of medicine

Animal: White rat both sex, weight as 120-150g each was supplied by medicinal institute of army

## 2.2 Method

White rat was randomly divided into 3 groups, 10 rat each, arranged following test study

| *Sl.No.* | *Groups* | *Test products orally administered* |
|---|---|---|
| 1. | Control | NaCl 0,9 per cent–1ml/100g |
| 2. | reference | Prednisolon 2mg/kg–1ml/100g |
| 3. | Extract 2:1 | Extract 2:1 equivalence 20g/kg–1ml/100g |

The first day, after orally administered test product, rats were Steptococcus pyogenes induced chronic polyarthritis by injecting 0.15ml solution consisting of 7.5mg Steptococcus pyogenes diluted in 1ml 0.9 per cent saline solution to rat left hind paw pad.

The rats were measured weight and orally administered test product at stable hour daily, rat paw volume was measured in periods from 1st day to 10th day ($V_{1-10}$), 11st day to 15th day ($V_{11-15}$), 16th day to 21st day ($V_{16-21}$)

Antipolyarthritic action of pharmacognosy was estimated basing on edema percentage and edema inhibitory percentage of test groups in comparison with control group

Edema percentage was calculated by following formula:

$$E = \frac{Vt - Vo}{Vo} x100$$

*where,*

E: Edema percentage of rat's paw at t time after inflamed

Vt: Volume of rat's paw after inflamed

Vo: Volume of rat's paw before inflamed

Edema inhibitory percentage of test groups in comparison with control group was calculated by following formula:

$$I = \frac{Ec - Et}{Ec} x100$$

*where,*

I: Edema inhibitory percentage of test group in comparison with control group

Ec: Medium edema percentage of rat's paw of control group

Et: Medium edema percentage of rat's paw of test group (H,B Lassman, 1977; HUM 1993; S,wong 1972)

Statistical analysis: Data was expressed as mean ± SEM. The statistical significant difference between test and control group were determined by Student's t-test with Anova Exel 2003

## 3. Results

Antipolyarthritic action of test products was estimated basing on rat right paw volume chance. Results were summarized in Table 29.1 and 29.2.

**Table 29.1: Rat Paw Edema Percentage of Test Groups**

| *Sl.No.* | *Group* | *Test product* | *Edema Percentage According to Time Period P in Comparison with Control Group* | | |
|---|---|---|---|---|---|
| | | | *E(1-10)* | *E(11-15)* | *E(16-21)* |
| 1. | Control | NaCl 0.9 per cent | 11.97 ± 3.86 | 16.73 ± 4.10 | 23.26 ± 4.26 |
| 2. | Reference | Prednisolon 2mg/kg | 0.69 ± 1.42 $P_{2-1} < 0.05$ | 2.48 ± 2.18 $P_{2-1} < 0.01$ | 5.72 ± 2.06 $P_{2-1} < 0.01$ |
| 3. | Extract 2:1 | Extract 2:1 equivalence 20g/kg | 5.80 ± 2.06 P > 0.05 | 6.78 ± 2.38 P > 0.05 | 11.03 ± 2.48 P < 0.05 |

*Rhizoma cibotii* reduced edema at all three time period but only 3rd period, reduction was statistical significance (p<0.05 in comparison with control group. Edema reduction due to prednisolon was stronger that of *Rhizoma cibotii* and in all periods

**Table 29.2: Edema Inhibitory Percentage of Test Groups**

| *Sl.No.* | *Group* | *Orally Administered Test Product* | *Edema Inhibitory Percentage (%)* | | |
|---|---|---|---|---|---|
| | | | *I (1-10)* | *I (11-15)* | *I (16-21)* |
| 1. | Control | Prednisolon 2mg/kg | 94.20 | 85.17 | 75.41 |
| 2. | Extract 2:1 | Extract 2:1 equivalence 20g/kg | 51.59 | 59.45 | 52.57 |

*Rhizoma cibotii* at dose 20g/kg w.m inhibited polyarthritis at all three time period as 51.59; 59.45; 52.57 per cent respectively but only edema inhibition of 3rd period was statistical significance (p<0.05 in comparison with control group. Prednisolon at dose 2mg/kgw.m inhibited strong polyarthritis at all 3 periods p<0.05.

## 4. Discussion

In control group, rat right hind paw begun swelling on 3rd day to 5th day after being induced inflammation by injecting inflamed agent to rat left hind paw pad, rat right hind paw volume closely increased from 7th day to 21st day. In addition to swelling of right hind paw, there is that of paw before. Some rats further were injured in neck and arm pits at the end of study period, these correspond with pathological mechanism caused by Steptococcus pyogenes (HUM, 1993)

Antipolyarthritic activity of Rhizoma cibotii expressed no strong and after orally administered a long duration (16-21 day) which corresponds with herbal medicine action often exhibiting slowly and after orally administered a long duration. However it is necessary to continue study to conclude exactly.

Rats were orally administered prednisolon at dose 2mg/kg, performed strong antipolyarthritic activity at all 3 stage because prednisolon was strong antiarthritic drug in modern medicine, which demonstrated that use Steptococcus pyogenes induced polyarthritic model was based on science

## 5. Conclusion

Liquid extract 2:1 of *Rhizoma cibotii* inhibited polyarthritis in stage 2 (after being inflamed from 16th to 21st days) with $p<0.05$ at dose 20g dry material/kg w.r on S. pyogenes induced polyarthritis model.

Prednisolon at dose 2mg/kg b.w exhibited strongly antipolyarthritic activity in all 3 stage on this model, therefore this model can be suitable for experimental antipolyarthritis and prednisolon can also be suitable for referential drug.

## References

Lassman, H. B. *et al.*, 1977. Pharmacology of a New non–steroidal, anti–inflammatory agent: 6, 11–dihydro–11–oxodibenz[b,e] oxepin–2–aceticacid (HP 549), Arch. Int. Pharmacodyn, 227, pg 142–154.

Microbiological department of Hanoi University of Medicine, 1993. Medimicrobiological lectures, Medical publishing house Hanoi.

Pharmacological department of Hanoi University of Medicine, 1999. Pharmacology, Medical publishing house Hanoi.

Tat, Loi Do, 1999. Vietnam medicinal plants and pharmacognosies. Medical publishing house Hanoi.

Wong, S., *et al.*, 1972. "Pharmacologic evaluation of tolectin (Tolmetin, McN–2559) and McN–2891, two anti–inflammatory agents", The journal of pharmacology and experimental therapeutics, Vo l 185, No 1, Pg 127–138.

## Chapter 30

# Study on Chemical Composition and Some Bio-activities of *Herba piperis* Lolot

*Dien Vu Van*[1]* *and Hung Le Quoc*[2]

[1]*Hanoi University of Pharmacy, Vietnam*

[2]*Centre of Drug Quality Control of Army, Vietnam*

**E-mail vandien1951@vnn.vn*

## ABSTRACT

The alkaloid, flavonoid, antranoid, tanin, reduce sugar and amine acid in dried aerial part of piper lolot were found. The content of total alkaloid, flavonoid and essential oil were showed such as 1.11 per cent, 1.54 per cent and 0.49 per cent respectively. The 14-beta pregnane (1), 4 hydroxybenzyl-8-0-β-D-glucopyranosid (2) and 3,4-dihydroxy-4(1hydroxyethyl)-3,5,5-trimethylxyclohexyl hexopyranoside (3) from fraction of ethyl acetate were isolated and structure identified by MS, NMR spectroscopic data.

The antioxidant activity of ethanol 90 per cent extract 2:1 and 5 per cent solution of total flavonoid on suspension of liver cell and brain cell were demonstrated that the ethanol 90 per cent extract 2:1 inhibited 40.60 per cent on liver cell, 47.60 per cent on brain cell, 5 per cent solution of total flavonoid inhibited 56.90 per cent on liver cell, 41.10 per cent on brain cell, The free radical scaveging, stimulating choleresis, acute anti-inflammatory and analgesic activities of both ethanol 90 per cent extract 2:1 and 5 per cent solution of total flavonoid were demonstrated that free radical scaveging activities were 46.18 per cent and 46.76 per cent, stimulating choleresis effect were 18.03 per cent and 25.50 per cent, acute anti-inflammatory activities were 69.15 per cent and 58.21, analgesic activities by hot plate method were 62.50 per cent and 42.60 per cent, by Koster method were 64.05 per cent and 54.92 per cent. *Herba piperis* lolot was demonstrated to be no toxicity by oral administration with dose 200g/kg w.m

***Keywords:*** *Antioxidant, Piper lolot, Free radical scavenging, Flavonoid.*

## 1.0 Introduction

*Herba piperis* lolot was very commonly utilized in Vietnam and over world as medicinal plant and spicy plant, means for cultivation, collection and use was very easy, some disease as rheumatitis, indigestion, toothache, diarrhea, headache due to cold was used to treat. The research about this plant remains a little, no system, especially plant growing in Vietnam. Therefore we were carried out plant cultivated in Vietnam to contribute guiding rationally, safely and efficiently use.

## 2.0 Materials and Methods

### 2.1 Materials

The aerial part of *Piper lolot* C.DC was collected in Hanoi region, cut into segment, dried and conserved for research, botanically, sample of plant was controlled its authenticity by comparison with specimens being deposited in the herbarium of institute of material medica of Vietnam and controlled by botanically specialists

**Products for Test**

Decoction (2:1) (sign NS), 90 per cent ethanol extract (2:1)(sign DC), 5 per cent solution of total flavonoid (sign DF), substance for reference as 5 per cent astiso extract contained in film coated tablet named chophytol.

Chemicals, solvent, pre-coated silicagel plates which reached to standards for analysis was supplied by Merck supplier.

Animals for experiments: white mice belong to Swiss strain, weight of each one is 18-22g, weight of each white rat is 120-140g, both kind reached to standards for experiments.

### 2.2 Methods

Quantitative analysis total alkaloid, flavonoid: Gravimetry and essential oil: steam distillation (Dan N,V, 1985; Thu N,V, 1990).

Extract, isolation, identification constituents: constituents were extracted by ethyl acetate, residue after evaporating was isolated by column chromatography with the solvent system to elute as methanol–cloroform in gradually increasing polarity, isolated constituents were controlled purity by thin layer chromatography. Pure constituents were determined structure by spectroscopic (IR, MS,1H-NMR,13C-NMR (Dan N,V, 1985; De oliveira Chaves MC 2002; Thu N,V, 1990).

Acute toxicity assay: according to methods of World Health Organization Region office for the Western Pacific. (WHO Manila1993).

Test for cholereteric effect: according to method of (Pesson M, J.Salle, C.Auffret,1965).

Anti-inflammatory test: according to method of (Winter *et al.*, 1962).

Test for antioxidant activity: cited in Biol. Pharm. Bull 23(3) 2000 of Aniya Y., M. Shimabukuro, Mshimoji *et al.* and Imanari, T., Hirota, M. and Miyazaki, M.,1977); Karthikeyan J., Rani P., 2003).

Test for analgesic effect: according to method' Koster and hot plate (Koster, Anderson, EJ De Berr 1959; 10. Turner R.A 1965).

**Statistical Analysis**

Data were expressed as the mean ± SD and analyzed by one or two way ANOVA. Difference with $p<0.05$ were considered significant.

## 3.0 Results

### 3.1 Chemicals

***Qualitative Analysis of Phytochemical Groups**

Common solvents, reagents and special solvents, reagents of each phytochemical group were used for qualitative analysis of phytochemical groups. Result, substance groups as flavonoid, alkaloid, antranoid, tanin, free reduce sugar, acid amine, essential oil were found in *Herba piperis* lolot

*** Quantitative Analysis Total Alkaloid, Flavonoid and Essential Oil**

*Alkaloid*

Quantitative analysis 5 samples were carried out, result, medium content of total alkaloid was 1.11 per cent calculating according to dry absolutely material

*Flavonoid*

Quantitative analysis 5 samples were carried out, result, medium content of total flavonoid was 1.54 per cent calculating according to dry absolutely material

*Essential Oil*

Quantitative analysis 5 samples were carried out, result, medium content of essential oil was 0.49 per cent calculating according to dry absolutely material

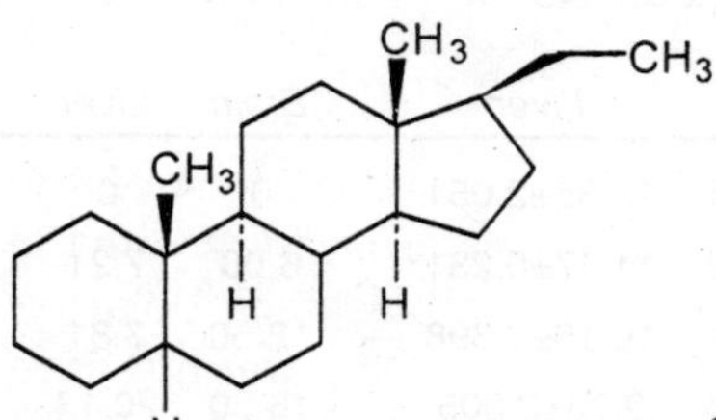

(1)

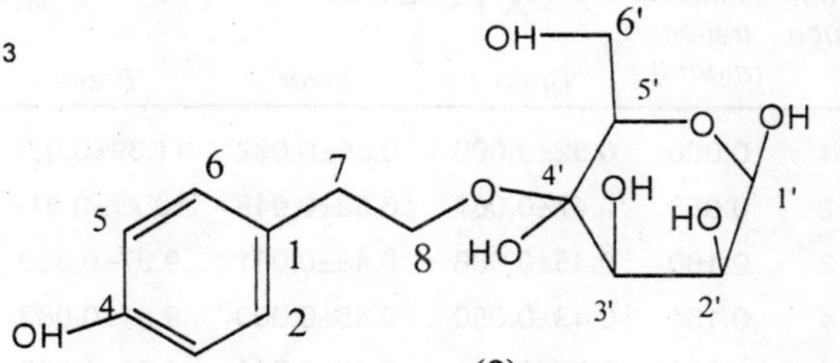

(2)

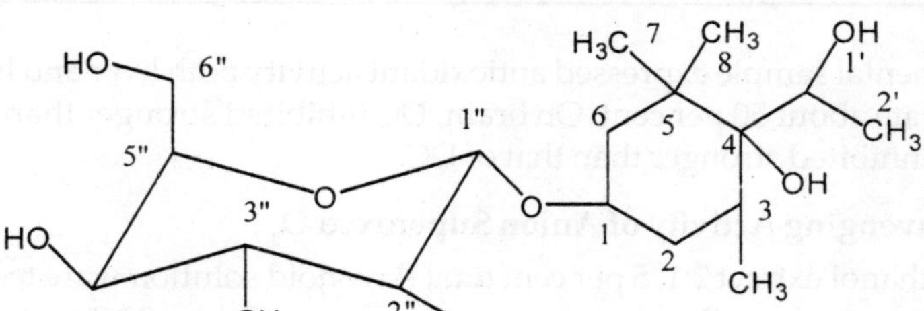

(3)

***Extract, Isolation and Identification of Some Compounds**

3 compounds as H2,T1,T2 were isolated and preliminary identified being 14-beta pregnane (1), 4-hydroxybenzyl–8-0-β-D-glucopyranoid (2) and 3,4-dihydroxy-4(1hydroxyethyl)-3,5,5-trimethylxyclohexyl hexopyranoside (3)

## 3.2 Bio-assay

*** Antioxidant Activity**

90 per cent ethanol extract 2:1, 5 per cent total flavonoid solution of ware tested on homogenous liver cell and brain cell of white mice. Results were summarized in Table 30.1 and 30.2.

**Table 30.1: Results of Antioxidant Activity of 90 per cent Ethanol 2:1**

| Test Tube | Concentration (mg/ml) | $\overline{X}_E$ ± SD n=5 | | $\overline{X}_{MDA}$ ± SD n=5 | | % Inhibition | |
|---|---|---|---|---|---|---|---|
| | | Brain | Liver | Brain | Liver | Brain | Liver |
| 1 | 0.000 | 0.62±0.008 | 0.49±0.009 | 13.78±2.207 | 10.96±0.780 | 0 | 0 |
| 2 | 0.050 | 0.48±0.008 | 0.44±0.011 | 10.63±1.640 | 9.73±0.782 | 22.91 | 1.24 |
| 3 | 0.100 | 0.46±0.010 | 0.44±0.004 | 10.16±2.510 | 9.60±0.581 | 26.33 | 12.56 |
| 4 | 0.150 | 0.43±0.092 | 0.42±0.007 | 9.23±0.921 | 9.28±0.530 | 33.16 | 15.38 |
| 5 | 0.200 | 0.40±0.042 | 0.39±0.003 | 8.89±0.632 | 8.71±1.008 | 35.54 | 20.53 |
| 6 | 0.250 | 0.33±0.009 | 0.29±0.002 | 7.22±0.541 | 6.51±0.842 | 47.66 | 40.69 |

**Table 30.2: Results of Antioxidant Activity of Total Flavonoid**

| Test Tube | Concentration (mg/ml) | $\overline{X}_E$ ± SD n=5 | | $\overline{X}_{MDA}$ ± SD n=5 | | % Inhibition | |
|---|---|---|---|---|---|---|---|
| | | Brain | Liver | Brain | Liver | Brain | Liver |
| 1 | 0.000 | 0.52±0.009 | 0.56±0.082 | 11.39±0.021 | 12.35±2.051 | 0 | 0 |
| 2 | 0.050 | 0.47±0.067 | 0.52±0.045 | 10.71±0.012 | 11.47±0.231 | 6.00 | 7.21 |
| 3 | 0.100 | 0.45±0.008 | 0.46±0.051 | 9.97±0.820 | 10.15±0.398 | 12.50 | 7.81 |
| 4 | 0.150 | 0.43±0.050 | 0.45±0.060 | 9.51±0.083 | 9.78±2.005 | 16.50 | 20.13 |
| 5 | 0.200 | 0.36±0.021 | 0.42±0.041 | 7.97±1.008 | 9.63±2.005 | 30.10 | 22.15 |
| 6 | 0.250 | 0.35±0.023 | 0.24±0.004 | 6.71±2.000 | 5.32±0.019 | 41.11 | 56.92 |

Both experimental sample expressed antioxidant activity both liver and brain of mice, inhibitory rate about 50 per cent. On brain, DC inhibited stronger than that of DF. On liver, DF inhibited stronger than that of DC.

***Free Radical Scavenging Activity of Anion Superoxyd $O_2$**

90 per cent ethanol extract 2:1, 5 per cent total flavonoid solution ware tested on Xanthine\ xanthine oxydase. Results were summarized in Tables 30.3 and 30.4.

**Table 30.3: Results of Free Radical Scavenging Effect of Ethanol Extract 2:1 (per cent)**

| *Group* | *Samples Added (μl)* | *PBS Added (μl)* | *C Sample for Test (μg/ml)* | $\overline{E}$ ±SD | *(%) Inhibition* |
|---|---|---|---|---|---|
| 1 | 0 | 50 | 0 | 0.340±0.012 | 0 |
| 2 | 30 | 20 | 60 | 0.212±0.002 | 37.65 |
| 3 | 40 | 10 | 80 | 0.187±0.005 | 45.00 |
| 4 | 50 | 0 | 100 | 0.183±0.012 | 46.18 |

**Table 30.4: Results of Free Radical Scavenging of 5 per cent Total Flavonoid Solution**

| *Group* | *Samples Added (μl)* | *PBS Added (μl)* | *C Sample for Test (μg/ml)* | $\overline{E}$ ±SD | *(%) Inhibition* |
|---|---|---|---|---|---|
| 1 | 0 | 50 | 0 | 0.340±0.012 | 0 |
| 2 | 30 | 20 | 60 | 0.257±0.006 | 24.42 |
| 3 | 40 | 10 | 80 | 0.249±0.004 | 26.77 |
| 4 | 50 | 0 | 100 | 0.181±0.006 | 46.76 |

PBS: Phosphate-Buffered Solution; Concentration: C.

Two experimental sample inhibited form of anion superoxyd $0_2$ (about 50 per cent) at dose 100μg/ml. Inhibition of DC at lower dose (60μg/ml) was gradually increased but at higher dose(100μg/ml) was not increased

***Test for Choleretic Effect**

Herba piperis lolot weakly expressed choleretic effect, DC as 18.03 per cent, DF as 25.50 per cent in comparison with control group

***Anti-inflammatory Activity**

White rats were inflamed by injecting 1 per cent carrageenin suspension to their right hind paw pad then orally administered test products and observed degree their inhibition

Results were presented in Table 30.5.

**Table 30.5: Anti-inflammatory Effect of Tested Groups (per cent)**

| *Groups* | *1st hour* | *2nd hour* | *3rd hour* | *4th hour* | *5th hour* | *6th hour* | *24th hour* | *30th hour* |
|---|---|---|---|---|---|---|---|---|
| Control | – | – | – | – | – | – | – | – |
| Aspirin | 31.07 | 53.81 | 60.94 | 62.63 | 57.59 | 55.52 | 15.92 | 20.13 |
| DC | 41.79 | 44.92 | 41.63 | 39.63 | 46.55 | 45.27 | 51.12 | 69.15 |
| DF | 55.00 | 52.03 | 50.43 | 41.08 | 47.93 | 51.11 | 47.76 | 58.21 |

DC (2:1) and DF inhibited inflammation from 1st hour to 30th as 41.79 per cent and 55.00 per cent respectively in comparison with group received normal saline with $p<0.05$ and time was longer and inflammatory inhibition was stronger too, which corresponds with effect of herbal medicine, often happens slower and longer than that of modern drugs after oral administration. While, exhibiting time of effect of aspirin was shorter that of two experimental samples, closely effect expressed time of aspirin was from 2nd hour to 4th, time was longer and action was lower, too.

***Test for Analgesic Effect**

Method' koster:

White mice was divided into 4 groups, 10 mice each one:

Group 1 was orally administered normal saline at dose 0.1ml/10g w.m

Group 2 was orally administered mixture of 4 per cent aspirin at dose 0.1ml/10g w.m

Group 3 was orally administered DC at dose 0.1ml/10g w.m

Group 4 was orally administered DF at dose 0.1ml/10g w.m

The mice were orally administered test samples in three day, then caused pain by intraperitoneal injection of 1 per cent acid acetic solution and observed number of stomach-ache fits in 5 minutes of each period with time sum observed as 30 minutes.

Results of analgesic action was presented in Table 30.6.

**Table 30.6: Analgesic Effect of Tested Groups (per cent)**

| *Groups* | *Analgesic Effect (per cent)* | | | | | |
|---|---|---|---|---|---|---|
| | *5–10'* | *10–15'* | *15–20'* | *20–25'* | *25–30'* | *TB* |
| 1–Control | – | – | – | – | – | – |
| 2–Aspirin | 74.59 | 52.82 | 51.79 | 32.89 | 38.39 | 50.20 |
| 3–DC | 69.67 | 68.31 | 57.14 | 55.26 | 70.37 | 64.05 |
| 4–DF | 64.75 | 61.27 | 62.50 | 24.21 | 51.85 | 54.92 |

Group 3,4 expressed analgesic action was stronger that of group 1 and 2. Analgesic action of group 3,4 was 64.15 per cent and 54.92 per cent respectively in comparison with control and referent group with $p<0.05$.

*Method' Hot Plate*

The mice that were sensitive with temperature during time from 6 to 20 second were selected for experiment and divided 4 groups, 8 mice each one and oral administered test products at dose as heading over mentioned. Results were presented in Table 30.7

The mice that were oral administered DC at dose 20g/kg w.m and DF at dose 4g/kg w.m closely expressed analgesic action in comparison with control group $P<0.05$. This action was similar that of aspirin at dose 400mg/kg w.m.

**Table 30.7: Hot Withstanding Time of Mice (second)**

| *Number of Mice* | *Hot Withstanding Time of Mice* | | | |
|---|---|---|---|---|
| | *Control Lot* | *Aspirin Lot* | *DC Lot* | *DF Lot* |
| 1 | 17.5 | 28.0 | 24.9 | 18.5 |
| 2 | 6.5 | 17.5 | 15.1 | 22.0 |
| 3 | 8.7 | 19.6 | 18.4 | 38.3 |
| 4 | 6.5 | 23.5 | 11.5 | 16.1 |
| 5 | 17.6 | 14.2 | 14.5 | 19.6 |
| 6 | 18.1 | 21.8 | 26.0 | 17.4 |
| 7 | 15.2 | 16.0 | 18.6 | 16.4 |
| 8 | 19.2 | 23.4 | 16.7 | 19.3 |
| Medium time (second) | 13.11 | 20.81 P< 0.05 | 21.31 P< 0.05 | 18.69 P< 0.05 |
| Medium Analgesic activity | | 58.7 | 62.5 | 42.6 |

Two experimental products had analgesic effect in both test methods, in that, sample of ethanol 2:1 exhibited stronger effect that of aspirin at tested dose with $p<0.05$

*Test for Acute Toxicity*

White mice was orally administered decoction 4:1 with gradually increasing dose to maximum dose could be administered up to 200g/kg w.m, 1000 folding higher than common dose for human. Result, the mice did not express acute toxicity. That mean that herba piperis lolot had very low toxicity.

## 4.0. Conclusion

The alkaloid, flavonoid, antranoid, tanin, reduce sugar and amine acid were found in dried aerial part of piper lolot. The content of total alkaloid, flavonoid and essential oil were determined being 1.11 per cent, 1.54 per cent and 0.49 per cent respectively.

The 14-beta pregnane, 4 hydroxybenzyl-8-0-β-D-glucopyranosid and 3,4-dihydroxy-4(1hydroxyethyl)-3,5,5-trimethylxyclohexyl hexopyranoside from fraction of ethyl acetate extract were isolated and structure identified by MS, NMR spectroscopic data.

The antioxidant activity of ethanol 90 per cent extract 2:1 and 5 per cent total flavonoid solution on homogeneous suspension of liver cell and that of brain cell were demonstrated, the ethanol 90 per cent extract 2:1 inhibited 40.60 per cent on liver cell, 47.60 per cent on brain cell, 5 per cent total flavonoid solution inhibited 56.90 per cent on liver cell, 41.10 per cent on brain cell.

The free radical scavenging, stimulating choleresis, acute anti-inflammatory and analgesic activities of both ethanol 90 per cent extract 2:1 and 5 per cent total flavonoid solution were demonstrated. The free radical scavenging activities were 46.18 per cent and 46.76 per cent, stimulating choleresis effect were 18.03 per cent and 25.50 per cent, acute anti-inflammatory activities were 69.15 per cent and 58.21, analgesis activities by hot plate method were 62.50 per cent and 42.60 per cent, by Koster method were 64.05 per cent and 54.92 per cent successively. *Herba piperis* lolot was demonstrated to be no toxicity by oral administration with dose 200g/kg w.m.

## References

Bao Dam Trung, Huyen Hoang Tich, Vinh Pham Nguyen, 1999. Antioxidants to prevent disease and antiaging, Medical publishing house Hanoi.

Biochemical department of Hanoi University of Medicine, 1991. Biochemicology. Medical publishing house Hanoi.

Dan Nguyen Van, Tuu Nguyen Viet, 1985. Methods for phytochemical research of medicinal plant, Medical publishing house Hanoi.

De oliveira Chaves MC; De oliveira santos BV, 2002. Contituents from piper marginatum fruits, Fitoterapia 73(6) 547-9.

Imanari, T., Hirota, M. and Miyazaki, M., 1977. Improved assay method for superoxide dismutase. Igaku no Ayumi 101, 496–497.

Karthikeyan, J. and Rani P., 2003. Enzymatic and non–enzymatic antioxydants in selected Piper species, Indian J Exp Biol, 41(2), 135–40.

Koster, Anderson, EJ De Berr, 1959. Acid acetic for analgesic screening, pp. 412.

Pluger, M. Weber, N. X. Dung, V. T. Luu, D. D. Rang, D. T. Tuong, P. H. Ngoc, 2002. The Crystal Structure of 3-(4'–Methoxyphenyl) propanoyl pyrrole of Piper lolot C.DC from Vietnam.

Thu Ngo Van, 1990. Chemistry of saponine, Edition by Ho Chi Minh University of Medicine and Pharmacy.

Turner, R.A., 1965. Sreening methods in pharmacology, Academic

Winter, C.A, Risley E.A, Nus GW (1962): Carrageenin-induced edema in hind paw of the rat as an assay for anti-inflammatory drug, Proc Soc.Exp, Biol. Med, No.111, 547.

World health organization region office for the western pacific. Manila, 1993. Research guideline for evaluating the safety and efficacy of herbal medicines.

# Chapter 31

# Study on Antioxidant Activities and Principles of Vietnamese Bitter Tea *Ilex kudingcha*

*Phuong Thien Thuong*[1], *Nguyen Hai Dang*[2], *Tran Minh Ngoc*[3], *Tran Manh Hung*[1], *Nguyen Duy Thuan*[4] *and Won Keun Oh*[1]*

[1] *College of Pharmacy, Chosun University, Gwangju 501–759, Korea*

[2] *Institute of Natural Product Chemistry, 18 Hoang Quoc Viet, Hanoi, Vietnam*

[3] *College of Pharmacy, Chungnam National University, Daejon 305–764, Korea*

[4] *Vietnam Institute of Medicinal Materials, 3B Quang Trung, Hanoi, Vietnam*

**E-mail: wkoh@chosun.kr.ac*

## ABSTRACT

In an ongoing project aimed at discovery of natural antioxidants, a MeOH extract of Vietnamese kudingcha (*Ilex kudingcha*) was found to contain abundantly phenolic content (with garlic acid equivalent level of 58.9 mg/g extract) and exhibit significant antioxidant activity. The MeOH extract and EtOAc-soluble fraction displayed remarkable free radical scavenging activity against DPPH ($IC_{50}$ = 28.7 and 16.3 μg/ml, respectively) and superoxide anion ($IC_{50}$ = 3.4 and 1.3 μg/ml, respectively). These extracts also significantly protected LDL oxidation mediated by either an ion $Cu^{2+}$ or a free radical AAPH, evidenced by the suppression of the conjugated diene formation and dose-dependent inhibition the extent of TBARS production with $IC_{50}$ values of 2.0 and 1.4 μg/ml, respectively (when LDL was oxidized by $Cu^{2+}$), and $IC_{50}$ values of 7.8 and 4.8 μg/ml, respectively (when LDL was treated with AAPH). Repeated chromatographic processes including HPLC with UV detector was employed for the identification and quantification of active constituents of *Ilex kudingcha*. The result indicated that the major phenolic compounds are caffeoyl derivatives caffeic acid (1), chlorogenic acid (2), 3,4-dicaffeoylquinic acid (3), 3,5-dicaffeoylquinic acid (4) and 4,5-

dicaffeoylquinic acid (5), and flavonoids quercetin (6), kaempferol (7), and rutin (8). This finding suggests that the dietary consumption of kudingcha tea may provide beneficial effects on reducing cardiovascular and oxidative stress-related diseases.

***Keywords:*** *Ilex kudingcha, Aquifoliaceae, Antioxidant activity, Phenolic compounds.*

## 1.0 Introduction

The plant *Ilex kudingcha* C. J. Tzeng (synonym *Ilex kudincha*, Aquifoliaceae), native to Southern China and Northern Vietnam, has long been used indigenously as a tea for headache, cold, hypertension, fever and diabetes. The tea is called kudingcha, which means bitter tea, because of having bit taste. Previous studies have revealed that kudingcha is a rich source of triterpenoids, triterpenoid saponins, and flavonoids that exhibit various biological effects, for example anti-inflammatory, anti-ulcer, antioxidant, and enzyme inhibitory activities (Ouyang *et al.*, 1996a; Ouyang *et al.*, 1996b; Nishimura *et al.*, 1999a; Nishimura *et al.*, 1999b; Ouyang *et al.*, 2001; Tang *et al.*; 2005). Studies on *Ilex* species have reported that the herbs showed antioxidant activity (Schinella *et al.*, 2000; Nahar *et al.*, 2005; Gugliucci, 1996; Filip, 2003), cardiovascular effects (Mosimann *et al.*, 2006; Paganini *et al.*, 2005; Gorgen *et al.*, 2005; Schinella *et al.*, 2005), antiparkinsonian property (Milioli *et al.*, 2007), intestinal propulsion (Filip, 2003; Gorzalczany *et al.*, 2001), and cytotoxicity (Gonzalez *et al.*, 2005). Therefore, *Ilex* species, especially *I. paraguariensis*, have been reputed to be a have protective properties against heart diseases, brain dysfunction and maintaining proper body weight. Although some *Ilex* species have been reported as antioxidant source, the antioxidant activities of kudingcha and its principles have only partially been determined so far. In our continuation research for antioxidant from medicinal plants, we found that an aqueous extract of this bitter tea exhibited significant antioxidant activities. This study evaluates the antioxidant activity of Vietnamese kudingcha and characterizes its principles.

## 2.0 Materials and Methods

### 2.1 General Experimental Procedure

Optical rotations were determined on a JASCO P-1020 polarimeter using a 100 mm glass microcell. NMR spectra were obtained on Varian Inova 500 MHz spectrometer with TMS as the internal standard. EIMS and HREI-MS data were performed on a Micromass QTOF2 (Micromass, Wythenshawe, UK) mass spectrometer. For column chromatography, silica gel (Merck, 63-200 µm particle size) was used. TLC was carried out with silica gel 60 $F_{254}$ and RP-18 $F_{254}$ plates from Merck.

### 2.2 Materials

#### 2.2.1 Plant Material

Leaves of *Ilex kudingcha* C. J. Tzeng were collected at Caobang province, Northern Vietnam in spring, 2004. The voucher specimen was identified by Prof. Pham Thanh Ky, Department of Pharmacognosy, Hanoi University of Pharmacy.

### 2.2.2 Chemicals and Reagents

The common solvents used for extraction and isolation were purchased from commercial resources in Korea. All chemicals and reagents used for bioassays were of analytical grade obtained from Sigma-Aldrich Corp. (USA) and Junsei Co. Ltd. (Japan).

## 2.3 Preparation of Extracts and Assay Samples

The dried leaves were (2 kg) extracted with boiled MeOH (10 : l) and repeated twice. The extracts were combined and exhaustively concentrated *in vacuo* to dryness (680 g). The powdery extracts were dissolved in $H_2O$ (2 : l) and partitioned with Hexane, EtOAc, and BuOH (each 2 l, repeated five times) and then the solvents were removed under reduced pressure to get Hx (226 g), EA (113 g), and BuOH (171 g) fractions, respectively. The MeOH extract (IK) and organic solvent fractions (Hx, EA, BuOH) were used for study, (+)–catechin and α–tocopherol were used as reference compounds.

## 2.4 Determination of Total Phenolic Content

Total phenolic compounds of plants were performed according to the Folin-Ciocalteu method (Cai *et al.*, 2004). Briefly, 20 μl of sample (1 mg/ml) and 930 μl of 2 per cent $Na_2CO_3$ were seeded in a tube, and then 50 μl of Folin-Ciocalteu's reagent was added. The reaction mixture was incubated at 40°C for 60 min and the absorption of the mixtures was read at 760 nm. Each sample was tested at final concentration of 20 μg/ml in triplicate, and calibration graph with 4 data points for gallic acid. Total phenolic content of each plant was expressed in mg of gallic acid equivalents (GAE) per 1 g of extract.

## 2.5 Isolation of Phenolics in *I. kudingcha* by HPLC

For this study, a part of the EA fraction (50 g) was subjected to silica gel column chromatography (2 kg) and eluted with hexane–EtOAc (10:1, 7.5:1, 5:1, 2.5:1, 1:1, and 1:2, each 5 l) and then EtOAc–MeOH (1:1, 5 l). The selected fraction (9.7 g, eluted with EtOAc–MeOH) was used for isolation by HPLC. The phenolic compounds in kudingcha were isolated by a Gilson HPLC system with UV detector, ODS-H80 column (150×20 mm, particle size 4 μm, Japan), using a gradient of MeOH (solvent A) and 0.1 per cent formic acid in $H_2O$ (solvent B) as mobile phase. The gradient program was as follows: 0–30 min (50 per cent A), 30–50 min (50?75 per cent A) and 50–60 min (75?100 per cent A). The UV absorptions were detected at 254 and 320 nm.

## 2.6 Free Radical Scavenging Assays

### 2.6.1 DPPH Radical Scavenging

DPPH radical scavenging activity was performed according to a described method (Thuong *et al.*, 2007). Briefly, 5 μl of each sample, dissolved in DMSO, was added to 195 μl of 150 μM DPPH in methanol in 96 well plates. The solution was mixed for 1 min and incubated at room temperature for 30 min. The absorbance of the reaction mixture was measured at 520 nm on a microplate reader. The scavenging activity is expressed by the degree of radical reduction of a test group in comparison with that of the control.

### 2.6.2 Hydroxyl Radical Scavenging

*Non-site Specific Assay*

Hydroxyl radical scavenging activity was evaluated by a method reported (Mahakunakorn *et al.*, 2004). The mixture, in a total volume of 500 µl, contained PBS $FeCl_3$ (100 µM), ascorbic acid (100 µM), EDTA (100 µM), $H_2O_2$ (10 mM), deoxyribose (2.8 mM), and test sample was incubated at 37°C for 1 h and then stopped by addition 250 µl of TCA (10 per cent, w/v). After adding 250 µl of TBA (1 per cent w/v), the reaction mixture was boiled for 15 min in a water bath. The colour development was measured at 532 nm and the scavenging activity of test sample was expressed as percentage inhibition of the deoxyribose degradation to malonaldehyde.

*Site-Specific Assay*

This was performed similarly to non-site-specific assay described above, except that EDTA was discarded.

### 2.6.3 Superoxide Radical Scavenging

Superoxide was generated by xanthine/xanthine oxidase and measured by the NBT reduction method (Thuong *et al.*, 2007). In brief, 5 µl of xanthine oxidase was added to 495 ml of 20 mM phosphate buffer (pH 7.8) containing 100 µM NBT and 50 µM xanthine and test sample. The absorbance of the reaction mixture was read at 550 nm after 5 min. Superoxide radical scavenging activity was expressed by the degree of NBT reduction of a test group in comparison with that of the control.

## 2.7 Lipid Peroxidation Assay

Inhibitory activity of kudingcha against mitochondrial lipid peroxidation was measured by thiobacbituric acid reactive substance (TBARS) method. The preparation of mitochondrial and measurement of lipid peroxidation were reported previously (Thuong *et al.*, 2007).

## 2.8 LDL Oxidation Assay

*Preparation of human LDL*: LDL was isolated from fasted healthy human plasma as reported previously (Thuong *et al.*, 2007; Hung *et al.*, 2006). In brief, plasma was flotation ultracentrifuged at the density ranged between 1.019-1.063 g/ml. LDL was dialyzed extensively at 4°C against 10 mM phosphate saline buffer (PBS, pH 7.4). Before the oxidation experiment, LDL protein was determined by BCA method (Smith *et al.*, 1985).

*Assay for inhibitory effect on LDL oxidation*: LDL (0.1 mg protein/ml) was incubated with 5 µM $Cu^{2+}$ ($CuSO_4$) or 5 mm AAPH in the absence or present of bitter tea in 10 mM PBS buffer (pH. 7.4) at 37°C (Thuong *et al.*, 2007; Hung *et al.*, 2006). The extent of LDL oxidation was assayed by measurements of conjugated dienes formation and TBARS methods (Thuong *et al.*, 2007; Hung *et al.*, 2006).

## 3.0 Results

## 3.1 Free Radical Scavenging Activity of *Ilex kudingcha*

The antioxidant abilities of MeOH extract of *I. kudingcha* (IK) and its fractions were first tested using free radical scavenging assays against DPPH, $OH^\bullet$, and $O_2^{-\bullet}$

The results were presented in Table 31.1. The MeOH extract exhibited a strong bleaching effect on DPPH with an $IC_{50}$ value of 28.7 μg/ml, indicating that the extract possesses antioxidant-constituents. Among the fractions tested, the EA fraction (EA) displayed a significant scavenging activity ($IC_{50}$ = 16.3 μg/ml), stronger than that of α-tocopherol ($IC_{50}$ = 19.1 μg/ml). Next, the hydroxyl radical scavenging activities of IK against hydroxyl radical were evaluated using non-site-specific hydroxyl radical-generating system. It was found that EA fraction is substantially efficient in quenching hydroxyl radical formation, expressed an $IC_{50}$ value of 87.5 μg/ml, while (+)-catechin was less active ($IC_{50}$ > 100 μg/ml). A related assay in which the effect of IK on site-specific hydroxyl radical system was evaluated, the IK and EA were found to demonstrate a remarkable hydroxyl radical scavenging activity ($IC_{50}$ = 37.6 and 27.3 μg/ml, respectively), comparable to that of (+)-catechin ($IC_{50}$ = 34.9 μg/ml) under the same experimental condition. Further, the scavenging effects of IK and its fractions on xanthine/xanthine oxidase-generated superoxide anion, based on the reduction of NBT, were determined. The IK appeared to be less effective in quenching superoxide anion production ($IC_{50}$ = 3.4 μg/ml), but the EA displayed a significant bleaching ability ($IC_{50}$ = 1.3 μg/ml), when compare to that of catechin ($IC_{50}$ = 2.0 μg/ml).

## 3.2 Anti-lipid Peroxidation Activity of IK

The ability of IK to prevent lipid peroxidation of mice liver mitochondrial induced by $Fe^{3+}$/ascorbate was investigated. Table 31.1 demonstrates that IK and EA showed strong protection against lipid peroxidation ($IC_{50}$ = 17.4 and 7.1 μg/ml, respectively). When the anti-lipid peroxidation ability of these extracts was compared with α-tocopherol and catechin, the order of potency was (+)-catechin > EA > IK > α-tocopherol.

## 3.3 Suppressive Effect of IK on Conjugated Dienes Formation during LDL Oxidation

In an attempt to evaluate protective effect of IK on LDL oxidation, LDL was exposed to 5 μM $Cu^{2+}$ in the absence or absence of IK and EA. The formation of conjugated dienes, early product of lipid peroxidation, was monitored by measurement of absorbance at 234 nm. Figure 31.1A depicts the suppressive effect on conjugated diene produced during LDL was oxidation induced by $Cu^{2+}$ in the presence of IK and EA. The lag time of $Cu^{2+}$-induced LDL oxidation (blank) was calculated as 30 min, and it was significantly prolonged when test samples were added. In the presence of IK and EA at the concentration 2 μg/ml, the lag time was increased to 205 and 290 min, respectively. Meanwhile, (+)-catechin and α-tocopherol prolonged the lag time to 280 and 85 min, respectively, at the same condition. Therefore, IK was significantly more potent in preventing LDL oxidation than α-tocopherol, an antioxidant present in LDL particles, while EA exhibited an equivalent activity to that of (+)-catechin.

Figure 31.1B shows the kinetic profiles of conjugated dienes formation in the presence or absence of test samples when LDL was incubated with 5 mM AAPH. The effect of test samples could be characterized by the rate of the oxidation, which expressed the slope of the kinetic. When the slope of the blank was defined as 1, the suppression upon LDL oxidation in the presence of IK or EA at 1 μg/ml was evidenced

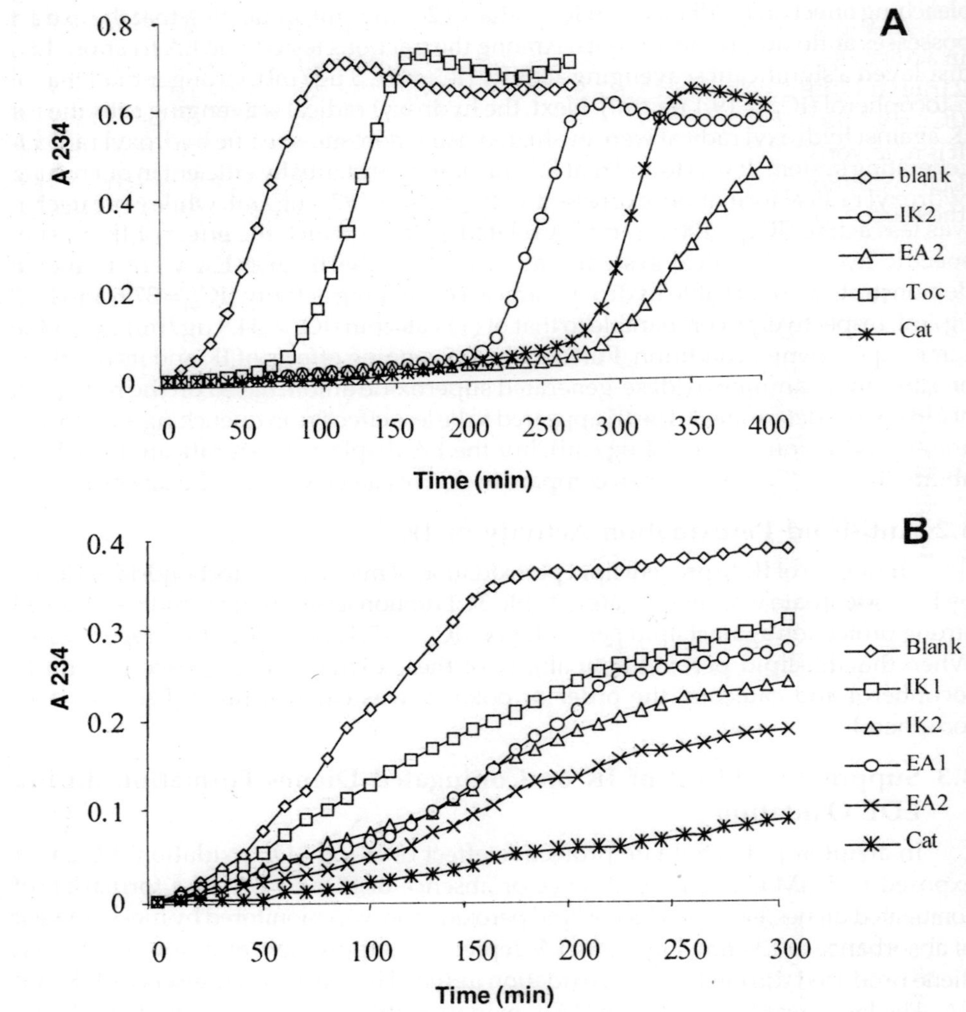


**Figure 31.1: Suppressive Effect of IK on Conjugated Dienes Formation during LDL Oxidation induced by $Cu^{2+}$ (A) and AAPH (B)**

by the slope value of 0.76. In the presence of IK, EA and (+)-catechin at 2 µg/ml, the slope values are 0.62, 0.50, and 0.22, respectively. Hence, IK and EA are weaker inhibitors of LDL oxidation initiated by AAPH than (+)-catechin.

LDL (50 µg/ml) in PBS was incubated with 5 µM $CuSO_5$ or 5 mM AAPH at 37°C in the presence or absence of test sample. Kinetic profiles of conjugated diene formation were measured at 234 nm every 10 min. Values are mean from two different experiments. (+)-Catechin and $\alpha$-tocopherol were used as reference compounds and tested at the concentration of 2 µg/ml. IK1: IK at 1 µg/ml, IK2: IK at 2 µg/ml, EA1: EA at 1 µg/ml, EA2: EA at 2 µg/ml.

## 3.4 Inhibitory Effect of IK on TBARS Production of LDL Oxidation

As shown in Figure 31.2A, IK markedly inhibited $Cu^{2+}$-induced LDL oxidation in a dose-dependent fashion, reaching the 50 per cent inhibition at concentration of 2.0 μg/ml. The protective action of IK was significant stronger than that of α-tocopherol ($IC_{50}$ = 9.4 μg/ml, data not shown), further reaffirming the antioxidant potency of IK. It is noteworthy that AE ($IC_{50}$ = 1.4 μg/ml) was comparably effective in preventing the LDL oxidation to (+)-catechin ($IC_{50}$ = 1.5 μg/ml). This was in a good agreement with those observed in conjugated diene assay.

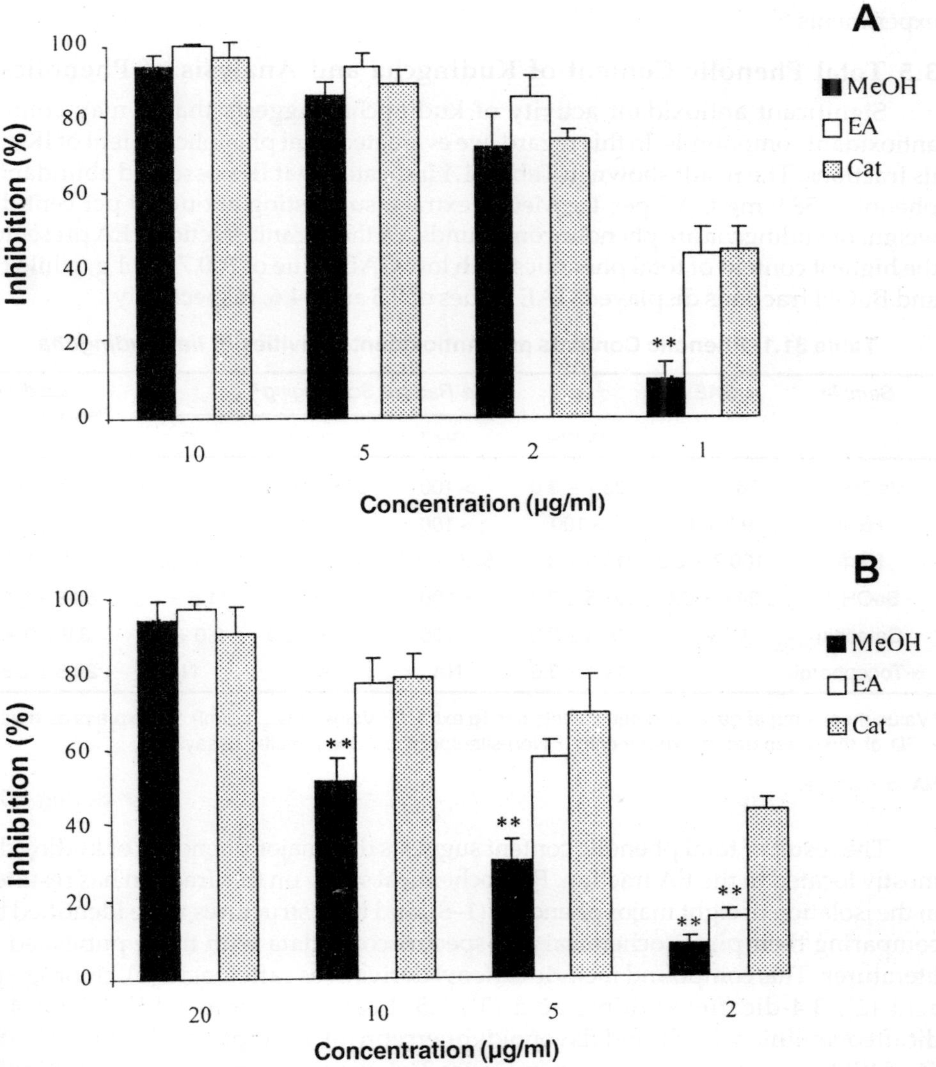


**Figure 31.2: Inhibitory Action of IK upon TBARS Production of LDL Oxidation induced by $Cu^{2+}$ (A) and AAPH (B)**

Figure 31.2B reveals a dose-dependently protective effect on LDL oxidation caused by AAPH of IK and EA, achieving 94 per cent protection at concentration as low as 20 µg/ml. The concentration ($IC_{50}$) of IK and EA required to achieve 50 per cent protection was 7.8 and 4.8 µg/ml, respectively, while (+)-catechin showed an $IC_{50}$ value of 3.1 µg/ml. In this assay, α-tocopherol was observed to exhibit no effect on AAPH-mediated LDL oxidation, probably due to the lipophilic property.

LDL (50 µg/ml) in PBS was incubated with 5 µM $CuSO_5$ or 5 mM AAPH at 37°C in the presence or absence of test sample. After incubation for 3 h, the extent of LDL oxidation was assayed by TBARS method. Values are mean from three different experiments.

## 3.5 Total Phenolic Content of Kudingcha and Analysis of Phenolics

Significant antioxidant activity of kudingcha suggests that it may contain antioxidant compounds. In this regard, we evaluated total phenolic content of IK and its fractions. The result shown in Table 31.1 indicated that IK possessed abundantly phenolics 58.9 mg GAE per 1 g MeOH extract, suggesting about 2.0 per cent dry weight of kudingcha are phenolic compounds. Of the organic fractions, EA presented the highest content of total phenolics with low GAE value of 100.7 per 1 g, while Hx and BuOH fractions displayed GAE values of 9.5 and 34.6, respectively.

**Table 31.1: Phenolic Contents and Antioxidant Activities of *Ilex kudingcha***

| *Sample* | *GAE* [1] | *Free Radical Scavenging* [2] | | | | *Lipid Peroxidation* [2] |
|---|---|---|---|---|---|---|
| | | *DPPH* | *OH•* [3] | *OH•* [4] | $O_2^{\cdot -}$ | |
| MeOH ex | 58.9 ± 3.8 | 28.7 ± 3.0 | > 100 | 37.6 ± 10.7 | 3.4 ± 0.4 | 17.4 ± 2.3 |
| Hx fr | 9.5 ± 1.1 | > 100 | > 100 | > 100 | > 20 | > 100 |
| EA fr | 100.7 ± 2.3 | 16.3 ± 0.1 | 87.5 ± 9.6 | 27.3 ± 3.7 | 1.3 ± 0.4 | 7.1 ± 1.3 |
| BuOH fr | 34.6 ± 2.0 | 67.5 ± 7.7 | > 100 | > 100 | 11.6 ± 1.9 | 60.8 ± 9.3 |
| Catechin | – | 10.6 ± 2.0 | > 100 | 34.9 ± 5.3 | 2.0 ± 0.3 | 3.9 ± 0.9 |
| α-Tocopherol | – | 19.1 ± 3.6 | NA | NA | NA | 29.5 ± 2.8 |

[1] Value means mg of gallic acid equivalents per 1g extract; [2] Values ($IC_{50}$, µg/ml) are express as means ± SD of three separated experiments; [3] Non-site-specific; [4] Site-specific assays.

NA: not active.

The result of total phenolic content suggests that major phenolics of kudingcha mostly located in the EA fraction. Phytochemical study on this fraction has resulted in the isolation of eight major phenolics (1–8), and their structures were identified by comparing their physicochemical and spectroscopic data with those published in literatures. This compound include caffeoyl derivatives caffeic acid (1), chlorogenic acid (2), 3,4-dicaffeoylquinic acid (3), 3,5-dicaffeoylquinic acid (4) and 4,5-dicaffeoylquinic acid (5), and flavonoids quercetin (6), kaempferol (7), and rutin (8). The HPLC chromatogram shown in Figure 31.4 was performed during isolation of these phenolics with the condition described in the Materials and methods section.

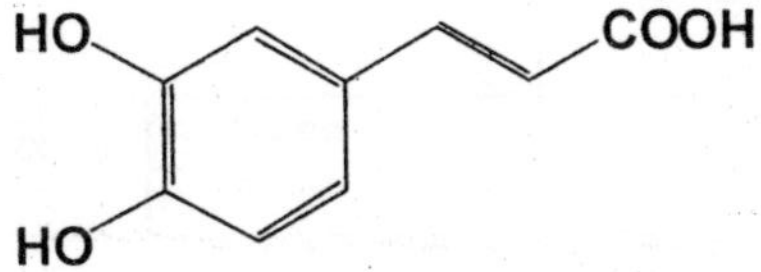


**1** Caffeic acid

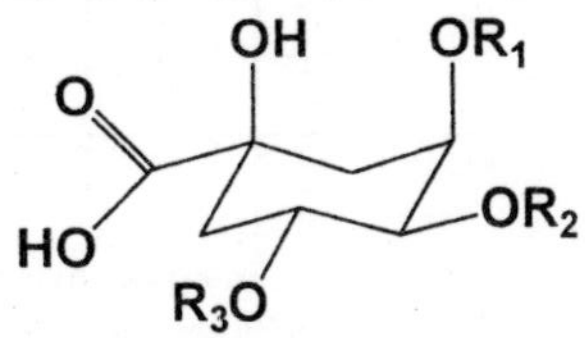


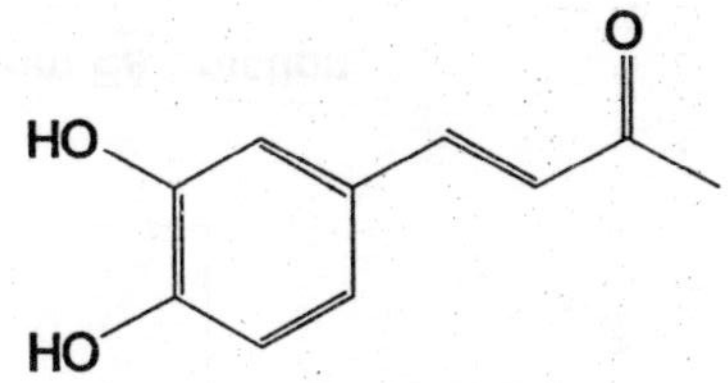


Caffeoyl

| Compound | $R_1$ | $R_2$ | $R_3$ |
|---|---|---|---|
| **2** | H | H | Caffeoyl |
| **3** | Caffeoyl | Caffeoyl | H |
| **4** | Caffeoyl | H | Caffeoyl |
| **5** | H | Caffeoyl | Caffeoyl |

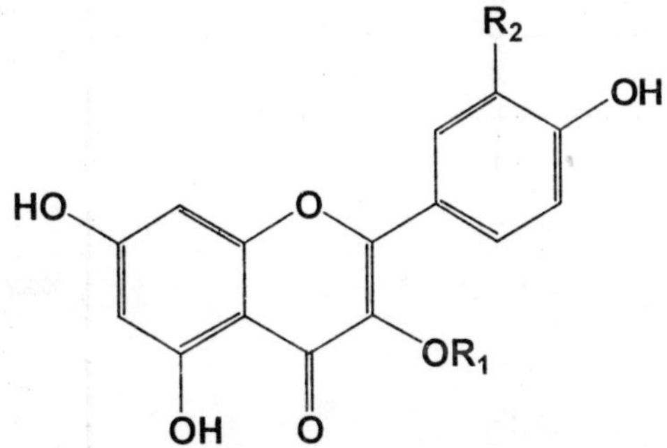


| Compound | $R_1$ | $R_2$ |
|---|---|---|
| **6** | H | OH |
| **7** | H | H |
| **8** | Rutinose | OH |

**Figure 31.3: Chemical Structures of Major Antioxidants in *I. Kudingcha***

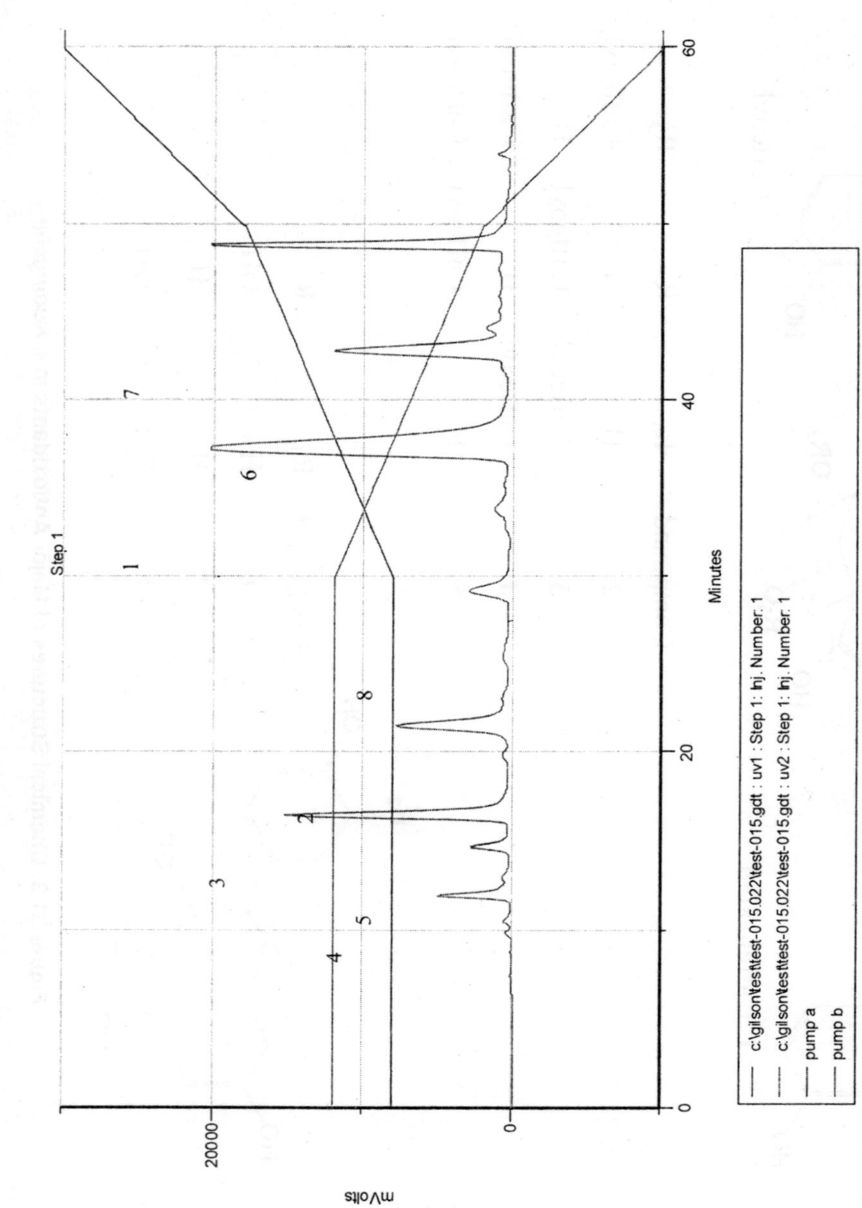


**Figure 31.4: A Representative HPLC Profile of Phenolics (1–8) from EA Fraction**

## 4.0 Discussion

Phytochemical investigations on the *Ilex* species have revealed several phenolics (Nahar *et al.*, 2005; Filip *et al.*, 2003; Filip *et al.*, 2001; Zhang *et al.*, 2005; Yang *et al.*, 2006) and these major phenolics are caffeoyl derivatives and flavonols. In this study, an evaluation for total phenolic content showed that a Vietnamese species *I. kudingcha* is an abundant source of natural phenolics and these compounds are mostly located in the EA fraction. It was demonstrated to contain similarly major phenolics from *Ilex* species growing in South America (Filip *et al.*, 2001). The major phenolics of *I. kudingcha* include caffeic derivatives (1–5), and flavonols (6–8). Except for 7, other compounds possess catechol (*o*-hydroxyl) group(s).

It is extensively known that phenolics have wide impacts on living system and the most interested one of phenolics in food industry is antioxidant property (Karakaya, 2004). In this study, we examined the antioxidant property of IK using several *in vitro* assay systems. First, a methanol extract (IK) and ethyl acetate fraction (EA) exhibited potent scavenging action against a stable radical DPPH due to the presence of large phenolic compounds. The IK and EA extracts also showed inhibitory activity against hydroxyl radical, generated by Fenton reaction, in the presence or absence of EDTA. In comparison, both extracts, as well as (+)-catechin, displayed much higher trapping activity in the absence of EDTA, indicating that IK and EA exhibited a strong chelation of iron ion (Mahakunakorn *et al.*, 2004). This is in good agreement with previous predication that characterized the catechol group play a major role in chelation of metal ions (Pietta, 2000; Rice *et al.*, 1996). Next, IK and EA were also demonstrated to have a significant quenching effect on superoxide anion generated by an enzyme system xanthine/xanthine oxidase, not only due to the radical scavenging but also result from suppressive action against xanthine oxidase of phenolic compounds (Pietta, 2000; Rice *et al.*, 1996).

In further study to confirm the protective action of IK against lipid oxidation, the inhibitory effect of IK was determined by measurements of conjugated diens formation and TBARS, which are early product and end fatty acid-derived product, respectively. The result indicated the strong anti-lipid peroxidation activity of IK and EA against mitochondrial oxidation initiated by hydoroxyl radical generated from Fenton reaction. Furthermore, it was also demonstrated that these extract also showed significant inhibitory effect on LDL oxidation induced by either a metal ion $Cu^{2+}$ or free radical AAPH. The protective action against lipid oxidation of kudingcha derives from both chelation of metal ions and quenching effect on free radical (hydroxyl, lipid peroxyl, lipid alkoxyl) of phenolics presented (Pietta, 2000; Rice *et al.*, 1996).

Although there have been several reports on antioxidant activity of *Ilex* species, especially *I. paraguariensis*, this study investigated for the first time the significant antioxidant activity and the principles of *I. kudingcha*. Considerable evidence has indicated that reactive oxygen species (ROS) play an important contributory role in various diseases such as inflammation, atherosclerosis, aging, and cancer. ROS are known to be capable of chemically altering all major classes of biomolecules including lipids, protein, and nucleic acids, leading to change their structure and function (Halliwell, 2000; Valko, 2007). The oxidation of LDL induced by free radicals and metal ions has been proposed as a major contributor in the development of atherosclerosis, the most cause of mobility in the developed world (Berliner, 1996). In supported of this, the oxidized form of LDL was detected in atherosclerotic lesions from both animal and human (Glass, 2001). Particularly, it is important to note that kudingcha has been used traditionally in Vietnam for the treatment of hypertension and diabetes, the diseases link with oxidative process in the body (Halliwell, 2000; Valko, 2007). Furthermore, the healthy diet of natural phenolics is believed to reduce the risk of cancer, heart disease, diabetes, ageing, attributing to their antioxidant, anticancer, anticarcinogenic, antimutagenic, and cytotoxic activities (Cai *et al.*, 2004; Karakaya, 2004, 26, Halliwell, 2000; Valko, 2007). Therefore, IK is expected to be used beneficially in protecting atherosclerosis and its complications, as well as reducing oxidative stress. This is well identical with the consumption of Mate (*I. paraguariensis*) that is used for the treatment of heart diseases, brain dysfunction in South America.

In conclusion, *I. kudingcha* was demonstrated to possess significant antioxidant activity due to its abundantly antioxidant phenolics content. This finding suggests that kudingcha tea is a rich source of natural antioxidants and could be used for the prevention and treatment of cardiovascular and oxidative stress-related diseases.

## References

Berliner, J. A., Heinecker, J. W., 1996. The role of oxidized lipoprotein in atherosclerosis. *Free Radic. Biol. Med.* (20); pp.707–727.

Cai, Y., Luo, Q., Sun, M., Corke, H., 2004. Antioxidant activity and phenolic compounds of 112 traditional Chinese medicinal plants associated with anticancer. *Life Sci.* (74); pp.2157–2184.

Filip, R., Lopez, P., Giberti, G., Coussio, J., Ferraro, G., 2001. Phenolic compounds in seven South American *Ilex* species. *Fitoterapia* (72); pp.774–778.

Filip, R., Ferraro, G. E., 2003. Researching on new species of "Mate": *Ilex brevicuspis*: phytochemical and pharmacology study. *Eur. J. Nutr.* (42); pp.50–54.

Glass, C. K., Witstum, J. L., 2001. Atherosclerosis: the road ahead. *Cell* (104); pp.503–516.

Gonzalez de Mejia, E., Song, Y. S., Ramirez-Mares, M. V., Kobayashi, H., 2005. Effect of yerba mate (*Ilex paraguariensis*) tea on topoisomerase inhibition and oral carcinoma cell proliferation. *J. Agric. Food Chem.* (53); pp.1966–1973.

Gorgen, M., Turatti, K., Medeiros, A. R., Buffon, A., Bonan, C. D., Sarkis, J. J., Pereira, G. S., 2005. Aqueous extract of *Ilex paraguariensis* decreases nucleotide hydrolysis in rat blood serum. *J. Ethnopharmacol.* (97); pp.73–77.

Gorzalczany, S., Filip, R., Alonso, M. R., Mino, J., Ferraro, G. E., Acevedo, C., 2001. Choleretic effect and intestinal propulsion of 'mate' (*Ilex paraguariensis*) and its substitutes or adulterants. *J. Ethnopharmacol.* (75); pp.291–294.

Gugliucci, A., 1996. Antioxidant effects of *Ilex paraguariensis*: induction of decreased oxidability of human LDL in vivo. *Biochem. Biophys. Res. Commun.* (224); pp.338–344.

Halliwell, B., Gutteridge J. M. C., 2000. Free radicals in biology and medicine. Oxford University Press (3).

Hung, T. M., Na, M. K., Thuong, P. T., Su, N. D., Sok, D. E., Song, K. S., Seong, Y. H., Bae, K. H., 2006. Antioxidant activity of caffeoyl quinic acid derivatives from the roots of *Dipsacus asper* Wall. *J. Ethnopharmacol.* (108); pp.188–192.

Karakaya, S., 2004. Bioavailability of phenolic compounds. *Critical Rev. Food Sci. Nutr.* (44); pp.453–464.

Mahakunakorn, P., Tohda, M., Murakami, Y., Matsumoto, K., Watanabe, H., 2004. Antioxidant and free radical-scavenging activity of choto-san and its related constituents. *Biol. Pharm. Bull.* (27); pp.38–46.

Milioli, E. M., Cologni, P., Santos, C. C., Marcos, T. D., Yunes, V. M., Fernandes, M. S., Schoenfelder, T., Costa-Campos, L., 2007. Effect of acute administration of hydroalcohol extract of *Ilex paraguariensis* St Hilaire (Aquifoliaceae) in animal models of Parkinson's disease. *Phytother. Res.* (21); pp.771–776.

Mosimann, A. L., Wilhelm-Filho, D., da Silva E. L., 2006. Aqueous extract of *Ilex paraguariensis* attenuates the progression of atherosclerosis in cholesterol-fed rabbits. *Biofactors* (26); pp.59–70.

Nahar, L., Russell, W. R., Middleton, M., Shoeb, M., Sarker, S. D., 2005. Antioxidant phenylacetic acid derivatives from the seeds of *Ilex aquifolium*. *Acta Pharm.* (55); pp.187–193.

Nishimura, K., Fukuda, T., Miyase, T., Noguchi, H., Chen, X. M., 1999a. Activity-guided isolation of triterpenoid acyl CoA cholesteryl acyl transferase (ACAT) inhibitors from *Ilex kudincha*. *J. Nat. Prod.* (62); pp.1061–1064.

Nishimura, K., Miyase, T., Noguchi, H., 1999b. Triterpenoid saponins from *Ilex kudincha*. *J. Nat. Prod.* (62); pp.1128–1133.

Ouyang, M. A., Yang, C. R., Chen, Z. L., Wang, H. Q., 1996a. Triterpenes and triterpenoid glycosides from the leaves of *Ilex kudincha*. *Phytochemistry* (41); pp.871–877.

Ouyang, M. A., Wang, H. Q., Chen, Z. L., Yang, C. R., 1996b. Triterpenoid glycosides from *Ilex kudincha*. *Phytochemistry* (43); pp.443–445.

Ouyang, M. A., Yang, C. R., Wu, Z. J., 2001. Triterpenoid saponins from the leaves of *Ilex kudincha*. *J. Asian Nat. Prod. Res.* (3); pp.31–42.

Paganini Stein, F. L., Schmidt, B., Furlong, E. B., Souza-Soares, L. A., Soares, M. C., Vaz, M. R., Muccillo Baisch, A. L., 2005. Vascular responses to extractable fractions of *Ilex paraguariensis* in rats fed standard and high-cholesterol diets. *Biol. Res. Nurs.* (7); pp.146–156.

Pietta, P. G., 2000. Flavonoids as antioxidants. *J. Nat. Prod.* (63); pp.1035–1042.

Rice-Evans, C. A., Miller, N. J., Paganga, G., 1996. Structure-antioxidant relationships of flavonoids and phenolic acids. *Free Radic. Biol. Med.* (20); pp.933–956.

Schinella, G. R., Troiani, G., Davila, V., de Buschiazzo, P. M., Tournier, H. A., 2000. Antioxidant effects of an aqueous extract of *Ilex paraguariensis*. *Biochem Biophys Res Commun.* (269); pp.357–360.

Schinella, G., Fantinelli, J. C., Mosca S. M., 2005. Cardioprotective effects of *Ilex paraguariensis* extract: evidence for a nitric oxide-dependent mechanism. *Clin. Nutr.* (24); pp.360–366.

Smith, P. K., Krohn, R. I., Hermanson, G. T., Mallia, A. K., Gartner, F. H., Provenzano, M. D., Fujimoto, E. K., Goeke, N. M., Olson, B. J., Klenk, D. C., 1985. Measurement of protein using bicinchoninic acid. *Anal. Biochem.* (150); pp.76–85.

Tang, L., Jiang, Y., Chang, H. T., Zhao, M. B., Tu, P. F., Cui, J. R., Wang, R.Q., 2005. Triterpene saponins from the leaves of *Ilex kudingcha*. *J. Nat. Prod.* (68); pp.1169–1174.

Thuong, P. T., Kang, H. J., Na, M. K., Jin, W. Y., Youn, U. J., Seong, Y. H., Song, K. S., Min, B. S., Bae, K. H., 2007. Anti-oxidant constituents from *Sedum takesimense*. *Phytochemistry* (In press, Doi: 10.1016/j.phytochem.2007.05.031).

Valko, M., Leibfritz, D., Moncol, J., Cronin, J., Mazur, M., Telser, J., 2007. Free radicals and antioxidants in normal physiological functions and human disease. *Int. J. Biochem. Cell Biol.* (39); pp. 44–84.

Yang, X., Ding, Y., Sun, Z. H., Zhang, D. M., 2006. Studies on chemical constituents from *Ilex pubescens*. *J. Asian Nat. Prod. Res.* (8); pp.505–510.

Zhang, A. L., Ye, Q., Li, B. G., Qi, H. Y., Zhang, G. L., 2005. Phenolic and triterpene glycosides from the stems of *Ilex litseaefolia*. *J. Nat. Prod.* (68); pp.1531–1535.

*Chapter 32*

# Protein Tyrosine Phosphatase-1B Inhibitory Constituents from *Erythrina* spp.

**Long Cui[1], Zacharias Tanee Fomum[2], Phuong Thien Thuong[3] and Won Keun Oh[3]***

[1]*Korea Research Institute of Bioscience and Biotechnology (KRIBB), 52 Eoun-dong, Yuseong-gu, Daejeon 305-806, Korea*

[2]*Faculty of Science, University of Yaounde I, P.O. Box 812 Yaounde, Cameroon*

[3]*College of Pharmacy, Chosun University, 375 Seosuk-dong, Dong-gu, Gwangju 501-759, Korea*

**E-mail: wkoh@chosun.ac.kr*

## ABSTRACT

As part of an ongoing project searching for PTP1B inhibitors, we found that the stem bark and root bark of *Erythrina* spp., including *E. mildbraedii, E. addisoniae,* and *E. abyssinica,* had a potent PTP1B inhibitory activity. Our investigation on the PTP1B inhibitory principles from these plants has resulted in the isolation of a series of prenylated compounds, including 38 new (twelve from *E. addisoniae* 1–12, six from *E. mildbraedii* 13–18, and twenty from *E. abyssinica* 19–38) and 70 known compounds. Their structures were elucidated on the basis of physicochemical and spectroscopic analyses. In addition, the inhibitory effect on PTP1B of these compounds was evaluated in vitro. From the structure-activity relationships, it is suggested that the prenyl group plays an important role in enhancing inhibitory activity.

***Keywords**: Erythrina sp., Leguminosae, Prenylated flavonoid, PTP1B inhibitors, Diabetes.*

## 1.0 Introduction

The enzyme protein tyrosine phosphatase-1B (PTP1B) has been considered as a major negative regulator of insulin signalling (Johnson *et al.*, 2002; Bialy and Waldmann, 2005). As with the insulin-signaling pathway, the leptin signaling pathway can be also regulated by PTP1B. Therefore, it has been suggested that compounds that reduce PTP1B activity or expression levels can be used for treating type-2 diabetes and obesity (Johnson *et al.*, 2002; Bialy and Waldmann, 2005; Elchebly *et al.*, 1999). Although there have been a number of reports on the design and development of PTP1B inhibitors, new types of PTP1B inhibitors with suitable pharmacological properties remain to be discovered (Johnson *et al.*, 2002; Bialy and Waldmann, 2005). Since plant kingdom is a promising source for the development of new PTP1B inhibitors, we have undertaken the screening of plant extracts for PTP1B inhibitory activity.

As part of an ongoing project searching for PTP1B inhibitors, we found that the stem bark of *Erythrina* spp., including *E. mildbraedii*, *E. addisoniae*, and *E. abyssinica*, had a potent PTP1B inhibitory activity. The genus *Erythrina* of the family Leguminosae comprises over 110 species of trees and shrubs, those are widely distributed in tropical and subtropical regions, and representative species have been used in indigenous medicine (Oliver-Bever, 1986). The chemical constituents such as alkaloids, pterocarpans, flavonoids, and other benzofurans have been isolated from this genus and reported to possess a wide range of biological activities that include antioxidant, antimicrobial and estrogenic activities (Cui *et al.*, 2007). Despite a number of studies on the chemical constituents and biological activities of the genus *Erythrina*, there has been no report on its PTP1B inhibitory constituents. Our investigation on the PTP1B inhibitory principles from these plants has resulted in the isolation of a series of prenylated compounds, including 38 new (twelve from *E. addisoniae* 1–12, six from *E. mildbraedii* 13–18, and twenty from *E. abyssinica* 19–38) and 70 known compounds. In this seminar, we will discuss the isolation, structure elucidation, evaluation the inhibitory effect on PTP1B of these compounds and their structure-activity relationships.

## 2.0 Materials and Methods

### 2.1 General Experimental Procedure

Optical rotations were determined on a JASCO P-1020 polarimeter using a 100 mm glass microcell. UV spectra were taken in MeOH using a Shimadzu spectrophotometer. The CD spectrum was recorded in MeOH on a JASCO J-715 spectrometer. Nuclear magnetic resonance (1D–and 2D-NMR) spectra were obtained on Varian Unity Inova 400 MHz spectrometer with TMS as the internal standard. All accurate mass experiments were performed on a JMS-700 (Jeol, Japan) mass spectrometer. Column chromatography was conducted using silica gel 60 (40-63 and 63-200 μm particle size, Merck), and RP-18 (150 μm particle size, Merck). Precoated TLC silica gel 60 $F_{254}$ and RP-18 plates from Merck were used for thin-layer chromatography. HPLC were carried out using a Shimadzu System LC-10AD pump equipped with a model SPD-10Avp UV detector, and an Optima Pak® $C_{18}$ column (10×250 mm, 10 μm particle size, RS Tech, Korea) for semipreparative runs.

## 2.2 Plant Material

The root bark of *E. mildbraedii* was collected in July 1997 in Buea, Southwest Province, and the stem bark of *E. addisoniae* was collected in April 1996 in Etoug-Ebe, Yaounde, Cameroon Cameroon. The stem bark of *E. abyssinica* was collected in June 2005 in Mukono, Uganda. The botanical samples were identified and authenticated at the Cameroon National Herbarium (Yaounde, Cameroon) where voucher specimens have been deposited.

## 2.3 Extraction and Isolation

The dried stem bark or root bark of three samples were extracted separately with MeOH at room temperature. After the solvent was removed under reduced pressure, each residue was suspended in $H_2O$ and then partitioned with EtOAc and *n*-BuOH successively. Among the solvent fractions, all three EtOAc-soluble fractions were found to be the most active (> 80 per cent inhibition at 30 μg/ml). This fraction was first separated by silica gel column chromatography (63-200 μm particle size) using a gradient of hexane-EtOAc, or gradient of then $CHCl_3$-MeOH, to yield primary fractions. These fractions were further purified by reversed phase RP-18 column chromatography using a stepwise gradient of MeOH-$H_2O$, and/or by semipreparative HPLC [column RS Tech Optima Pak® $C_{18}$, mobile phase gradient of AcCN-$H_2O$, flow rate 2 mL/min; UV detection at 254 nm] resulted in the isolation of 38 new (1–38) and about 70 known compounds.

## 2.4 Assay for PTP1B Inhibitory Activity

PTP1B (human, recombinant) was purchased from BIOMOL® International LP (Plymouth Meeting, PA). The inhibitory effect of test compounds on enzyme activity was measured by a method described previously (Na *et al.*, 2006). To each 96 well (final volume: 100 μL) was added 2 mM *p*NPP and PTP1B (0.05 - 0.1 μg) in a buffer containing 50 mM citrate (pH 6.0), 0.1 M NaCl, 1 mM EDTA, and 1 mM dithiothreitol (DTT), with or without test compounds. Following incubation at 37 °C for 30 min, the reaction was terminated with 10 M NaOH. The amount of produced *p*-nitrophenol was estimated by measuring the absorbance at 405 nm. The nonenzymatic hydrolysis of 2 mM *p*NPP was corrected by measuring the increase in absorbance at 405 nm obtained in the absence of PTP1B enzyme.

# 3.0 Results and Discussion

Phytochemical study on EtOAc fraction of the MeOH extract of stem bark and root bark of three *Erythrina* spp. resulted in the isolation of a series phenolics and alkaloids. Their structures were identified by physicochemical ($[\alpha]_D$, mp) and spectroscopic analyses (UV, CD, NMR, MS, HR-MS), and by comparing their physical and spectroscopic data with reported values. The structures of new compounds (1–38) were identified as shown in Figure 32.1–32.4 (Bae *et al.*, 2006; Na *et al.*, 2006; Na *et al.*, 2007; Cui *et al.*, 2007a,b; Jull *et al.*, 2007; Cui *et al.*, 2007).

The isolates were examined for their inhibitory effect on enzyme PTP1B in vitro. The result showed that the compounds that possess prenyl group exhibited positive activity. Table 32.1 presents the $IC_{50}$ values of some most active compounds among the isolates.

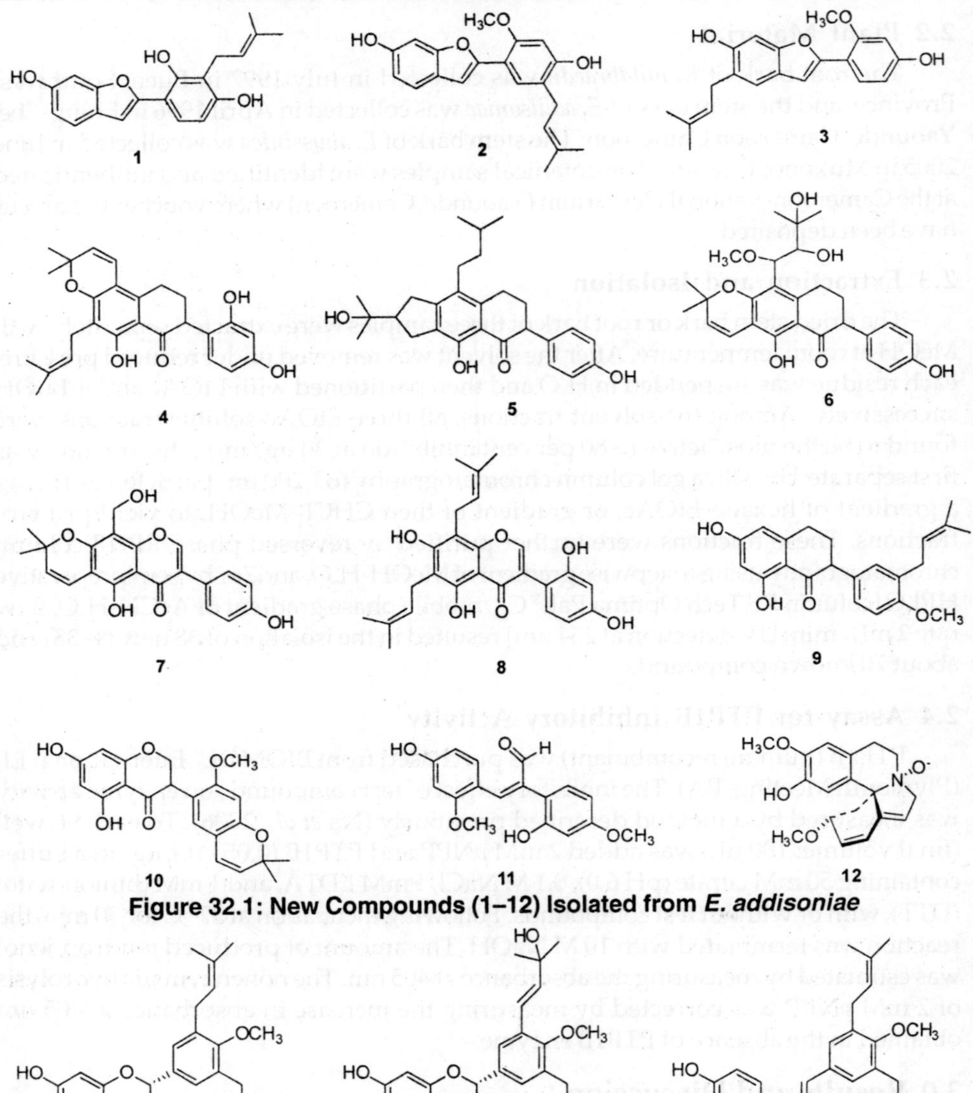


**Figure 32.1: New Compounds (1–12) Isolated from *E. addisoniae***

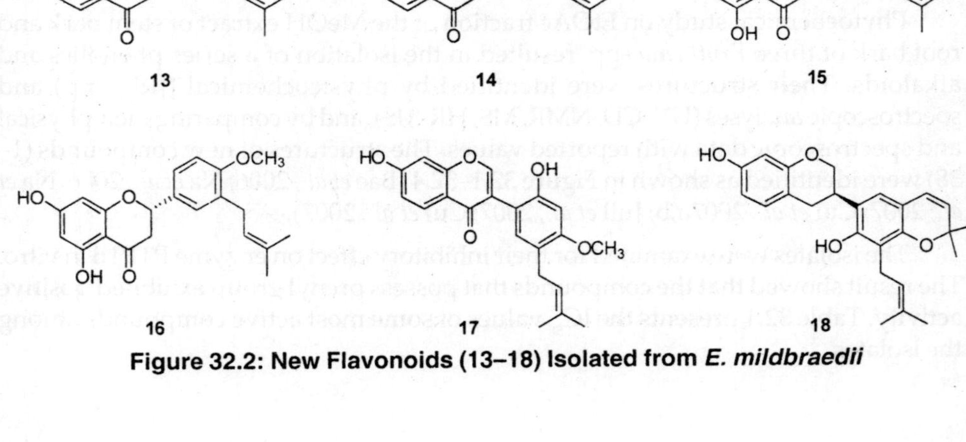


**Figure 32.2: New Flavonoids (13–18) Isolated from *E. mildbraedii***

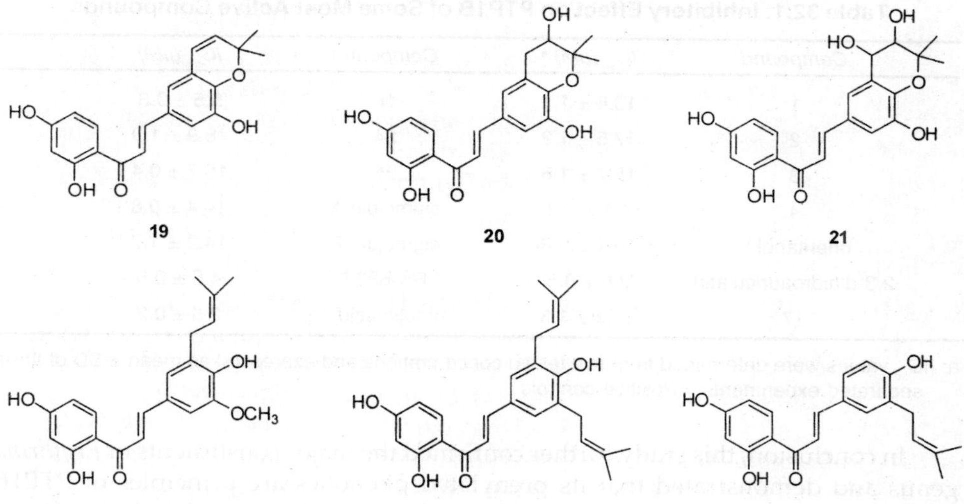


**Figure 32.3: New Chalcones (19–22) Isolated from *E. abyssinica***

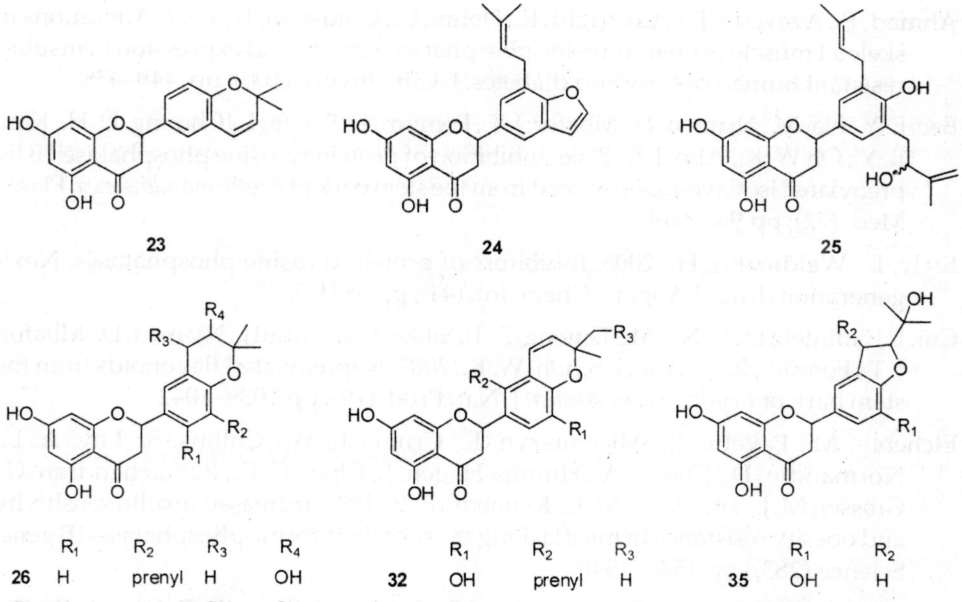


| | $R_1$ | $R_2$ | $R_3$ | $R_4$ |
|---|---|---|---|---|
| **26** | H | prenyl | H | OH |
| **27** | H | prenyl | OH | OH |
| **28** | H | H | OH | OH |
| **29** | prenyl | OH | OH | OH |
| **30** | H | $OCH_3$ | H | OH |
| **31** | H | OH | =O | H |

| | $R_1$ | $R_2$ | $R_3$ |
|---|---|---|---|
| **32** | OH | prenyl | H |
| **33** | OH | H | OH |
| **34** | $OCH_3$ | H | OH |

| | $R_1$ | $R_2$ |
|---|---|---|
| **35** | OH | H |
| **36** | $OCH_3$ | H |
| **37** | prenyl | H |
| **38** | prenyl | OH |

**Figure 32.4: New Flavanones (23–38) Isolated from *E. abyssinica***

**Table 32.1: Inhibitory Effect on PTP1B of Some Most Active Compounds**

| *Compound* | *$IC_{50}$ (μM)* [a] | *Compound* | *$IC_{50}$ (μM)* |
|---|---|---|---|
| 1 | 13.6 ± 1.1 | 18 | 5.5 ± 0.3 |
| 2 | 17.5 ± 1.2 | 24 | 18.9 ± 1.9 |
| 3 | 15.7 ± 1.6 | 25 | 15.7 ± 0.4 |
| 4 | 4.1 ± 0.2 | sigmoidin A | 14.4 ± 0.8 |
| orientanol E | 10.1 ± 0.3 | sigmoidin F | 14.2 ± 1.7 |
| 2,3-dihidroauriculatin | 2.6 ± 0.5 | RK-682 [b] | 4.5 ± 0.5 |
| 17 | 21.3 ± 1.3 | ursolic acid [b] | 2.5 ± 0.2 |

a: $IC_{50}$ values were determined from five tested concentrations and expressed as mean ± SD of three separated experiments; [b] Positive controls

In conclusion, this study further confirmed the major constituents of *Erythrina* genus and demonstrated that its prenylated phenolics are principles of PTP1B inhibitors. The result suggests that *Erythrina* plants could be considered as a natural source for the development of anti-diabetes drug.

## References

Ahmad, F., Azevedo, J. J., Cortright, R., Dohm, G., Goldstein, B., 1997. Alterations in skeletal muscle protein-tyrosine phosphatase activity and expression in insulin-resistant human obesity and diabetes. J. Clin. Invest. (100); pp. 449–458.

Bae, E. Y., Na, M., Njamen, D., Mbafor, J. T., Fomum, Z. T., Cui, L., Choung, D. H., Kim, B. Y., Oh W. K., Ahn, J. S., 2006. Inhibition of protein tyrosine phosphatase 1B by prenylated isoflavonoids isolated from the stem bark of *Erythrina addisonea*. Planta Med. (72); pp.945–948.

Bialy, L., Waldmann, H., 2005. Inhibitors of protein tyrosine phosphatases: Next-generation drugs? Angew. Chem. Int. (44); pp.3814-3839.

Cui, L., Ndinteh, D. T., Na, M., Thuong, P. T., Silike-Muruumu, J., Njamen, D., Mbafor, J. T., Fomum, Z. T., Ahn, J. S., Oh, W. K., 2007. Isoprenylated flavonoids from the stem bark of *Erythrina abyssinica*. J. Nat. Prod. (70); pp.1039–1042.

Elchebly, M., Payette, P., Michaliszyn, E., Cromlish, W., Collins, S., Loy, A. L., Normandin, D., Cheng, A., Himms-Hagen, J., Chan, C. C., Ramachandran, C., Gresser, M. J., Tremblay, M. L., Kennedy, B. P., 1999. Increased insulin sensitivity and obesity resistance in mice lacking the protein tyrosine phosphatase-1B gene. Science (283); pp.1544–1548.

Jang, J., Na, M., Thuong, P. T., Njamen, D., Mbafor, J. T., Fomum, Z. T., Woo, E. R., Oh, W. K., 2007. Prenylated flavonoids with PTP1B inhibitory activity from the root bark of *Erythrina mildbraedii*. Chem. Pharm. Bull. In press.

Johnson, T. O., Ermolieff, J., Jirousek, M. R., 2002. Protein tyrosine phosphates 1B inhibitors for diabetes. Nat. Rev. Drug. Discov. (1); pp.696–709.

Na, M., Jang, J., Njamen, D., Mbafor, J. T., Fomum, Z. T., Kim, B. Y., Oh, W. K., Ahn, J. S., 2006. Protein tyrosine phosphatase-1B inhibitory activity of isoprenylated flavonoids isolated from *Erythrina mildbraedii*. J. Nat. Prod. (69); pp.1572–1576.

Na, M., Hoang, D. M., Njamen, D., Mbafor, J. T., Fomum, Z. T., Thuong, P. T., Ahn, J. S., Oh, W. K., 2007. Inhibitory effect of 2-arylbenzofurans from *Erythrina addisoniae* on protein tyrosine phosphatase-1B. Bioorg. Med. Chem. Lett. (17); pp.3868–3871.

Oliver-Bever, B., 1986. Medicinal plants in tropical West Africa. Cambridge University Press, New York, USA.

## Chapter 33

# Management of Difficult Fistula in Ano by Ksharasutra (Chemical Seton)

***Manoranjan Sahu***

*Department of Shalya Tantra, Institute of Medical Sciences,*
*Banaras Hindu University, Varanasi – 5, UP, India*
*E-mail: msahuvns@gmail.com*

## ABSTRACT

Anal fistula is a tract, which communicates with the anal canal or rectum by means of an internal opening and usually is in continuity with one or more external opening in the perianal, perineal or ischiorectal areas commonly resulted after suppuration of anal gland. Though numerous techniques of surgery have been laid down, it is of great importance to note that all these procedures are associated with a dishonourable repute of causing recurrence of the disease, faecal incontinence and anal stricture. The treatment sometime results in complications far severe than the disease it self. There fore the disease posses a great challenge to both the patients as well as to the surgeons. The disease has been described in Ayurveda under the heading of *Bhagandara* and has been consider one of the most difficult diseases to cure. For the treatment of this disease an alternative minimal invasive procedure has been described in the classics of Ayurveda, which is known as *Ksharasutra* therapy, was re-established by the Department of Shalya Tantra in Banaras Hindu University. The therapy is in practice since 1964 and over 20,000 patients have been treated successfully by this method of treatment. The therapy is also found highly effective even in recurrent and difficult types of Fistula in ano.

***Keywords:*** *Difficult fistula in ano, Recurrence, Incontinence, Ksharsutra therapy, Effective, Safe.*

## 1.0 Introduction

Among diseases of ano rectal region fistula in ano is one of the commonest ailment associated with persistent physical discomfort along with psychological stress due to chronicity of the disease and limited treatment modalities with high failure rates. "Fistula" term is derived from a Latin word meaning 'pipe'. In medical terminology it implies a chronic granulating tract connecting two epithelial surfaces. In Ayurvedic classics the diseased is named as *Bhagandara*. It is named so as it causes *"darana" i.e.,* destruction of *bhaga pradesha* (perineal and perianal region). Sushruta (1500-1000 BC), the father of ancient Indian surgery, for the first time has described in detail the causative factors, signs and symptoms, classification and management of *bhagandara* (fistula in ano). Hippocrates tried apolinose (a plain thread) in cases of fistula in ano. Sainio and Helsinki provided data in favour of male predominance of the disease. Raymond J. Jackman (1944) and J.E. Dumphy (1955) analysed their treated cases and shown very high recurrence rates after surgical intervention.

The disease was widely prevalent and numerous concoctions of treatment were tried for its management. However, none of them could provide solace to the suffering humankind. Even today in spite of advancement in the field of surgery still the disease poses a challenge to the surgeons. The complications like faecal incontinence, stricture etc. following treatments are sometimes far more severe than the disease itself.

The high recurrence rate and many other serious complications of treatment stimulated for search of an alternative method of treatment and researchers attracted towards *ksharasutra* treatment, an alternative minimal invasive procedure described in Ayurveda. The great task to rediscover the old forgotten legacy and bring back this treatment modality into practice was done by Dr P.S. Shankaran and Prof. P.J. Deshpande in the Department of Shalya Tantra, Banaras Hindu University in the year 1964. More than 20,000 patients have been treated successfully by this noble method of treatment till date, with a very high success rate (97 per cent) even in difficult and failure cases after surgery.

## 2.0 Preparation of Ksharsutra

For preparation of Ksharsutra (chemical seton) the following raw materials are needed:

1. Guggulu–*Commiphora mukul* (Hook ex Stocks) resin extracted in ethyl alcohol
2. Apamarga (*Achyranthes aspera*) kshara (caustic material) anhydrous powder prepared by burning of the whole plant.
3. Fine powder of haridra (*Curcuma longa*)
4. Barbour's surgical thread No. 20.

### 2.1 Preparation of Apamarg Kshar

The whole plant (from root to seeds) of Apamarga *(Achyranthes aspera)* was collected during summer, washed well to remove dust, mud etc., and was dried under shade. Once completely dry, the plants were burnt in a clean place to obtain greyish ash. Once cool, the ash was stored in clean containers. Ash was dissolved in distilled water in 1:6 ratios and allowed to stay overnight. After 24 hours the content was filtered through double *Wartman's* filter paper and the collected clear filtrated, was carefully boiled over mild heat. After complete evaporation of water the dried caustic material (*Apamarg Kshar*) was collected and stored in airtight glass container for preparation of Ksharsutra.

For preparation of Ksharsutra surgical thread no 20 was spreaded over a specially designed hanger for application of various contents of Ksharsutra. Applications of various ingredients were made as follows:

- First 11 coatings of Guggulu
- Followed by 7 coatings of Guggulu and *Apamarga kshara*
- Followed by 3 coatings of Guggulu and *Haridra*
- Average length of each thread = 32.07± 0.06 cm
- Average thickness of each thread = 0.97± 0.06 mm
- Average weight of each thread = 113.63±1.70 mg
- Amount of Guggulu smeared on each thread after 11 coatings = 35.46 mg

The pH of the final Guggulu based ksharasutra was 9.188, at 26.8ºC, using 100 ml of double distilled water.

## 3.0 Clinical Study

Patients attending to anorectal clinic of Sir Sunderlal Hospital between August 2004 and December 2005 with symptoms of fistula in ano were taken in the study. 100 cases of fistula in ano, only of cryptoglandular origin were selected for study. All

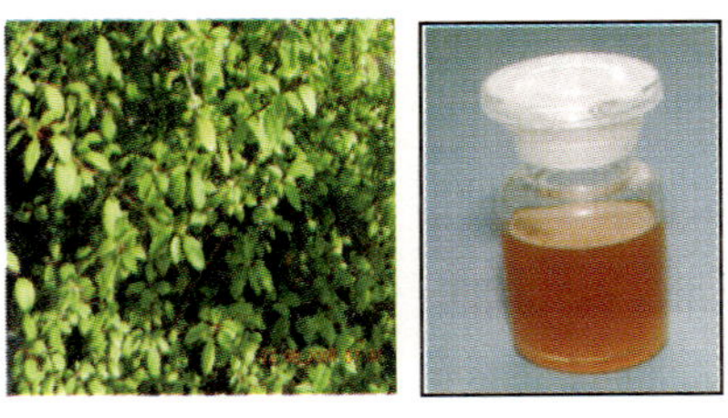

***Commiphora mukul* and Resin Extracted in Ethyl Alcohol**

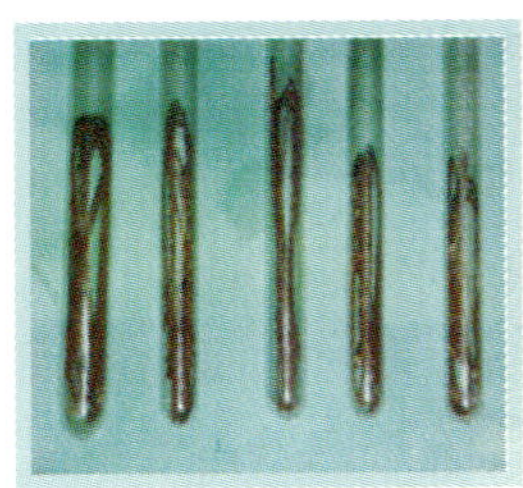

**Kshar Sutra**

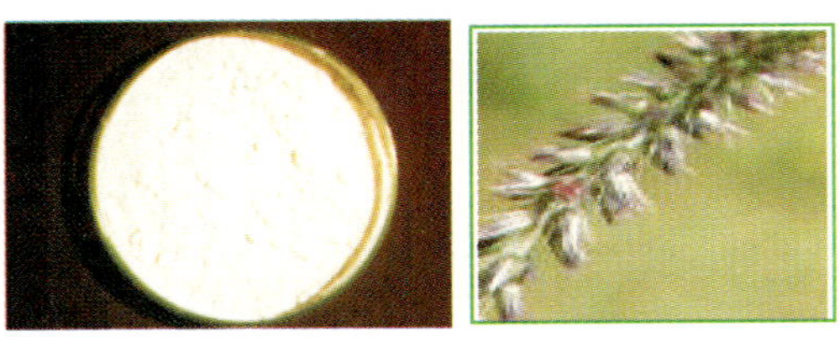

**Alkaline Ash of *Achyranthes aspera***

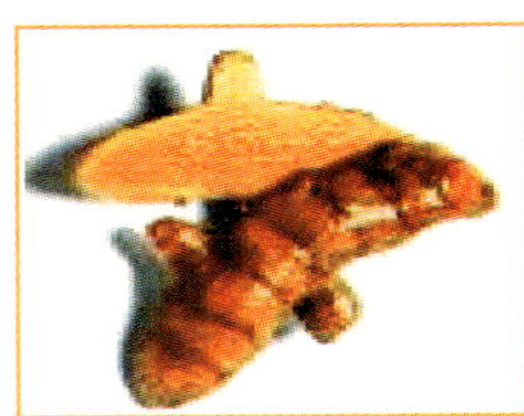

**Dry Powder of *Curcuma longa***

**Figure 33.1: Raw Material Required for Preparation of Kshar Sutra and Kshar Sutra Sealed in Glass Tube**

had history of previous perianal suppuration drained either surgically or spontaneously.

### 3.1 Inclusion Criteria

All the patients included in this study were high anal types with or without abscess cavity. High transphincteric, multiple track and high horseshoe fistula were also included in this study.

### 3.2 Exclusion Criteria

Patients with uncontrolled diabetes mellitus, tuberculosis, malignancy, HIV, gross anaemia and hypo proteinemia were excluded from this study.

### 3.3 Procedure of Ksharsutra Application

Prior to application of Ksharsutra all the patients were thoroughly examined and investigated. The history and findings were recorded in a specially designed case record sheet. Bowel and local part preparation of the patients were done prior to application of kshar sutra. Once prepared, the patient was placed in lithotomy position comfortably. Patient was reassured and the procedure was explained. The perianal skin was prepared with antiseptic solutions. Once the patient was comfortable and cooperative, gloved, lubricated index finger was inserted into the anal canal and the findings were rechecked. Local anaesthesia in the form of Surface or Infiltration was given as per the requirement of the patient. Then a suitable probe was selected and introduced into the external opening of the tract and carefully advanced along the path of least resistance. The finger in the anal canal supported the advancement of the probe towards the internal opening. The probe was advanced, brought out of the internal opening and then carefully manipulated to come outside the anal canal. Initially a suitable length of plain thread was placed in the eye of the probe and the probe was pulled out in order to position the thread in the tract. The two ends of the thread were tied loosely outside the anal orifice. This procedure is termed the "primary threading." In children and sensitive patients the process requires general anaesthesia.

### 3.4 Replacement of Ksharsutra

New one on weekly interval replaced the Kshar sutra that was already placed in the fistulous tract. New ksharasutra was tied to the lateral side of the knot (of old thread), the thread was cut between the knot and clipped by artery forceps, the artery forceps was gently pulled out along with the old thread such that the thread came out leaving behind the new ksharasutra the fistulous track. The old thread was cut and the ends of the new ksharasutra were tied firmly outside the anal orifice. This procedure of change of the thread was done by *"Rail-Road technique"*.

At each changing of the thread, the length of the previously changed thread was measured and recorded in the Performa. This provides information regarding the amount of tissue already excised and the length of the tract that still needs to be excised.

## 3.5 Adjuvant Therapies, Diet and Precautions

1. *Laxatives*: like Isapgool husk or other suitable Ayurvedic preparations were advised to the patients during the course of treatment.
2. *Anu taila vasti*: enema of medicated oil also used 15 to 20 minutes before defecation to minimize pain and inflammation.
3. Sitz bath was advised routinely, twice daily after defecation, to maintain local hygiene and reduce pain and inflammation.
4. *Jatyadi ghrita(Wound healing ointment)*: For local application, over the wound (once the fistulous track was completely excised or cut through)–enhanced early healing of the wound.
5. *Analgesics*: Oral analgesics and anti-inflammatory drugs are required in some cases to control pain.
6. Patient was advised to do his normal routine work but was advised against riding vehicles or sitting on hard surfaces for long periods of time.
7. *Diet*: Green leafy vegetables, nutritious and easy digestible food were advised where as non-vegetarian, fried and spicy foods to be avoided.

## 3.6 Follow Up

Once the tract was completely excised or "cut through", the patient was advised to visit the clinic once every month for 3 months to recheck the status of the excised area or wound. Then onwards patient was advised to visit once in 3 months for two times to assess the untoward effects of treatment like faecal incontinence (if present).

The incontinence was assessed based on the St. Mark's Continence Scoring System (Table 33.1)

**Table 33.1**

| *Observation* | *Never* | *Rarely (< once a month)* | *Sometime (< Once a week)* | *Usually (< Once a day)* | *Always/ Daily* |
|---|---|---|---|---|---|
| Leakage of solid stool | 0 | 1 | 2 | 3 | 4 |
| Leakage of liquid stool | 0 | 1 | 2 | 3 | 4 |
| Leakage of flatus | 0 | 1 | 2 | 3 | 4 |
| Lifestyle alteration because of faecal incontinence | 0 | 1 | 2 | 3 | 4 |

| *Observations* | *No* | *Yes* |
|---|---|---|
| Need to wear a pad/plug or change underwear because of soiling | 0 | 2 |
| Need to take constipating medicines | 0 | 2 |
| Inability to defer for < 15 minutes | 0 | 4 |
| Total score | 24 | |

## 4.0 Observations

In the study majority of the cases were males (84 per cent) as compared to females (16 per cent) and were from 20-60 years age group with peak incidence in 31-40 years. Study showed 52.50 per cent patients belonged to the rural areas and 47.50 per cent belonged to urban areas. It was observed that 66 per cent patients were non-vegetarians and 34 per cent of the patients were vegetarians and majority of the patients of fistula in ano led a sedentary life, among whom the patients belonging to the business community were the largest (30.00 per cent) followed by those doing various office jobs (21.67 per cent). Socio economic status of these patients suggested that 50 per cent patients belonged to the middle class families followed by 41 per cent to poor class, whereas 9 per cent patients were from upper class. Chronicity of the disease varied from 1week to 15 years. Majority of the patients had fistula in ano with a chronicity ranging from 1 to 3 years (64 per cent). Patients having a history of chronicity of greater than 3 years were in a minority. Majority of the tracts of fistula in ano in the study had a length ranging between 5.1-10 cm (48.8 per cent) and only (3.2 per cent) of cases had a tract length greater than 15 cm. About 25.8 per cent patients were operated elsewhere before they came for Kshar sutra therapy, where as rest 74.2 per cent patients attended as a primary case of fistula in ano. Among the operated cases it was observed that majority of the cases (64.52 per cent) had undergone surgery once before coming for Kshar sutra treatment. 24.19 per cent of the patients had undergone surgery twice and 11.29 per cent of the patients had undergone surgery more than twice for the same tract of fistula, elsewhere.

## 5.0 Response of Therapy

Present study showed that Kshar sutra therapy is highly effective in the treatment of difficult and recurrent fistulae with a success rate of 98 percent. The patients were meticulously followed up for regarding failure of treatment in the form of recurrence of the diseases or causation of any form of incontinence for a period of one year. After one year of follow up the rate of recurrence rate was only 2 per cent and none of the patients developed incontinence in this study. The cure rate by this method of treatment is very high in comparison to conventional surgery.

## 6.0 Conclusion

The therapy has many advantages over the conventional therapy surgery. It is an ambulatory form of treatment does not require hospitalisation. During the course of treatment patient can continue his or her routine work therefore the source of income is not affected. The treatment was well tolerated by almost all the patients and rate of recurrence is very negligible. One of the major disadvantages of surgery in high fistula in ano is that it invariably damages the muscles around the anal canal leading to anal incontinence but in Ksharasutra therapy chance of incontinence is very negligible and does not cause extensive damage of the tissue around the anal canal. The therapy is also suitable for those patients of fistula in ano who are other wise unsuitable or high risk for surgery like old age and cardiac patients etc. The cost of treatment is also very less and does not require high-tech sophisticated equipments.

This method of treatment is very much popular in India and well accepted to both patients as well as surgeons.

## References

Ammon, H. P., Wahl, M. A., 1991. Pharmacology of Curcuma longa, Planta Med.; pp. 57.

Banerjee, A., Nigam, S.S., 1977. Antibacterial efficacy of the essential oil derived from the various species of the genus–Curcuma linn. J of Res in Ind Med Yoga and H (XII).

Belliveau, P., Thompson, J.P., Parks, AG, 1983. Fistula in ano: A manometric study. Dis Colon Rectum (26): pp. 152-4.

Datta, C., Bhagandara, A., Chakradatta, 1959. Sri Laxmi Venkateshwara steam press, Bombay (2): pp. 206-208.

Deshpande, P.J. and Sharma, K.R., 1973. Treatment of fistula-in-ano by a new technique, review and follow up of 200 cases. Am J Proctol (24): pp. 49.

Deshpande, P.J. and Sharma, K.R., 1976. Successful nonoperative treatment of high rectal fistula. Am J Proctol (39).

Goligher, J., 1984. Surgery of the anus, rectum and conlon. Baillier Tindall, London (5): pp. 181.

Goligher, J., 1900. Surgery of the anus, Rectum and Colon. London: Longmans (5).

Kumar, P., *et al.*, 1998. Study of *Guggulu based kshara sutra* in the management of *bhagandara* (fistula in ano). Thesis submitted for M.S (Shalyatantra), Dept. of Shalya Shalakya, IMS, and BHU.

Sharma, A., Mehta, M., Handa, S.S. *et al*. Standardization of kshara sutra–yurvedic medicated thread used in the management of fistula in ano, CMR Centre for Advanced Pharmacological Research on Traditional Remedies.

Sushruta; Nidana, Sharira, Chikitsa sthana, 1997. Sushruta Samhita with Nibandha sangraha vyakya of Dalhana and Nyaya chandrika Panjika of Gayadasacharya, Chowkhamba Orientalia, Varanasi. 6th Edition.

Yadav, A.K., *et al.*, 1999. Study of *Guggulu based kshara sutra* in the management of high anal fistula. Thesis submitted for M.S (Shalyatantra), Dept. of Shalya Shalakya, IMS, and BHU.

## Chapter 34

# Studies on Breast Cancer in Relation to Prakriti (Constitution)

**Mridula Singh[1]* and G.C. Prasad[2]**

[1]*Consultant, Swami Harshankaranand Hospital and Research Centre, Sunderpur, Varanasi – 221005, India*

[2]*Former Head, Department of Shalya Tantra, IMS, BHU, Varanasi – 221005, India*

**E-mail: msinghvns@gmail.com*

## ABSTRACT

Cancer in general and breast cancer in particular is one of the serious concerns in heath care. The cause of this disease is still unknown and management is concentrated mainly by improving the result of local treatment through detection of the disease while it is still localized. As no cure of the disease is yet known, risk factors like age, parity, diet, benign breast diseases etc. has been emphasized so that early detection is possible for a better survival. In recent times data from several human epidemiological studies suggest positive correlation with relative body size and weight with high breast cancer incidence. The above fundamental observations indicate that there is relationship between the physical structure the body with breast cancer incidence and prognosis. Not only the physical characters but also mental status is important in development, progress and prognosis of this disease.

In Ayurveda physical and mental constitution has been described under the heading of *Prakriti*, occupies a special position as it has been considered one of the important factors involved in initiation and progress of diseases including breast cancer. Due to wide involvement of human constitution (*Prakriti*) in health and different stages of disease the relation of *Prakriti* is found important and a clinical study was carried out to study the constitution of breast cancer patients to evaluate the following:

(*i*) The risk of breast cancer and its association with human constitution (*Prakriti*) (*ii*) Variation of clinical presentation and its relation with constitution (*Prakriti*)

(*iii*) The course of breast cancer and its relation with constitution (*Prakriti*)

(*iv*) Response of treatment in different human constitution (*Prakriti*)

***Keywords:*** *Prakriti (Human constitution), Breast cancer, Risk factor.*

## 1.0 Introduction

The word *Prakriti* has been widely applied in different *Darshanas* and many other Hindu classics including Ayurveda with the meaning of–making, placing and original or natural form. It has been defined as a state of body and mind, which is unchangeable and not harmful to the individual concern through out the life, develops at the time of fertilization. It denotes the constitution of a person. The constitution or the Prakriti of a person has been analyzed from different angle like body built, natural and acquire character, mental temperaments, attitudes and orientations, urges and inclination, capacity and weakness, liking and disliking etc. Ayurveda is based on humeral theory. According to Ayurveda three humours like *Vata, Pitta* and *Kapha* are responsible for state of health and disease. Similarly predominance of any one of these above humours is responsible for development three different types of somatic and psychic *Prakriti* or constitutions *viz. Vata Prakriti, Pitta Prakriti* and *Kapha Prakriti.* In ancient classics various physical and mental characters have been described to determine these constitutions as mentioned in Table 34.1. *Prakriti* has been considered intimately linked with health and disease process and also responsible for individual differences.

**Table 34.1: Characters of Different *Prakriti* as Described in Ayurveda**

| *Sl.No.* | *Qualities* | *Vata* | *Pitta* | *Kapha* |
|---|---|---|---|---|
| 1. | Conscience | Wavering conscience, lack of conscience | Follows to some extent dictates of his conscience | Follows the dictates of his conscience |
| 2. | Control over mind | No control over mind | Fairly good control | Good control |
| 3. | Mind | Weak mind | Moderately strong mind | Strong mind with good qualities |
| 4. | Forgiving nature | Poor | Moderate | Forgiving nature |
| 5. | Tolerance | Poor | Moderate | Well Tolerant |
| 6. | Friendship | Has very few friends, friendship does not last long | Very few friends | Many friends, lasting friendship |
| 7. | Intellect | Wavering intellect, intellect not well organized | Intelligent, brilliant | Good intellect |
| 8. | Memory | Poor memory wavering memory | Fair | Good memory |

*Contd...*

**Table 34.1–Contd...**

| *Sl.No.* | *Qualities* | *Vata* | *Pitta* | *Kapha* |
|---|---|---|---|---|
| 9. | Concentration | Unsteady, inability to concentrate | Fairly steady, can concentrate fairly well | Steady mind, good concentration |
| 10. | Grasping power | Quick grasping power | Moderate | Takes long time to grasp |
| 11 | Knowledge | Poor | Moderate | Learned |
| 12. | Attention | Absent | Attentive on one subject at a time | Simultaneously attentive every where |
| 13. | Truthful-ness | Very less | Less | Truthful, trustworthy |
| 14. | Quarrel-some | Quarrelsome | Quarrelsome | Calm |
| 15. | Gratitude | Ungrateful | Often grateful | Grateful |
| 16. | Kindness | Harsh to people | Kind only to friendly people | Kind |
| 17. | Helping attitude | Less | Helping those who ask for help | Helping nature |
| 18. | Desires and likes | Music, laughter, hunting, arts, hot and humid climate, massage | Flowers, application of pastes, cold environment | Scientific, philosophical literature, sleep, music, warm environment, warm food items |
| 19. | Irritability | Very quickly excited | Quickly excited | Calm, not crying excessively even in infancy |
| 20. | Anger | Angry quickly | Gets angry quickly, gets angry in excess | Does not get angry quickly, and anger is of mild degree, but lasts log |
| 21. | Greed | Greedy | Greedy | Not greedy even during childhood |
| 22. | Fear | Fearful | Frightened quickly, but is not coved down by fear | Minimum |
| 23. | Moods | Changing moods | Gets happy quickly, changing moods | Steady moods, in general happy |
| 24. | Love | Falls a prey to sex instinct | Moderate control over sex urge | Fair control over sex urge |
| 25. | Ladies | Disliked by ladies | Not appreciated by ladies | Liked by ladies |
| 26. | Speech | Incoherent speech, talkative | Insulting speech | Does not use harsh language, consistent and thoughtful speech |
| 27. | Courage | | Courageous | |
| 28. | Brave | | Brave | |
| 29. | Ability to tolerate exertion | Can hardly tolerate exertion | Cannot tolerate mental or physical exertion | Tolerates both physical and mental strain |

*Contd...*

**Table 34.1–Contd...**

| *Sl.No.* | *Qualities* | *Vata* | *Pitta* | *Kapha* |
|---|---|---|---|---|
| 30. | Activities | Unsteady and fast movements, gait is quick and fast, likes to wander | | Slow movements, slow activity, steady, heavy |
| 31. | Energy | Moderate | Moderate | Energetic |
| 32. | Life span | Short life span | Medium | Long life |
| 33. | Built | Tall thin and poorly built, parts of the body not well placed, dry rough and weak | Delicate, medium built, flabby, medium strength and soft | Large, well built, steady, strong, proportionate and well placed parts of the body |
| 34. | Strength | Weak | Moderate | Strong |
| 35. | General appearance | Not beautiful, dry and emaciated | | Pleasant appearance |
| 36. | Voice | Rough, high pitched, unclear, monotonous, weak, low tones and fast speech | Clear, high pitched | Deep, pleasant, resonating |
| 37. | Colour | Dark | White complexion, with reddish or yellowish tinge | Fair colour (white complexion) |
| 38. | Face | Rough | Delicate | Delicate and pleasing |
| 39. | Limbs | Thin rough, well differentiated, not well placed in relation to each other | Red palms and soles | Long unctuous smooth limbs |
| 40. | Veins, tendons and lines on soles | Prominent, unclear | Not prominent | Well covered |
| 41. | Weight | Light | Medium | Heavy |
| 42. | Joint | Not well placed | Soft loose ligaments of joints | Strong and well organized ligaments and joints, joints deep and well covered |
| 43. | Skin | Dry, rough, thin cracked, prominent veins | Soft, thin, warm, wrinkled skin with pink, reddish, numerous moles and skin eruptions | Sort luster, wet and cold skin |
| 44. | Hair | Dry, rough, smoky, thin and cracked hair, less in number and cracked | Early greying of hair, baldness, pinkish or reddish, soft and thin hair and less in number | Strong, dark, long, dark blue, thick growth of good quality |
| 45. | Nails | Dry, small, rough, discoloured and cracked nails | Pinkish | Soft, oily, smooth, white and steady |

*Contd...*

**Table 34.1–Contd...**

| Sl.No. Qualities | Vata | Pitta | Kapha |
|---|---|---|---|
| 46. Appetite | Irregular, eating small quantities frequently | Good, Eating large quantity of food, eating frequently | Less appetite |
| 47. Thirst | Thirsty | Thirsty | Less Thirsty |
| 48. Sleep | Less, disturbed, wakeful | Moderate sleep | Sleepy, loves sleep |
| 49. Pulse | Thready, fast | Warm and fast | Slow and heaving |
| 50. Bowels | Constipation | Large quantity of stool and tendency for diarrhoea | Normal |
| 51. Perspiration | Less | Excessive | Less |
| 52. Menstrual flow | Scanty and dark flow | Profuse, red and foul smelling, foul smell of body, sweat and mouth also | Moderate flow |

The present clinical study was carried out in S.S. hospital; BHU and 100 cases were included in this study. In each case detail history like age, sex, religion, dietary habit, occupation, socio economic status and chief complains were recorded. Menstrual and reproductive history was also recorded carefully.

### Criteria of Inclusion

Only histopathologically confirmed cases of breast cancer were included in this study.

### Determination of *Prakriti*

For determination of *Prakriti* or individual constitution patients were examined or interrogated on the basis of 52 points parameters of determination of Prakriti as mentioned in Table 34.1. The findings were recorded in a specially designed Performa. Scoring of the characters was made and final determination of *Prakriti* was done after calculating highest score characters related to a particular *Prakriti*.

## 2.0 Observation

All the patients of breast cancer were assessed care fully as per the Table 34.1 and *Prakriti* of every patient was recorded. It was observed that among the 100 patients 69 per cent patients belong to *Kaphaja Prakriti* where as 22 per cent belong to *Pittaja Prakriti* and only 9 per cent belong to *Vataja Prakriti*. The clinical presentation of breast cancer patient and there relation with *Prakriti* was also recorded (Table 34.2) and it was found that breast mass is the common most clinical presentation of breast caner followed by palpable auxiliary lymph node. Mastalgia is a late clinical presentation is more frequent among *Vataja Prakriti* patients. It may be one of the reasons that *Vataja Prakriti* patients report early to hospital.

**Table 34.2: Clinical Presentation of Breast Cancer in Relation to *Prakriti***

| Sl.No. | Clinical Presentation | No of Patients | Prakriti | | |
|---|---|---|---|---|---|
| | | | Vataja | Pittaja | Kaphaja |
| 1. | Breast lump | 98 | 9 | 22 | 67 |
| 2. | Palpable auxiliary lymph node | 71 | 9 | 15 | 47 |
| 3. | Mastalgia | 53 | 7 | 10 | 36 |
| 4. | Change in nipple character | 45 | 5 | 1 | 29 |
| 5. | Dimple over breast | 23 | 4 | 2 | 47 |
| 6. | Discharge | 12 | 1 | 1 | 10 |
| 7. | Ulcer | 8 | 0 | 2 | 6 |
| 8. | Lymph edema of arm | 7 | 1 | 1 | 5 |
| 9. | Miscellaneous | 18 | 3 | 4 | 11 |

The duration of illness and their relation with *Prakriti* was studied and it was observed that majority of the patients attended hospital after 4 to 6 months of self detection of the disease and only a few (13 per cent) came for treatment within 3 months of onset of breast lump. It was found that majority of *Vataja Prakriti* patients (78 per cent) consulted a doctor within 6 months of self detection of the disease in compare to 46 per cent in *Kaphaja Prakriti* patients and 47 per cent in *Pittaja Prakriti* patients. *Vataja Prakriti* patients by virtue of their poor tolerance to pain and discomfort they attended early to hospital.

Two third of the patients came for treatment at a very advance stage of breast cancer and so far no case of breast cancer attended at the early stage of the disease *i.e.* in stage I. It was found that 12 per cent of breast cancer came in a very late stage of the disease that is in stage IV. It was further observed that the progress of the disease was highest in *Kaphaja Prakriti* patients followed by *Pittaja Prakriti* and *Vataja Prakriti* patients. The response of therapy and five-year survival of breast cancer patients were studied according to their constitution. It was observed that patients who are treated by surgery + chemotherapy + radiation were survived longer than who are treated only by surgery + chemotherapy or Surgery + radiation. The response of therapy in relation to *Prakriti* suggests that the highest percent of survival was observed in *Vataja Prakriti* patients (43 per cent) in comparison to *Kaphaja* (34 per cent) and *Pittaja Prakriti* (23 per cent) patients.

Aetiopathogesis of breast cancer and its management is a global scientific interest because of its high incidence, mortality and morbidity. Though in our country breast cancer incidence is relatively low but it is the second commonest cause of death in female after uterine cancer. The over all result of present available treatment is not very encouraging in our country because most of the patients attend hospital at a very late stage of disease. Late reporting of the disease is a known factor as the disease is chronic and painless in nature. In our country late reporting of disease is still more as major part of our population lives in rural area where health services are poor. Other factors for late reporting are less education, fear of loss of feminity and low socio economical condition. Study suggested that late reporting of the disease is very common and only 15 per cent of the patients attended for medical advice when the disease is localized.

There is a growing interest that mental and physical characters linked with the development of cancer. The inborn physical and mental character has been described in Ayurveda under the heading of *Prakriti*. The incidence of different types of cancer like leukaemia and lymphoma are common in *Kaphaja Prakriti* has been reported.

## 3.0 Conclusion

The present study suggests that inborn physical and mental characters have link in the development of breast cancer also. The disease is prevalent in *Kaphaja Prakriti* patients. Thus, like many other risk factors of breast cancer development, *Kaphaja Prakriti* also may be considered as a risk factor for the development of the disease and it may be taken as a useful guideline in mass screening programme of breast cancer among the females above the age of 35 years. The response of therapy in different Prakriti suggests that *Vataja Prakriti* patients responded well to the treatment and survived for longer period in comparison to the patients of *Pittaja* and *Kaphaja Prakriti*. Therefore *Prakriti* as described in Ayurveda may be useful not only in early detection of breast cancer but also it may be helpful for assessment of prognosis of the disease.

## References


Astanga Hridaya, Chaukhamba Shanskrit Series, Varanasi (1975). Edited by-Atridev Gupta.

Bacon, G.L. *et al.*, 1952. A psychosomatic survey of the cancer of the breast. Psychosom Med (14): pp. 453.

Carroll, K.K., Khor, H.T, 1975. Experimental evidence of dietary factors and hormone dependent cancer. Can Res. (33): pp. 3374.

Charak Samhita, Chaukhamba Shanskrit Series, Varanasi (1962). Edited by–Rajeswar Dutta Shastri.

Donegan, W.L., *et al.*, 1988. Association of body weight and recurrent cancer of breast. WB Saunderson Company, Philadelphia.

Handerson, I.C., *et al.*, 1989. Cancer principal and practice of oncology. J.B. Lippincott Company.

Jussawala, D.J., *et al.*, 1981. Breast cancer incidence in Bombay and Poona. Ind J. cancer (18): pp. 91-98.

Sushruta Samhita, Chaukhamba Sanskrit Series, Varanasi (1976). Edited by–Ambikadutt Shastri.

Sarangadhar Samhita, Chaukhamba Sanskrit Series, Varanasi (1993). Edited by–Daya Shankar Pande.

Tannenbaum, A., 1986. Relationship of body weight to cancer incidence. ArchPatho (30): pp. 509–17.

## *Chapter 35*

# Studies on Hepato-protective Action of *Terminalia chebula*, *Terminalia bellerica* and *Emblica officinalis* (Triphala)

**O.P. *Singh*[1]*, *N. Sujatha*[1], *P.K. Rai*[1], *N.P. Rai*[1] *and S.K. Singh*[2]**

*[1]Department of Kayachikitsa Faculty of Ayurveda, Institute of Medical Sciences, Banaras Hindu University, Varanasi, India*

*[2]Centre of Experimental Medicine and Surgery, Institute of Medical Sciences, Banaras Hindu University, Varanasi, India*

**E-mail: dr_om@bhu.ac.in, dropsingh67@gmail.com*

## ABSTRACT

Liver is one of the extensively explored areas in Modern Medicine. Among the various diseases affecting it, Hepatitis-B virus infection is very important one because of its potential to cause life-threatening complications like cirrhosis, ascites, and hepatocellular carcinoma. More than 400 million people worldwide are chronically infected by the hepatitis B virus (HBV) (WM Lee, 1997). 82 per cent of the world's 530000 cases of liver cancer per year are caused by viral hepatitis infection, with 316 000 cases associated with hepatitis B and 118000 with hepatitis C (WHO, World Health Report 1996). It is the $10^{th}$ leading cause of mortality. Western Medicine, despite its enormous success does not offer any promising cures and the role of traditional systems of medicine cannot be overlooked. The clinical symptoms of Hepatitis-B are similar with those described under *Kamala roga* in Ayurveda and various herbal and herbomineral drugs have been described for its management (Caraka Samhita, 2005; Ashtanga Hridaya of Vagbhata, 1997; Susruta Samhita with Dalhanas, 1994). A trial has been conducted to evaluate the role and efficacy of the fruits of *Terminalia chebula, Terminalia bellerica and Emblica officinalis* popularly known as *Triphala* (Three fruits) described in classics of Ayurveda for the management of Hepatitis-B (*Kamala*).

***Keywords:*** *Hepatitis B (Kamala), Triphala, Hepatoprotective, and Antioxidant.*

## 1.0 Introduction

Evaluation of a jaundice patient is one of the frequent challenges encountered by a physician in general practice and one of them is acute viral hepatitis. Hepatitis B virus is an important cause of acute viral hepatitis. Hepatitis B virus is a DNA virus with a unique enzyme *i.e.* the DNA Polymerase that has the capacity to synthesize DNA by reverse transcription. The clinical features produced by HBV virus may range in one hand from asymptomatic to fulminating fatal infection on the other hand sub clinical persistent infection to rapidly progressive chronic liver disease with cirrhosis and hepatocellular carcinoma (Harrisons Principles of Internal Medicine).

Triphala, a polyherbal formulations containing *Haritaki* (*Terminalia chebula*), *Vibhitaki* (*Terminalia bellerica*), and *Amalaki* (*Emblica officinalis*) have been tried both experimentally as well as clinically in the in the cases of hepatitis B.

## 2.0 Clinical Study

A total of 44 cases from the O.P.D. and I.P.D. of Kayachikitsa, B.H.U, Varanasi, were registered for this study and out of which 38 cases completed the trial.

### 2.1 Inclusion Criteria

1. Age between 20-50 years of either sex
2. Symptoms and signs of acute viral hepatitis
3. Abnormal Liver Function Tests
4. Presence of HbsAg and other viral markers for HBV in blood.

### 2.2 Exclusion Criteria

1. Chronic hepatitis (>6 months duration)
2. Viral markers of hepatitis 'B' negative
3. Other causes of viral hepatitis like HAV, HCV, HDV and HEV.
4. Complications like obstructive jaundice, cirrhosis, fulminating hepatitis, liver failure, hepatocellular carcinoma etc.

### 2.3 Study Design

This was a double blind, placebo controlled study where the observer and subjects were unaware of the study medication. The institution Ethical Review Committee of B.H.U approved the study. All patients underwent complete general examination to rule out any gross abnormalities and were evaluated clinically and biochemically to confirm the diagnosis.

### 2.4 Grouping

Subjects were divided into groups as follows:

(*i*) *Treated group*: (n=30): received 80 ml of decoction (*kwath*) of Triphala orally in two divided doses along with honey.

(*ii*) *Control group* (n=8): received oral glucose and normal diet.

## 2.5 Selection and Preparation of Drug

The dried fruits of *Terminalia chebula, Terminalia bellerica and Emblica officinalis* popularly called as *Triphala* (three fruits) were selected for this study. The pulp of all the three fruits was taken in equal proportion, mixed together and course granule was prepared. 5 grams of course granules of Triphala was boiled in 250 ml of water and allowed it to dry until it reached approximately 80 ml. The whole content was filtered and the prepared decoction was advised to take in two equal doses in a day.

**Follow-up and Assessment**

(*a*) All subjects were evaluated weekly for the initial one month and thereafter once in a month up to 6 months. Efficacy of trial drug was assessed by:

Relief in symptoms on a point rating score:

0- Free from symptoms

1- Mild and intermittent

2- Moderate and constant

3- Severe and progressive

(*b*) Normalization of abnormal liver function tests and disappearance of Australia Antigen from the blood. The bio chemical tests were carried out at enrolment and thereafter weekly for 1 month and once in a month up to 6 months. Hepatitis 'B' surface antigen was done at enrolment and at the end of 3rd and 6th month.

## 3.0 Statistical Analysis

Both the groups were compared by "Students unpaired 't' test". Changes in the various biochemical parameters were evaluated at the end of 1st, 2nd, 3rd and 4th weeks and later assessed by *"Students paired 't' test"* for statistical significance.

**Table 35.1**

| *Variable* | *Treated Group (n=30)* | | *Control Group (n= 8)* | | *Unpaired 't'* |
|---|---|---|---|---|---|
| | *BT* *Mean ± SD* | *AT* *Mean ± SD* | *BT* *Mean ± SD* | *AT* *Mean ± SD* | |
| Sr. Bilirubin | 17.03±3.82 | 1.64±0.82 P<. 001 HS | 11.49±1.23 | 7.5±0.76 P< 0.01 S | 15.52 P<.001 |
| ALT | 832.53±141.27 | 52.6±16.92 P<. 001HS | 838.7±37.39 | 650.0±30.6 P<0.01S | 22.4 P<0.001 |
| AST | 723.94±57.53 | 40.4±24.5 P<0.001 HS | 562.0±34.8 | 380.12±30.86 P<0.01S | 25.69 P<0.001 |
| Alk. Phosphatase | 648.8±60.13 | 120.5±26.52 P<. 001 HS | 593.0±40.38 | 380.0±25.65 P<0.1S | 16.94 P<0.001 |

## 4.0 Observations and Results

In the treated group the scores of the symptoms like yellow sclera and urine, anorexia, nausea and fatigue were significantly reduced at the end of

1 month (80 per cent). On the other hand the control group showed only moderate relief 50 per cent in anorexia and nausea but only mild relief in symptoms like yellow discolouration of sclera and urine. Moreover some of the patients became associated with pain in abdomen and constipation.

The improvement of symptoms was supported by biochemical parameters like level of total serum bilirubin, ALT, AST and Alkaline phosphatase. The mean difference of bilirubin, ALT, AST and ALP were found to be statistically significant in the fourth follow-up of treated group as compared to control group.

An inter group comparison between treated and control groups was statistically highly significant in the unpaired't' values $P<0.001$ for all the above parameters. Among 30 patients of *treated group*, 26 became negative for Australia antigen at the end of $4^{th}$ month, while in the *control group (n=8)* 6 of them became negative when administered trial drug after the completion of trial period.

## 5.0 Experimental Study

The study was carried out to evaluate the hepatoprotective activity and Antioxidant properties of Triphala.

### Grouping of Animals

A total of 24 rats were included in the study and was divided into 4 groups of 6 animals in each group.

**Group I**

Control

**Group II**

Animals received 1.3ml/g wt., of Triphala orally for seven days.

**Group III**

Animals were given 1 per cent carboxy methylcellulose (CMC) in distilled water for seven days with paracetamol at 2g/kg body wt. P.O. suspended in 1 per cent CMC administered on the fifth day (Asha and Pushpangadan, 1997). (Paracetamol treated)

**Group IV**

Animals received 1.3ml/g wt., of triphala orally for seven days with paracetamol at 2g/kg body wt. orally given on the fifth day (Triphala treated)

At the end of the experiment (48 hrs. after paracetamol administration), under ether anesthesia, blood samples were collected in centrifuge tubes via cardiac puncture, and the serum was separated. The abdomen was then cut open and liver samples were removed. In order to prevent RBC contamination, samples were cut into small slices, rinsed thoroughly in ice-cold normal saline and blotted by with blotting paper. Serum samples were frozen immediately in a deep freezer at–20°C and enzyme assays were performed on the next day.

The Enzyme assays were done by collecting the serum samples and subjected to assay for hepatic marker enzymes such has Aspartate transaminase (AST) Alanine transaminase (ALT) and Alkaline phosphatase (ALP). Activities of AST and ALT were assayed according to the 2-4 DNPH methods. Values are expressed as IU/dl ALP activity was measured using the method of Kind and King (1954) and results are expressed as K.A. units/L.

The histopathological examination was done by preserving liver pieces in 10 per cent formaldehyde solution and embedding them in paraffin wax. Sections of about 4-6μm thicknesses were taken and stained with hematoxylin eosin and photographed.

## 6.0 Results and Observations

The following tables show the effect of Triphala on serum Liver Transaminases enzymes (AST, ALT, ALP) and MDA and SOD levels in paracetamol (PCT) induced hepatotoxicity. Inter group comparison was made between Group I and Group II, Group III and Group I (y), and Group IV and Group III (z)

All statistical analysis are done by student unpaired 't' test 'P' values < 0.01 were considered to be statistically significant.

**Table 35.2**

| *Sl.No* | *Group* | *AST (IU/L) Mean±S.E* | *ALT (IU/L) Mean±S.E* | *ALP (IU/L) Mean±S.E* | *M.D.A Mean±S.E (nmol/ml serum)* | *S.O.D Mean±S.E (nmol/ml serum)* |
|---|---|---|---|---|---|---|
| 1. | Control | 51.33±1.75 | 17.67±0.76 | 39.33±1.05 | 0.347±0.06 | 0.181±0.002 |
| 2. | Triphala Perse | 51.50±0.96(ax) | 19.50±0.67(a,x) | 38.50±1.34(a,x) | 0.374±0.006(a,x) | 0.171±0.005 (a,x) |
| 3. | Paracetamol Treated | 90.17±0.98(ax) | 70.00±0.86(c,y) | 70.00±0.68(c,y) | 0.671±0.005(c,y) | 0.392±0.036 (c,y) |
| 4. | Triphala Treated | 72.83±1.33(cz) | 50.50±0.89(c,z) | 40.67±0.88(c,z) | 0.539±0.042(b,z) | 0.145±0.004 (c,z) |

The results are summarized in Tables 35.1 and 35.2. As compared to the control group, the animals in the paracetamol-treated group showed a significant increase in lipid peroxidation (LPO) as revealed by raised M.D.A and SOD activity with an equal increase in serum levels of hepatic marker enzymes. Prevention was significant in animals receiving Triphala and paracetamol. Animals given only Triphala did not show any alteration in LPO and SOD without any significant effect on other parameters.

Liver section from control rats showed normal lobular architecture and normal hepatic cells with a well-preserved cytoplasm and well-defined nucleus and nucleoli (Photos 1-A, 1-B).

Histopathological examination of the livers of animals given only Triphala showed no significant morphological changes, as compared to animals in the control group. Photos 2-A, 2-B showed cloudy swelling and ballooning degeneration, and loss of lobular architecture and Liver sections from animals given paracetamol marked regenerative activity in the form of binucleation, nuclear enlargement and prominent nucleoli. Some cells showed loss of nucleus and nucleoli, kupffer cells were hyperplastic (Photos 3-A, 3-B)

Pretreatment with Triphala showed normal lobular structure with less cloudy swelling and hardly ascertainable ballooning degeneration and less regenerative activity in paracetamol challenged animals (Photos 4-A, 4-B).

## 7.0 Discussion

Triphala is a polyherbal Ayurvedic formulation containing ingredients Haritaki *(Terminalia chebula)*, Amalaki *(Emblica officinalish)* (Jose, J. K. and Kuttan, R., 2000) and Vibhitaki *(Terminalia bellerica)* (Padam S.K. *et al.*, 1995). Among them Haritaki is a laxative (Tamhane, MD., *et al.* , 997; Hamada, S.I., *et al.*, 1997) and a popular remedy for constipation. It also possesses chologogue and cholerectic activities. Amalaki (Bhattacyarya, A., *et al.*, 1999) is well known drug for its Antioxidant and hepatoprotective properties. Amalaki and Haritaki have antioxidant, immuno modulatory and membrane stabilizing properties by increasing the levels of Glutathione and SOD enzymes present in the hepatocytes (Rege, NN., *et al.*, 1999; Vani T. *et al.*, 1997)

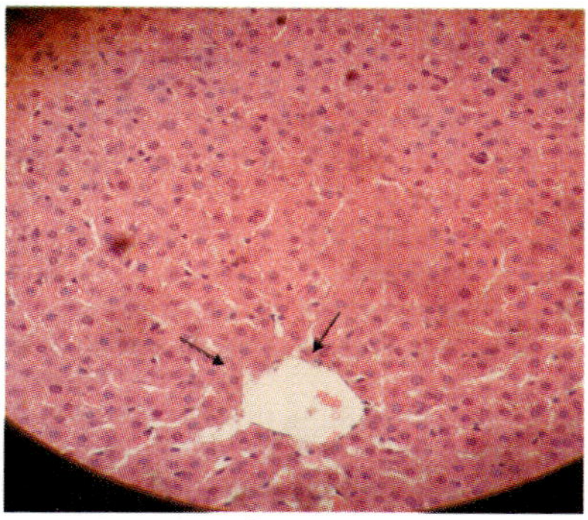

Photo 1A

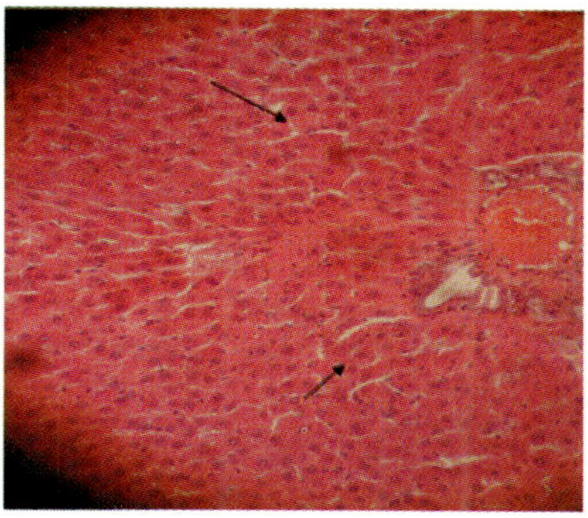

Photo 2A

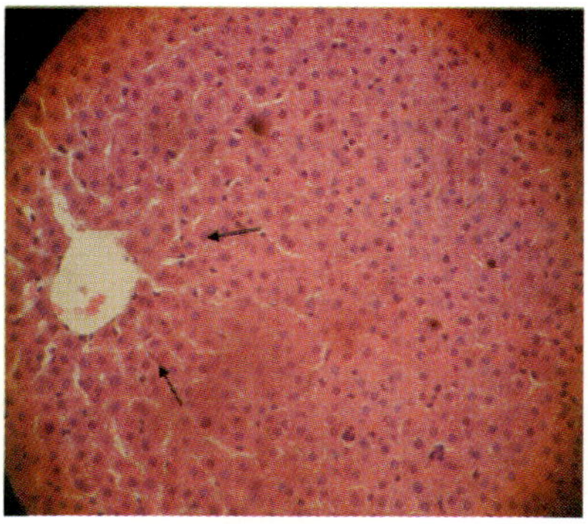

Photo 1B

Histology of Liver–Control Group

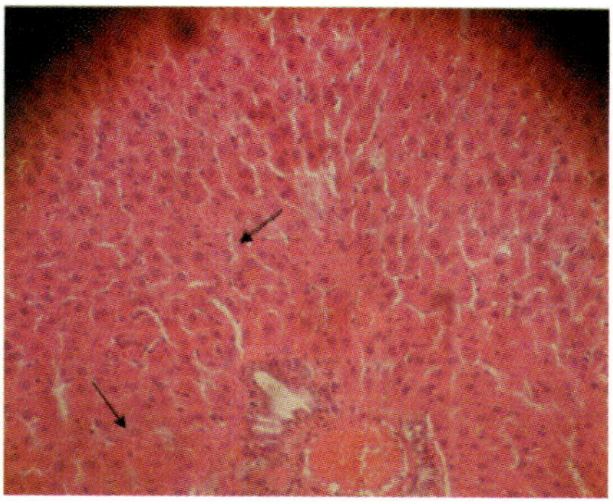

Photo 2B

Histology of Liver–Triphala Group

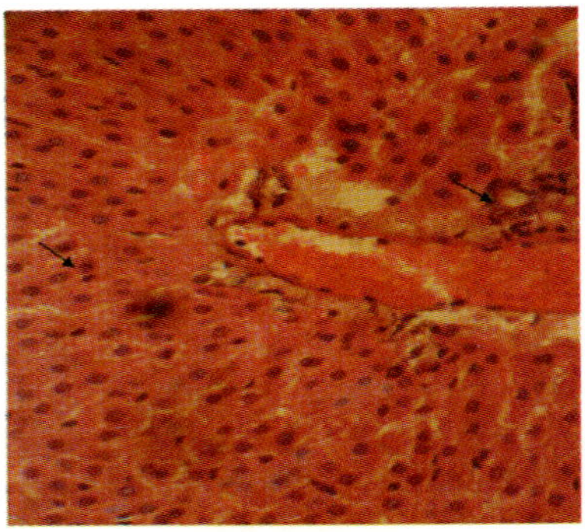

*Photo 3A*

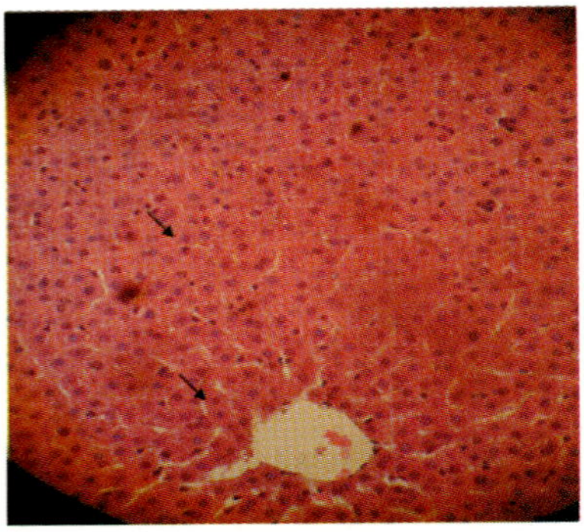

*Photo 4A*

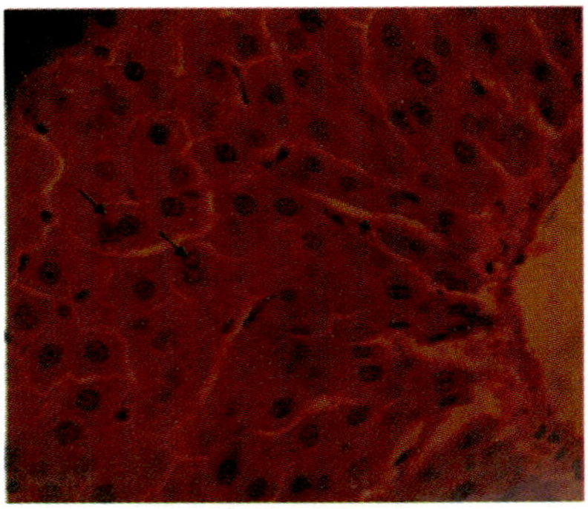

*Photo 3B*

**Histology of Liver–
Paracetomal Group**

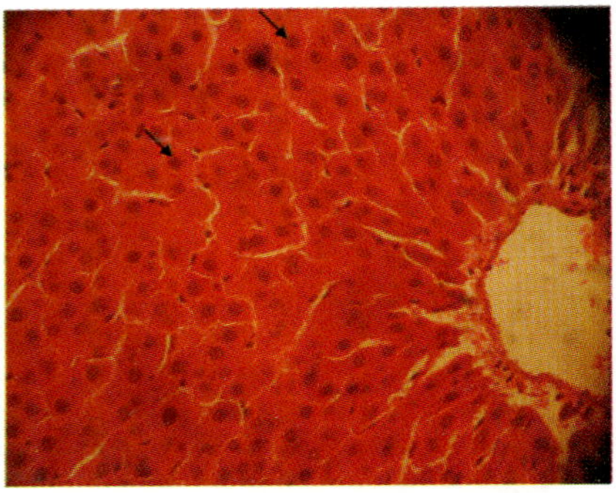

*Photo 4B*

**Histology of Liver–
Pre treatment with Triphala**

## 8.0 Conclusion

Hepatitis B is a disease, which clinically resembles with kamala described in Ayurveda and several herbal and herbomineral preparations has been described for its management. Triphala is one such polyherbal formulation commonly used in for the treatment of kamala. Double blind placebo controlled clinical study of Triphala decoction in cases of Hepatitis B have shown improvement in 80 per cent cases of Hepatitis B findings were supported by experimental study also drug was proved to have hepatoprotective and antioxidant activity. The drug was also found safe in clinical and experimental studies.

## References

Ashtanga Hridaya of Vagbhata with commentaries of Sarvanga sundara, 1997. By Yadunandan Upadhyay, edited Kaviraja Atridev Gupta, Published by Chowkamba Sanskrit Series, Nidana Sthana, and chapter 13, pp. 363.

Bhattacharya, A. Chatterjee, A. Ghosal, S., Bhattacharya, S.K., 1999. Antioxidant activity of active tannoid principles of *Emblica officinalis* (amla) 2. Indian J. Exp. Biol. 37 (7): pp.676-80.

http://www.newcrops.uq.edu.au/listing/emblicaofficinalis.htm

Caraka Samhita of Agnivesha, 2005. By Kashinath Shastri *et al.*, Part II, Chapter-16, pp. 423, 8th Edition.

Hamada, S.I., Kataoka, T., *et al.*, 1997. Immunosuppressive effects of gallic acid and chebulagic acid on CTL-mediated cytotoxicity. Biological and Pharmaceutical Bulletin 20(9), pp.1017-1019. {a} Dep. Bioeng., Tokyo Inst. Technol., 4259 Nagatsuta-cho, Midori-ku, Yokohama 226, Japan.

http://www.newcrops.uq.edu.au/listing/terminaliachebula.htm

Harrisons Principles of Internal Medicine. By Braunwald, Kasper *et al.*, 16th Edition Vol. II, pp.1840-1841.

Jose, J. K. and Kuttan, R., 2000. Hepatoprotective activity of *Emblica officinalis* and Chyavanaprash. Journal of Ethnopharmacology (72(1-2)), pp.135-140. {a} Amala Cancer Research Centre, Amala Nagar PO, Thrissur, KER, 680 553, India

http://www.newcrops.uq.edu.au/listing/emblicaofficinalis.htm

Lee, WM, 1997. Hepatitis B infection virus. N Engl J Med (337), pp. 1733–1745.

Padam, S.K. *et al.*, 1995. Antimutagenic effects of polyphenols isolated from *Terminalia bellerica* myroblan in Salmonella typhimurium. Indian J Exp Bio 34(2), pp. 98-102.

https://oa.doria.fi/bitstream/handle/10024/27195/traditio.pdf?sequence

Rege NN *et al.*, 1999. Adaptogenic properties of six Rasayana herbs used in Ayurvedic medicine (including E officinalis). Phytother Res. (13 (4)).

http://www.oneearthherbs.com/OneEarthReferences.html

Susruta Samhita with Dalhanas. By Kaviraja Ambika Datta Shastri, edited and Reprinted 1994 published by Chowkamba Sanskrit Series, Part-II, Chikitsa Sthana, pp.288-290.

Tamhane, MD., Thorat, SP, Rege, NN, Dahanukar, SA, 1997. Effect of oral administration of *Terminalia chebula* on gastric emptying; an experimental study. J. Postgrad Med. (43), pp.12-3.

http://www.wjgnet.com/1007-9327/14/1491.pdf

Vani T. *et al*, 1997. Antioxidant properties of the Ayurvedic formulation Triphala and its constituents. J. Pharmacognosy (35), pp.313-317.

http://www.iisc.ernet.in/currsci/apr252006/1100.pdf

WHO, World Health Report, 1996. Fighting disease, fostering development, World Health Organization, Geneva.

## *Chapter 36*

# Status of AYUSH and Need for Standardization of Medicinal Plants

**A. *Saraswathy***

*Captain Srinivasa Murti Drug Research Institute for Ayurveda,*
*(CCRAS, Dept of AYUSH, Ministry of Health and Family Welfare, Govt. of India),*
*Arumbakkam, Chennai – 106, Tamil Nadu, South India*
*E-mail: csmdria@gmail.com, saraswathy20042000@yahoo.co.in*

## ABSTRACT

The drugs used in Indian System of Medicine are mainly derived from plants and plant products, besides metals/minerals and marine origin. These plant drugs are subjected to wide variation with respect to their chemical composition, due to the influence of climatic conditions, nature and properties of soil, geographical distribution, age of plant, source of collection, altitude and period of harvesting. There are other factors, which do contribute to the variations *viz.*, method of storage, influence of heat, humidity and light during preservation, type of drying process, method of purification of raw materials and method of manufacturing of compound formulations which are specific to individual manufacturer.

WHO has prescribed parameters along with the testing methods for deciding the identity, purity and strength and safety of the herbal medicinal plant materials. For identification, macroscopy, microscopy, colour test, fluorescence test, thin layer chromatographic techniques are employed.

Microbial load heavy metals, aflatoxins and pesticide residues are to be estimated to determine the safety aspect of the drugs. Acute, sub-acute and chronic toxicity studies in animal models are to be performed as per Organization of Economic Co-operation and Development (OECD)/WHO guidelines.

The efficacy of the drug is to be determined through pharmacological and anti-microbial means.

***Keywords***: *Indian System of Medicines, Standardization, Quality control.*

## 1.0 Department of AYUSH in a Nutshell

A separate department *viz.* Indian Systems of Medicine and Homeopathy (ISM and H) has been established in 1995 under the Ministry of Health and Family Welfare, Govt. of India. This has been now named as the Department of Ayurveda, Yoga and Naturopathy, Unani, Siddha and Homoeopathy (AYUSH). A Secretary and system wise technical officers headed by Advisers are heading the Department. The overall governance of regulation, development and growth of AYUSH systems in the country and abroad is seen by the Department. It has 3 subordinate offices and 15 autonomous bodies in the form of research councils, national institutes, and pharmacopoeia laboratories. 23 states have Directorate of Indian systems of medicine. Department of AYUSH administers the Acts relating to rules, regulations of education, practice and drugs of Ayurveda, Siddha, Unani and Homoeopathy through concerned state departments. The details can be had from the AYUSH website www.indianmedicine.nic.in

### 1.1 Recognized Systems

The following six systems are officially recognized systems by the government of India: Ayurveda, Siddha, Unani, Yoga, Naturopathy and Homoeopathy.

Ayurveda the most ancient system is practiced since ancient India. It is of natural modes and modalities of preventive, promotive, mitigative and curative health care that is believed to be originated with human life. It is, documented in Vedic literature. Siddha is one of the oldest therapeutic systems akin to Ayurveda in fundamental principles, prevalent predominantly in Southern part of India. It makes use of minerals and herbo-mineral preparations to a larger extent. Unani was originated in Greece during the 4-5th century BC under the patronage of Hippocrates and Khan and enriched in Arabian countries. It was brought to India during medieval period. Now it is inseparably assimilated as a part of traditional Indian medicine. These systems have many fundamental common principles. Yoga is a way of life and drugless therapy based on ancient Indian approach to attain eternal peace of mind. It is now culminated into a complete science and art for healthy living with roots of psychosomatic harmony. Naturopathy is a system of man building in harmony with constructive principles of nature on physical, mental, moral and spiritual planes of living. Homoeopathy means treating the diseases with remedies, usually prescribed in minute doses, which was capable of producing symptoms similar to the diseases when taken by healthy people. It was evolved by the German physician Dr. Samuel Hahnemann.

### 1.2 Infrastructure

The infrastructure of AYUSH comprises of teaching institutions, registered medical practitioners, hospitals and dispensaries and drug manufacturing units available in the country are as under:

(*a*) Registered practitioners: 7,17,860

(*b*) Total number of Colleges: 456

(*c*) Admission Capacity per annum for degree course: 24,880

(*d*) Postgraduate colleges: 105

(*e*) Admission Capacity for Postgraduate courses: 2,128
(*f*) Ayurveda Universities: 2
(*g*) Licensed Drug Manufacturing Units: 9,493
(*h*) Hospitals: 3,100
(*i*) Beds in hospitals: 53,296
(*j*) Dispensaries: 22,635

## 2.0 Regulation and Quality Control of Drugs

The regulatory Act and the rules there under are common for Allopathic and Indian Medicines and Homoeopathic drugs. There is a separate Chapter IVA in the Drugs and Cosmetics Act, 1940 with provisions for regulation of manufacture, packaging, labelling and sale of ASU drugs. The Act is enforced through the State Drug Licensing and Drug Control Authorities. A separate Ayurveda, Siddha and Unani Technical Advisory Board (ASUTAB) has been constituted by the Central Government comprising of officials and nominees of Central Government, pharmacognosists, phytochemists and Members of the respective ASU Pharmacopoeia committee and representatives of teachers, practitioners and ASU drugs industry nominated by the Central Government to advise the Governments on technical matters relating to regulation. The Central Government has also constituted an Ayurveda, Siddha and Unani Drugs Consultative Committee (ASUDCC) under the Act to advise the Central and State Government and the ASUDTAB on any matter for the purpose of securing uniformity throughout India in the administration of Drugs and Cosmetics Act, 1940.

As a first step of, laying down of pharmacopoeial standards the Pharmacopoeial Laboratory of Indian Medicine (PLIM) was set up in 1970 and the Homoeopathic Pharmacopoeial Laboratory (HPL) in 1975 to facilitate drug standardization and testing of ASU drugs. In addition, 13 other reputed laboratories have been engaged to lay down pharmacopoeial standards, preparation of monographs and for evolving Standard Operating Procedures (SOPs) for ASU drugs. Pharmacopoeial Committees have been constituted separately for ASU systems. It is the responsibility of these Committees to lay down standards of quality, purity and strength of drugs and approve drug formularies. So far, 424 monographs of Ayurveda drugs in 5 volumes have been published. Formularies of Ayurveda, Siddha and Unani containing 636, 248 and 745 multi-ingredient classical formulations, respectively have been published to facilitate manufacture of drugs with uniform composition and manufacturing procedures.

### 2.1 Parameters Adopted for Quality Control and Standardization

Ayurveda, Siddha and Unani drugs, which are mainly poly-herbals, depend on the quality and availability of raw materials of botanical origin. National Medicinal Plants Board (NMPB) was established in the year 2000 with the objectives of *in situ* conservation and *ex situ* cultivation of quality medicinal plants raw materials.

The following major initiatives have been taken by the Central Government for ensuring safety and quality control of ASU drugs:

## 2.2 GMP for ASU Medicines

Schedule T–GMP for ASU medicines was notified in the Gazette of India on 23rd June 2000 for new units and became mandatory for old ASU units.

**Objectives**

- To ensure authentic and good quality raw materials are used in ASU drugs.
- To ensure proper manufacturing process and quality control measures during processing.
- To ensure the acceptable quality of finished ASU medicines.

**Space Requirements**

The manufacturing units should have space for, receiving and storing raw material, manufacturing process areas, quality control section, finished goods store, office, and rejected goods/drugs store. Minimum manufacturing space required is 1200 Sq. ft. covered area. Plus 200 sq.ft. for furnace section.

**Hygienic Conditions**

- The general requirements have been made to avoid contamination from open sewerage, drain, public lavatory etc.
- Raw-material Store and finished Goods store should be free from rodent and insect infestation and the raw materials be kept in suitable cabins and finished Goods in finished Goods stock area.
- Workers employed should be free from contagious diseases, yearly medical check up and in proper uniform.
- Machinery and equipments can be either manually operated or automatically operated.
- Batch to Batch manufacturing records of all the steps, Sale and Distribution records, and Market complaints records should be properly maintained.
- Facility for quality control section can be provided in the premises of manufacturing unit, alternatively through a Government approved testing Laboratory.

**GMP Benefits**

- Wide acceptability of ASU medicines to the consumers
- To boost the export potential of ASU drugs
- To supply the ASU medicines in Central and State Government hospitals and dispensaries, GMP is very much essential.

## 3.0 Need of Standardization of Herbal Medicinal Plants

The use of plants for treating various diseases predates human history and forms the origin of much of the modern medicine. Plants were the mainstream remedies for nearly all ailments before the advent of modern medicine. Plant drugs are also being used increasingly as dietary supplements to treat or prevent ailments like cancer, heart attacks and depression. Plant remedies are unpurified extracts containing several active constituents, which often work together synergistically (Nadkarni, 1976).

India is one of the richest nations in terms of biological diversity, with vast array of species of plants, animals, insects and microorganisms, inhabiting the earth (Anonymous, 2004). It stands quite high in the wealth of the total number of species. India has 16 agro-climatic zones, more than 47,000 different plant species and 15000 medicinal plants. ISM has identified 1500 plants, of which 500 species are mostly used in the preparation of drugs. Medicinal plants contribute to cater 75 per cent of the raw materials used in the preparation of ASU compound drugs. The effectiveness of these medicines mainly depends upon the proper use and sustained availability of genuine raw materials. Demand for natural products like drugs, food supplements, cosmetics and domestic market is increasing day by day.

Further India has a tremendous passion for medicinal plants. Traditionally, local communities in every ecosystem right from the trans Himalayan down to the coastal plains have discovered the medicinal uses of thousands of local plants found in their surroundings. India probably has one of the richest plant medicine cultures in the world. Several formulations are available in the indigenous medical texts, many of which are sufficiently to be tapped.

**Table 36.1: Biodiversity in India and World**

| *Group* | *India* | *World* |
|---|---|---|
| Flowering plants | 15000 | 250000 |
| Insects | 60000 | 800000 |
| Fishes | 1693 | 23400 |
| Amphibians | 181 | 2000 |
| Birds | 1175 | 8400 |
| Reptiles | 399 | 5375 |
| Mammals | 372 | 4231 |

*Source*: Wildlife Institute of India (1993), Biodiversity in India (1994).

India stands one among the world's top twelve mega-diverse nations. The drugs used in Indian Systems of Medicine are mainly derived from plants and plant products besides metals/minerals and marine origin. These plant drugs are subjected to wide variation with respect to their chemical composition, due to the influence of climatic conditions, nature and properties of soil and fertilizer, geographical distribution, age of plant, source/season/time of collection, altitude, and period of harvesting. There are other factors, which do contribute to the variations *viz.*, method of storage, influence of heat, humidity and light during storage and preservation, type of drying process, method of purification of raw materials and method of manufacture, which are specific to individual manufacturer.

Break up details of raw materials of plant origin used in ISM based on life forms is as follows. Analyses of habit wise distribution revealed that one-third of the medicinal plants are trees with herbs and shrubs sharing equal amount.

**Table 36.2: Plants Used in ISM**

| *Plants* | *Per cent* | *Plants* | *Per cent* |
|---|---|---|---|
| Trees | 36 | Shrub | 21 |
| Herbs | 28 | Lianas | 3 |
| Climbers (W) | 5 | Climbers (H) | 7 |

The raw materials consists of a variety of anatomical part of the plant ranging from root, rhizome, stem, heartwood, bark, leaves, flowers, fruits, seeds, gum/resin/oil and whole plant. Break up of the plants parts used is reported to be as detailed below.

**Table 36.3: Plant Parts Used in ISM**

| *Plants Parts* | *Per cent* | *Plants Parts* | *Per cent* |
|---|---|---|---|
| Flowers | 10 | Stem | 6 |
| Fruit | 7 | Wood | 3 |
| Bark | 14 | Whole plant | 16 |
| Rhizome | 4 | Root | 29 |
| Leaves | 6 | Seeds | 5 |

The drugs of plant origin are being used in different forms as:

- Plant powder (uni–and poly herbals)
- Essential Oils
- Tinctures
- Extracts
- Phytopharmaceuticals

## 4.0 Harvesting of Medicinal Plants

About 95 per cent of the plant materials are harvested from the wild sources. Increasing population, Urbanization, Shrinking forest and unsustainable harvesting have brought many plants to extinction. Hence conservation of threatened medicinal plants is the most important responsibility of bio-diverse rich nations. An analysis of plant species in use by Traditional medicine pharmacies and industries shows that more than 70 per cent of these involve destructive harvesting. The crude drugs are available in different forms *viz.*, entire plant or broken form, cut forms, shredded forms, powdered form and peeled form.

Quality assurance implies certification in respect of authentication, standardization, composition, stability and safety. It also ensures that the herbal medicines are free from adulterants and contaminants. Authentication of some plant is difficult because of the confusion created by the vernacular names used by the drug dealers. In fact local names of several plants have different botanical identity. Therefore there is need to adopt uniform binomial names for medicinal plants. Adulteration of drugs is prevalent due to ignorance, carelessness and economic reasons. Examples: *Ailanthus, Phytolacca and Scopolia* leaves for *belladonna*; *Xanthium* leaves for *Stramonium*; *Dandelion* for henbane; *Echinacea purpurea* is adulterated with similar looking plant .*Parthenium integrifolium*. Pepper is adulterated with *Carica pappaya* seeds, *Abies webbiana* leaves substituted with the leaves of *Taxus buccata*, *Swetia chirata* leaves is substituted with the leaves of *Andrographis paniculata*, rhizome of *Alpinia officinarum* is substituted with *A. galangal* (Anonymous, 2003).

## 4.1 Plants Need to be Identified Pharmacognostically

The potency of the active chemicals in herbals is dependent on how and where the herbs are grown, when they are harvested, how they are processed and stored, what anatomical parts of the plants are used, and how these plant parts are subjected to extraction (Harborne, 1973). Thus there will be variation even within the same herbal drugs in terms of the amount and strength of the active constituents. Standardization implies that the active chemicals must be identified to ensure that all brands and batches have the same amount of that particular chemical (*i.e.*) Marker chemical. WHO guidelines entitled "Quality Control Methods for Medicinal Plant Materials" (Anonymous, 1998; The Ayurvedic Pharmacopoeia of India, 1986), has prescribed parameters along with the testing methods for deciding the identity, purity and strength and safety of the herbal medicinal plant materials. The parameters include ash: acid-insoluble ash, water soluble ash, water soluble extractive, alcohol soluble extractive, loss on drying at 105°C. For identification, macroscopy, microscopy (Johansen, 1940; Wallis, 1967), colour test, fluorescence test (Trease and Evans, 1989), assay for chemical marker by thin layer chromatography (Igon Stahl, 1969; Wagner and Bladt) and HPTLC techniques are employed (Gupta, Gupta and Sushil Kumar; Singh *et al.*; Sethi, 1996).

Microbial load (bacterial, fungal, *Enterobacteriaceae*, *Salmonella* spp., *Escherichia coli* and *Staphylococcus aureus*), heavy metals (lead, cadmium, mercury and also arsenic), aflatoxins $B_1$, $B_2$ and $G_1$, $G_2$ (Anonymous, 1998) and pesticide residues (Sharma, 2007) such as organochlorine and organophosphorus are to be estimated to determine the safety aspect of the drugs. Acute, sub-acute and chronic toxicity studies in animal models are to be performed as per Organization of Economic Co-operation and Development (OECD)/WHO guidelines.

The efficacy of the drug is to be determined through pharmacological and anti-microbial means. The pharmacological activity such as analgesic, antipyretic, anti-inflammatory, anti-hepatotoxic, anti-fertility, anti-oxidant, wound healing, immunomodulatory, anti-diabetic are to be performed by approved methods. Herbal drug research should be directed towards establishing the safety and efficacy using modern techniques.

## 5.0 Conclusion

The herbal drug industry is growing at an astounding rate all over the world. Herbal remedies are now available not only in drug stores, but also, in food stores and supermarkets. Therefore, the efficacy and efficacy of herbals is very essential. Thus through multi-disciplinary approach (as detailed below), they must undergo well planned systematic pre-clinical and ethical clinical trials so as to establish their therapeutic value and to make them acceptable world over.

- Right plant material with correct botanical identity
- Growing in original ecological situation
- Harvesting at the right time
- Drying and storage at controlled conditions
- Absence of pesticide, aflatoxin and heavy metal contamination
- Absence of bacterial and fungal contamination
- Evidence on presence of certain marker compounds
- A minimum percentage of availability of secondary metabolites
- Meeting the requirements of GAP, GMP, GLP and GSP
- Packing, labelling and documentation, are required to be adopted/checked for, to obtain quality medicines for global acceptance.

## Acknowledgements

I thank the Director, Central Council for Research in Ayurveda and Siddha, New Delhi and Department of AYUSH, Ministry of Health and Family Welfare, Govt. of India, New Delhi for nomination and financial support.

## References

Anonymous 1998, Quality Control Methods for Medicinal Plant Materials, World Health Organisation, Nonserial Publication: Geneva.

Anonymous 2003, WHO Guidelines on Good Agricultural and Collection Practices (GACP) for Medicinal Plants Nonserial Publication World Health Organization

Anonymous 2004, The Wealth of India: A Dictionary of Indian Raw Materials and Industrial Products: First Supplement Series (Raw Materials), Vol. 5: R-Z. New Delhi, National Institute of Science Communication and Information Resources, xxv, 468 p. (Vol. V). ISBN 81-7236-309-5.

Gupta, A. P., Gupta, M. M. and Sushil Kumar. High Performance Thin Layer Chromatography of Asiaticoside in *Centella asiatica*. *J. Ind. Chem. Soc.* 76: 321-322

Harborne, J.B.. 1973. Phytochemical Methods. Jackman H. (Ed.), London, P 70.

Igon, Stahl. 1969. Thin Layer Chromatography, A Laboratory Hand Book (Student Edition). Springer-Verlag, Berlin. p. 52-86; 127-128, 900.

Johansen, O.A.. 1940. Plant Microtechniques. Mc.Grow Hill, New York, P 182-203.

Nadkarni, K.M.. 1976. Indian Materia Medica. Popular Prakashan Pvt. Ltd., Bombay, II[nd] Edn., P 284-285.

Sethi, P.D.. 1996. High Performance Thin Layer Chromatography (1[st] Edition). CBS Publishers and Distributors, New Delhi, Vol X. p. 1-56.

Singh, D.V., Verma, R. K., Gupta, M. M. and Sushil Kumar. HPTLC quantification of Oleane derivatives in *Terminalia arjuna*. Phytochemical Analysis, 13(4), 207-210, 2002.

Sharma, K. K. Pesticide Residue Analysis Manual. Indian Council of Agricultural Research, Directorate of Information and Publications of Agriculture, New Delhi; 2007.

The Ayurvedic Pharmacopoeia of India, Part–1, vol-I. 1st edn. New Delhi: Government of India, Ministry of Health and Family Welfare, Department of Indian System of Medicine and Homoeopathy; 1986; p. 29

Trease, G.E. and Evans, W.C.. 1989. Pharmacognosy (13th Edition). Bailliere Tuidall, London, p. 799-803.

Wagner, H. and Bladt, S. Plant Drug Analysis, A Thin Layer Chromatography Atlas (2nd Edition). Springer-Verlag, Germany.

Wallis, T.E.. 1967. Text Book of Pharmacognosy (15th Edition). T.A. Churchill, London, p. 571-575.

## Chapter 37

# The Research of Bioactive Components from Different Plants: Case of Rwanda

*Kabera N. Justin* and Nyetera Polycarpe*
*IRST/Research Centre in Phytomedicines and Life Sciences, Butare, Rwanda*
**E-mail: kajust68@yahoo.fr*

## ABSTRACT

In Rwanda, the first scientific work on the pharmacopoeia and traditional medicine started in the year 1972, at the National University of Rwanda (UNR), more precisely within the Faculty of Medicine by a small group of researchers-teachers.

In 1975, this group is reinforced by a few teachers of the Faculty of Science, in particular those from the department of chemistry.

In the years 1980, these researchers put in place the University Research Centre on the Pharmacopoeia and Traditional Medicine known as CURPHAMETRA. In 1989, this centre became the centre Pharmacopoeia of the Institute of scientific and technological research (IRST) by law Nr 06/1989 of March 15, 1989. Very recently, this centre was named "Research Centre in Phytomedicines and Life sciences" (CRP and SV).

Since 1989, several drugs containing plant extracts were developed, components with new structures were isolated and were given names inspired by the vernacular names of the plants; such as for example: Idomaïn de Gutenbergia coridifolia (vernacular name: Idoma).

The studies undertaken on the medicinal plants are mainly based on information provided by traditional healers during ethno-botanic investigations. First, these plants are the subject of a botanical study for the exact scientific identification. Then, the extracts of these plants prepared using various solvents are subjected to a series of biological and pharmacological tests in order to detect one or the other biological activity. The plants having revealed a particularly interesting activity are the subject of a chemical study including isolation, purification and structural identification of active ingredients having the initially detected biological activity. The isolation of the active ingredients is generally carried out using various methods of extraction, column and thin layer chromatography, preparative chromatography and purification by crystallization. The determination of chemical structures is carried out, in collaboration with foreign laboratories better equipped than ours, by various techniques of spectrometry: infra-red (IR), ultraviolet (UV), gas chromatography coupled with mass spectrometry (GC-MS) and by nuclear magnetic resonance (NMR). The biological and pharmacological tests are mainly carried out on laboratory mice, in our "Research centre in Phytomedicines and Life Sciences" (CRP and SV).

Essential oils are extracted by the method of steam distillation. Their chemical composition is established by gas chromatography coupled with mass spectroscopy. The antimicrobial activity is tested by the traditional biological methods.

The results of this research led to the manufacture of drugs containing the local plants extracts and also aroused the interest to continue research because the potentialities are enormous.

***Keywords:*** *Medicinal plants, Bioactive components, Phytomedecine, Rwanda.*

## 1.0 Introduction

The Research centre in Phytomedicines and Life sciences (CRP and SV) founded in the years 1980 under the name of CURPHAMETRA (University Research Centre on the Pharmacopoeia and Traditional Medicine) has the following main objectives:

- The promotion of research in the field of medicinal plants in order to produce drugs from local vegetal material;
- The valorization of the phytomedicine in all its aspects while collaborating narrowly with the traditional healers;
- The contribution to the development of a NATIONAL PHARMACOPOEIA.
- The achievement as of these objectives is carried out through the following 4 departments:
- Phytomedicines and Traditional Medicine;
- Essential Oils;
- Agro forestry, Land Rehabilitation, Conservation and Protection of the biodiversity;
- Biotechnologies.

During the last few years, several Phytomedicines were developed following the discovery of new molecules considered as active ingredients.

## 2.0 Material and Methods

A very deep bibliographic study made it possible to highlight the various methodologies used in previous research which we also use currently.

The studies undertaken on the medicinal plants are mainly based on information provided by the traditional healers during ethno-botanic investigations. These plants are at first the subjects of a botanical study for the exact scientific identification. After that, the extracts of these plants prepared using various solvents are subjected to a series of biological and pharmacological tests in order to detect one or the other biological activity according to the methods of Fong *et al.* (1997); Harbonne (1984). The plants having revealed a particularly interesting activity are the subject of a chemical study including isolation, purification and structural identification of active ingredients having the initially detected biological activity.

The active ingredients isolation is generally carried out using various methods of extraction, column and thin layer chromatography, preparative chromatography and purification by crystallization. The determination of the chemical structures is done in collaboration with the foreign laboratories (France, Belgium, the United States), better equipped than ours. The methods used are infra-red (IR)and ultraviolet (UV)spectrometry techniques, gas chromatography coupled with mass spectrometry (GC-MS)and the nuclear magnetic resonance (NMR) according to Benn *et al.* (1983); Morris, (1986). The biological and pharmacological tests are mainly carried out on laboratory mice, in our "Research centre in Phytomedicines and Life sciences" (CRP and SV).

The essential oils extracted by the method of steam distillation are analyzed by gas chromatography described by Arpino (1995); Adams(1995)

The anti-diarrhoeal activity consists in testing, in vitro, the inhibiting action of the plants extracts on bacteria such as Salmonella and Shigella cultivated on gelose of Triptic-soy (Difco) at 40°C. The bacteria are then inoculated on a bubble of Mueller-Hinton and are incubated at 37°C during 24 hours. The activity is observed and measured in the mice, whose diarrhea is induced with the castor oil. A similar experiment is carried out by replacing this oil by one of the bacteria responsible for the diarrhea. The antibacterial and antimycotic activities tests are carried out according to the traditional methods called dilution and diffusion methods, described by Rasoanaivo *et al.* (1993); Paris *et al.* (1976).

The anti-scabies activity study is made by setting in contact the mites *Psoroptes cuniculi* with the plant extracts. The liver protection activity is tested in the CRP and SV laboratory on mice whose liver is previously poisoned by carbon tetrachloride or paracetamol.

The anti-amoebic activity is evaluated in vitro, by observing the growth inhibition of *Entamoeba hystolitica*, in contact with the product to be tested, in the Jones liquid medium containing a little starch. The observation is carried out using a microscope.

The study of essential oils from aromatic plants was also the subject of research. The plants (leaves and inflorescences) collected in various localities of the country are treated by steam distillation. The essential oil obtained, after purification, is subjected to the physicochemical studies and to biological and pharmacological tests according to one or the other of the previously described techniques. These studies are also supported by our collaborators from French and American Universities.

## 3.0 Results of Research

### 3.1 Biological, Pharmacological and Phytochemical Results

The various techniques described previously made it possible to obtain interesting results for the plants having any biological or therapeutic wanted activity as well as for the products having an economic interest such as essential oils. The major part of these results is presented in the two following tables and illustrated by figures showing the chemical structures of some of the identified products.

Table 37.1 gives the results obtained with pharmacological tests (screening) on several medicinal plants. In this table, one will find the studied activity, the number of the plants tested and some plants with interesting activity. In the same table, we give, for each activity, the interesting plants without claiming that in fact they are the only plants of the Rwandan flora having this capacity. The screening was not undertaken on the entire Rwandan vegetal flora. Some plants are endowed with several biological activities so that it is not astonishing to see a plant being in front of several biological activities. Rwangabo (1993).

**Table 37.1: Biological Activity of Some Plants Used in Rwandan Traditional Medicine**

| *Sl.No.* | *Activity* | *Tested Plants Number* | *Interesting Active Plants* | |
|---|---|---|---|---|
| | | | *Vernacular Name* | *Scientific Name* |
| 1. | Against malaria | 18 | Bambuwa | *Conyza sumantrensis* |
| | | | Umutagara | *Seneccio manii* |
| | | | Umubilizi | *Vernonia amygdalina* |
| | | | Umusave | *Markhamia lutea* |
| | | | Umutarama | *Gardenia ternifolia* |
| 2. | Against diarrhoea | 20 | Isubyo | *Myrica kandtiana* |
| | | | Igonde | *Sesanum angolense* |
| | | | Umugote | *Syzygium zambalaw* |
| 3. | Antivirus | 200 | Umubilizi | *Vernonia amygdalina* |
| | | | Madwedwe | *Euphorbia grantii* |
| | | | Umukunde | *Cajanus cajan* |
| 4. | Antibacterial | | | |
| 4.1. | Against gonorrhoea | 25 | Idoma | *Vernonia aenulans* |
| | | | Igifumba | *Rumex abyssicus* |
| | | | Umukunde | *Cajanus cajan* |
| | | | Umuhengeli | *Lantana trifolia* |

*Contd...*

**Table 37.1–Contd...**

| *Sl.No.* | *Activity* | *Tested Plants Number* | *Interesting Active Plants* | |
|---|---|---|---|---|
| | | | *Vernacular Name* | *Scientific Name* |
| 4.2. | In general | 100 | Umuravumba | *Tetradenia riparia* |
| | | | Inyabarasanya | *Bidens pilosa* |
| | | | Umwishywa | *Momordica foetida* |
| | | | Umutamatama | *Helichrysum hochstetteri* |
| | | | Igifumba | *Rumex abyssicus* |
| | | | Umwenya | *Ocimum gratissimum* |
| | | | Isonga | *Ocimum urticifolium* |
| 5. | Kills dust mites | 42 | Igitembetembe | *Neorautanenia mitis* |
| | | | Igitoborwa | *Solanum dasyphyllum* |
| 6. | Against scabies | 16 | Igitembetembe | *Neorautanenia mitis* |
| | | | Isagara | *Pentas zanzibarica* |
| 7. | Protects liver | 6 | Magaru/ | *Hypoestes triflora* |
| | | | Umubilizi | *Vernonia amygdalina* |

Table 37.2 shows the active ingredients identified with the corresponding biological activity of the plants which were the subject of a thorough chemical study. Figure 37.1 is an example of some interesting molecules isolated from the Rwandan medicinal plants.

## 3.2 Development and Production of Some Drugs Containing Medicinal Plants Extracts, Already Described in Various Pharmacopeias

The drugs containing medicinal plants extracts have an important therapeutic value against a great number of diseases and thus the interest for this kind of drugs does not cease growing. That's why the Research centre in Phytomedicines and Life sciences developed the culture of medicinal plants used in Rwandan traditional medicine and introduced in Rwanda the culture of medicinal plants used in other countries for the local production of various extracts (dyeing, fluid extracts) and essential oils.

The production of drugs started preferably from the plants already known and described in different pharmacopeias, for the only reason that this process is faster and does not require thorough research. Gradually, as our research develops, we introduce new drugs coming from plants which were not used before. It is the case of castamibe (Nkurunziza, 2004). A unit for plant extraction and essential oils distillation was installed to this end. This unit is also used for ethanol production, ethanol being our main solvent for plant extraction.

**Figure 37.1: Chemical Structures of Some Interesting Molecules Isolated from Rwandan Medicinal Plants**

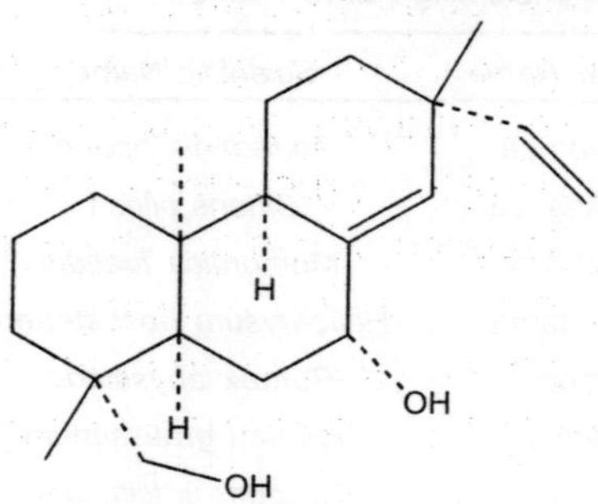

**8 (14),15-SANDARACOPIMARADIEN-7α,18-DIOL (*Tetradenia riparia*)**

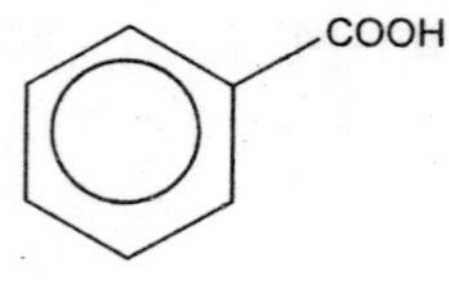

ACIDE BENZOIQUE
**(*Hypoestes triflora*)**

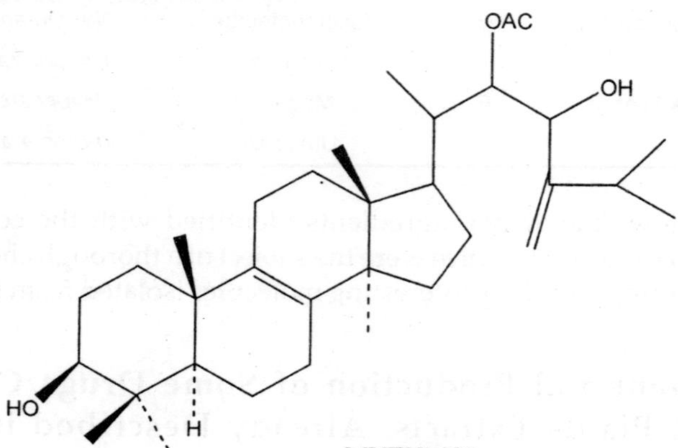

MUTUMOL
**(*Pisolithus arhizus*)**

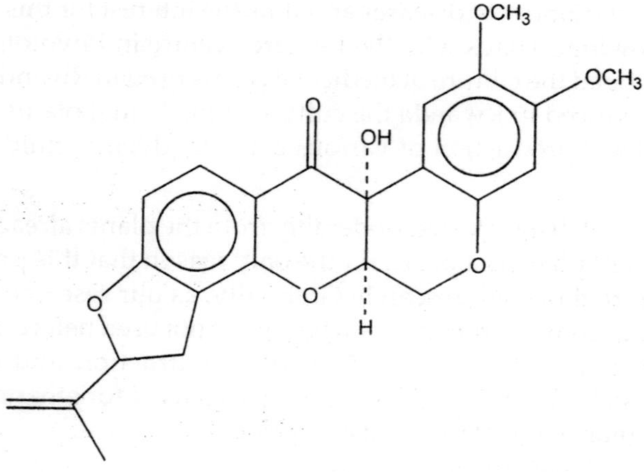

**12α-HYDROXYROTENON (*neorautanenia mitis*)**

*Contd...*

**Figure 37.1–Contd...**

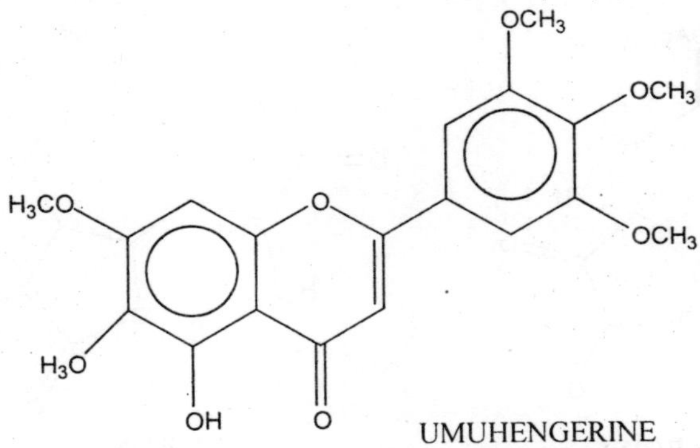


UMUHENGERINE
(***Lantana triflora***)

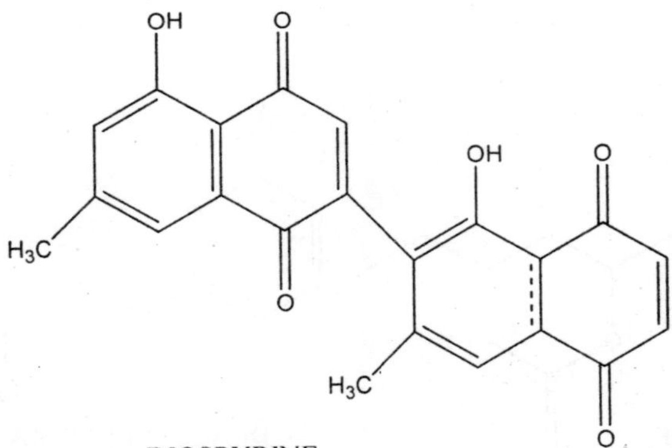


DIOSPYRINE
(***Lantana triflora***)

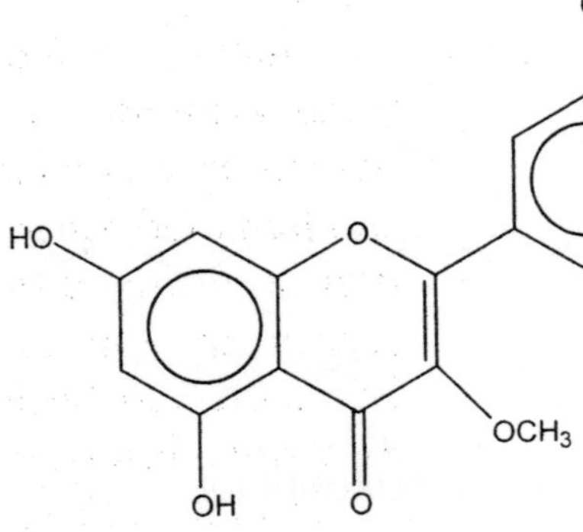


3-O-METHYLQUERCETINE
(***Helichrysum odoratissimum***)

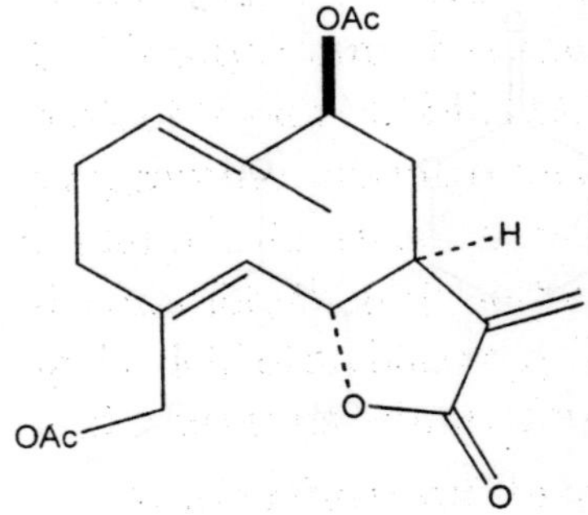


IDOMAINE
(***Gutenbergia cordifolia***)

Contd...

**Figure 37.1–Contd...**

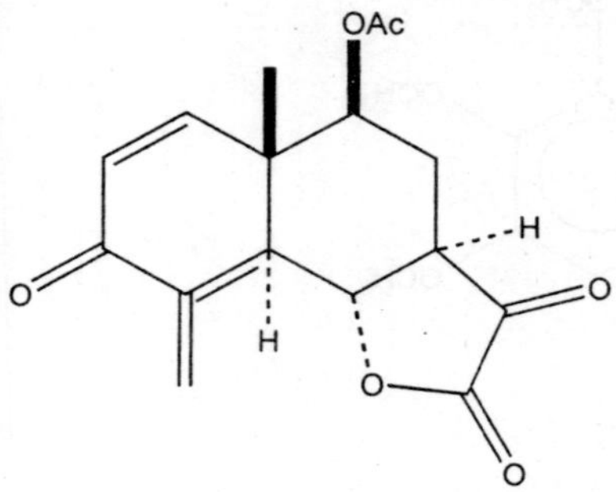

GUTENBERGINE
***(Gutenbergia cordifolia)***

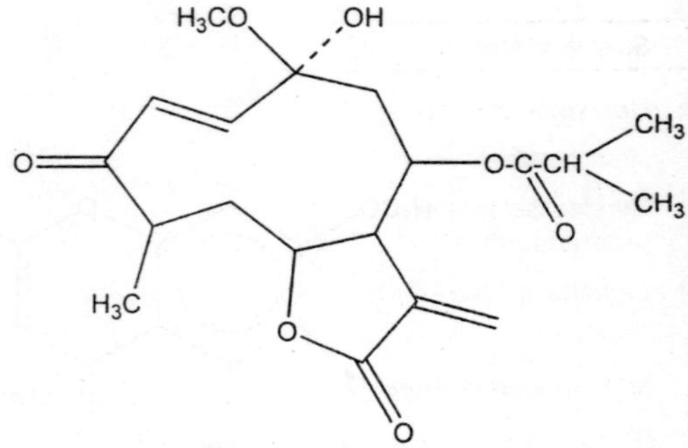

TAGITININE C
**(*Thitonia diversifolia*)**

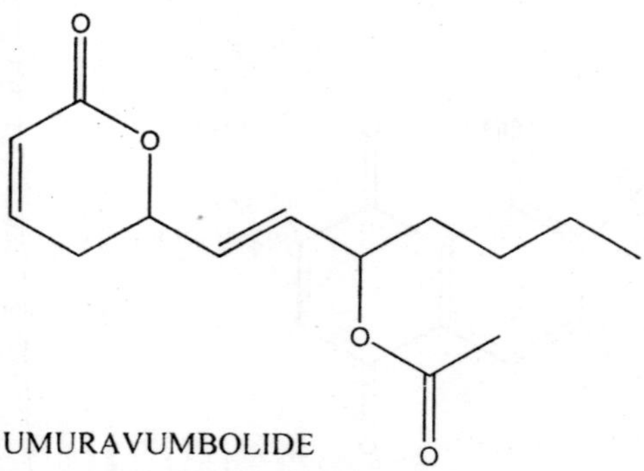

UMURAVUMBOLIDE
**(*Tetradenia riparia*)**

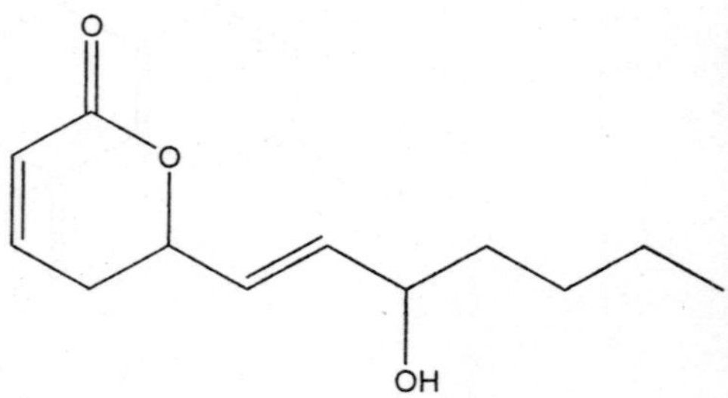

DEACETYLUMURAVUMBOLIDE
**(*Tetradenia riparia)***

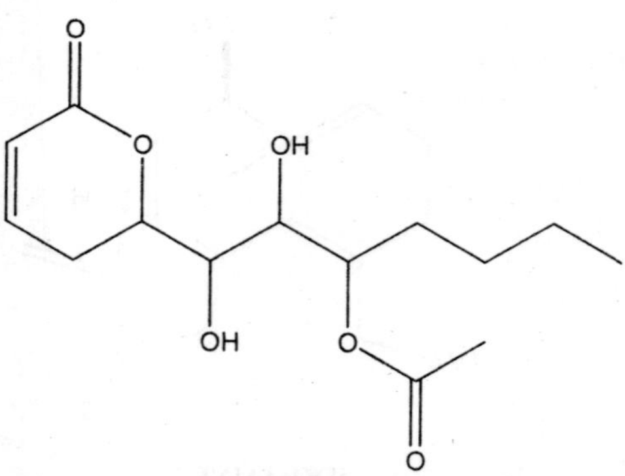

**1', 2'-DIDEACETYLBORONOLID**
**(*Tetradenia riparia)***

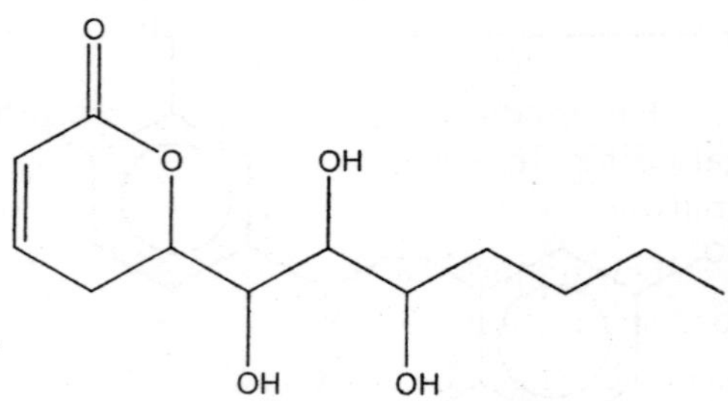

DEACETYLBORONOLIDE

***(Tetradenia riparia)***

**Table 37.2: Active Ingredients of the Medicinal Plants of Rwanda from which the Structure was given in Figure 37.1**

| *Scientific Name* | *Isolated Active Ingredient* | *Activity* |
|---|---|---|
| *Helichrysum odoratissimum* | 3-0-Methylquercetin Helichrysetin | Antimicrobial |
| (Asteraceae) | 3,5-Dyhdroxy-6,7,8-trimethoxy-flavon | |
| *Hypoestes triflora* (Acanthaceae) | Benzoic acid | Protects liver |
| *Lantana triflora* (Verbenaceae) | Umuhengerin | Antibacterial |
| | Diospyrin | Antibacterial |
| *Neorautanenia mitis* | 12&-Hydroxyrotenon | Kills dust mites |
| (Fabaceae) | Neotonon, Pachryrrhizin | Antiscabies |
| | Dolineon, Neodulin | |
| | Dehydroneotenon | |
| | 12&-Hydroxydoliceon | |
| *Rumex abyssinica* | Eodin | Antibacterial |
| (Polygonaceae) | Chrysophanol, Physcion | |
| *Tetradenia riparia* | 8(14),15-Sandaracopimaradien-7&, 18-diol | Antimicrobial |
| | 8(14),15-Sandaracopimaradien-2&, 18-diol | Against trichomonas |
| | Akhdardiol | |
| | Umuravumbolid | |
| | Déacétylumuravumbolid | |
| | Déacétylboronolid | |
| | 1',2'-Didéacétylboronolid | |
| *Gutenbergia cordifolia* | Idomaìn | Antileukemic |
| | Guitenbergin | Antileukemic |

The methodology of drug production proceeds in seven stages: culture–gathering, drying, crushing, first analysis, extraction, second analysis and control analysis.

During the first analysis, the various batches of medicinal plants are analyzed to meet the pharmacopeias' standards concerning:

- The macro and microscopic aspect;
- The dry weight;
- The active ingredient dosage.

Plants like *Plantago lanceolata, Calendula officinalis, Thymus vulgaris* and *Mentha sacchalinensis* are introduced plants and their analyses show that they meet the pharmacopeias' standards.

After extraction, a second analysis is required to conform to the pharmacopeias' standards:

- Organoleptic test;
- Dry Weight,
- Alcoholic content;
- Active ingredient dosage.

A control analysis is mandatory after the drugs conditioning. Finally, from the dyeing, extracts and essential oils we manufacture various drugs as presented in Table 37.3.

**Table 37.3: Phytomedicines Produced in the CRP and SV**

| *Used Plant* | *Medicine Name* | *Pharmaceutical Form* | *Therapeutic Properties* |
|---|---|---|---|
| *Plantago lanceolata* | Batancor | Syrup | Expectorant, bronchial secretions fluidizing, anti-inflammatory, anti-prurigo |
| *Datura stramonium* | Gifurina | Syrup | Against hypo-acid gastritis and glaucoma |
| *Syzygium Parvifolium* | Castamibe | Capsules | Against amoebiasis and other forms of bleeding diarrhoea |
| *Neorautanenia mitis* | Tembatembe | Ointment | Against scabies caused by *Sarcoptes scabei* |
| *Calendula officianalis* | Calendular | Ointment | Against burns, infected wounds and irritation |
| *Capsicum frutescens* | Rusendina | Ointment | Against rheumatic fever, progressive chronic arthritis, arthropathy, sciatic neuralgia, myalgia |
| *Eucaryptus globulus labili* | Tusinkor | Syrup | Against acute and chronic bronchitis with sputum, pulmonary abscess, adjuvant in the pulmonary tuberculosis treatment |
| *Tetradenia riparia* | Umuravumba | Capsules | Antibiotic |

It should be noted that *Datura stramonium* (Rwiziringa) showed a high percentage of alkaloids, in certain areas of the country, very important (0.6 per cent) in comparison with that is found elsewhere in the world (0.3 per cent). Thus, from this plant, it is possible to plan the exploitation of atropine marketable outside the country.

## 3.3 Results of Research on Essential Oils

An ethnobotanic study of the plants of Rwanda yielding essential oils made it possible to inventory 649 aromatic species (Ntezurubanza, 2000; Kajangwe, 2001).

Species such as *Pelargonium graveolens, Mentha officinalis, Artemisia annua,* Eucalypti (62 species), Ocimum (8 species), Helichrysum (3 species), Citrus (2 species), Cupressus, *Cymbopogon citratus, Tagetes minuta, Satureja pseudosimensis* were the subject of an extraction and analyses of the chemical composition and their testing for antimicrobial activity is still going on.

Table 37.4, hereafter, indicates the main components of the essential oils extracted from some aromatic plants of Rwanda and their uses.

**Table 37.4**

| *Aromatic Plant Used* | *Main Components* | *Uses* |
|---|---|---|
| *Ocimum canum* | Linalool | Perfumery, Insecticide |
| *Ocimum kilimandscharicum* | 1,8-cinerol | Respiratory tract disinfection |
| *Ocimum trichodon* | Eugenol | Food, Dentistry |
| *Ocimum urticifolium* | Eugenol, Methyleugenol and methylisoeugenol | Dentistry, Perfumery |
| *Ocimum gratissimum* | Thymol | Pulmonary antiseptic |
| *Satureja pseudosimensis* | Piperitone epoxyde<br>Menthone, isomenthone | Piperitone production<br>Menthol production |

## 4.0 Conclusion

It appears very clearly that, throughout these various studies, the results obtained by the CRP and SV are focused on three main axes. These are the valorization of the national heritage in therapeutic material, the research of medicinal active ingredients in the Rwandan flora as well as the local production of useful drugs. The centre thus continues its activities within the framework of the mission assigned by the Government, meeting a real need felt by the Rwandan people in the health field.

About the valorization of traditional medicine, the results reached mark an important step especially when we consider the collaboration between traditional and modern medicine. In fact, the research organized initially in the forms of ethnobotanic investigation and the meeting with the healers within clinical units such as the traditional dispensary set up at Butare by the CRP and SV, had shown that the traditional healers, being wary and secretive about their knowledge, could not agree to work quite sincerely with researchers coming from modern medicine. But, the ambiguity is removed since collaboration is currently excellent. That contributes to the concretization of the national policy of legitimating and organizing the traditional medicine and integrating it in the health services. Everything is certainly not finished in this sector; In particular, the methods and conditions of exercise of this art still need to be improved, the intoxications likely to result from it must be prevented and the hygienic requirements have to be scrupulously respected.

The search for new products with biological activity in the plants of Rwanda served two main goals: to prove the merits of the plants used by the traditional healers in the treatment of different diseases and to show that the national flora constitutes a reliable source for the research of new and better drugs.

The various results achieved by the centre prove sufficiently the real importance of the Rwandan plants in the development of the medical and pharmaceutical national sectors. These results are, inter alia, the chemical screening and the biological tests, and the varied and interesting activities of products isolated from the plants which sometimes showed effectiveness in fields where even modern medicine lacks drugs.

The production of drugs and other related products, developed within the CRP and SV, especially started with known plants, already described in pharmacopeias. These plants are either of Rwandan origin, or introduced from outside the country.

The progressive disappearance of some plant species having medicinal interest reduced the vegetal potential, source of the traditional healers' drugs and justifies the need for botanical gardens installation.

As the majority of the traditional healers exerting individually or in association have neither financial resources nor scientific knowledge necessary for the creation of such gardens, it is necessary to find how to assist them.

Lastly, the availability of a law governing the exercise of traditional medicine in Rwanda proves to be urgent and should be accompanied by a whole set of measures aiming at facilitating the collaboration between the two therapeutic systems.

## References

Arpino, P., Prévôt, A. Serpinet, J., Tranchant, J., Vergnol, A., Wittier, P., 1995. *Manuel pratique de chromatographie en phase gazeuse*–Ed: Masson, Paris,

Adams, R.P., 1995. Identification of essential oil components by Gas Chromatography/ Mass Spectroscopy. Allured Stream,IL.

Benn, R. and Gunther, H., 1983. Modern Pulse Methods in High-resolution NMR Spectrometry, Angew; Chem. Int. Ed. Engl., 1983, 22, pp.350–380.

Morris, G.A., 1986. Modern NMR technics for structure Elucidation. Department of Chemistry, vol.24, pp. 371–403.

Fong, H.H., Tin-wam and Farnsorth, R., 1997. Phytochemical Screening Plants, Documents of Department of Pharmacognosy and Pharmacology; University of Illinois.

Harbonne, J.B., 1984. Phytochemical Method. Academie Press London.

Paris, R.R. and Moyse, H., 1976. Précis de Matière médicale Masson et Cie, Paris.

Rasoanaivo, P. and Ratsimamanga, U.S., 1993. Biological evaluation of plants with reference to the Malagasy Flora, Monographie NAPRECA-Madagascar.

Rwangabo, P.C., 1993.La Médecine traditionnelle au Rwanda. ACCT, Ed. Karthala, 253p.

Nkurunziza, J.P., 2004. Biological and chemical screening of syzygium species of Rwanda. Isolation and identification of secondary metabolites of *Syzygium parvifolium*, Univ. of Koblenz Landau, Germany

Ntezurubanzal, 2000. Les Huiles essentielles du Rwanda, Ed. Laseve, UQUAC, Québec, Canada.

Kajangwe, V. and Mukarusine, E., 2001. Etude comparative de la teneur en huiles essentielles de 61 espèces d'Eucalyptus de l'arboretum de Ruhande. Bulletin de l'IRST n°1, pp24-30.

Chapter 38

# Identification of Interaction of Mosquito Larvicidal Compounds from *Lantana viburnoides* ssp. *viburnoides* var. *kisi* by Using Subtraction Bioassay

*Ester Innocent[1]*, Nicholas K. Gikonyo[2], M.J. Moshi [1], Mayunga H.H. Nkunya [3], Joseph C. Cosam[3] and Ahmed Hassanali[4]*

[1]*Institute of Traditional Medicine, Muhimbili University of Health and Allied Sciences, P.O. Box 65001, Dar es Salaam, Tanzania*

[2]*Department of Pharmacology and Complementary/Alternative Medicine, Kenyatta University, P.O. Box 43844-00100, Nairobi, Kenya*

[3]*Department of Chemistry, University of Dar es Salaam, P.O. Box 35061, Dar-es–Salaam, Tanzania*

[4]*The International Centre of Insect Physiology and Ecology, P.O. Box 30772-00100, Nairobi, Kenya*

*E-mail: minza@talk21.com, innocent@chem.udsm.ac.tz*

## ABSTRACT

Bioassay-guided fractionation and subtraction bioassays of the dichloromethane extract of the root barks of *Lantana virbunoides* ssp. *viburnoides* var. *kisi* (A. Rich) Verdc. (Verbenaceae) were used in order to identify the bioactive components for controlling *Anopheles gambiae s.s* larvae. Different blended and unblended fractions were tested in the laboratory and their mean mortalities compared to the effect of the extract (Dunnetts test, $p<0.05$). Subtraction of some fractions resulted in activity enhancement. Fractions that demonstrated some activity were subjected to chromatography in order to isolate and identify structures of the compounds, which could have contributed to larvicidal activities.

The active fractions contained furanonaphthaquinones ($LC_{50}$ = 5.48–5.70 ppm in 72 h.) and the lantadene triterpenoid camaric acid ($LC_{50}$ = 6.19 ppm in 72 h) as active principles while the lupane triterpenoid betulinic acid (LC50 < 10 ppm in 72 h) was obtained from the least active fraction. These compounds could be used as distinct markers in the active extracts or plant materials belonging to the genus *Lantana*.

***Keywords:*** *Bioassay-guided fractionation, Subtraction bioassay, Lantana viburnoides ssp. virbunoides var. kisi, Larvicide, Anopheles gambiae s.s.*

## 1.0 Introduction

*Lantana viburnoides* ssp *viburnoides* var. *kisi* (A. Rich) Verdc. belongs to the family Verbenaceae which comprises 100 genera and 2,600 species that grow as herbs, shrubs or trees. The genus *Lantana* consists of about 150 species occurring in tropical and sub-tropical countries (Gilbert, 1989; Verdcourt, 1992; Ghisalberti, 2002). *L. viburnoides* ssp *viburnoides* var. *kisi* is indigenous to Tanzania whereby ethno botanically, the leaves are used as mosquito repellents and sometimes chewed for stomach relief. The fruits are used as famine food by the Zulu in South Africa while the Luo of Northern Tanzania regard the plant as poisonous if eaten in large amount but non-poisonous to sheep and goats (Watt, M.J. and Breyer-Brandwijk, G.M., 1962). There is no phytochemical and biological studies have been done on *L. viburnoides* ssp *viburnoides* var. *kisi*. However, phytochemical studies of other plants of the genus *Lantana* have indicated presence of triterpenoids as main constituents (Siddiqui *et al.*, 1995; Begum *et al.*, 1995; John *et al.*, 1983; Misra *et al.*, 1997a; Hart *et al.*, 1976). Presence of flavanoids and phenylpropanoid glycosides (Begum *et al.*, 2000; Mahato *et al.*, 1994; Barre *et al.*, 1997), volatile oils (Misra *et al.*, 2000), furanonaphthaquinones (Ghisalberti, 2002; Abeygunawardena *et al.*, 1991; Perry *et al.*, 1997; Diminguez *et al.*, 1983) and some hydrocarbons have also been, documented (Watt, M.J. and Breyer-Brandwijk, G.M., 1962). In this communications, the bioassay-guided fractionation and subtraction bioassays of the dichloromethane root extract to isolate and identify the bioactive components will be discussed. The prospect of using purified and/or semi-purified compounds from *Lantana viburnoides* ssp. *viburnoides* var. *kisi* (Verbenaceae) in the management of *Anopheles gambiae s.s, i.e.* the main vector of malaria parasites in Africa has also been discussed.

## 2.0 Experimental Study–Plant Material and Extraction

Plant materials of *Lantana viburnoides* ssp. *viburnoides* var. *kisi* (A. Rich.) Verdc. (Verbenaceae) were collected from Iringa Region, Tanzania. The plant specimens were identified and deposited at the department of Botany, University of Dar es Salaam, Tanzania. The plant materials were air-dried in shade, pulverised and soaked sequentially in n-hexane, dichloromethane and methanol for 72 h and then filtered. Soaking was done twice for every solvent. The crude filtrates were concentrated *in vacuo* using a rotary evaporator while maintaining the bath temperature at 40 °C in order to avoid thermal decomposition of labile compounds. The crude fractions were stored at–4 °C until time for bioassay or chromatography.

## 2.1 Bioassay Guided Fractionation and Subtraction Bioassay of Fractions (Blends)

Bioassay guided fractionation to isolate bioactive compounds was done on silica gel (230-400 mesh size) or sephadex® LH 20. Vacuum liquid chromatography (VLC) of the dichloromethane extract of the root bark of *L. viburnoides* ssp *viburnoides* var. *kisi* (LRRD) was carried out on silica gel using a glass column (15 cm i.d x 25 cm) eluting with the mixture of n-hexane, ethyl acetate and methanol. The extract (LRRD) yielded six VLC fractions namely LF1 (5 per cent ethyl acetate/n-hexane), LF2 (20 per cent ethylacetate/n-hexane), LF3 (40 per cent ethylacetate/n-hexane), LF4 (70 per cent ethylacetate/n-hexane), LF5 (20 per cent methanol/ethyl acetate/) and LF6 (100 per cent methanol). Percentage yield of each fraction was calculated and used in estimating the amount to be included in formation of blends. Subtraction bioassay was carried out by omitting one fraction at a time and its contribution with respect to the activity of the extract compared. Thus, Blend one (LB1) was prepared by omitting fraction one (LF1), Blend two (LB2) was prepared by omitting fraction two (LF2), likewise for LB3, LB4, LB5 and LB6.

## 2.2 Mosquito Larvae

*Anopheles gambiae s.s* (Ifakara strain) were used in this study. The species originated from Ifakara, Tanzania and it has been reared since 1996 at the International Centre of Insect Physiology and Ecology (ICIPE) insectary. Larvae were allowed to emerge in plastic containers filled with distilled water. At the second instar stage, the larvae were transferred to large plastic pans (37 cm x 31cm x 6 cm) at densities of 200-300. Larvae were fed on tetramin® fish food, and water temperature was maintained at 26± 2 °C throughout larval development.

## 2.3 Larvicidal Assay

Larvicidal assay was carried out by exposing 20 late 3rd or early 4th instar larvae of *An. gambiae s.s* to various concentrations of the plant extracts, fractions, blends and pure compounds by adding a known volume of pre-prepared of stock solution in beakers to make up 100 ml of water-sample solution (water temperature 26 ± 2 °C). Samples were dissolved with known volume of acetone to make up a desired concentration of stock solutions. The control experiment contained only acetone (blank). The test was triplicated from separately reared batches of larvae. The number of larval death were recorded every 24 h. During the experiment, larvae were fed on tetramin® fish food at 1 mg per beaker per day.

## 2.4 Data Analysis

Data was subjected to analysis of variance (ANOVA) and mean percentage mortality were compared using Dunnetts' test of the SAS package (SAS, 2000). Probit analysis to compute $LD_{50}$ was done using the Lackfit Inversel procedure of the SAS program (SAS, 2000).

## 3.0 Results and Discussion

The cumulative mean percentage mortality due to the effect of exposure of the larvae to the extracts, fractions, blends and pure compounds were used to compare larvicidal activity among the fraction and hence identification of various interactions of compounds within the extract (Figure 38.1 and Table 38.1). Larvicidal activity of fraction four (LF4) and fraction five (LF5) of the dichloromethane extract of the root bark of *L. viburnoides* ssp *viburnoides* var. *kisi* compared well with the parent extract (LRRD) suggesting that, the active compounds were in LF4 and LF5. There was no significant difference between the extract (LRRD) and blend three (LB3) while significant difference was observed with fraction three (LF3) (Figure 38.1). These observations suggest presence of less active compounds in LF3. Both LF2 and LB2 had lower activity compared to the extract showing the contribution of the active compounds in LF2, which were present only in trace amounts. Similarly, there was no larvicidal activity for fraction six (LF6) probably because the fraction was obtained by washing the chromatographic column with methanol (residue). Consequentially, blend six (LB6) showed high larvicidal activity because it was enriched blend of the extract. Low larvicidal activity was followed by fraction one (LF1) and blend one (LB1) especially at 24 h post exposure time.

**Table 38.1: Larvicidal Activity ($LC_{50}$) of Extract LRRD, Fractions and Blends against *Anopheles gambiae s.s* in 72 h**

| *Sample Code* | *$LC_{50}$ (CI) in ppm* | *SAMPLE CODE* | *$LC_{50}$ (CI) in ppm* |
|---|---|---|---|
| LF1 | 73.61 (61.03-106.18) | LB1 | 22.62 (19.95-25.76) |
| LF2 | 60.97 (54.04-75.46) | LB2 | 20.21 (17.77-23.35) |
| LF3 | 60.73 (50.03-80.72) | LB3 | 7.72 (6.70-8.98) |
| LF4 | 15.14 (13.98-16.36) | LB4 | 10.60 (9.52-11.88) |
| LF5 | 9.11 (8.21-10.11) | LB5 | 10.55 (9.75-11.84) |
| LRRD | 7.70 (7.09-8.29) | LB6 | 10.01 (9.11-11.23) |
| Lantadene triterpenoid, camaic acid | 6.19 (5.50-6.99) | Furanonaphth-aquinones | 5.48-5.48 |
| Lupane triterpnoid, betulinic acid | 10.43 (9.21-12.11) | | |

Value in parentheses represent lower and upper confidence limit, values are significant at $p < 0.05$ by Lackfit Inversel.

Columns with the same letter at a particular time are not significantly different ($p < 0.05$) by Dunnett's test.

Bioassay-guided fractionation lead to isolation of camaric acid from LF4 and LF5 as the active principle exhibiting $LC_{50}$ values of 6.19 ppm after 72 h of exposure (Table 38.1). Camaric acid is the lantadene type triterpenoid that have been isolated from many *Lantana* species. Other compounds isolated from LF4 were the mixture of regio-isomeric prenylated naphthaquinones that were not active. However,

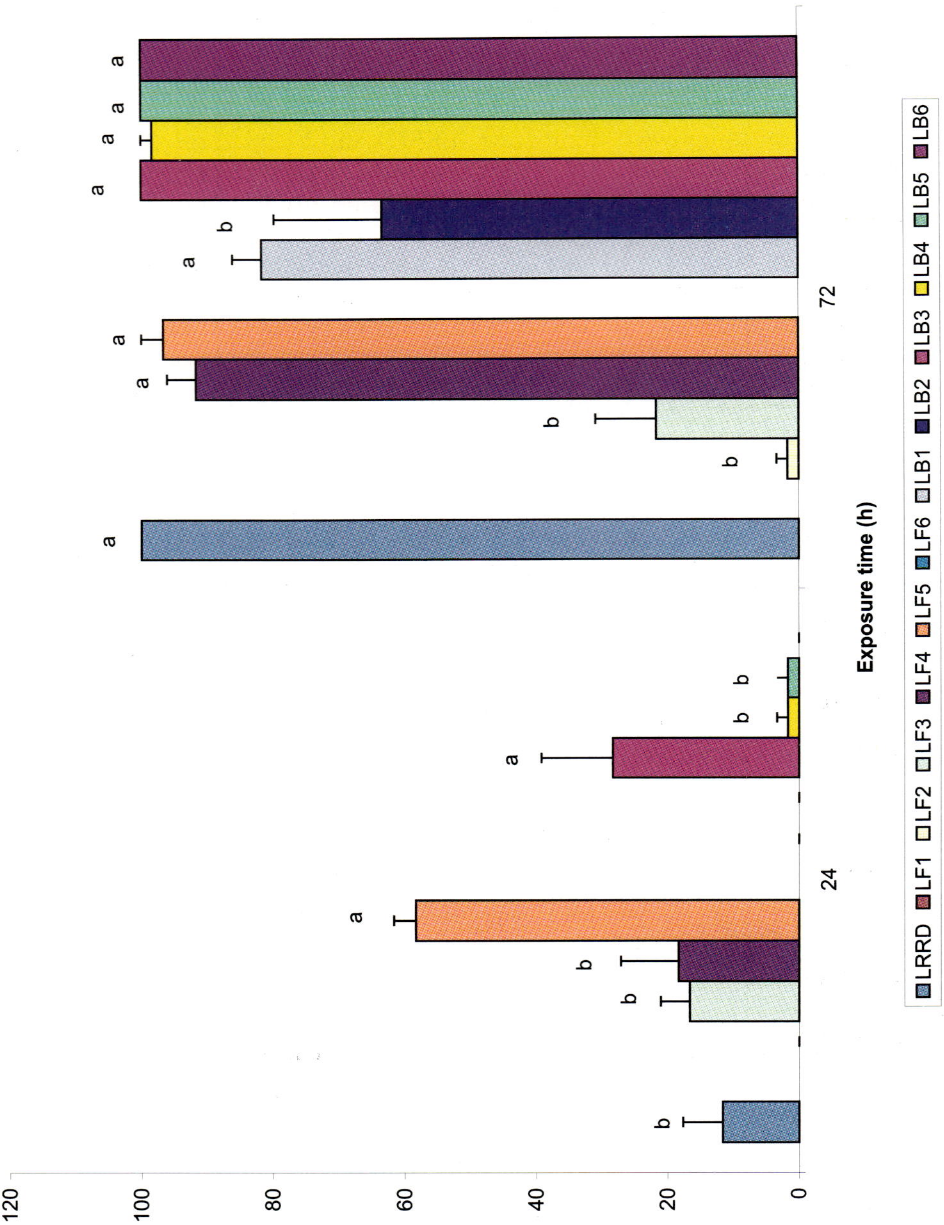


**Figure 38.1: Larvicidal Efficacy of the Extract, Faction and Blends of the Dichloromethane Extract of the Root Bark of *L. viburnoides* ssp *Viburnoides* var. *kisi* at 20 ppm**

compounds isolated from LF2 as mixtures of regio-isomers furanonaphthaquinones were more active compared to the mother fraction. The $LC_{50}$ values of the mixtures of the furanonaphthaquinone were 5.48-5.48 ppm, after 72 h exposure (Table 38.1). The compounds were obtained in small quantities and this may have contributed to the observed low activity of the fraction (LF2). The larvicidal activity of LF2 may also have been obscured by a lupanoid triterpenoid, betulinic acid. Betulinic acid was the major constituent in LF3 and exhibiting only mild activity ($LC_{50}$ >10 ppm in 72 h). Due to the small amounts of the compounds obtained from fraction two (LF2), synergistic studies with compounds obtained from fraction four (LF4) could not be carried out.

## 4.0 Recommendation

Eco-friendly chemicals are recommended in larviciding mosquito breeding sites. In this case, plants that are used by the communities in rural areas in management of mosquitoes and other insects were analyzed. Plants being a natural resource are known to contain larvicidal agents, which may act jointly or independently (Ndugu *et al.*, 2004; Hostettmann, K. and Potterat, O., 1997; Gershenzon and Dudareva, 2007) hence necessity to study their interactions. In this study, the crude extracts and some fractions had higher or comparable larvicidal activity to the pure compounds. These results demonstrating that *L. viburnoides* ssp *viburnoides* var. *kisi* may serve as source of larvicide for managing various mosquito habitats in field ecosystems even in their semi-purified form. Similarly, presence of lantadene tritepenoids and furanonaphthaquinones in *Lantana* species may serve as an indicator for mosquito larvicidal agents. Previously, lantadene A and lantadene B were found to exhibit insecticidal (Wachter *et al.*, 2001). However, in the present investigations, neither lantadene A nor latandene B was isolated but a related compound, camaric acid.

## Acknowledgement

This study was funded through a grant from the WHO Special Programme for Research and Training in Tropical Diseases (Grant No. U19A145511-01) and Singerberg Foundation. We thank Mr. F.M. Mbago from the Herbarium of the Botany Department at the University of Dar-es–Salaam, Tanzania for the identification of the investigated plant species. The Muhimbili University of Health and Allied Sciences and the Centre for Science and Technology of the Non–aligned and other developing countries (NAM S&T) are acknowledged for the opportunity they rendered to enable me present this paper.

## References

Abeygunawardena, C., Vijaya, K., Marshall, D.S., Thomson, R.H. and Wickramaratne, D.B.M. 1991. Furanonaphthoquinones from two *Lantana* species. Phytochemistry (30); pp. 941-945.

Barre, J.T., Bowden, B.F., Coll, J.C., De Jesus, J., De La Fuente, V.E., Janairo, G.C. and Ragasa, C.Y., 1997. A bioactive triterpene from *Lantana camara*. Phytochemistry (45); pp. 321-324.

Begum, S., Raza, S.M., Siddiqui, B.S. and Siddiqui, S., 1995. Triterpenoids from the aerial parts of *Lantana camara.* J. Nat. Prod. (58); pp. 1570-1574.

Begum, S., Wahab, A., Siddiqui, B.S. and Qamar, F., 2000. Nematicidal constituents of the aerial parts of *Lantana camara.* J. Nat. Prod. (63); pp. 765-767.

Diminguez, X.A., Franco, R., Cano, G., Consue, L.O., Garcia, F.M., Dominguez, Jr. X.A. and Pena, M.L., 1983. Isolation of a new furano-1,4-naphthaquinone, diodantunezone from *Lanthana achyranthifolia.* Planta Med. (49); pp. 63.

Gershenzon J. and Dudareva, N., 2007. The function of terpene natural products in the natural world. Nature Chemical Biology (3); pp. 408-414.

Ghisalberti, E.L., 2000. *Lantana camara* L (Verbenaceae). Fitoterapia (71); pp. 467-486.

Gilbert, M.G., 1989. *Flora of Ethiopia, Rutaceae.* University of Ethiopia and Uppsala University Press, Sweden.

Hart, N.K., Lamberton, J.A., Sioumis, A.A., Suares, H. and Seawright, A.A., 1976. Triterpenes of toxic and non-toxic taxa of *Lantana camara.* Experimentia, (32); pp. 412-413.

Hostettmann, K. and Potterat, O., 1997. Strategy for the isolation and analysis of antifungal, molluscicidal, and larvicidal agents from tropical plants. In Phytochemicals for Pest Control, Hedin, P. A., Hollingworth, R.M., Masler, E.P., Miyamoto, J. and Thompson, D.G (eds), ACS symposium (658); pp. 14-26. American Chemical society, Washington D.C., USA.

Johns, S.R., Lamberton, J.A., Morton, T.C., Suares, H. and Willing, R.I., 1983. Triterpenes of *Lantana tiliaefolia*: 24-Hydroxy-3-oxours-12-en-28-oic acid, a new triterpene. *Austr.* J. Chem. (36); pp. 2537-2547.

Mahato, S.B., Sahu, N.P., Roy, S.K. and Sharma, O.P., 1994. Potential antitumor agents from *Lantana camara*; Structures of flavonoid and phenylpropanoid glycosides. Tetrahedron (50); pp. 9439-9446.

Misra, L.N., Dixit, A.K. and Sharma, R.P., 1997. High concentration of hepatoprotective oleanolic acid and its derivatives in *Lantana camara* roots. Planta Med. (63); pp. 582.

Misra, L. and Laatsch, H., 2000. Triterpenoids essential oil and photo-oxidative 2813–lactonization of oleanolic acid from *Lantana camara.* Phytochemistry (54); pp. 969-972.

Ndung'u, M., Torto, B., Knols, B.G.J. and Hassanali, A. 2004. Laboratory evaluation of some eastern African Meliaceae as sources of botanicals for *Anopheles gambiae.* International Journal of Tropical Insect Science (24); pp. 311-318.

Perry, P.J., Pavlidis, V.H. and Hadfield, J.A., 1997. Synthesis of cytotoxic furonaphthoquinones: Regiospecific synthesis of diodantunezone and 2–ethylfuronaphthoquinones. Tetrahedron (53); pp. 3195-3204.

SAS Institute, 2000. SAS procedures guide for personal computers, version 8.01. SAS Institute, Cary, NC, USA.

Siddiqui, B.S., Begum, S., Raza, S.M. and Siddiqui, S., 1995. Pentacyclic triterpenoids from *Lantana camara*. Phytochemistry (38); pp. 681-685.

Verdcourt, B., 1992. Flora of Tropical East Africa. Vebenaceae. A.A. Balkema, Rotterdam, Netherlands.

Wachter, G.A., Valcin, S., Franzblau, S.G. and Timmermann, B.N., 2001. Antitubercular activity of triterpenoids from *Lippia turbinate*. Journal of Natural Products (64); pp.37–41

*Chapter 39*

# Chemoprofiling and Bioefficacy Evaluation of Herbal Drugs and Formulations Pre-treated by Gamma Radiation for Microbial Decontamination

***Bishan Datt Gupta***

*Natural Product Chemistry Division, Indian Institute of Integrative Medicine, Jammu-Tawi – 180 001, India*

*E-mail: bdgupta2003@rediffmail.com*

## ABSTRACT

The use of drugs of biological origin has increased many folds during the last one decade. People all over the world have realized that vast plant wealth has much to offer in the shape of new and effective remedies, which are safe and accessible to masses. Besides their use as such, medicinal plants continue to provide new and important leads against various pharmacological targets including cancer, HIV/AIDS, Alzheimer's, malaria, and pain. Several natural product drugs of plant origin have recently been introduced to the market and some are currently involved in late-phase clinical trials. One of the quality control parameters, which make herbs and herbal preparations unacceptable in the world market, is heavy microbial load. Microbial contamination of botanical raw materials occurs in all stages of plant production like growth, harvesting and post-harvest handling. The microbial decontamination of herbal raw materials, usually carried out by fumigation with ethylene oxide or ether is not acceptable under FDA regulations. Another procedure commonly employed for the purpose is use of hot air treatment, which generally results in decomposition of thermo labile constituents and thus therapeutic properties of herbs get compromised. Recently use of gamma irradiation is being made in microbial decontamination of food products as well as herbs and herbal preparations. Treatment by irradiation is particularly suitable measure to be integrated into processing of biological materials for microbial safety. The aim of the proposed study was to evaluate some selected medicinal plants/formulations for their chemical constituents as well as bio efficacy after subjecting them to gamma radiations of suitable dose for bioload decontamination and compare with the unirradiated control samples.

*Keywords: Herbs and herbal preparations, Bioload, Microbial decontamination, Gamma irradiation.*

## 1.0 Introduction

Traditional medicine systems all over the world use herbs or herbal products as medicines. In India also the medicines mostly used in the Ayurvedic and Unani systems largely comprise of powdered herbs and plant parts either alone or in mixtures. Many Ayurvedic formulations contain extracts of herbs and other plant parts in different proportions, often in combination with other organic or inorganic materials (Premila, 2006). Herbal medicine is becoming increasingly popular around the world (Sami, 2007; Pal, 2003). A majority of herbs, herbal teas and plant products come from tropical areas.

During their long journey from forests to formulation herbs are exchanged in several hands. Improper handling, like drying in open, inadequate packaging and storage result in contamination of herbs and plant products with microbes, soil and dust. These biotic factors are mostly responsible for deterioration of spices and herbs. Contamination with biotic agents not only risks spoilage of the valuable commodity but also poses risk to human health due to the presence and outgrowth of pathogens and toxin producing molds. Due to low water activity herbs and plant parts are inherently resistant to bacterial spoilage but may sustain fungal growth and mycotoxin production (Sharma, 2005).

Radiation processing, which has been approved world over for food commodities and spices, involves controlled application of the energy of ionizing radiations such as gamma rays, X-rays, and accelerated electrons to food commodities including spices and herbal teas for achieving disinfestations, shelf-life extension, hygienization, and sterilization (Nair, 1994; Josephson, 1983) can also be used for decontamination of herbs and herbal products. It offers a very effective and safe method for disinfestations and microbial decontamination of food materials including spices and dry ingredients (Sharma, 2005; Sharma, 2000; WHO, 1994; Subbulakshami, 1991; Sharma, 1989; Farkas, 1988; Padwal-Desai, 1987; Munasiri, 1987; Sharma, 1984). It is a cold process, sometimes also referred to as cold pasteurization, therefore, is less likely to affect the bioactive compounds in herbs and plant drugs and their formulations. Radiation processing can be carried out in pre-packed material without running the risk of post-treatment contamination. The process is very effective compared to fumigants, environment friendly and does not leave any harmful residues (Sharma, 2005; Farkas, 1988).

The present study was undertaken to evaluate the efficacy of gamma radiation for microbial decontamination of Ayurvedic herbs, plant drugs and a hepatoprotective formulation and to assess effects, if any, on their chemical composition and bioefficacy.

## 2.0 Plan of Work

- Selection and Collection of authentic plant material
- Suitable packing of material
- Irradiation of the packed materials
- Bioload determination (Control and Irradiated)
- Chemoprofiling by HPLC/HPTLC
- Storage of control and irradiated materials at 20-25°C
- Analysis of stored samples after 90 and 180 days
- Bio-evaluation of Hepatoprotective formulation

## 2.1 Plants and Formulations Selected

1. *Andrographis paniculata*
2. *Aegle marmelos*
3. *Adhatoda vasica*
4. *Bunium persicum*
5. *Butea monosperma*
6. *Cuminum cyminum*
7. *Curcuma longa*
8. *Ferula narthex*
9. *Phyllanthus emblica*
10. *Piper longum*
11. *Piper nigrum*
12. *Ricinus communis*
13. *Terminalia chebula*
14. *Terminalia belerica*
15. *Tinospora cordifolia*
16. *Vitex negundo*
17. *Withania somnifera*
18. *Zingiber officinale*

**Formulation**

Hepatoprotective formulation. Coded as Formulation–H

## 2.2 Packing of Plant Materials and Irradiation

Powdered plant material (100g) each was packed in triple seal laminated aluminums bags. The bags were properly sealed to make them airtight.

For each plant material the packets were labeled as:

1. 2 packets as Control

2. 4 packets as Sample–5
3. 4 packets as Sample–10

## 2.3 Irradiation

Samples labeled as Sample-5 were given gamma radiation of 5 kGy and Samples labeled as Sample-10 was given gamma radiation of 10 kGy at BARC, Mumbai and brought to IIIM, Jammu. Two Sealed packets of Hepatoprotective formulation were also given gamma radiation, one packet at 5 kGy and another at 10 kGy.

## 2.4 Bioload Determination

Three samples from each plant material labeled as Control (1 packet), Sample-5 (1 packet) and Sample-10 (1 packet) were given for bioload determination. All the eighteen plants and the hepatoprotective formulation were analyzed for total bacterial load and total yeast and mould counts. Results of the bioload analysis indicate that irradiation at 10 kGy completely decontaminates the material from bioload. Irradiation at 5kGy also brings the bioload down to permissible limits.

## 2.5 Chemical Studies and HPLC Analysis

Suitable methods were developed for the HPLC analysis of the above plants using marker compounds. Results of the irradiated and control samples were compared on the basis of contents of the marker compounds. Relative peak areas of HPLC peaks other than those for marker compounds were also compared to find any change in chemical profiles of the samples.

### 2.5.1 Standard Operating Procedure for Chemoprofiling

1. Extraction: Each sample (in duplicate, 5 gm each) was extracted in Soxhlet apparatus using methanol or other suitable solvent.
2. Coding: Samples were coded as:

| | | |
|---|---|---|
| (*a*) Control as: | Control-1 | Control-2 |
| (*b*) Irradiated at 5 kGy as: | S-5(1) | S–5 (2) |
| (*c*) Irradiated at10 kGy as: | S-10(1) | S-10(2) |

3. Whole extract or a small weight of extract was dissolved in HPLC grade methanol and diluted as required.
4. Marker compounds were used to draw standard curves and suitable amount of extract was injected to determine the concentration of markers in extract.
5. To compare the contents of constituents other than marker compounds in the control and irradiated samples relative area per cent of the peaks in HPLC was also compared.

The studies carried out reveal that gamma irradiation of 5 kGy as well as 10 kGy had no effect on the chemical constituents of the plants. Details of studies on three commonly used medicinal plants are described below.

## A. Name of the Plant: *Andrographis paniculata*

### HPLC Analysis after Irradiation

### Samples

Three plant samples were taken in duplicate:

1. Control-1 and control-2
2. Irradiated at 5 kGy coded as S5 (1) and S5 (2)
3. Irradiated and 10 kGy coded as S10 (1) and S10 (2)

*Andrographis paniculata* has been analysed on the basis of three markers andrographolide, neoandrographolide and deoxydidehydroandrographolide by HPLC

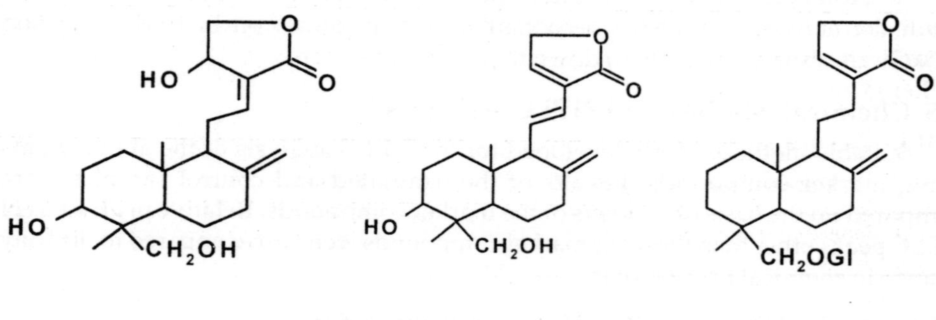


1. Andrographolide 2. Neoandrographlide 3. Deoxydidehydro-andrographolide

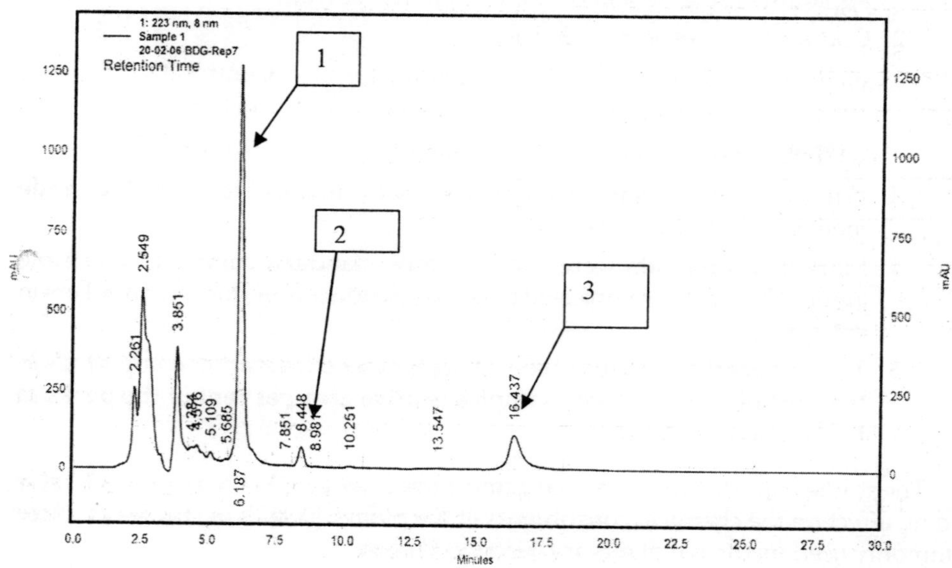


**HPLC Graph of *Andrographis paniculata* Extract**

**Preparation of Extracts**

Extracts were prepared by Soxhlet extraction with methanol

Extractive values per cent:

1. Control-1 = 13.2 2. Control-2 = 12.92 3. Sample-5 (1)= 12.48
4. Sample-5 (2) = 12.2 5. Sample10 (1) = 12.84 6. Sample10 (2)= 12.64

**Preparation of Standard Solution**

Standards used:

Weight of andrographolide = 4.4 mg/5 ml methanol

Weight of neoandrographolide = 7.5 mg/5 ml methanol

Weight of deoxydidehydroandrographolide = 3.5 mg/5 ml methanol

1 ml of each standard was mixed to give 3 ml mixture, which was diluted to 6ml with methanol to give reference standard solution. 2, 4, 6, 8, and 10 µl of reference standard was used for making standard curve. Each extract was diluted to 50 ml, filtered and 3 µl of each sample solution was injected for HPLC.

**HPLC Results after Irradiation**

**Percentage of Marker Compounds in Plant Material (Plant Basis)**

| *Sample Code* | *Extractive Value* | *Andro-grapholide %* | *Neoandro-grapholide %* | *Deoxydidehydro-andrographolide %* |
|---|---|---|---|---|
| Control–1 | 13.20 | 1.0308 | 0.3996 | 0.2101 |
| Control-2 | 12.92 | 1.0386 | 0.4416 | 0.2288 |
| S 5 (1) | 12.48 | 0.9913 | 0.3789 | 0.2110 |
| S 5 (2) | 12.20 | 0.9923 | 0.3697 | 0.2120 |
| S 10 (1) | 12.84 | 1.0770 | 0.4507 | 0.2737 |
| S 10 (2) | 12.64 | 1.0379 | 0.4422 | 0.2382 |

**Relative Areas of Major Peaks in the HPLC Graphs of Samples**

| | *Area Per cent of Major Peaks* | | | | | |
|---|---|---|---|---|---|---|
| *Major Peaks* | *Sample Codes* | | | | | |
| *Retention Time (min)* | *Control–1* | *Control–2* | *5-(1)* | *5-(2)* | *10(1)* | *10(2)* |
| 1.88 | 33.43 | 32.698 | 32.736 | 32.663 | 31.046 | 31.828 |
| 2.28 | 4.336 | 4.854 | 4.075 | 4.462 | 3.986 | 4.246 |
| 3.057 | 9.061 | 9.191 | 9.922 | 10.036 | 9.483 | 9.781 |
| 3.803 | 1.097 | 1.114 | 1.528 | 1.497 | 1.117 | 1.260 |
| 4.960 | 26.311 | 26.93 | 27.008 | 26.844 | 27.779 | 26.544 |
| 5.287 | 5.114 | 5.059 | 5.085 | 5.049 | 5.171 | 5.035 |
| 6.858 | 2.543 | 2.838 | 2.574 | 2.503 | 2.878 | 2.803 |
| 12.435 | 5.292 | 5.854 | 5.668 | 5.656 | 6.979 | 6.018 |

## Comparative Results after Storage for 90 Days

### Percentage of Marker Compounds in Plant Material (Plant Basis)

| *Sample Code* | *Extractive Value* | *Andro-grapholide %* | *Neoandro-grapholide %* | *Deoxydidehydro-andrographolide %* |
|---|---|---|---|---|
| Control–1 | 12.86 | 1.055 | 0.349 | 0.300 |
| Control-2 | 12.60 | 1.055 | 0.327 | 0.342 |
| S 5 (1) | 13.10 | 1.111 | 0.315 | 0.362 |
| S 5 (2) | 12.18 | 0.953 | 0.263 | 0.335 |
| S 10 (1) | 12.24 | 1.00 | 0.278 | 0.337 |
| S 10 (2) | 11.98 | 1.072 | 0.302 | 0.367 |

### Relative Areas of Major Peaks in the HPLC Graphs of Samples

| *Major Peaks* | *Area Per cent of Major Peaks — Sample Codes* | | | | | |
|---|---|---|---|---|---|---|
| *Retention Time (min)* | *Control–1* | *Control–2* | *5-(1)* | *5-(2)* | *10(1)* | *10(2)* |
| 1.830 | 37.762 | 39.544 | 39.424 | 32.053 | 32.345 | 32.557 |
| 3.070 | 8.174 | 8.136 | 8.206 | 8.354 | 8.231 | 8.190 |
| 3.760 | 3.158 | 3.085 | 3.022 | 3.243 | 3.489 | 3.238 |
| 4.157 | 1.918 | 1.859 | 1.838 | 2.088 | 1.992 | 2.000 |
| 4.945 | 34.901 | 34.464 | 34.992 | 39.577 | 39.201 | 39.178 |
| 6.737 | 3.091 | 2.864 | 2.664 | 2.938 | 2.934 | 2.964 |
| 12.687 | 6.948 | 7.708 | 7.983 | 9.725 | 9.242 | 9.291 |

## Comparative Results after Storage for 180 Days

### Percentage of Marker Compounds in Plant Material (Plant Basis)

| *Sample Code* | *Extractive Value* | *Andro-grapholide %* | *Neoandro grapholide %* | *Deoxydidehydro-andrographolide %* |
|---|---|---|---|---|
| Control–1 | 13.84 | 1.151 | 0.210 | 0.318 |
| Control-2 | 12.60 | 1.030 | 0.183 | 0.286 |
| S 5 (1) | 13.78 | 1.106 | 0.193 | 0.283 |
| S 5 (2) | 12.84 | 1.007 | 0.178 | 0.280 |
| S 10 (1) | 12.86 | 0.880 | 0.158 | 0.240 |
| S 10 (2) | 13.44 | 0.916 | 0.175 | 0.254 |

**Relative Areas of Major Peaks in the HPLC Graphs of Samples**

| | Area Per cent of Major Peaks | | | | | |
|---|---|---|---|---|---|---|
| *Major Peaks* | *Sample Codes* | | | | | |
| *Retention Time (min)* | *Control–1* | *Control–2* | *5-(1)* | *5-(2)* | *10(1)* | *10(2)* |
| 2.261 | 2.750 | 2.272 | 1.953 | 1.482 | — | — |
| 2.549 | 25.602 | 22.631 | 22.548 | 21.690 | 40.460 | 40.509 |
| 3.851 | 12.583 | 13.080 | 12.826 | 12.301 | 14.0333 | 15.201 |
| 6.187 | 45.048 | 47.559 | 48.664 | 49.534 | 34.586 | 33.282 |
| 8.448 | 2.264 | 2.339 | 2.353 | 2.423 | 1.728 | 1.686 |
| 16.437 | 10.211 | 10.473 | 9.844 | 10.758 | 7.331 | 7.171 |

The percentage of the three marker compounds in the irradiated samples as well as in the control samples was found to be same. There seems to be no effect of the gamma radiation on the chemical composition of the samples.

## B. Name of the Plant: *Aegle marmelos* (Bark)

### HPLC Analysis

### Samples

Three plant samples were taken in duplicate:

1. Control-1 and control-2
2. Irradiated at 5 kGy coded as S5 (1) and S5 (2)
3. Irradiated and 10 kGy coded as S10 (1) and S10 (2)

*Aegle marmelos* bark extract has been standardized on the basis of two coumarins marmesin and marmin by HPLC.

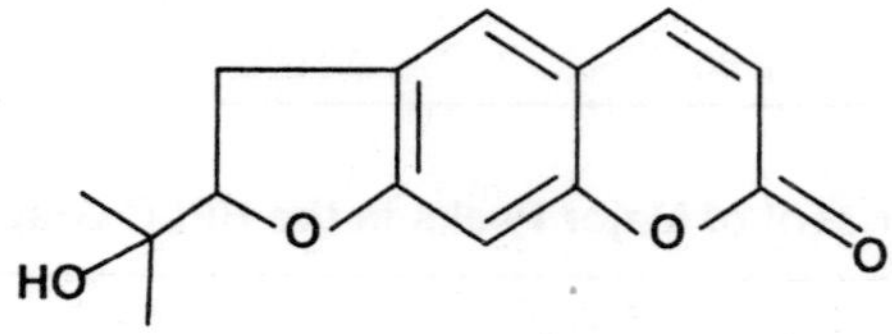


**1. Marmesin**

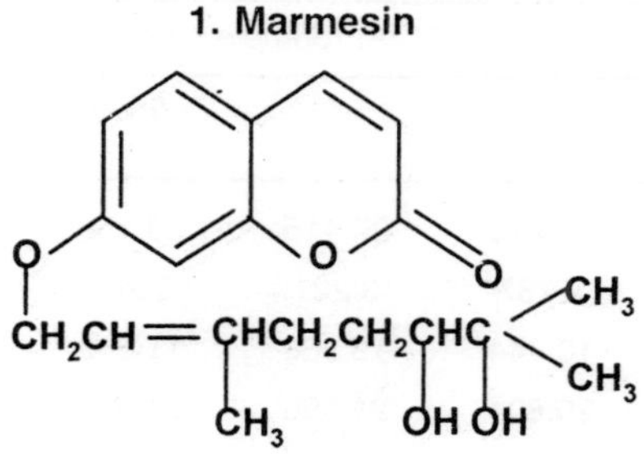


**2. Marmin**

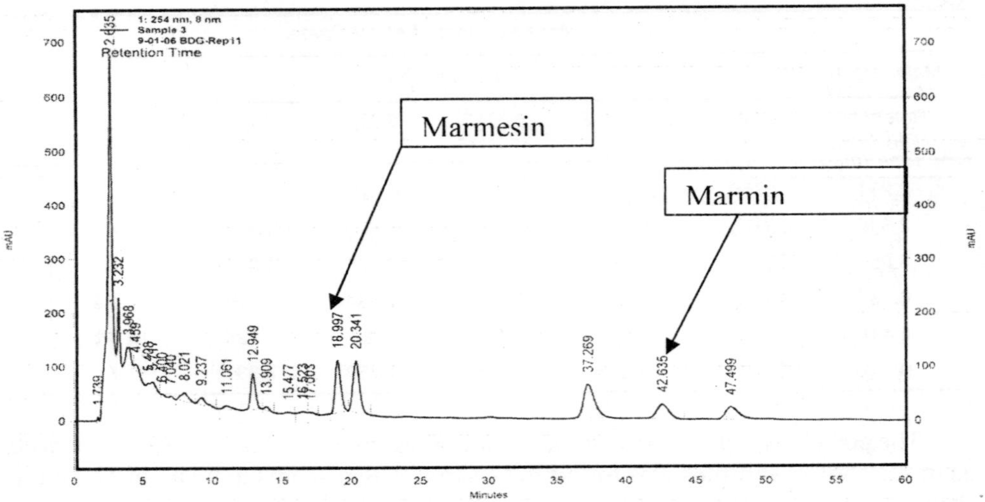


**HPLC Chromatogram of *Aegle marmelos***

## HPCL Results of Samples Analyzed after Irradiation

**Percentage of Marker Compounds in Plant Material (Plant Basis)**

| *Sample Code* | *Extractive Value* | *Percentage of Marmesin in Plant* | *Percentage of Marmin in Plant* |
|---|---|---|---|
| Control–1 | 12.44 | 0.1672 | 0.1831 |
| Control-2 | 13.12 | 0.1225 | 0.1414 |
| 5 (1) | 12.62 | 0.1525 | 0.1825 |
| 5 (2) | 12.58 | 0.1488 | 0.1804 |
| 10 (1) | 12.24 | 0.1505 | 0.1895 |
| 10 (2) | 12.80 | 0.1505 | 0.1833 |

**Relative Areas Per cent of Major Peaks in the HPLC Graphs of Samples**

| *Major Peaks* | *Area Per cent of Major Peaks* | | | | | |
|---|---|---|---|---|---|---|
| | *Sample Codes* | | | | | |
| *Retention Time (min)* | *Control–1* | *Control–2* | *5-(1)* | *5-(2)* | *10(1)* | *10(2)* |
| 2.065 | 20.980 | 19.276 | 27.415 | 23.152 | 24.371 | 20.472 |
| 2.358 | 2.558 | 2.787 | 3.221 | 3.395 | 3.904 | 3.000 |
| 2.580 | 11.080 | 10.744 | 13.968 | 11.889 | 13.693 | 11.012 |
| 3.120 | 20.904 | 20.804 | 21.096 | 21.978 | 23.231 | 20.364 |
| 4.090 | 13.218 | 12.933 | 4.376 | 11.300 | 7.109 | 13.072 |

*Contd...*

**Contd...**

| Major Peaks | Area Per cent of Major Peaks | | | | | |
|---|---|---|---|---|---|---|
| | Sample Codes | | | | | |
| *Retention Time (min)* | *Control–1* | *Control–2* | *5-(1)* | *5-(2)* | *10(1)* | *10(2)* |
| 5.707 | 2.636 | 2.457 | 0.126 | 1.413 | - | 2.280 |
| 6.247 | 5.562 | 5.622 | 1.217 | 2.450 | .660 | 5.421 |
| 7.053 | 3.067 | 2.963 | 0.420 | - | .077 | 3.077 |
| 9.047 | 3.238 | 2.633 | 4.112 | 3.552 | 3.947 | 3.115 |
| 11.740 | 5.775 | 6.810 | 8.275 | 7.261 | 7.946 | 6.316 |
| 12.962 | 4.725 | 5.414 | 6.824 | 5.979 | 6.430 | 5.270 |
| 20.853 | 3.887 | 4.594 | 5.676 | 4.812 | 5.348 | 4.165 |
| 28.887 | 1.592 | 1.347 | 2.205 | 1.920 | 2.231 | 1.698 |

## Comparative Results after Storage for 90 Days

**Percentage of Marker Compounds in Plant Material (Plant Basis)**

| *Sample Code* | *Extractive Value* | *Percentage of Marmesin in Plant* | *Percentage of Marmin in Plant* |
|---|---|---|---|
| Control–1 | 12.8 | 0.175 | 0.192 |
| Control-2 | 13.3 | 0.149 | 0.182 |
| 5 (1) | 12.0 | 0.134 | 0.191 |
| 5 (2) | 12.5 | 0.167 | 0.235 |
| 10 (1) | 12.3 | 0.154 | 0.219 |
| 10 (2) | 12.9 | 0.157 | 0.198 |

## HPLC Results of Analysis after Storage for 90 Days

**Relative Areas Per cent of Major Peaks in the HPLC Graphs of Samples**

| Major Peaks | Area Per cent of Major Peaks | | | | | |
|---|---|---|---|---|---|---|
| | Sample Codes | | | | | |
| *Retention Time (min)* | *Control–1* | *Control–2* | *5-(1)* | *5-(2)* | *10(1)* | *10(2)* |
| 2.645 | 37.639 | 39.337 | 39.734 | 32.021 | 37.981 | 35.487 |
| 3.232 | 3.449 | 3.628 | 3.616 | 3.837 | 3.865 | 4.054 |
| 3.957 | 2.923 | 2.955 | 2.879 | 2.900 | 2.896 | 2.736 |
| 12.939 | 6.157 | 5.720 | 5.340 | 6.276 | 5.538 | 6.056 |
| 18.976 | 9.577 | 8.945 | 9.091 | 10.226 | 8.683 | 9.481 |
| 20.341 | 11.130 | 10.716 | 10.616 | 11.591 | 10.826 | 11.264 |
| 37.269 | 11.748 | 11.769 | 11.757 | 13.171 | 12.098 | 12.152 |
| 42.656 | 4.677 | 4.760 | 5.152 | 5.915 | 5.328 | 5.181 |
| 47.509 | 5.171 | 4.830 | 4.649 | 5.517 | 4.731 | 5.295 |

## Comparative Results after Storage for 180 Days

**Percentage of Marker Compounds in Plant Material (Plant Basis)**

| *Sample Code* | *Extractive Value* | *Percentage of Marmesin in Plant* | *Percentage of Marmin in Plant* |
|---|---|---|---|
| Control–1 | 13.0 | 0.172 | 0.227 |
| Control-2 | 13.4 | 0.149 | 0.193 |
| 5 (1) | 12.2 | 0.153 | 0.186 |
| 5 (2) | 12.8 | 0.125 | 0.153 |
| 10 (1) | 13.3 | 0.160 | 0.199 |
| 10 (2) | 12.6 | 0.167 | 0.208 |

## HPLC Results after Storage for 180 Days

**Relative Areas Per cent of Major Peaks in the HPLC Graphs of Samples**

| *Major Peaks* | *Area Per cent of Major Peaks* | | | | | |
|---|---|---|---|---|---|---|
| | *Sample Codes* | | | | | |
| *Retention Time (min)* | *Control–1* | *Control–2* | *5-(1)* | *5-(2)* | *10(1)* | *10(2)* |
| 2.517 | 6.397 | 7.035 | 5.389 | 7.332 | 5.463 | 4.850 |
| 2.688 | 8.402 | 8.161 | 9.577 | 9.103 | 10.526 | 10.320 |
| 3.317 | 4.161 | 4.365 | 3.788 | 4.139 | 3.617 | 3.639 |
| 3.957 | 4.039 | 3.898 | 8.248 | 8.101 | 3.432 | 8.197 |
| 7.904 | 3.459 | 3.103 | 3.022 | 2.982 | 3.176 | 3.025 |
| 12.096 | 8.477 | 8.373 | 8.074 | 7.955 | 8.474 | 8.127 |
| 17.397 | 12.690 | 13.028 | 13.018 | 12.871 | 13.668 | 13.023 |
| 18.656 | 14.931 | 14.944 | 14.576 | 14.400 | 15.310 | 14.604 |
| 33.451 | 16.435 | 16.432 | 15.175 | 14.952 | 16.053 | 15.422 |
| 38.187 | 7.550 | 7.309 | 6.669 | 6.604 | 7.142 | 6.874 |
| 42.368 | 7.506 | 7.428 | 7.510 | 7.360 | 7.963 | 7.771 |

The percentage of the marker compounds in the irradiated samples as well as in the control samples was found to be same. Besides the quantification of the marker compounds, comparison of extractive values and relative peak areas of peaks of other constituents in the HPLC graphs also indicated no variation in all the samples. There seems to be no effect of the gamma radiation of the chemical composition of the samples.

## C. Name of the Plant: *Withania somnifera*

### Samples

Samples were taken in duplicate and extracted in methanol in Soxhlet

1. Control-1 and control-2
2. Irradiated at 5 kGy coded as S5 (1) and S5 (2)
3. Irradiated and 10 kGy coded as S10 (1) and S10 (2)

## HPLC Analysis After Irradiation

Each extract was dissolved in 50 ml HPLC grade methanol, filtered and was given for HPLC. Volume used for each injection = 10.0 µl

## Markers Used

1. WSC (Withastramonolide)
2. WSCO (27-hydroxywithanone)
3. WSG3 (Withanoside-IV)
4. WS-1 (Withanolide-A)
5. WS-3 (Withaferin-A)
6. WS12 D (12-Deoxywithastramonolide)

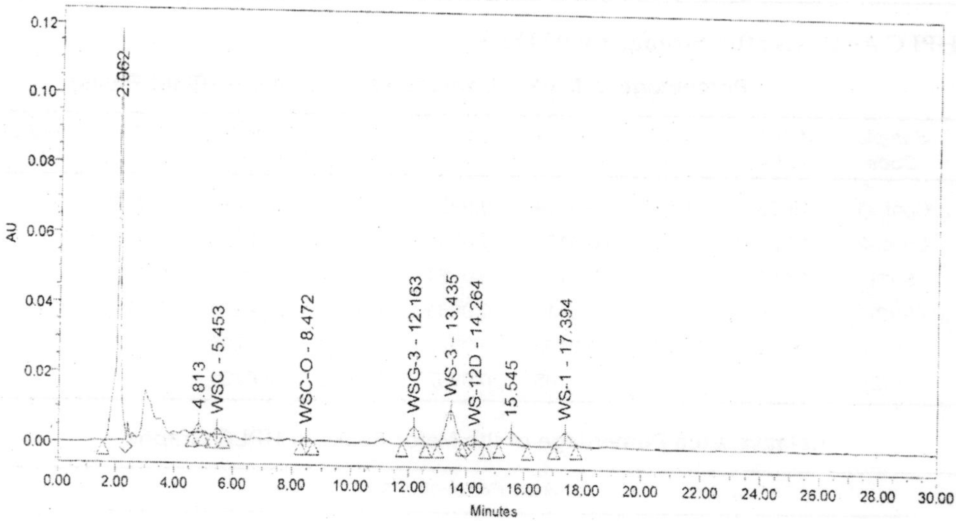


**HPLC Graph of *Withania somnifera* Extract**

**Percentage of Marker Compounds in samples (Plant basis)**

| *Sample Code* | *Extractive Value* | *WSC %* | *WSC-O %* | *WSG-3 %* | *WS-3 %* | *WS12-D %* | *WS-1 %* |
|---|---|---|---|---|---|---|---|
| Cont.–1 | 16.62 | 0.0088 | 0.0019 | 0.1083 | 0.0166 | 0.0627 | 0.0194 |
| Cont.-2. | 17.52 | 0.0087 | 0.0020 | 0.1098 | 0.0172 | 0.0639 | 0.0206 |
| 5 (1) | 17.22 | 0.0076 | 0.0019 | 0.1058 | 0.0148 | 0.0607 | 0.0181 |
| 5 (2) | 16.98 | 0.0093 | 0.0020 | 0.1405 | 0.0207 | 0.0773 | 0.0284 |
| 10 (1) | 17.06 | 0.0065 | 0.0027 | 0.1104 | 0.0150 | 0.0576 | 0.0182 |
| 10(2) | 16.50 | 0.0067 | 0.0023 | 0.1092 | 0.0172 | 0.0671 | 0.0202 |

**Relative Area Percentage of the Major Peaks in HPLC Graphs**

| *Major Peaks* | *Area Per cent of Major Peaks* | | | | | |
|---|---|---|---|---|---|---|
| | *Sample Codes* | | | | | |
| *Retention Time (min)* | *Control–1* | *Control–2* | *5-(1)* | *5-(2)* | *10(1)* | *10(2)* |
| 3.115 | 37.432 | 28.516 | 20.648 | 25.731 | 26.404 | 26.157 |
| 3.392 | 2.293 | 3.291 | 5.613 | 1.539 | 2.454 | 2.551 |
| 4.160 | 1.479 | 1.723 | 1.429 | 1.365 | 1.460 | 1.348 |
| 5.749 | 1.567 | 2.010 | 1.731 | 2.037 | 1.639 | 1.740 |
| 6.592 | 4.242 | 4.644 | 4.685 | 3.779 | 3.763 | 3.562 |
| 9.973 | 0.685 | 0.778 | 0.848 | 0.603 | 1.112 | 0.914 |
| 14.240 | 11.772 | 13.238 | 14.573 | 12.874 | 14.238 | 13.127 |
| 15.125 | 17.395 | 19.674 | 21.372 | 17.973 | 18.922 | 20.502 |
| 17.856 | 7.198 | 8.413 | 8.550 | 9.310 | 7.992 | 8.399 |
| 19.851 | 9.691 | 11.095 | 10.927 | 10.153 | 10.382 | 11.044 |

## HPLC Analysis after Storage for 90 Days

**Percentage of Marker Compounds in Samples (Plant Basis)**

| *Sample Code* | *Extractive Value* | *WSC %* | *WSC-O %* | *WSG-3 %* | *WS-3 %* | *WS12-D %* | *WS-1 %* | *WS-2 %* |
|---|---|---|---|---|---|---|---|---|
| Cont.–1 | 16.88 | 0.0117 | 0.0104 | 0.0932 | 0.0654 | 0.0212 | 0.0170 | — |
| Cont.-2 | 17.02 | 0.0087 | 0.0101 | 0.0905 | 0.0679 | 0.0245 | 0.0167 | — |
| 5 (1) | 17.16 | 0.0109 | 0.0103 | 0.0924 | 0.0661 | 0.0282 | 0.0180 | — |
| 5 (2) | 16.98 | 0.0124 | 0.0110 | 0.0963 | 0.0725 | 0.0320 | 0.0198 | — |
| 10 (1) | 16.62 | 0.0107 | 0.0105 | 0.0929 | 0.0697 | 0.0228 | 0.0179 | — |
| 10 (2) | 17.30 | 0.0101 | 0.0105 | 0.0897 | 0.0612 | 0.0201 | 0.0179 | — |

**Relative Area Percentage of the Major Peaks in HPLC Graphs**

| *Major Peaks* | *Area Per cent of Major Peaks* | | | | | |
|---|---|---|---|---|---|---|
| | *Sample Codes* | | | | | |
| *Retention Time (min)* | *Control–1* | *Control–2* | *5-(1)* | *5-(2)* | *10(1)* | *10(2)* |
| 1.888 | 39.03 | 25.37 | 56.06 | 61.59 | 61.26 | 61.2 |
| 4.717 | 3.87 | 0.71 | 4.42 | 2.51 | 1.79 | 2.26 |
| 5.663 | 2.49 | 2.56 | 1.32 | 1.74 | 1.40 | 1.38 |
| 8.535 | 0.97 | 0.39 | 0.55 | 0.94 | 0.74 | 0.83 |
| 12.185 | 10.67 | 6.12 | 6.53 | 6.92 | 7.22 | 7.74 |
| 13.462 | 19.00 | 11.75 | 11.82 | 13.31 | 13.85 | 13.36 |
| 14.282 | 2.35 | 1.96 | 1.61 | 2.00 | 2.16 | 1.37 |
| 15.572 | 8.29 | 2.44 | 3.72 | 5.05 | 6.43 | 6.28 |
| 17.430 | 6.59 | 3.73 | 4.73 | 5.95 | 5.13 | 5.76 |

### HPLC Analysis after Storage for 180 Days

**Percentage of Marker Compounds in Samples (Plant Basis)**

| *Sample Code* | *Extractive Value* | *WSC %* | *WSC-O %* | *WSG-3 %* | *WS-3 %* | *WS12-D %* | *WS-1 %* | *WS-2 %* |
|---|---|---|---|---|---|---|---|---|
| Cont.–1 | 17.26 | 0.0117 | 0.0104 | 0.0932 | 0.0654 | 0.0212 | 0.0170 | N.D. |
| Cont.–2 | 17.68 | 0.0087 | 0.0101 | 0.0905 | 0.0679 | 0.0245 | 0.0167 | — |
| 5 (1) | 18.06 | 0.0109 | 0.0103 | 0.0924 | 0.0661 | 0.0282 | 0.0180 | — |
| 5 (2) | 17.78 | 0.0124 | 0.0110 | 0.0963 | 0.0725 | 0.0320 | 0.0198 | — |
| 10 (1) | 17.66 | 0.0107 | 0.0105 | 0.0929 | 0.0697 | 0.0228 | 0.0179 | — |
| 10 (2) | 17.12 | 0.0101 | 0.0105 | 0.0897 | 0.0612 | 0.0201 | 0.0179 | — |

**Relative Area Percentage of the Major Peaks in HPLC Graphs**

| *Major Peaks* | *Area Per cent of Major Peaks* | | | | | |
|---|---|---|---|---|---|---|
| | *Sample Codes* | | | | | |
| *Retention Time (min)* | *Control–1* | *Control–2* | *5-(1)* | *5-(2)* | *10(1)* | *10(2)* |
| 4.599 | 3.4 | 3.03 | 3.10 | 2.97 | 3.13 | 2.90 |
| 5.296 | 6.64 | 6.84 | 6.80 | 5.78 | 3.87 | 5.73 |
| 5.805 | 2.96 | 2.71 | 2.20 | 2.03 | 3.56 | 2.94 |
| 7.656 | 2.32 | 1.64 | 1.74 | 2.26 | 1.86 | 1.4 |
| 9.246 | 0.71 | 4.35 | 1.18 | 1.19 | 3.13 | 2.44 |
| 10.469 | 15.21 | 16.79 | 16.21 | 14.54 | 12.69 | 14.02 |
| 11.634 | 39.60 | 38.48 | 39.57 | 39.15 | 34.95 | 36.00 |
| 13.109 | 16.26 | 13.51 | 16.16 | 16.89 | 13.54 | 15.97 |
| 14.266 | 12.46 | 11.30 | 13.09 | 14.55 | 13.46 | 12.92 |

## 2.0 Pharmacologiacl Studies of Hepatoprotective Formulation

Two sealed packets of the formulation–H (Prepared at IIIM, Jammu) consisting of nine plants, subjected to gamma radiations of 5 kGy and 10 kGy, were evaluated for hepatoprotective activity (curative, in *vivo*) in comparison to an unirradiated control sample.

### Results of *in vivo* Studies

#### Animals

The pharmacological studies were conducted on albino rats (Wistar, 150-180 g)) of either sex, colony–bred in the Institute's animal house

#### Models

Effect of different formulations on serum and hepatic biochemical parameters was determined using two models:

(*a*) D-Galactosamine induced hepatotoxicity

(*b*) Paracetamol induced hepatotoxicity

**Effect of different formulations on serum and hepatic biochemical parameters**

**Treatment of test material after hepatotoxin (Curative study, post treatment)**

**(*a*) D-Galactosamine Induced Hepatotoxicity**

Aqueous alcoholic (1:1) extracts (Extract code= A002) of the formulations: Formulation–(H)–control, formulation–(H)–5 and formulation–(H)–10, at single dose or in graded doses, and vehicle (normal saline) were fed to different groups of rats at 6 h, 24 h, and 48 h, after hepatotoxin (GalN, 300 mg/kg s.c.) intoxication. Blood was collected from the orbital sinus in all the animals 2 h after last treatment and serum separated for different estimations. All the animals were then killed by decapitation; their livers were quickly excised, cleaned of adhering tissue, weighed and homogenized in phosphate buffer saline for the analysis of hepatic parameters (Table 39.1).

**(*b*) Paracetamol Induced Hepatotoxicity**

**Treatment of test material after hepatotoxin (Curative study, post treatment)**

Aqueous alcoholic (1:1) extracts (Ext. Code =A002) of the formulations NMITLI–(H) control, NMITLI–(H)–5 and NMITLI–(H)–10, at single dose or in graded doses, and vehicle (normal saline) were fed to different groups of mice at 1 h, 24 h, 48 h, and 72h after hepatotoxin (paracetamol, 200 mg/kg, *i.e.*) intoxication. Blood was collected from the orbital sinus in all the animals 2 h after last treatment and serum separated for different estimations. All the animals were then killed by decapitation; their livers were quickly excised, cleaned of adhering tissue, weighed and homogenized in phosphate buffer saline for the analysis of hepatic parameters (Table 39.2).

## 3.0 Results and Discussion

Gamma Irradiation of the herbs and the formulation at a dose of 5 kGy was effective in bringing down the microbial population to acceptable safe levels in most of the herbs and plant products. A dose of 10 kGy was found to effectively eliminate all contamination making the herbs and plant products commercially sterile. The exposure to gamma radiation at the two dose levels (5 and 10 kGy) and subsequent storage up to 180 days did not have any significant effect on the yield of extractives or the oils when compared to control non-irradiated samples.

Gamma irradiation had no significant effect in gross properties of the herbs and plant products and it was observed that there was no change in the concentration of the marker compounds in comparison to the control sample. HPLC analysis after storage for 90 days and 180 days periods also showed no variations in the samples. Comparative studies on the hepatoprotective potential of the irradiadiated formulation-H with the unirradiated sample carried on rats also showed no difference in both Galactosamine (GalN) induced hepatic injury as well as Paracetamol (APAP) induced hepatic injury models. These studies clearly demonstrate the effectiveness of radiation processing in reducing microbial bioburden without affecting the bioefficacy of the herbs and formulation.

**Table 39.1: Hepato Protective Potential of Formulation–(H)–A002 (After $\gamma$ Radiation 5 and 10) and Normal Formulation–(H)-A002 against Galactosamine (GalN) Induced Hepatic Injury in Rats (Curative Study)**

| Treatment | Dose Mg/kg | Serum Parameters[a] | | | | | Hepatic Parameters | |
|---|---|---|---|---|---|---|---|---|
| | | ALT (Units) | AST (Units) | ALP[b] | Bilirubin (Mg%) | TG (mg%) | LP[c] | GSH[d] |
| Vehicle | - | 125.68±9.54 | 127.56±10.41 | 34.48±3.67 | 0.24±0.02 | 36.34±1.40 | 33.86±1.93 | 6.82±0.31 |
| Vehicle+ GalN | - | 1234.92±42.64 | 1074.27±41.96 | 84.81±2.87 | 0.52±0.02 | 69.26±1.75 | 65.42±2.42 | 3.22±0.16 |
| Formulation-(H)–A002 (5) + GalN | 200 | 360.92±43.14 (78.79) | 334.75±25.62 (78.11) | 48.38±3.56 (72.38) | 0.34±0.02 (64.28) | 42.96±2.04 (79.89) | 41.92±1.65 (74.46) | 5.68±0.22 (68.33) |
| Formulation (H)–A002 (10)+ GalN | 200 | 366.49±36.22 (78.29) | 338.90±21.08 (77.67) | 45.97±3.31 (77.17) | 0.33±0.01 (67.85) | 41.14±1.45 (85.41) | 41.83±1.46 (74.74) | 5.97±0.38 (76.38) |
| Formulation–(H)–A002 control+ GalN | 200 | 389.92±44.18 (76.17) | 336.08±26.50 (77.97) | 50.52±4.76 (68.13) | 0.35±0.01 (60.71) | 44.12±2.22 (76.36) | 41.24±2.72 (76.61) | 5.93±0.36 (75.27) |

a: Values represent mean ± SE of six animals in each group; parentheses represents per cent hepatoprotection; b: μ mole of p-nitrophenol formed/min/L; c: Lipid peroxidation (n mole MDA/g liver); d: Glutathione (μ mole GSH/g liver).

Units: Each unit is μ mole pyruvate/min/L.

**Table 39.2: Hepatoprotective Potential of Formulation–(H)–A002 (After γ Radiation 5 and 10) and Normal Formulation-(H)-A002 against Paracetamol (APAP) Induced Hepatic Injury in Rats (Curative Study)**

| *Treatment* | *Dose Mg/kg* | *Serum Parameters*[a] | | | | | *Hepatic Parameters* | |
|---|---|---|---|---|---|---|---|---|
| | | *ALT (Units)* | *AST (Units)* | *ALP*[b] | *Bilirubin (Mg%)* | *TG (mg%)* | *LP*[c] | *GSH*[d] |
| Vehicle | - | 127.36±8.37 | 136.33±11.73 | 26.82±2.88 | 0.24±0.02 | 38.19±2.55 | 33.99±2.64 | 7.86±0.24 |
| Vehicle+ GalN | - | 1645.92±44.89 | 1248.92±38.76 | 67.39±3.59 | 0.71±0.04 | 84.71±3.92 | 81.66±3.55 | 2.74±0.24 |
| Formulation-(H)–A002 (5) + GalN | 200 | 474.45±41.88 (77.14) | 444.77±66.88 (72.27) | 35.59±2.42 (78.38) | 0.34±0.02 (78.72) | 51.36±3.42 (71.68) | 41.34±2.86 (84.58) | 6.84±3.21 (80.07) |
| Formulation (H)–A002 (10)+ GalN | 200 | 468.39±37.46 (77.54) | 439.75±55.72 (72.72) | 36.38±1.58 (76.43) | 0.36±0.03 (74.46) | 49.38±2.72 (75.94) | 43.47±3.21 (80.11) | 6.98±4.31 (82.81) |
| Formulation–(H)–A002 control+ GalN | 200 | 476.99±22.43 (76.97) | 440.27±26.50 (72.68) | 37.42±2.32 (70.87) | 0.34±0.02 (78.72) | 50.14±3.41 (74.31) | 42.56±4.21 (82.02) | 6.86±4.21 (80.46) |

a: Values represent mean ± SE of six animals in each group; parentheses represents per cent hepatoprotection; b: μ mole of p-nitrophenol formed/min/L; c: Lipid peroxidation (n mole MDA/g liver); d: Glutathione (μ mole GSH/g liver).

Units: Each unit is μ mole pyruvate/min/L.

The results corroborate findings of several earlier studies on spices and dry ingredients (Sharma, 2005; Subbulakshami, 1991; Farkas, 1988; Munasiri,; Sharma, 1984). These findings are also consistent with those of Yu *et al.*, 2004, who irradiated a Korean medicinal herb, Paeoniae Radix, one of the most important ingredients of many Chinese drugs, a circulatory tonic and a diuretic, at a dose of 10 kGy, and found it to be chemically stable and toxicologically safe. There has been a steady scientific interest in using plants and plant products in treating diabetes mellitus as well as hepatic dysfunction (Soumyanath, 2006). This study shows that radiation processing could be used as a safe and effective tool for improving the microbiological quality of the herbs and their formulations without affecting the bioefficacy.

## References

Farkas, J., 1988. Irradiation of dry ingredients, CRC Press, Boca Raton, Florida.

Josephson, E.S., and Peterson, M.S. (Eds.). 1983. Preservation of food by ionizing radiations Vol.1, 2 and 3, CRC Press Inc., Boca Raton, Fl., USA.

McNeill, John, H., 1999. Experimental models of diabetes, Informa health Care, ISBN 0849316677.

Munasiri, M.A., Parte, M.N., Ghanekar, A.S., Sharma, A., Padwal-Desai, S.R, Nadkarni, G.B., 1987. Sterilization of ground pre-packed Indian spices by gamma irradiation. J. Food Sci. (52): pp. 823-825.

Nair, P.M., Sharma, A., 1994. Food Irradiation. Encyclopedia of Agricultural Sciences, Academic Press, New York.

Padwal-Desai, S.R., Sharma, A. and Amonkar, S.V., 1988. Disinfestation of whole and ground spices by gamma irradiation. J. Food Sci. and Technol. (24): pp.321-322.

Pal, S.K. and Shukla, Y.K., 2003. Herbal medicine Current status and the future. Asian Paci J Cancer Research (4(4)): pp. 281-88.

Premila, M.S., 2006. Ayurvedic Herbs: A clinical Guide to the healing Plants of Traditional Indian Medicine, Howarth Press, Inc., New York.

Sami, R.P., Gopalakrishnakone, P., 2007. Current status of herbals and their future perspective. Natyre Precedings: hdl:10101/npre.2007.1176.1.

Sharma, A., 2005. Radiation hygienization of spices and herbs, In Handbook of Spices and Herbs Volume III. (K.V. Peter ed.), Woodhead Publishing, London.

Sharma, A., Gautam, S., Jadhav, S.S., 2000. Spices as dose modifying factors in radiation inactivation of bacteria. J. Agric. Food Chem. (48); pp.1340-1344.

Sharma, A., Ghanekar, A.S., Padwal-Desai, S.R, Nadkarni, G.B., 1984. Microbiological status and antifungal properties of irradiated spices. J. Agric. Food Chem. (32); pp. 1061-1064.

Sharma, A., Padwal-Desai, S.R., Nair, P.M., 1989. Assessment of microbiological quality of some irradiated spices. J. Food Sci. (54): 489-490.

Soumyanath Amala 2006. Traditional Medicines and Modern Times, CRC Press, ISBN 0415334640.

Subbulakshami, G., Udipi, S., Raheja, R., Sharma, A., Padwal-Desai, S.R., Nair, P.M., 1991. Evaluation of sensory attributes and some quality indices of irradiated spices. J. Food Sci. and Technol. (28): pp. 396-397.

WHO. 1994. Safety and Nutritional Adequacy of Irradiated Food. World Health Organization, Geneva.

Young-Beob Yu, Ill-Yun Jeong, Hae-Ran Park, Haen Oh, Uhee-Jung, Sung-Kee Jo.,2004. Toxicological safety and stability of the components of an irradiated Korean medicinal herb Paeoniae Radix., Radiat. Phys. Chem. (71): pp. 115-119.

## Chapter 40

# *In vitro* Antioxidative Activity of some Medicinal Plants

*Nguyen Ngoc Hong*[1], *Ho Thi Cam Hoai*[2]*, *Ho Huynh Thuy Duong*[3] *and Tran Hung*[4]

[1]*Department of Applied Sciences, Ton Duc Thang University, Vietnam*

[2] *Department of Chemistry, College of Natural Sciences, Vietnam National University of Ho Chi Minh City, Vietnam*

[3] *Department of Biology, College of Natural Sciences, Vietnam National University of Ho Chi Minh City, Vietnam*

[4]*Faculty of Pharmacy, University of Medicine and Pharmacy-Ho Chi Minh City, Vietnam*

*E-mail: hocamhoai@gmail.com*

## ABSTRACT

The oxidation of biomolecules by toxic reactive oxygen species may cause a number of pathological conditions including aging, cancer, cardiovascular disease, motor neuron disease, Parkinson's disease, malaria, and viral infections. Synthetic antioxidants, such as butylated hydroxyanisole and butylated hydroxytoluene are strong antioxidants, however, they can be carcinogenic. Therefore, the use of natural antioxidants is favourable leading to an increase of interest in the study on plant antioxidants. In the course of finding potential antioxidants from natural resources, dichloromethane, methanolic, and aqueous extracts of 12 plant materials, which were selected by ethnopharmacological, pharmacological and chemical data were examined for their antioxidative activity on the ferric reducing/ antioxidant power assay (FRAP) and the 1,1-diphenyl-2-picryl-hydrazyl (DPPH) free radical scavenging assay. The results revealed that all of the extracts possess antioxidative activity. The FRAP range was from 378–4344 µmol $Fe^{2+}$/L, the DPPH inhibition range from 5.51 per cent to 93.09 per cent. Among the highly active samples, *Milletia sp.* possesses highest antioxidative ability in both testing models. The results of DPPH$^\bullet$ radical scavenging assay revealed that the crude methanolic extract of *Milletia sp.* ($IC_{50}$ = 3.19 mg/ml) has a better *in vitro* antioxidative activity than the pure natural antioxidant ascorbic acid ($IC_{50}$ = 3.46 mg/ml).

***Keywords:*** *Antioxidant, Antioxidative activity, DPPH assay, FRAP, Milletia sp., Medicinal plant extracts.*

## 1.0 Introduction

Reactive oxygen species (ROS) such as superoxide anions, hydrogen peroxide, and hydroxyl, nitric oxide, and peroxynitrite radicals, play an important role in oxidative stress related to various degenerative diseases including cancer, cataracts, cardiovascular disease and the aging process itself (Ames *et al.*, 1993, Halliwell *et al.*, 2000).

In recent years, synthetic antioxidants such as butylated hydroxyanisole and butylated hydroxytoluene are added to food preparations because they are good free radical scavengers. However, there were some experimental evidences that they induce DNA damage (Sasaki *et al.*, 2002). Therefore, the use of natural antioxidants is an effective way for the prevention of oxidative stress and treatment for various diseases (Liu and Wang 2000).

In finding potential antioxidants from natural resource, various *in vitro* antioxidative testing models have been used for screening the activity of extracts from selected plant materials. The bioassay guided chemical investigation will be carried out on the most active samples to find out most potential antioxidants from samples investigated. The aim of this study was to investigate the antioxidative capacity of thirty six extracts of 12 medicinal plants. For this purpose, the antioxidative activity on the ferric reducing/antioxidant power assay (FRAP) and the 1,1-diphenyl-2-picryl-hydrazyl (DPPH) free radical scavenging assay of 36 extracts from 12 plant samples will be reported.

## 2.0 Materials and Methods

### 2.1 Plant Material

12 plant materials (Table 40.1) were selected using their common use in traditional/folk medicine or pharmacological activities associated with antioxidative actions (such as liver protection, antibacterial, etc.) or by their chemical composition (polyphenolic compounds etc.). *Scutellaria barbata, Eleusine indica, Crescentia cujete, Tieghemopanax fruticosus, Momordica charantia, Equisetum debile* were freshly collected and carefully dried in shade or oven at temperatures not higher than 60°C. *Paeonia lactiflora, Milletia sp., Gentiana scabra, Periploca sepium, Dendrobium nobile, Tetrapanax papyriferus* were purchased from local herbal market in District 5, Ho Chi Minh City, Vietnam.

### 2.2 Sample Preparation and Extraction

Dried plant samples were grinded into coarse powders. 50 grams of each powder was extracted with dichloromethane, methanol 95 per cent and water successively to obtain dichloromethane, methanol 95 per cent and aqueous extracts, respectively, for use in antioxidative tests (Figure 40.1).

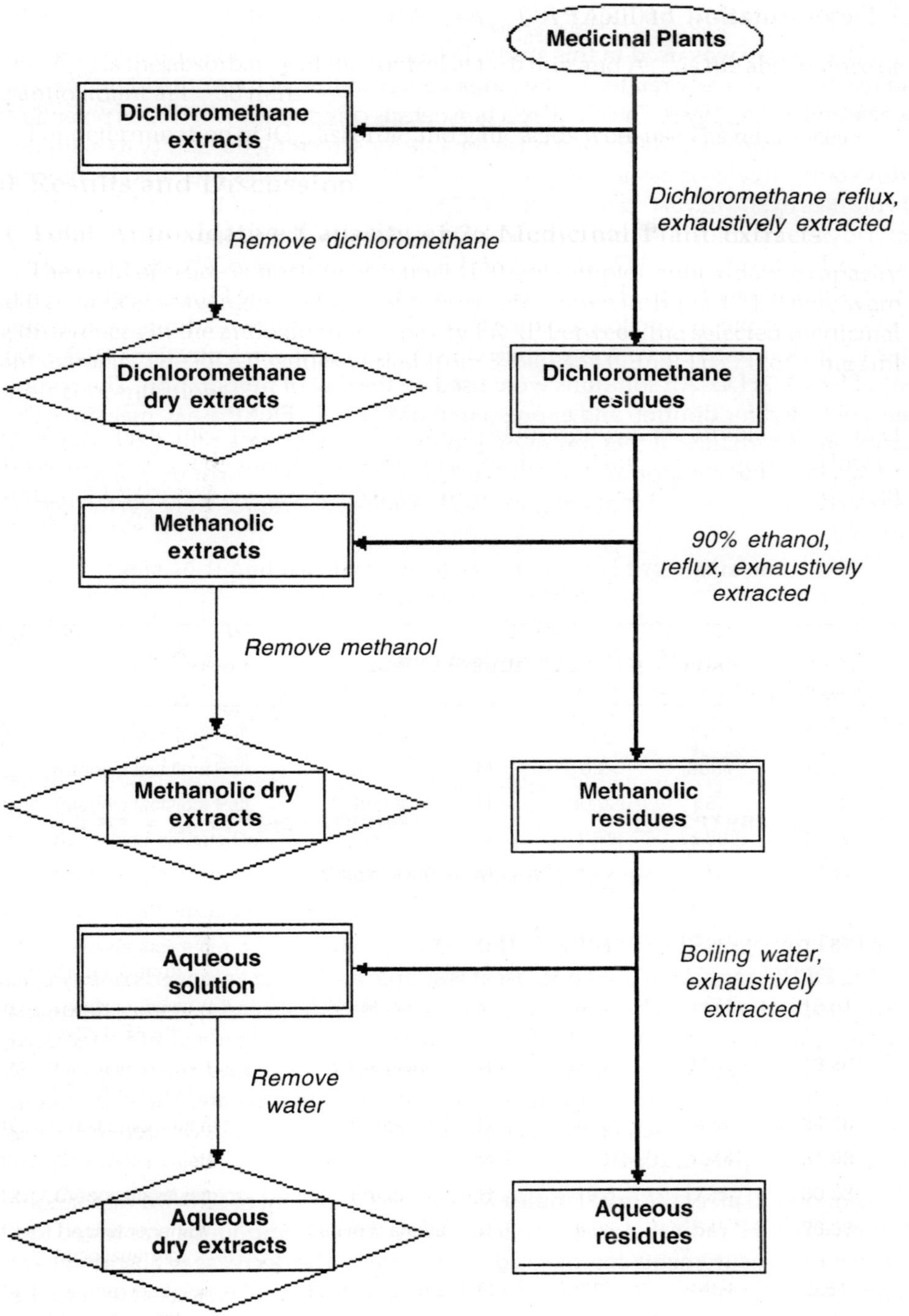


**Figure 40.1: Sample Preparation of Dichloromethane, Methanolic and Aqueous Extracts**

## 2.3 Determination of FRAP

FRAP assay was used in this study, because it is quick and simple to perform and reaction is linearly related to the molar concentration of the antioxidant present (Benzie and Strain, 1996). The FRAP reaction detects compounds with redox potentials of < 0.7V (Ronald *et al.*, 2005), so it is reasonable for screening the ability to maintain redox status in cells or tissues. The working FRAP reagent was prepared by mixing 10 volumes of 300 mM acetate buffer, pH 3.6, with 1 volume of 10 mM TPTZ (2,4,6-tripyridyl-s-triazine) in 40mM hydrochloric acid and with 1 volume of 20mM ferric chloride. Freshly prepared FRAP reagent (1.5ml) was warmed to 37°C. Subsequently, 50µl of sample and 150 µl of deionised water was added to the FRAP reagent. Final dilution of sample in reaction mixture was 1:34. Absorbance readings were taken after 1.5 h. Standard curve was prepared using different concentrations (100-1000 µM) of $FeSO_4.7H_2O$. All solutions were used on the day of preparation. The results were corrected for dilution and expressed in µM $Fe^{2+}$/L. FRAP assay measures the change in absorbance at 595 nm owing to the formation of a blue coloured $Fe^{II}$-tripyridyltriazine compound from colourless oxidized $Fe^{III}$ form by the action of electron donating antioxidants (Figure 40.2). All tested samples were performed in triplicate.

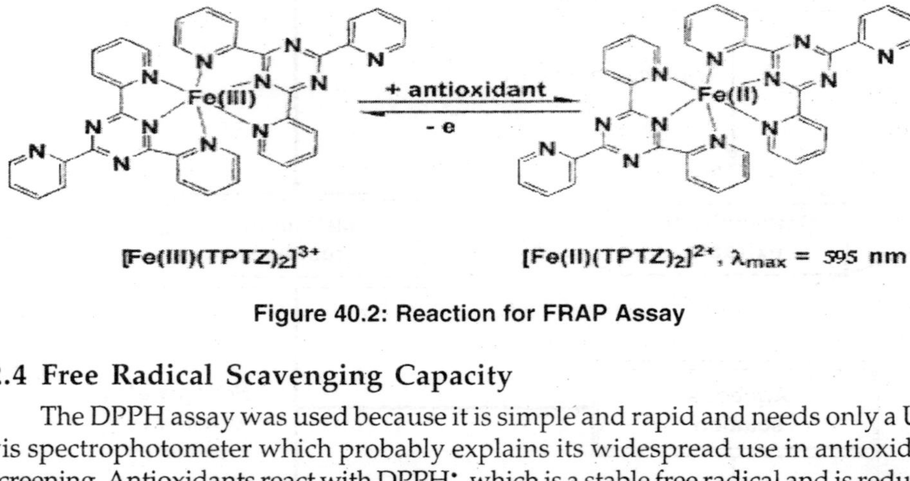


**Figure 40.2: Reaction for FRAP Assay**

## 2.4 Free Radical Scavenging Capacity

The DPPH assay was used because it is simple and rapid and needs only a UV-vis spectrophotometer which probably explains its widespread use in antioxidant screening. Antioxidants react with DPPH$^{\bullet}$, which is a stable free radical and is reduced to the DPPH-H and as consequence the absorbance's decreased from the DPPH$^{\bullet}$ radical to the DPPH-H form. The degree of discoloration indicates the scavenging potential of the antioxidant compounds or extracts in terms of hydrogen donating ability (Benabadji *et al.*, 2004).

Aliquots (50 µl) of the test samples were mixed with 2 ml of $6.10^{-5}$ M methanolic solution of DPPH$^{\bullet}$ radical. A methanolic solution of pure compounds was tested too. Absorbance measurements commenced immediately. The decrease in absorbance at 515 nm was determined after 30 min for all samples. Methanol was used to zero the spectrophotometer. All tested samples were performed in triplicate. The percentage of inhibition of the DPPH$^{\bullet}$ radical by the samples was calculated according to the formula proposed of Yen and Dul (1994):

$$\% \text{ Inhibition} = [(A_{C(0)} - A_{A(t)})/A_{C(0)})] \times 100$$

*where*, $A_{C(0)}$ is the absorbance of the control at t = 0 min and $A_{A(t)}$ is the absorbance of the antioxidant at t = 30 min

For determination of $IC_{50}$, ascorbic and galic acids were used as references.

# 3.0 Results and Discussion

## 3.1 Total Antioxidative Capacity of 36 Medicinal Plant Extracts

The yield of crude extracts (g of extract/100 g of sample), antioxidative capacity and free radical scavenging activity of extracts are shown in Table 40.1. There were big differences in the antioxidative capacity FRAP between the selected medicinal plant extracts. The FRAP values varied from 378 to 4344 µmol $Fe^{2+}$/L of 1 mg/ml sample concentrations.

According to their reducing ability/antioxidative power, the antioxidative effect of these thirty six medicinal plant extracts can be divided into four groups: (a) low (< 1 mM), n = 13; (b) average (1-2.5 mM), n = 18; (c) good (2.5-4 mM), n = 3; and (d) high (> 4 mM), n = 2.

**Table 40.1: Antioxidative Activities of Extracts of 12 plants on FRAP and DPPH• Free Radical**

| *Sl.No.* | *Names* | *Parts Used* | *Extracts* | *Extracted Yield* | *FRAP (µmolFe²⁺/L)* | *%DPPH Inhibition* |
|---|---|---|---|---|---|---|
| 1. | *Paeonia lactiflora* Pall. | Stems | D | 1.04 | 1492 | 17.60 |
| 2. | *Paeonia lactiflora* Pall. | Stems | M | 6.2 | 2684 | 90.57 |
| 3. | *Paeonia lactiflora* Pall. | Stems | H | 30.02 | 687 | 6.54 |
| 4. | *Scutellaria barbata* Don. | Whole plant | D | 1.51 | 656 | 44.77 |
| 5. | *Scutellaria barbata* Don. | Whole plant | M | 7.97 | 2349 | 67.41 |
| 6. | *Scutellaria barbata* Don. | Whole plant | H | 22.1 | 1868 | 48.79 |
| 7. | *Eleusine indica* (L.) Sweet Gaertn.f | Whole plant | D | 2.17 | 526 | 13.87 |
| 8. | *Eleusine indica (L.)* Sweet Gaertn.f | Whole plant | M | 8.53 | 1474 | 19.51 |
| 9. | *Eleusine indica* (L.) Sweet Gaertn.f | Whole plant | H | 20.56 | 1195 | 13.26 |
| 10. | *Crescentia cujete* | Fruits | D | 4.36. | 438 | 24.28 |
| 11. | *Crescentia* cujete | Fruits | M | 10.07 | 1344 | 31.93 |
| 12. | *Crescentia cujete* | Fruits | H | 19.3 | 725 | 30.53 |
| 13. | *Tieghemopanax fruticosus* Vig. | Leaves, stems | D | 6.03 | 645 | 26.33 |
| 14. | *Tieghemopanax fruticosus* Vig. | Leaves, stems | M | 9.87 | 1454 | 5.51 |
| 15. | *Tieghemopanax fruticosus* Vig. | Leaves, stems | H | 18.85 | 1888 | 16.39 |

**Table 40.1–Contd...**

| *Sl.No.* | *Names* | *Parts Used* | *Extracts* | *Extracted Yield* | *FRAP ($\mu$molFe$^{2+}$/L)* | *%DPPH Inhibition* |
|---|---|---|---|---|---|---|
| 16. | *Milletia sp.* | Stems | D | 0.83 | 1248 | 14.05 |
| 17. | *Milletia sp.* | Stems | M | 12.76 | 4344 | 93.09 |
| 18. | *Milletia sp.* | Stems | H | 21.27 | 3774 | 87.39 |
| 19. | *Gentiana scabra* Bunge | Roots | D | 4.95 | 729 | 64.66 |
| 20. | *Gentiana scabra* Bunge | Roots | M | 12.8 | 1893 | 69.23 |
| 21. | *Gentiana scabra* Bunge | Roots | H | 23.6 | 1104 | 40.85 |
| 22. | *Equisetum debile* Roxb. | Whole plant | D | 3.27 | 742 | 35.53 |
| 23. | *Equisetum debile* Roxb. | Whole plant | M | 8.93 | 1780 | 66.11 |
| 24. | *Equisetum debile* Roxb. | Whole plant | H | 23.1 | 1029 | 29.04 |
| 25. | *Momordica charantia* L. | Fruits | D | 1.23 | 378 | 38.98 |
| 26. | *Momordica charantia* L. | Fruits | M | 12.9 | 1079 | 31.79 |
| 27. | *Momordica charantia* L. | Fruits | H | 20.3 | 682 | 26.94 |
| 28. | *Periploca sepium* Bunge | Stem bark | D | 5.95 | 1045 | 21.24 |
| 29. | *Periploca sepium* Bunge | Stem bark | M | 14.56 | 4088 | 71.80 |
| 30. | *Periploca sepium* Bunge | Stem bark | H | 21.34 | 3393 | 36.51 |
| 31. | *Dendrobium nobile* Lindl. | Whole plant | D | 2.41 | 2056 | 81.00 |
| 32. | *Dendrobium nobile* Lindl. | Whole plant | M | 8.23 | 1655 | 39.03 |
| 33. | *Dendrobium nobile* Lindl. | Whole plant | H | 18.3 | 1573 | 29.69 |
| 34. | *Tetrapanax papyriferus* (Hook) K.Korch | Core of stems | D | 0.32 | 824 | 13.35 |
| 35. | *Tetrapanax papyriferus* (Hook) K.Korch | Core of stems | M | 2.5 | 882 | 26.61 |
| 36. | *Tetrapanax papyriferus* (Hook) K.Korch | Core of stems | H | 40.49 | 613 | 9.52 |

D: dicloromethane; M: methanol; H: aqueous extracts

As shown in Table 40.1 and Figure 40.3, the extracts with the strongest antioxidative properties when measured with the FRAP assay (in order) were: *Milletia sp.* (M extract) > *Periploca sepium* (M extract) > *Milletia sp.* (H extract) > *Periploca sepium* (H extract) > *Paeonia lactiflora* (M extract) > *Scutellaria barbata* (M extract) > *Dendrobium nobile* (D extract)

In general, values of methanolic or aqueous extracts were higher than those of dichloromethane ones. Depending on samples, the methanolic or aqueous extracts can be stronger than the other with the exception of *Paeonia lactiflora, Dendrobium nobile, Tetrapanax papyriferus* where the activity of the D extracts were stronger than their aqueous extracts.

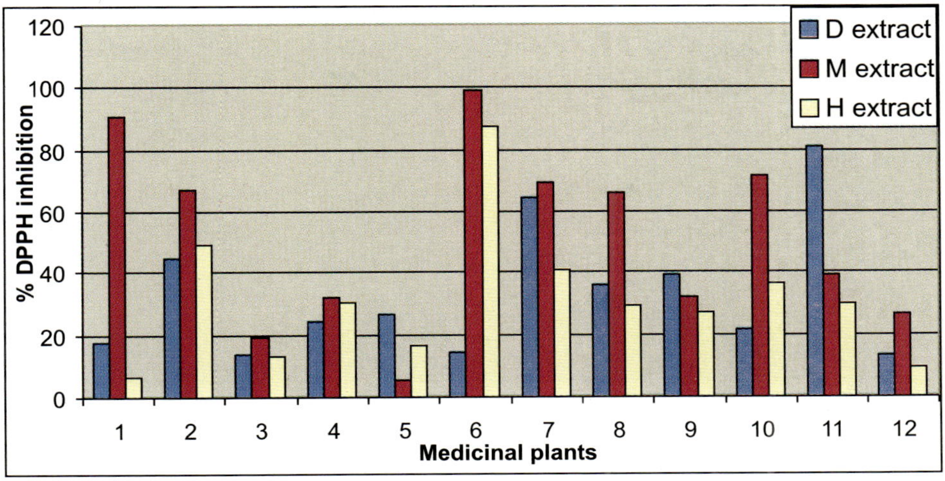


**Figure 40.3: Total Antioxidant Capacity Determined as FRAP of 36 Extracts of 12 Plants**

**1: *Paeonia lactiflora*; 2: *Scutellaria barbata*; 3: *Eleusine indica*; 4: *Crescentia cujete*; 5: *Tieghemopanax fruticosus*; 6: *Milletia* sp.; 7: *Gentiana scabra*; 8: *Equisetum debile*; 9: *Momordica charantia*; 10: *Periploca sepium*; 11: *Dendrobium nobile*; 12: *Tetrapanax papyriferus***

## 3.2 Free Radical Scavenging Ability of Medicinal Plant Extracts

As shown in Table 40.1 and Figure 40.4, there were three different kinds of extracts according to their activities: 9 plant samples showed activity of M extracts were stronger than that of D and H extracts. On the other hand, activity of D extracts of other 3 plant samples was stronger than that of M and H extracts.

$IC_{50}$ value is defined as the concentration of substrate that causes 50 per cent loss of the $DPPH^{\bullet}$ activity and was calculated by linear regression method of plots of the percentage of antiradical activity against the concentration of the tested compounds. The result was shown in Figure 40.5 and Table 40.2. Each $IC_{50}$ value was achieved from a linear regression analysis showing good correlation coefficient ($r^2 > 0.9$).

**Table 40.2: $IC_{50}$ Values of 5 Extracts and Reference Compounds**

| *Names* | *Extract* | *$IC_{50}$(μg/ml)* |
|---|---|---|
| *Paeonia lactiflora* | M | 3.61 |
| *Milletia sp.* | M | 3.19 |
| *Milletia sp.* | H | 4.34 |
| *Periploca sepium* | M | 15.65 |
| *Dendrobium nobile* | D | 15.3 |
| Ascorbic acid | | 3.46 |
| Galic acid | | 2.3 |

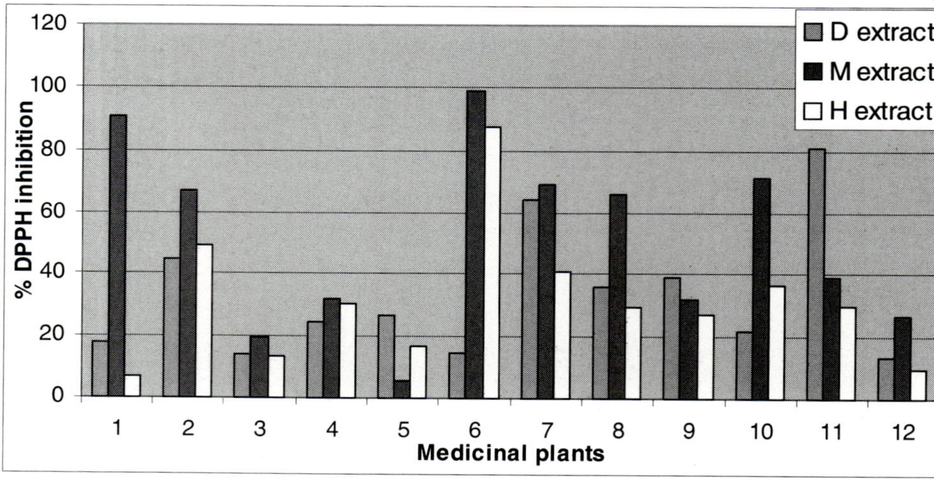


**Figure 40.4: Free Radical DPPH Scavenging Activity of 36 Extracts (Legend: as that of Figure 40.3)**

The highest 5 active extracts in DPPH assay among tested ones (in order) were: *Milletia sp.* (M extract) > *Paeonia lactiflora* (M extract) > *Milletia sp.* (H extract) > *Dendrobium nobile* (D extract) > *Periploca sepium* (M extract). These extracts were further determined their $IC_{50}$ values in comparison with reference ascorbic and galic acids.

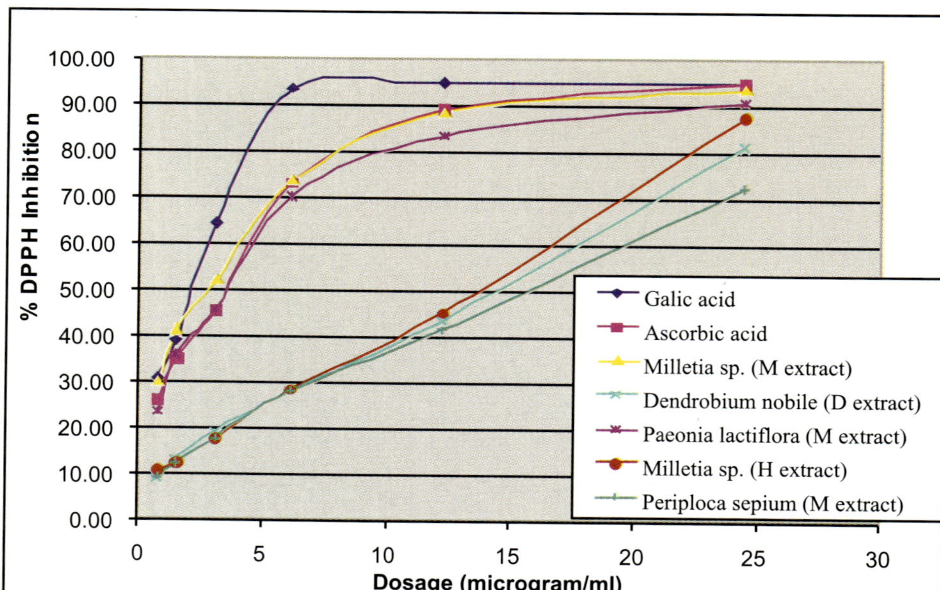


**Figure 40.5: Free Radical Scavenging Activities of 5 Most Active Crude Extracts on DPPH Test in Comparison with Ascorbic and Galic Acids as References**

$IC_{50}$ of crude *Milletia sp.* M extract which showed $IC_{50}$ of 3.19 µg/ml has better *in vitro* antioxidative activity than that of ascorbic acid ($IC_{50}$= 3.46 µg/ml)

### 3.3 Comparison of Total Antioxidant FRAP and DPPH• Radical Scavenging Properties

The FRAP mechanism is totally electron transfer. Hence, in combination with DPPH assay, the FRAP can be very useful in distinguishing dominant mechanisms with different antioxidants. The DPPH assay is considered to be mainly based on an electron transfer reaction and hydrogen atom abstraction is the marginal reaction pathway (Ronald *et al.*, 2005).

Some extracts had the different levels of antioxidative capability in each method: M extract of *Periploca sepium* ranked second in FRAP but ranked fifth in DPPH assay, M extract of *Paeonia lactiflora* ranked fifth in FRAP but ranked second in DPPH assay, D extract of *Dendrobium nobile* ranked seventh in FRAP but ranked fourth in DPPH assay or specially, H extract of *Periploca sepium* has weak DPPH• radical scavenging, ranked fifteenth in DPPH assay but ranked fourth in FRAP etc. This may be explained as being due to the FRAP reaction taking place in aqueous solution where the polarized compounds easily react while the others meet a problem when reaction is in a polarized solvent. In DPPH assay, reaction is in methanolic solvent, consequently, compounds that are not very polarized react well in this solution.

In both testing models, M extract of *Milletia sp.* was the strongest one of 36 medicinal plant extracts. This extract will be further studied in *in vivo* assay and on animal cells for isolating of active compounds.

## 3.0 Conclusion

The results of the study demonstrate that some medicinal plants are promising sources of natural antioxidants. The strongest antioxidative properties when measured with FRAP and DPPH assay among thirty six test samples were methanolic extracts of *Milletia sp., Periploca sepium,* and *Paeonia lactiflora.* Aqueous extracts of *Milletia sp., Periploca sepium,* and dichloromethane extract of *Dendrobium nobile.* The best results were obtained in this study was methanolic extract of *Milletia sp.* The work on *in vivo* antioxidative properties of *Milletia sp.* is in process.

## Acknowledgements

This work was partially supported by the Ministry of Education and Training of Vietnam for project B2006-18-04TD

## References

Ames, B. N., Shigenaga, M. K. and Hagen, T. M., 1993. Oxidants, antioxidants, and the degenerative diseases of aging. Proceeding of National Academy of Sciences of United States of America (90), pp. 7915-7922.

Benabadji S. H., Wen R, Zheng J-B, Dong X-C, Yuan S-G., 2004. Anticarcinogenic and antioxidant activity of diindolylmethane derivatives. Acta Pharmacol. Sin (25), pp. 666-671.

Benzie, J.F., and Strain, J. J., 1996. The ferric reducing ability of plasma (FRAP) as measurement of "antioxidant power": The FRAP assay. Analytical Biochemistry (239), pp. 70–76.

Halliwell, B. and Gutteridge, N.-J-C., 1999. Free radicals in Biology and Medicine, Oxford University Press, Oxford, U.K

Liu, F. T. B. N., and Wang, Z.T., 2000. Antioxidative activity of natural products from plant. Life Sciences (66 (8)), pp.709-723.

Priscilla, M. C. and Heather, S. T., 2000. Antioxidants what role do they play in physical activity and health, American Journal of Clinical Nutrition (72 (2)), pp. 637S-646S.

Ronald, L. P., Xianli, W., and Karen, S., 2005. Standardized methods for the determination of antioxidant capacity and phenolics in foods and dietary supplements. Agricultural and Food Chemistry (53 (10)), pp.4290-4302.

Sasaki, Y. F, Kawaguchi, S., Kamaya, A., Ohshita, M., Kabasawa, K., Iwama, K., Taniguchi, K., Tsuda S 2002. The comet assay with 8 mouse organs: Results with 39 currently used food additives. Mut Res-Gen Tox En (519), pp. 103-109.

Yen, G.C., and Duh, P.D., 1994. Scavenging effect of methanolic extracts of peanut hulls on free radical and active oxygen species. Agricultural and Food Chemistry (42), pp. 629-632

## Chapter 41

# Bioactivities of a Vietnamese Medicinal Plant Vang Se (*Jasminum subtriplinerve* Blume.)

*Dai Hue Ngan[1], Ho Thi Cam Hoai[1]*, Le Mai Huong[2], Poul Erik Hansen[3] and Ole Vang[3]*

[1] *Department of Chemistry, College of Natural Sciences, National University of HCM City, Vietnam*

[2] *Institute of Natural Products Chemistry, Vietnam Academy of Science and Technology, Hanoi, Vietnam*

[3] *Department of Science, Systems and Models, Roskilde University, P.O. Box 260, DK-4000 Roskilde, Denmark*

**E-mail: htchoai@hcmuns.edu.vn, hocamhoai@gmail.com*

## ABSTRACT

From the total crude ethanol extract of the leaves and stems of *Jasminum subtriplinerve* Blume. *(Vang se in Vietnamese)*, seven extracts were obtained using different solvents. These extracts were investigated for antimicrobial, antioxidant and cytotoxic activities. All extracts exhibited antimicrobial activity. Antioxidant activity was determined using the DPPH radical scavenging assay. All the extracts showed antioxidant activity except the petroleum ether extracts. The antioxidant activity of the ethyl acetate extract was even greater than that of the positive control ascorbic acid which has the $SC_{50}$ values of 123.82 µg/ml. Cytotoxic tests against three human cancerous cell lines, using SRB protocol, chloroform and petroleum ether extracts showed cytotoxic activity against both human cancer cell lines used. In cytotoxic tests against DLD-1 (human colon cancer) with cell proliferation protocol, the petroleum ether extract exhibited the most potential activity due to the reduction of DLD-1 cell survival percentage to 95 per cent at 25 ug/ml concentration after 48 hours of treatment. From the petroleum ether extracts, six compounds were isolated, including five triterpenes namely oleanolic acid (1), 3β-acetyl-oleanolic acid (2), lup-20-en-3β-ol (3), stigmast-5-en-3β-ol (4) and betulin (5); and an alcohol: dotriacontanol (6). The structures of those compounds were elucidated by spectrometric methods IR, MS, LC-MS, 1D–and 2D-NMR.

***Keywords***: *Jasminum subtriplinerve, Cytotoxic, Antimicrobial, Antioxidant, Triterpenes, Vang se.*

## 1.0 Introduction

Water extract of *Jasminium subtriplinerve* Blume *(Oleaceae)* has been widely used for tea, for bathing against impetigo and combined with other herbal plants in traditional therapy: for treatment of irregular menstruation and painful menstrual haematometra. Besides that, the decoction of fresh leaves is used as an antiseptic for wounds and fresh leaf poultice for abscesses and mastitis; the juice obtained by grinding the root in vinegar is used to cure suppurative boils (Do, 2003; Nguyen and Doan, 1986). Very little literature exists on the chemical constituents of this plant. Five glycosides were identified namely anatolioside A, 6-epi-anatolioside A, chevangin A, chevangin B, 6-epi-chevangin B, chevangin C, chevangin D (Do, 2004; Kraus, 2002).

In our previous work (Dai, 2007), a preliminary study evaluated the antibacterial, antioxidant, and cytotoxic activity of five crude extracts of *J. suptriplinerve* obtained by maceration method. It was found out that most of extracts exhibited antimicrobial as well as antioxidant activity and the petroleum ether extract was cytotoxic against both human cancer cell lines Hep-G2 and RD ($IC_{50}$ = 19.2 µg/ml and 20.0 µg/ml, respectively). This prompted our further research on bioactivities of *J. suptriplinerve*, especially on the cytotoxicity of the non-polar extract, the petroleum ether extract.

## 2.0 Materials and Methods

### 2.1 Tested Material and Extraction

*J. subtriplinerve* Blume *(Oleaceae)*, leaves and stems were collected in September 2005 in Cam Lo district, Quang Tri province. A sample was deposited in the Department of Botany and Ecology, College of Natural Sciences, National University of HCM city.

Desiccated and grinded sample (1 kg) was macerated with ethanol to give total crude ethanolic extract (26.8 g). This crude extract was dissolved in water/EtOH (3:1), stirred and filtered giving residue A and filtrate B. Petroleum ether was used to separate the soluble fraction in Residue A (S.A1-1), the residue A1 which completely dissolved in chloroform giving S.A2. Further liquid-liquid extraction was done on filtrate B consecutively using petroleum ether, chloroform, ethyl acetate and n-butanol giving five crude extracts S.B1-2, S.B2, S.B2-1, S.B3, S.B4 respectively. Distilled water extract S.B5 was obtained by refluxing the sample with water. The commercial water extract (S.CB5) was purchased from the local herbal market in Cam Lo district, Quang Tri province. Totally, nine extracts were prepared.

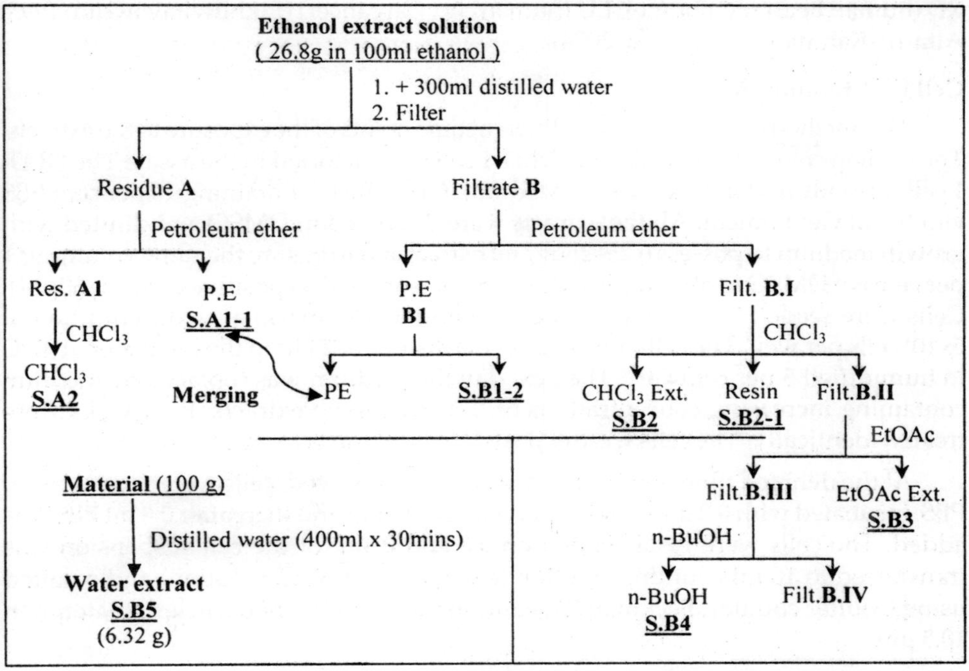


**Figure 41.1: Maceration and Refluxing Extraction Scheme**

## 2.2 Bioactivity Tests

### Antimicrobial Assay (Mensor, 2001)

The crude extracts were tested for antimicrobial activity against the following microorganisms: of gram (-) bacteria: *E. coli* and *P. aeruginosa.* of gram (+) bacteria: *B. subtilis* and *S. aureus.* of fungi: *A. niger, F. oxysporum,* and of yeasts: *C. albicans, S. cerevisiae.* The antimicrobial activity of the crude extracts was examined by use of dilution method. A stock solution of each compound was prepared in methanol. The necessary dilutions were made and plated into standard 96-well microtiter plates. Control wells received the appropriate solvents without the test compounds.

### Antioxidant Assay

The antioxidant activity of all extracts was determined according to the DPPH radical scavenging assay. The odd electron in the DPPH free radical gives a strong absorption maximum at 515 nm and was purple in color. When DPPH reacts with an antioxidant compound, which can donate hydrogen, it was reduced. The changes in colour (from purple to light yellow) were measured at 515 nm on a Lisa UV/visible light spectrophotometer.

### Assay for Cytotoxic Activity

Cytotoxicity assay was done as described (Dai, 2007) using the dye binding assay SRB (Sulforhodamine B) method on Hep-G2 (human hepatocellular carcinoma),

RD (human heart membrane), LU (human cervical cancer) (Likhitwitayawuid, 1993; Atta-ur-Rahman, 2001; Chau, 2004).

**Cell Proliferation Assay**

This method counts the cells at different time points of the exposure to the extracts. The human colon cancer cells line, DLD-1 cell was included in the assay. The DLD-1 cells are cultured in McCoy's 5A Medium (Gibco BRL) containing 10 per cent FBS and 0.5ml Gentamicin. All the extracts were dissolved in DMSO and diluted with growth medium to possess 6.25–25μg/ml extract and to ensure the same volume (0.1 per cent) of DMSO in all samples. Resveratrol was used as positive control (60μM). Cells were seeded into 24-well dishes (Technunc, Denmark) at a concentration of $5x10^4$ cells per well. The cells attached on the dishes for 24 hr in the incubator at 37°C in humidified 5 per cent $CO_2$. The next day the medium was replaced by medium containing increasing concentrations of *J. subtriplinerve* extracts. Four wells were treated identically. The cells were exposed to the extracts for 0, 24 or 48 hr.

At the denoted time points, the medium was removed, cells were washed with PBS, incubated with 0.2 ml Versene/trypsin for 20 min and thereafter 0.8 ml PBS was added. The cells were resuspended on ice and 0.8ml of the cell suspension was transferred to 10 ml counting solution (a 0.9 per cent NaCl solution) and counted using Coulter counter, Beckman Z2, counting the number of particles greater than 10,5 μm.

Calculation of the cell survival (per cent) value: The per cent of cell survival was calculated by

$$\text{cell survival } (\%) = \left[ \frac{NC_{\text{test sample}}}{NC_{\text{negative control}}} \right] \times 100\%$$

*where,* NC was the number of the cells.

The numbers of cells are expressed as average values for each time–and concentration points at 0hr, 24hr and 48hr.

## 2.0 General Experimental Procedures

Mass spectra were obtained using a Hewlett Packard 5989 HP MS spectrometer. $^{1}$H-NMR (500 MHz) and $^{13}$C-NMR (125 MHZ) were recorded on a Bruker–Advance–500MHz instrument include 1D: $^{1}$H, $^{13}$C-NMR, DEPT and 2D: HMQC, HMBC. Column chromatography was performed on silica gel (Kieselgel 60, 70-230 mesh and 230-400 mesh, Merck).

## 3.0 Results and Discussion

In our previous study (Dai, 2007), extracts of *J. subtriplinerve* were prepared by consecutively maceration of sample with increasing polarity solvent. In this present study, the total crude ethanol extract was liquid-to-liquid partitioned to obtain various crude extracts. The advantages of this method were that it was more selective and did not consume much time and solvent.

## 3.1 Bioactive Tests

### Antimicrobial Activity

The lowest concentrations of the antimicrobial agents inhibiting bacterial growth are reported as a minimum inhibitory concentration (MIC). The results are shown in Table 41.1. Most of the extracts exhibited antimicrobial activity against fungi except S.A1-1 and S.B4. The S.B2 and S.B2-1 showed remarkable activities with the MIC of 50 µg/ml against *A. niger* whereas the others showed activity at 100µg/ml. In addition, MIC on *F. oxysporum* ranged from 50 to 200µg/ml concentration with the lowest MIC for S.A2. None of the extracts inhibited the growing of *P. aeruginosa* and *C. albicans*.

**Table 41.1: The Minimum Inhibitory Concentration (MIC) (µg/ml) Values of Extracts**

| *Extracts* | *Samples* | *Gr(-)* | *Gr(+)* | | *Fungi* | | *Yeast* |
|---|---|---|---|---|---|---|---|
| | | *E. coli* | *B. subtilis* | *S. aureus* | *A. niger* | *F. oxysporum* | *S. cerevisiae* |
| P.E | S.A1-1 | 200 | – | 200 | – | – | – |
| $CHCl_3$ | S.A2 | – | 200 | – | 100 | 50 | – |
| EtOH | S.B1-2 | 200 | 50 | – | 100 | – | – |
| $CHCl_3$ | S.B2 | – | 50 | 200 | 50 | – | – |
| Resin | S.B2-1 | 200 | – | – | 50 | 200 | – |
| EtOAc | S.B3 | – | – | 200 | 100 | 200 | – |
| *n*-BuOH | S.B4 | 100 | 100 | 100 | – | – | 200 |
| DW | S.B5 | – | – | – | 100 | 100 | – |
| Com. DW | S.CB5 | 100 | 400 | – | 100 | 200 | – |

(–) indicates that no MIC could be established.

This was the first result indicating that *J. subtriplinerve* has inhibition on fungi. This result is in accordance with previous literature (Nguyen, 1986a; 1986b) which indicated that distilled-water and ethanol-water extracts of *J. subtriplinerve* (with 40, 50 and 90 per cent of ethanol) were less active against *P. aseruginosa* and displayed no effect on fungus *C. albicans*. In our previous work, significant anti-microbial effects of extracts of *J. subtriplinerve* was observed on *E. coli*, *B. subtilis* and *S. aureus* (Dai, 2007). Otherwise, the distilled water extract (S.B5) exhibited two fungi *A. niger* and *F. oxysporum* at MIC of 100 and 50 µg/ml, respectively. Ethyl acetate (S.B3) extract showed inhibitory activity against *S. aureus* with MIC of 200µg/ml as well as against two fungi *A. niger* and *F. oxysporum* at MIC value of 100 and 200 µg/ml.

The *n*-butanol extract (S.B4) was found out as the most potent antibacterial fraction which exhibited antimicrobial against bacteria *E. coli*, *B. subtilis*, *S. aureus* and yeast *S. cereviase*. This is the only extract which exhibited inhibitory effect against a yeast.

### Antioxidant Activity

Like other traditional beverages or teas, water extracts of *J. subtriplinerve* also contain significant antioxidant activity. In Table 41.2, extracts S.B1-2 and S.B3 displayed equally antioxidant activities. The S.B3 presented a remarkable $SC_{50}$ value at 99 μg/ml that was more potent than S.B1-2 (149 μg/ml). In accordance with the previous study, the ethyl acetate extract also showed the highest antioxidant activity.

The two water extracts S.B5 and S.CB5 have the same antioxidant activity. Therefore, we propose that water extract of *J. subtriplinerve* can be used as a beverage with good antioxidant activity like other traditional beverages or teas.

**Table 41.2: Antioxidant Activity of Extracts**

| | *Samples* | *SC (per cent)* | *$SC_{50}$ (μg/ml)* |
|---|---|---|---|
| (+) Control | Ascorbic Acid | 63.67 ± 0.00 | 124 |
| (–) Control | 5% DMSO/EtOH | 0 | – |
| P.E | S.A1-1 | 12.95 ± 1.60 | – |
| $CHCl_3$ | S.A2 | 41.01 ± 1.10 | – |
| EtOH | S.B1-2 | 56.35 ± 0.70 | 149 |
| $CHCl_3$ | S.B2 | 40.88 ± 1.00 | – |
| Resin | S.B2-1 | 41.01 ± 0.40 | – |
| EtOAc | S.B3 | 57.64 ± 0.20 | 99 |
| n-BuOH | S.B4 | 49.28 ± 0.80 | – |
| DW | S.B5 | 26.97 ± 0.30 | – |
| Com. DW | S.CB5 | 26.26 ± 0.70 | – |

**Table 41.3: Cytotoxic Activities of Extracts on Hep-G2, RD, and LU Cancerous Cell Lines**

| | *Samples* | *Cell Survival (%)* | | | *$IC_{50}$ (μg/ml)* | | |
|---|---|---|---|---|---|---|---|
| | | *Hep-G2* | *RD* | *LU* | *Hep-G2* | *RD* | *LU* |
| (+) control | Elipticine | 2.0 ± 0.0 | 1.5 ± 0.0 | 2.4 ± 0.1 | 2.0 | 0.1 | 0.3 |
| (–) control | DMSO | 100.0 ± 0.0 | 100.0 ± 0.0 | 100.0 ± 0.0 | >20 | >20 | >20 |
| P.E | S.A1-1 | 33.6 ± 0.2 | 26.0 ± 0.1 | 62.1 ± 0.9 | 10.7 | 12.6 | >20 |
| EtOH | S.B1-2 | 101.6 ± 0.6 | 82.8 ± 1.7 | 63.6 ± 2.3 | >20 | >20 | >20 |
| $CHCl_3$ | S.B2 | 95.4 ± 1.3 | 90.0 ± 1.4 | 84.7 ± 0.9 | >20 | >20 | >20 |
| Resin | S.B2-1 | 106.1 ± 0.7 | 72.1 ± 0.5 | 87.6 ± 0.3 | >20 | >20 | >20 |
| EtOAc | S.B3 | 103.0 ± 1.1 | 61.2 ± 0.4 | 79.4 ± 1.6 | >20 | >20 | >20 |
| n-BuOH | S.B4 | 80.8 ± 1.7 | 75.5 ± 0.5 | 71.2 ± 0.7 | >20 | >20 | >20 |
| DW | S.B5 | 108.1 ± 0.1 | 75.7 ± 1.2 | 80.8 ± 1.6 | >20 | >20 | >20 |
| $CHCl_3$ | S.A2 | 29.4 ± 0.4 | 49.5 ± 0.1 | 65.7 ± 0.9 | 6.9 | 19.0 | >20 |
| Com. DW | S.CB5 | 103.5 ± 1.4 | 109.2 ± 1.3 | 82.20 ± 0.4 | >20 | >20 | >20 |

## Cytotoxic Activity

All the extracts were tested for cytotoxic activity on Hep-G2, RD, and LU human cancerous cell lines. Only two out of the extracts, S.A1-1 and S.A2, showed strong cytotoxic activity against the cancerous cell lines used. The S.A2 extract exhibited the highest activity against Hep-G2 cell line with an $IC_{50}$ value at 6.9μg/ml, followed by the S.A1-1 extract ($IC_{50}$ 10.7 μg/ml). Conversely, on experiments with RD cell line, the influence of S.A1-1 on RD cell line was the highest, followed by S.A2 with the $IC_{50}$ at 12.6 and 19.0 μg/ml, respectively. This result showed that the cytotoxic activity compounds are in the non-polar phase of the plant's extracts.

**Cell Proliferation Assay**

All the extracts of *J. subtriplinerve* were initially tested at two concentrations (6.25 and 25μg/ml). Which extracts showed some inhibition of cell proliferation at 25μg/ml (S.A1-1, S.B2, S.B5 and S.CB5) would be additionally tested at 62.5 and 250μg/ml. The growth curves were shown below. Exposing the DLD-1 cells to 250μg/ml, the S.A1-1 extract reduced the percentage of number of cell to 22 per cent and 3 per cent of the control after 24hr and 48hr, respectively. In addition, the S.B2 was also present an enjoyable percentage of cell survival. At the concentration of 250μg/ml S.B2, the extract was four times than the 62.5μg/ml concentration but its ability to reduce the cell survival was stable about 2.3-2.4 times after 24hr or 48hr. The remaining extracts were also having activities but seem to be reducing the effectiveness after 24hr.

The number of cells was determined as described in the Material and Method section. The numbers are the relative number of cells at 62.5 and 250 μg/ml.

**Table 41.4: Dose and Time Effect of Various Extracts from *J. subtriplinerve* on the Cell Proliferation of DLD-1 Cells**

| *Samples* | *24hr* | | *48hr* | |
|---|---|---|---|---|
| | *62.5 μg/ml (%)* | *250 μg/ml (%)* | *62.5 μg/ml (%)* | *250 μg/ml (%)* |
| S.A1-1 | 111 | 22 | 89 | 3 |
| S.B2 | 83 | 36 | 71 | 29 |
| S.B6 | 72 | 68 | 91 | 78 |
| S.CB6 | 48 | 31 | 85 | 48 |

The results brought out the unforeseen data that indicated S.A1-1 was showing the highest activity by reducing the cell survival by 3 per cent at 250μg/ml concentration in 48hr experiment, after that was S.B2, then S.CB5 and S.B5 was the lowest with 29, 48 and 78 per cent, respectively. All these extracts presented activities, but only the percentages of cell survival of S.A1-1 and S.B2 were reduced when increasing concentration from 62.5μg/ml to 250μg/ml, together with increasing of time treatment. The others, S.B5 and S.CB5 were appearance that fading away their activities after 25 to 35hr treatment.

Among four higher concentration extracts, S.A1-1 was indicated that it was the most active extract in the DLD-1 cell assay and chosen for determining the $IC_{50}$. To determine the $IC_{50}$, five concentrations of S.A1-1 were prepared and tested: 15.625, 31.25, 62.5, 125 and 250μg/ml. After 24hr and 48hr, the value where the curves cross

**Figure 41.2 (a) and (b): Dose–and Time-dependent Inhibition of Cell Proliferation of DLD-1 Cells Exposed to Extract S.A1-1, S.B2, S.B6, and S.CB6; (c) Dose–and Time-dependent Inhibition of Cell Proliferation of DLD-1 Cells Exposed to Extract S.A1-1 to Determine IC50.**

**The numbers are mean and standard deviation of 4 numbers.**

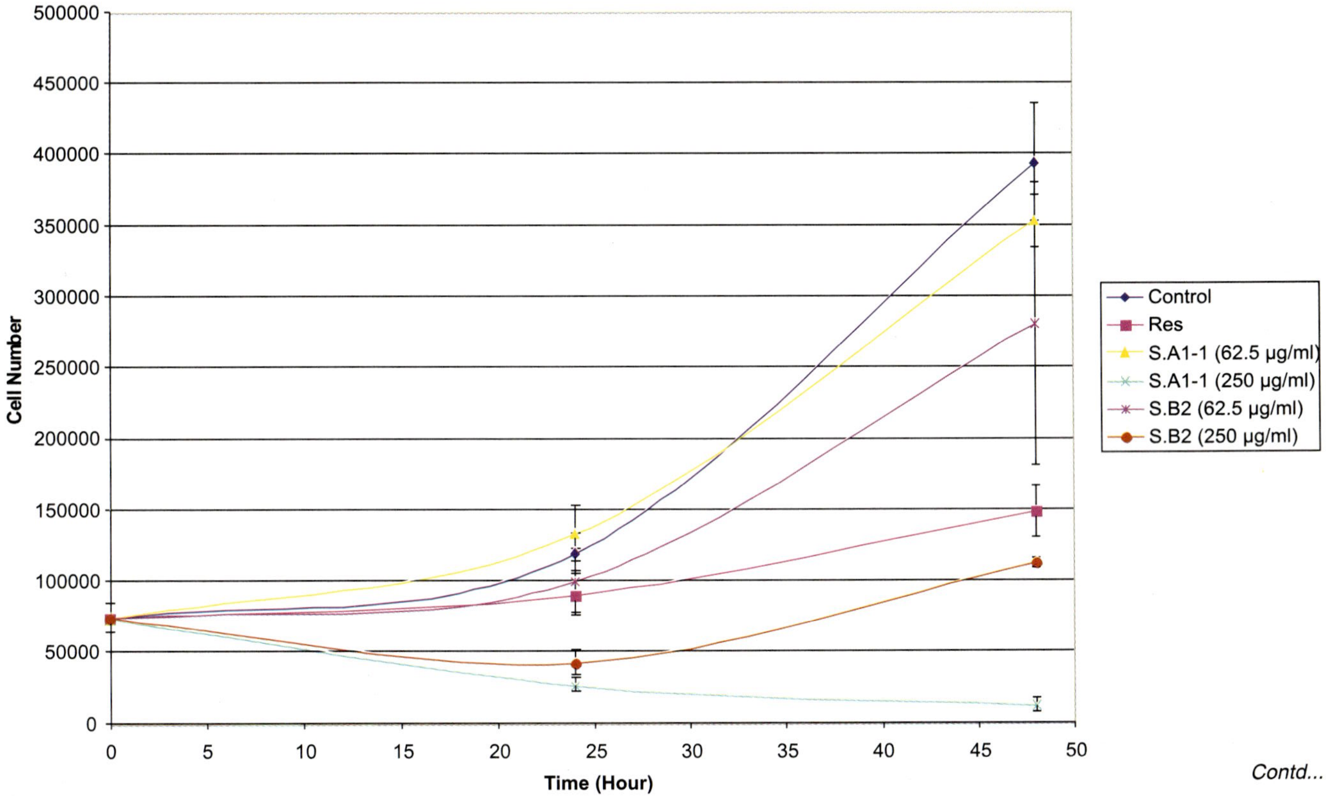


**(a)**

*Contd...*

**Figure 41.2–Contd...**

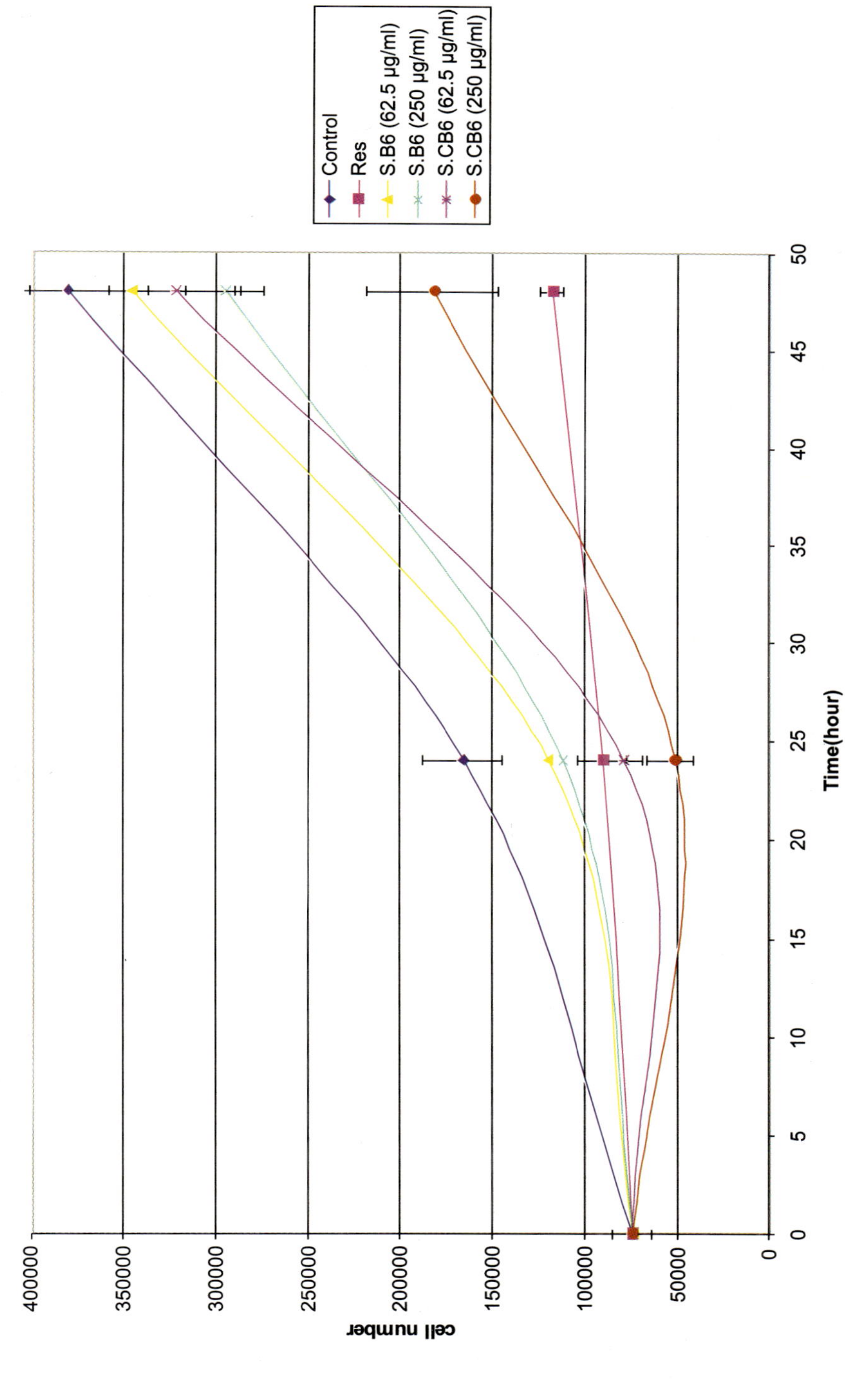


(b)

*Contd...*

**Figure 41.2–Contd...**

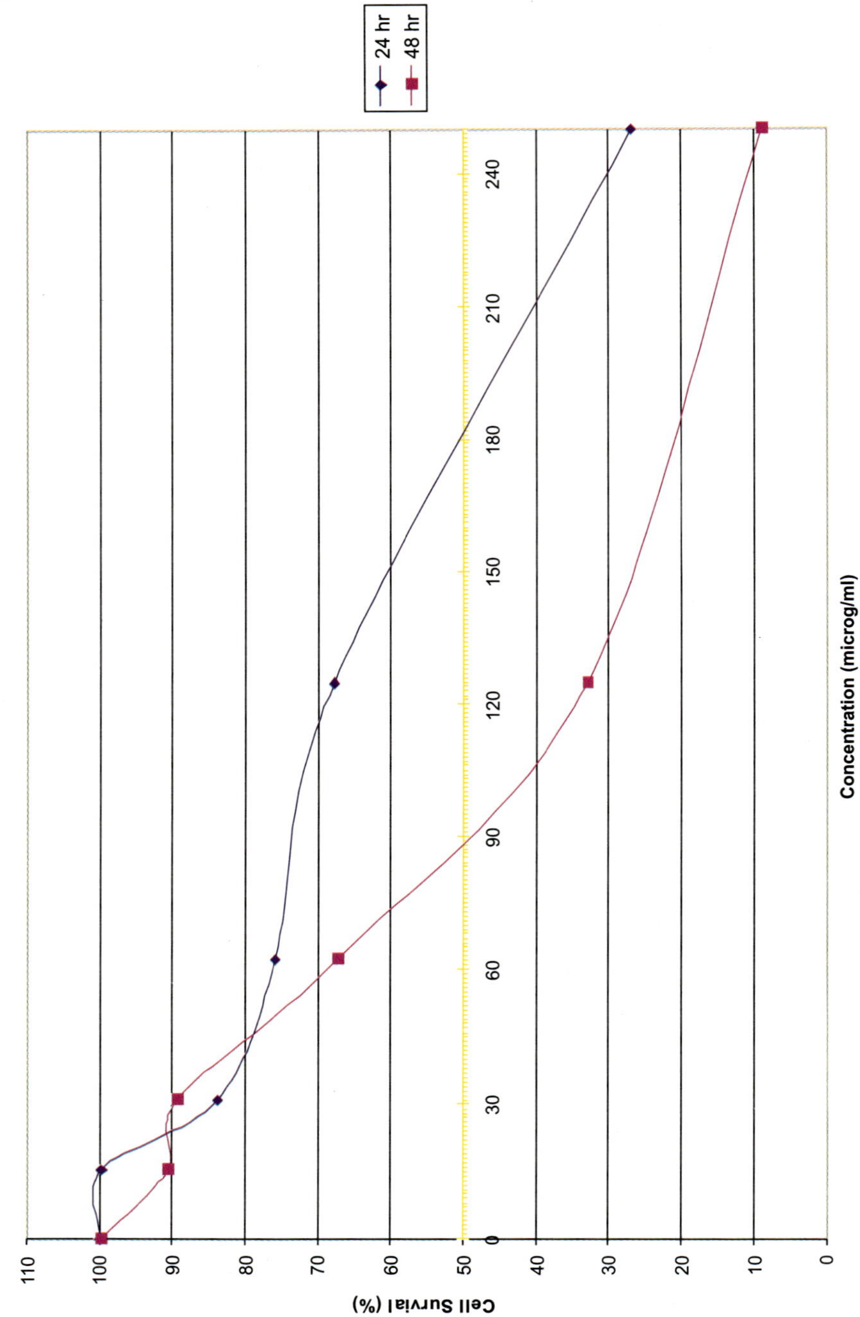


**(c)**

*Contd...*

the cell survival axis at 50 per cent was the $IC_{50}$. At 24hr, the $IC_{50}$ was 182μg/ml and at 48hr, the value was 88μg/ml.

**Table 41.5: Dose–and Time effect of S.A1-1 Extracts from *J. subtriplinerve* on the Cell Proliferation of DLD-1 Cells. The number of cells was determined as described in the Material and Method section. The numbers are the relative number of cells at 15.625, 31.25, 62.5, 125 and 250 μg/ml to define the $IC_{50}$**

| | *Res 60μM (%)* | *(-) control (%)* | *15.625 μg/ml (%)* | *31.25 μg/ml (%)* | *62.5 μg/ml (%)* | *125 μg/ml (%)* | *250 μg/ml (%)* |
|---|---|---|---|---|---|---|---|
| *24 hr* | 53 | 100 | 100 | 84 | 76 | 68 | 27 |
| *48 hr* | 33 | 100 | 91 | 89 | 67 | 33 | 9 |

Evidences represented in the Table 41.4 and 41.5 suggested that the extracts of *J. suptriplinerve* have both cytotoxic activity and depressive effect on cell proliferation. They exhibited not only inhibitory effect on Hep-G2, RD, and S.A1-1 extract but also on DLD-1.

## 3.2 Structure Determination

Due to the cytotoxic activity, the crude petroleum ether extract was chosen to be the main subject for further extraction and isolation together with the ethyl acetate extract. From these two extracts, six compounds were isolated, including five triterpenes namely oleanolic acid (1), 3β-acetyl-oleanolic acid (2), lup-20-en-3β-ol (3), stigmast-5-en-3β-ol (4) and betulin (5), and an alcohol: dotriacontanol (6). These compounds have been purified and their structures were determined using 1D, 2D-NMR: $^{1}H$, $^{13}C$, DEPT, (HMQC, HMBC spectrum only for compound (2)) and IR, UV, EI-MS for 3β-acetyl-oleanolic acid (2), lup-20-en-3β-ol (3) and stigmast-5-en-3β-ol (4), betulin (5); and dotriacontanol (6).

***Oleanolic acid* (1)**

White crystals; MS: *m/z* = 456 $[M]^+$ ($C_{30}H_{48}O_3$), 248, 233, 203, 207, 133.

***3ß–Acetyl-oleanolic acid* (2)**

White crystals

IR: $\nu_{max}$ ($cm^{-1}$) 3222 (OH), 2945 (CH), 1727 (C=O), 1680 (C=C), 1253 (C–O).

MS: m/z = 498 $[M]^+$ ($C_{32}H_{50}O_4$), 438, 248, 203, 175, 147, 133.

***Lup-20-en-3ß-ol* (3)**

White crystals; IR: $\nu_{max}$ ($cm^{-1}$) 3376 (OH), 2946 (CH), 2867 (CH), 1637 (C=C), 1293 (C–O).

MS: *m/z* = 426 $[M]^+$ ($C_{30}H_{50}O$), 411, 315, 257, 234, 218, 207, 189, 161, 135, 121.

***Stigmast-5-en-3ß-ol* (4)**

White crystals; IR: $\nu_{max}$ ($cm^{-1}$) 3422 (OH), 2944 ($CH_2$), 2865 (CH), 1646 (C=C);

MS: *m/z* = 414 $[M]^+$ ($C_{30}H_{50}O$), 396, 329 303, 273, 255, 213, 159, 145.

***Betulin* (5)**

MS: $m/z$ = 442 $[M]^+$ ($C_{30}H_{50}O_2$), 411, 234, 203, 189, 135.

***Dotriacontanol* (6)**

White crystals; MS: $m/z$ = 448 $[M-H_2O]^+$ ($C_{32}H_{66}O$), 83, 57.

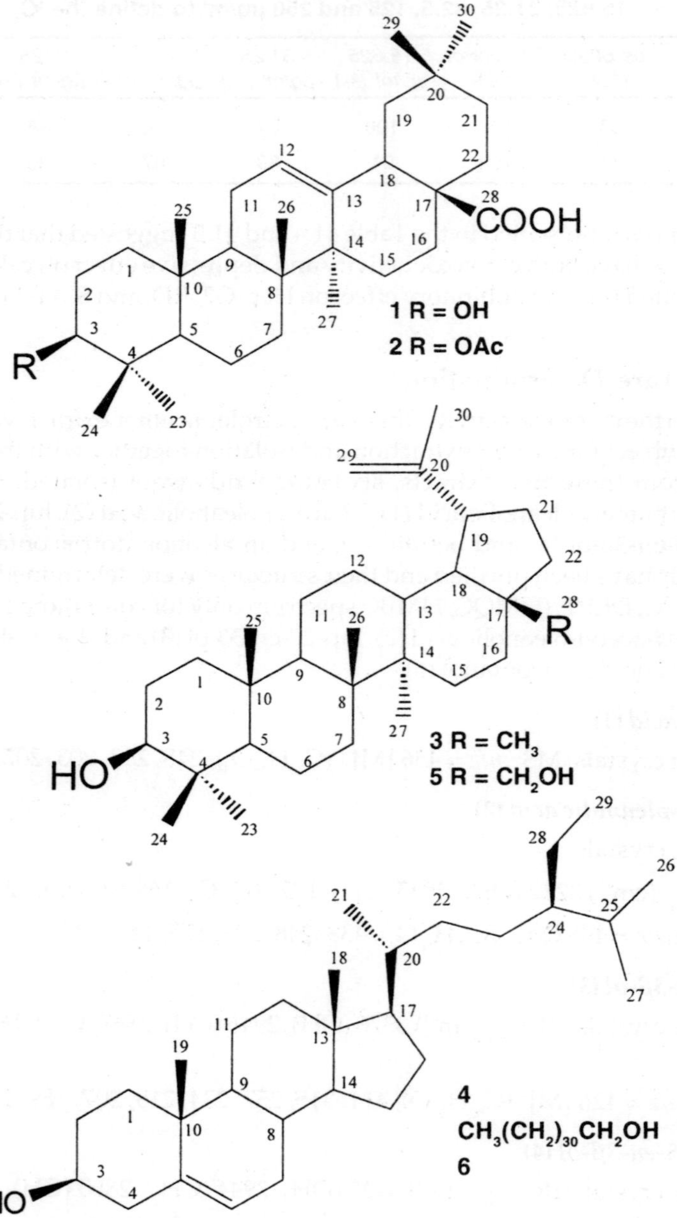


**Figure 41.3: Structures of 1-6**

**Table 41.6: $^{13}C$–NMR Data of Compounds 1–4 and 5**

| Position | Gr. | $\delta_C$ (ppm) | | Gr. | $\delta_C$ (ppm) | | Gr. | $\delta_C$ (ppm) | | Gr. | $\delta_C$ (ppm) | | Gr. | $\delta_C$ (ppm) | |
|---|---|---|---|---|---|---|---|---|---|---|---|---|---|---|---|
| | | *1* | *1a* | | *2* | *2a* | | *3* | *3a* | | *4* | *4a* | | *5* | *5a* |
| 1 | $CH_2$ | 38.50 | 38.1 | $CH_2$ | 38.10 | 38.5 | $CH_2$ | 40.64 | 38.33 | $CH_2$ | 37.28 | 37.23 | $CH_2$ | 38.73 | 38.8 |
| 2 | $CH_2$ | 26.57 | 27.2 | $CH_2$ | 27.70 | 23.6 | C | 27.46 | 27.35 | $CH_2$ | 31.69 | 29.48 | $CH_2$ | 27.41 | 27.2 |
| 3 | CH | 78.68 | 76.9 | CH | 81.96 | 81.1 | $CH_2$ | 79.04 | 78.91 | CH | 71.82 | 80.11 | CH | 79.00 | 78.9 |
| 4 | C | 38.31 | 38.4 | C | 37.70 | 37.7 | C | 38.76 | 38.8 | $CH_2$ | 42.33 | 38.95 | C | 38.88 | 38.9 |
| 5 | CH | 55.08 | 54.9 | CH | 55.30 | 55.2 | CH | 55.35 | 55.34 | C | 140.70 | 140.45 | CH | 55.32 | 55.3 |
| 6 | $CH_2$ | 18.13 | 18.0 | $CH_2$ | 18.20 | 18.3 | $CH_2$ | 18.36 | 18.26 | CH | 121.72 | 122.20 | $CH_2$ | 18.32 | 18.3 |
| 7 | $CH_2$ | 32.55 | 33.4 | $CH_2$ | 32.06 | 32.6 | $CH_2$ | 34.33 | 34.21 | $CH_2$ | 31.69 | 31.96 | $CH_2$ | 34.26 | 34.3 |
| 8 | C | 39.06 | 39.2 | C | 39.20 | 39.3 | C | 40.88 | 40.8 | CH | 31.93 | 31.90 | C | 40.95 | 40.9 |
| 9 | CH | 47.45 | 47.1 | CH | 47.60 | 47.6 | CH | 50.49 | 50.44 | CH | 50.17 | 50.23 | CH | 50.43 | 50.4 |
| 10 | C | 36.80 | 33.6 | C | 37.02 | 37.0 | C | 37.22 | 37.14 | C | 36.52 | 36.75 | C | 37.19 | 37.2 |
| 11 | $CH_2$ | 22.85 | 22.9 | $CH_2$ | 23.40 | 23.1 | $CH_2$ | 20.97 | 20.90 | $CH_2$ | 21.10 | 21.06 | $CH_2$ | 20.86 | 20.9 |
| 12 | –CH = | 122.10 | 121.5 | CH | 122.6 | 122.1 | $CH_2$ | 25.09 | 25.09 | $CH_2$ | 39.80 | 39.78 | $CH_2$ | 25.24 | 25.3 |
| 13 | –C = | 143.69 | 143.7 | C | 143.6 | 143.4 | CH | 38.89 | 36.97 | C | 42.33 | 42.36 | CH | 37.34 | 37.3 |
| 14 | C | 41.55 | 41.3 | C | 41.50 | 41.6 | C | 42.87 | 42.60 | CH | 56.79 | 56.81 | C | 42.74 | 42.7 |
| 15 | $CH_2$ | 27.48 | 26.9 | $CH_2$ | 27.70 | 27.7 | $CH_2$ | 27.49 | 27.44 | $CH_2$ | 24.37 | 24.30 | $CH_2$ | 27.07 | 27.0 |
| 16 | $CH_2$ | 23.19 | 22.6 | $CH_2$ | 23.55 | 23.4 | $CH_2$ | 34.31 | 34.31 | $CH_2$ | 28.25 | 28.24 | $CH_2$ | 29.20 | 29.2 |
| 17 | C | 46.25 | 45.5 | C | 46.60 | 46.6 | C | 42.87 | 42.95 | CH | 56.09 | 56.12 | C | 47.81 | 47.8 |
| 18 | CH | 41.06 | 40.9 | CH | 40.96 | 41.3 | CH | 40.88 | 40.29 | $CH_3$ | 11.86 | 11.86 | CH | 48.80 | 48.8 |
| 19 | $CH_2$ | 45.80 | 45.87 | $CH_2$ | 45.87 | 45.8 | CH | 29.89 | 29.77 | $CH_3$ | 19.40 | 19.35 | CH | 47.81 | 47.8 |
| 20 | C | 30.44 | 30.4 | C | 30.68 | 30.6 | C | 48.36 | 46.85 | CH | 36.52 | 36.14 | C= | 150.5 | 150.6 |

*Contd...*

**Table 41.6–Contd...**

| Position | Gr. | $\delta_C$ (ppm) | | Gr. | $\delta_C$ (ppm) | | Gr. | $\delta_C$ (ppm) | | Gr. | $\delta_C$ (ppm) | | Gr. | $\delta_C$ (ppm) | |
|---|---|---|---|---|---|---|---|---|---|---|---|---|---|---|---|
| | | 1 | 1a | | 2 | 2a | | 3 | 3a | | 4 | 4a | | 5 | 5a |
| 21 | $CH_2$ | 33.68 | 32.4 | $CH_2$ | 33.80 | 33.8 | $CH_2$ | 48.02 | 48.76 | $CH_3$ | 18.79 | 18.79 | $CH_2$ | 29.78 | 29.8 |
| 22 | $CH_2$ | 32.37 | 32.4 | $CH_2$ | 32.47 | 32.3 | $CH_2$ | 28.02 | 27.98 | $CH_2$ | 33.98 | 33.99 | $CH_2$ | 33.99 | 34.0 |
| 23 | $CH_3$ | 27.77 | 28.2 | $CH_3$ | 28.06 | 28.1 | $CH_3$ | 15.38 | 15.33 | CH2 | 26.14 | 26.15 | $CH_3$ | 28.00 | 28.0 |
| 24 | $CH_3$ | 16.58 | 15.9 | $CH_3$ | 16.67 | 15.6 | $CH_3$ | 16.13 | 16.06 | CH | 45.88 | 45.91 | $CH_3$ | 15.36 | 15.4 |
| 25 | $CH_3$ | 15.01 | 15.1 | $CH_3$ | 15.40 | 15.3 | $CH_3$ | 16.01 | 15.92 | CH | 28.91 | 29.23 | $CH_3$ | 16.11 | 16.1 |
| 26 | $CH_3$ | 15.32 | 16.8 | $CH_3$ | 17.20 | 16.8 | $CH_3$ | 14.58 | 14.48 | $CH_3$ | 19.80 | 19.06 | $CH_3$ | 16.00 | 16.0 |
| 27 | $CH_3$ | 25.62 | 25.9 | $CH_3$ | 25.90 | 26.0 | $CH_3$ | 18.03 | 19.74 | $CH_3$ | 18.79 | 19.81 | $CH_3$ | 14.80 | 14.8 |
| 28 | COOH | 180.77 | 178.6 | C | 184.03 | 181.0 | $CH_3$ | 150.97 | 150.71 | $CH_2$ | 23.10 | 23.12 | $CH_2$ | 60.58 | 60.2 |
| 29 | $CH_3$ | 32.80 | 32.9 | $CH_3$ | 33.06 | 33.1 | $CH_2$ | 109.3 | 109.32 | $CH_3$ | 11.99 | 11.99 | $CH_2$= | 109.7 | 109.6 |
| 30 | $CH_3$ | 23.27 | 23.4 | $CH_3$ | 23.60 | 23.6 | $CH_3$ | 19.33 | 19.57 | – | – | – | $CH_3$ | 19.10 | 19.1 |
| 31 | – | – | – | $CH_3$ | 21.29 | – | – | – | – | – | – | – | $CH_2$ | 38.73 | 38.8 |
| 32 | – | – | – | C | 171.04 | – | – | – | – | – | – | – | $CH_2$ | 27.41 | 27.2 |

1a: Oleanolic acid /pyridine-$d_5$ (Fayçal, 2003); 2a: Oleanolic acid/$CDCl_3$ (Seebacher, 2003); 3a: Lupeol/$CDCl_3$ (Reynolds, 1986); 4a: Stigmast–5–en–3–O–$\beta$–glucoside/$CDCl_3$ (Faizi, 2001); 5a: Betulin/$CDCl_3$ (Kadriya, 2001).

**Table 41.7: $^1$H–NMR Data of Compounds 1–4 and 5**

| Position | Gr. | $\delta_C$ (ppm) | | Gr. | $\delta_C$ (ppm) | | Gr. | $\delta_C$ (ppm) | | Gr. | $\delta_C$ (ppm) | | Gr. | $\delta_C$ (ppm) | |
|---|---|---|---|---|---|---|---|---|---|---|---|---|---|---|---|
| | | 1 | 1a | | 2 | 2a | | 3 | 3a | | 4 | 4a | | 5 | 5a |
| 3 | –CH–OH | 3.20 | 3.23 | CH | 4.45 | 3.44 | CH | 3.2? | 3.23 | CH | 3.52 | 3.98 | CH–OH | 3.19 | 3.13 |
| 4 | – | – | – | – | – | – | – | – | – | $CH_2$ | 2.24<br>2.28 | 2.49<br>2.72 | – | – | – |
| 5 | – | – | – | – | – | – | CH | 0.68 | 0.68 | – | – | – | – | – | – |
| 6 | – | – | – | – | – | – | – | – | – | CH | 5.36 | 5.35 | – | – | – |
| 8 | – | – | – | – | – | – | – | – | – | CH | 1.67 | 1.36 | – | – | – |
| 12 | CH= | 5.27 | 5.28 | CH | 5.27 | 5.49 | – | – | – | | | | – | – | – |
| 16 | – | – | – | – | – | – | – | – | – | $CH_2$ | –<br>1.84 | 1.25<br>1.85 | – | – | – |
| 18 | CH– | 2.84 | 2.87 | – | – | – | – | – | – | $CH_3$ | 0.68 | 0.66 | – | – | – |
| 19 | – | – | – | – | – | – | – | – | – | $CH_3$ | 1.02 | 0.94 | CH–C= | 2.39 | 2.30 |
| 20 | – | – | – | – | – | – | CH | 2.38 | 2.31 | – | – | – | – | – | – |
| 21 | – | – | – | $CH_2$ | 1.65<br>– | 1.46<br>1.23 | – | – | – | $CH_3$ | 0.94 | 0.98 | – | – | – |
| 22 | – | – | – | CH | 2.82<br>– | 2.04<br>1.82 | $CH_3$ | 1.03 | 1.23 | – | – | – | – | – | – |
| 23 | $CH_3$ | 0.98 | 0.89 | $CH_3$ | 0.87 | 1.24 | $CH_3$ | 0.96 | 1.06 | – | – | – | $CH_3$ | 1.01 | 0.96 |
| 24 | $CH_3$ | 0.93 | 0.87 | $CH_3$ | 0.85 | 1.02 | $CH_3$ | 0.76 | 0.83 | – | – | – | $CH_3$ | 0.98 | 0.76 |

*Contd...*

**Table 41.7–Contd...**

| Position | Gr. | $\delta_C$ (ppm) | | Gr. | $\delta_C$ (ppm) | | Gr. | $\delta_C$ (ppm) | | Gr. | $\delta_C$ (ppm) | | Gr. | $\delta_C$ (ppm) | |
|---|---|---|---|---|---|---|---|---|---|---|---|---|---|---|---|
| | | *1* | *1a* | | *2* | *2a* | | *3* | *3a* | | *4* | *4a* | | *5* | *5a* |
| 25 | $CH_3$ | 0.77 | 0.91 | $CH_3$ | 0.94 | 0.93 | $CH_3$ | 0.94 | 0.99 | CH | 1.65 | 1.68 | $CH_3$ | 0.76 | 0.81 |
| 26 | $CH_3$ | 0.79 | 0.75 | $CH_3$ | 0.74 | 1.04 | $CH_3$ | 0.82 | 0.97 | $CH_3$ | 0.85 | 0.84 | $CH_3$ | 0.97 | 1.07 |
| 27 | $CH_3$ | 1.14 | 1.12 | $CH_3$ | 1.13 | 1.30 | $CH_3$ | 0.79 | 0.86 | $CH_3$ | 0.83 | 0.86 | $CH_3$ | 0.83 | 0.98 |
| 28 | – | – | – | – | – | – | $CH_2$ | 4.56<br>4.69 | 4.69<br>4.59 | – | – | – | $CH_2$ | 3.80<br>3.34 | 2.25<br>3.27 |
| 29 | $CH_3$ | 0.91 | 0.90 | $CH_3$ | 0.90 | 0.97 | – | – | – | $CH_3$ | 0.86 | 0.88 | $CH_2$= | 4.68<br>4.58 | 5.53<br>5.56 |
| 30 | $CH_3$ | 0.90 | 0.96 | $CH_3$ | 0.93 | 1.02 | $CH_3$ | 1.69 | 1.65 | – | – | – | $CH_3$ | 1.68 | 1.68 |
| 31 | – | – | – | $CH_3$ | 2.04 | – | – | – | – | | | | | | |

1a: Oleanolic acid/$CDCl_3$ (Fayçal, 2003); 2a: Oleanolic acid/$CDCl_3$ (Mahato, 1994); 3a: Lupeol/$CDCl_3$ (Reynolds, 1986); 4a: Stigmast–5–en–3–O–$\beta$–glucoside/$CDCl_3$ (Faizi, 2001); 5a: Betulin/$CDCl_3$ (Kadriya, 2001).

Oleanolic acid and its derivatives were identified as potent anti-HIV agents (Kashiwada, 1998) and 3β-acetyl-oleanolic acid (2) showed inhibitory activity against *Porphyrormonas ginggivalis* (Kim, 1999). Lupeol (3) is a well-known anti-inflammatory triterpene (Akihisa, 1996) and did not show a noticeable cytotoxic activity against human tumor cell lines such as HT-29, Hep-G2, MCF-7 and MKN-45 using the MTT assay (Cordero, 2004), but is found to reduce the proliferation of HL-60 cells (Hata, 2003) and AsPC-1 cells likely by induction of apoptosis (Saleem, 2005). Beside this, lupeol suppress chemical induced oxidative stress (Saleem, 2001) and improve the antioxidant status of the liver (Sunitha, 2001). Betulin and its derivatives exhibit anti-malarial, anti-inflammatory and anti-HIV activity as well as showing cytotoxicity towards a number of tumour cell lines (Hanne, 2003). Stigmast-5-en-3β-ol (4) also showed a selective cytotoxic activity on Bowes cells (Nguyen, 2004). Lupeol (3) as well as stigmast-5-en-3β-ol (4) were identified as the two main compounds present in the most active antimicrobial fractions prepared from the methanol extract of *Buchholzia coriacea* stem bark (Ajaiyeoba, 2003). Alcohols which have 28 to 34 carbons like Dotriacontanol (6) exhibit anti-inflammatory activity.

## 4.0 Conclusion

The results of antimicrobial assay demonstrated that *J. suptriplinerve* possesses abilities of inhibition against *E. coli*, *S. aureus* and *B. subtilis* bacterial strains; *A. niger* and *F. oxysporum* fungi; and *S. cerevisiae* yeast but cannot affect the *P. aeruginosa* and *C. albicans*. In addition, using DPPH radical scavenging assay to investigate the antioxidant activity of crude extracts of *J. suptriplinerve*, we found out that antioxidant active compounds should be present in ethyl acetate and ethanol. This extract exhibited remarkably antioxidant activity ($SC_{50}$ = 99.0 µg/ml). Moreover, the evidence of cytotoxic assays clearly demonstrated that the petroleum ether extracts has strong effect on three human cancerous cell lines: Hep-G2, RD and DLD-1. However, the water extract showed non-toxic activity and therefore, we assume that the exposure by drinking *J. suptriplinerve* as tea will have no significant toxic effect. In addition, the proposed pharmacological activity of *J. suptriplinerve* extracts for its use in traditional medicine, is supported by the activities shown in here. The most active extract was found to contain oleanolic acid (1), 3β-acetyl-oleanolic acid (2), lup-20-en-3β-ol (3), stigmast-5-en-3β-ol (4), betulin (5), and an alcohol: dotriacontanol (6).

## Acknowledgements

This work was supported by the Ministry of Education and Training, Vietnam for project B2006-18-04TD. The authors are grateful to Prof. Le Cong Kiet and Mr. Nguyen Tran Quoc Trung (Department of Botany and Ecology, College of Natural Sciences, National University of HCM City) for sample identification. We thank to Prof. Tran Hung (Department of Pharmacognosy, School of Pharmacy, HCM City) for his helpful advice and Dr. Chu Dinh Kinh (Institute of Chemistry, VAST, Hanoi) for the mass and NMR spectra.

Ms. Dai Hue Ngan acknowledges DANIDA for a grant via the ENRECA program.

## References


Ajaiyeoba, E. O., Onocha, P. A., Nwozo, S. O., Sama, W., 2003. Antimicrobial and cytotoxicity evaluation of Buchholzia coriacea stem bark. Fitoterapia, 74, pp. 706-709.

Akihisa, T., Yasukawa, K., Oinuma, H., Kasahara, Y., Yamanouchi, S., Takido, M., Kumaki, K., Tamura T., 1996. Triterpene alcohols from the flowers of compositae and their anti-inflammatory effects. Phytochemistry, 43, pp. 1255-1260.

Atta-ur-Rahman, M. 1., Choudhary, W.J., Thomasen, 2001. Bioassay Techniques for Drug Development. Harwood Academic Publishers, pp. 28-31.

Chau, V. M., Phan, V. K, Le, M. H., Kim, Y. H., 2004. Cytotoxic constituents of *Diadema setosum*. Arch.Pham.Res., 27, pp. 734-737.

Cordero, C. P., Gomez-Gonzalez, S., Leon-Acosta, C.J., Morantes-Medina, S.J., Aristizabal, F.A., 2004. Cytotoxic activity of five compounds isolated from Colombian plants. Fitoterapia, 75, pp. 225-227.

Dai, H. N., Ho, T. C. H, Le, M. H, Hansen, P. E, Vang, O., 2007. Bioactivities and chemical constituents of a Vietnamese medicinal plant Che Vang, *Jasminum subtriplinerve* Blume (*Oleaceae*), Natural Product Research, accepted.

Do, H. B., Dang, Q. T., Bui, X. D., Nguyen, T. D., Do, T. D., Pham, V. H., Vu, N. L., Pham, D. M., Pham, K. M., Doan, T. N., Nguyen, T., Tran, D., 2004. Selected Medicinal Plants in Vietnam. Serdang: Science and Technology Publishing House, pp. 40-42.

Do, T. L., Y., 2003. Medicinal Plants and Drugs from Vietnam. Serdang: Hanoi Science and Technology Publishing House, pp. 121-122.

Fayçal, H., Hichem, B. J., Jihen, C., Samir, J., Zine, M., 2003. Antibacterial activities of a few prepared derivatives of oleanolic acid and of other natural triterpenic compounds. *Comptes rendus*. Chimie 6, pp. 473–483.

Faizi, S., Ali, M., Saleem, R., Irfanullah, Bibi, S., 2001. Complete $^{1}H$ and $^{13}C$ NMR assignments of stigma-5-en-3-*O*-$\beta$-glucoside and its acetyl derivative. Magn.Reson.Chem., 39, pp. 399-405.

Hata, K., Hori, K., Ogasawara, H., Takahashi, S., 2003b. Anti-leukemia activities of lup-28-al-20(29)-en-3-one, a lupane. Triterpene. Toxicol Lett, 143, pp. 1-7.

Kadriya, S. E. D., Rwaida, A. A., Jaber, S. M., Abel-Monem, A., 2003. Phytochemical and pharmacological studies of Maytenus forsskaoliana–Saudi Pharmaceutical Journal, 11, pp. 4.

Kashiwada, Y., Wang, H. K., Nagao, T., Kitanaka, S., Yasuda, 1., Fujioka, T., Yamagishi, T., Cosentino, L. M., Kozuka, M., Okabe, H., Ikeshiro, Y., Hu, C-Q, Yeh, E., Lee, K-H., 1998. Anti-AIDS Agents. 30. Anti-HIV Activity of Oleanolic Acid, Pomolic Acid, and Structurally Related Triterpenoids. J.Nat.Prod., 61, pp. 1090-1095.

Kim, N. C., Desjardins, A.E., Wu, C. D., Kinghorn, A. D., 1999. Activity of triterpenoid glycosides from the root bark of Mussaenda macrophylla against two oral pathogens. J.Nat.Prod., 62, pp. 1379-1384.

Kraus, W., Luu, H. N., Conrad, J., Klaiber, I., Reeb, S., Vogler, B., 2002. Investigation of biologically active natural products using online LC-bioassay, LC-NMR, and LC-MS techniques. Phytochem.Rev., 1, pp. 409-411.

Likhitwitayawuid, K., Angerhofer, C. K., Cordell, G. A., Pezzuto, J. M., 1993. Cytotoxic and antimalarial bisbenzylisoquinoline alkaloids from Stephania erecta. J.Nat.Prod., 56, pp. 30-38.

Mahato, S. B., Kundu, A. P., 1994. $^{13}$C NMR spectra of pentacyclic triterpenoids–a compilation and some salient features. Phytochem., 37, pp. 1517-1575.

Mensor, L. L., Menezes, F.S., Leitão, G. G., Reis, A.S., Santos, T. C., Coube, C. S., Leitão, S.G., 2001. Screening of Brazilian Plant Extracts for Antioxidant Activity by the Use of DPPH Free Radical Method. *Phytotherapy.Res.* 15, pp. 127-130.

Nguyen, T.A., Malonne, H., Duez, P., Vanhaelen, R., Fontaine, J., 2004. Cytotoxic constituents from Plumbago zeylanica. Fitoterapia, 75, pp. 500-504.

Nguyen, T. N. H., 1986a. PhD. Thesis of Pharmacy.

Nguyen, T. N. H., Doan, N. T., 1986b. Vietnamese J. Pharm. 1, pp. 17-18.(in Vietnamese)

Reynolds, W. F., McLean, S., Poplawski, J., 1986. Total assignment of [13]C and [1]H spectra of three isomeric triterpenol derivatives by 2D NMR: an investigation of the potential utility of [1]H chemical shifts in structural investigations of complex natural products. Tetrahedron, 42, pp. 3419-3428.

Saleem, M., Alam, A., Arifin, S., Shah, M.S., Ahmed, B., Sultana, S., 2001. Lupeol, a triterpene, inhibits early responses of tumor promotion induced by benzoyl peroxide in murine skin. Pharmacol.Res., 43, pp.127-134.

Saleem, M., Kaur, S., Kweon, M. H., Adhami, V. M., Afaq, F., Mukhtar, H., 2005. Lupeol, a fruit and vegetable based triterpene, induces apoptotic death of human pancreatic adenocarcinoma cells via inhibition of Ras signaling pathway. Carcinogenesis, 26, pp. 1956-1964.

Seebacher, W., Simic N., Weis, R., Saf, R., Kunert, O., 2003. Complete assignments of $^{1}$H and $^{13}$C NMR resonances of oleanolic acid, 18$\alpha$-oleanolic acid, ursolic acid and their 11-oxo derivatives. Magn.Reson.Chem., 41, pp. 636-638.

Sunitha, S., Nagaraj, M., Varalakshmi, P., 2001. Hepatoprotective effect of lupeol and lupeol linoleate on tissue antioxidant defence system in cadmium-induced hepatotoxicity in rats. Fitoterapia, 72, pp. 516-523.

Ziegler H.L., Franzyk H., Sairafianpour M., Tabatabai M., Tehrani M.D., Bagherzadeh K., Hagerstrand H., Staerk D., Jaroszewski J.W, 2004. Erythrocyte membrane modifying agents and the inhibition of *Plasmodium falciparum* growth–structure-activity relationships for betulinic acid analogues. Bioorganic and Medicinal Chemistry, 12, pp. 119-127.

## Chapter 42

# Use of Acetylcholinesterase Activity for the Quantitative Determination of Organophosphate Pesticides

*Le Minh Tri[1], Nguyen Quoc Khang[1] and Ngo Thi Thuy Phuong[2]*

[1]*Faculty of Biology Hanoi College of Science, Hanoi, Vietnam*

[2]*Institute of Chemistry and Material, Central for Military Science and Technology, Hanoi, Vietnam*

## ABSTRACT

Acetyl cholinesterase (EC 3.1.1.7) is a widely distributed enzyme, particularly in excitable tissues such as muscle, nerve that is also found in erythrocytes and serum. AChE is inhibited by neurotoxins, which include not only Organophosphate pesticides but also carbamate pesticides and many other compounds. Biosensors based on acetyl cholinesterase (AChE) inhibition have been an active research area over the last decade. The degree of inhibition of acetyl cholinesterase activity of the serum of perching duck by different concentrations of pesticides was studied. The results indicated that the optimum pH for activity of AChE is around 8.0 and the decrease of acetyl cholinesterase activity at 30°C is concentration dependent and concentration of 0.007mg/l could reduce the activity up to 99 per cent. As a first step a test kit using a biosensor to determine OP concentration is being developed.

***Keyword:*** *Acetyl cholinesterase, Organophosphate, Perching duck, Biosensor.*

## 1.0 Introduction

Every time you move a muscle and every time you think, your nerve cells are hard at work. They are processing information: receiving signals, deciding what to do with them, and dispatching new messages off to their neighbouring cells. Some nerve cells communicate directly with muscle cells, sending them the signal to contract.

Other nerve cells are involved solely in the bureaucracy of information, spending their lives communicating only with other nerve cells. But unlike our human bureaucracies, this processing of information must be fast in order to keep up with the ever-changing demands of life.

Nerves communicate with one another and with muscle cells by using neurotransmitters. These are small molecules that are released from the nerve cell and rapidly diffuse to neighbouring cells, stimulating a response once they arrive. Many different neurotransmitters are used for different jobs: glutamate excites nerves into action; GABA inhibits the passing of information; dopamine and serotonin are involved in the subtle messages of thought and cognition. The main job of the neurotransmitter acetylcholine is to carry the signal from nerve cells to muscle cells. When a motor nerve cell gets the proper signal from the nervous system, it releases acetylcholine into its synapses with muscle cells. There, acetylcholine opens receptors on the muscle cells, triggering the process of contraction. Of course, once the message is passed, the neurotransmitter must be destroyed, otherwise later signals would get mixed up in a jumble of obsolete neurotransmitter molecules. The clean up of old acetylcholine is the job of acetyl cholinesterase (Brimijoin, 1992).

Acetyl cholinesterase has one of the fastest reaction rates of any of our enzymes, breaking up each molecule in about 80 microseconds. Cholinesterases (ChEs) are widely distributed in the animal kingdom but have been studied in only a few groups of invertebrates.

In mammals, ChEs are typically separated into two major groups, the true cholinesterases (*i.e.*, acetylcholinesterases: AChEs; E.C. 3.1.1.7) and the pseudocholinesterases, namely the butyrylcholinesterases (BuChEs; E.C. 3.1.1.8). AChEs preferentially hydrolyze acetylcholine as substrate and are very sensitive to eserine inhibition, whereas BuChEs preferentially hydrolyze butyrylcholine, are sensitive to eserine, and are selectively inhibited by iso-OMPA (tetraisopropyl pyrophosphoramide). The ChEs of invertebrates appear to be a group of related enzymes with widely varying properties, that are also distinct from those of mammalian ChEs; substrate specificity and patterns of inhibition are especially variable. As a consequence, invertebrate ChEs cannot be separated into AChEs and pseudocholinesterases, as mammalian ChEs are, so the term 'pseudocholinesterase' is irrelevant to invertebrates (Abernathy, 1988).

The nerve toxin sarin and insecticides such as Malathion directly attack the active site machinery of acetylcholinesterase.

Synthetic organophosphates (OP), amongst the most toxic substances known, are widely used as pesticides, insecticides, and chemical warfare agents. A large volume of wastewaters contaminated with these neurotoxin compounds, generated at both the producer and consumer levels, requires treatment before being released to the environment. Because currently available abiotic treatment methods, chemical hydrolysis, and incineration are considered inadequate, biotic methods based on enzymes and microorganisms are being investigated in many research laboratories. The successful use of any laboratory developed technology for detoxification of the organophosphate neurotoxins will require analytical tools for monitoring concentrations of these neurotoxins (Sultatos, 1994). Biosensors based on acetylcholinesterase (AChE) inhibition have been an active research area over the last decade. AChE is inhibited by neurotoxins, which include not only OP pesticides but also carbamate pesticides and many other compounds

Organophosphorus hydrolase (OPH), a biological catalyst, has been shown to effectively hydrolyze a range of organophosphate esters, pesticides such as parathion, coumaphos and acephate, and chemical warfare agents such as soman, sarin, VX, and tabun (Ballantyne, 1992).

## 2.0 Materials and Methods

### 2.1 Materials

Perching duck blood samples were collected from various locations around Hanoi. The ratio between anti-agglutinating and blood is 1:10 in each sample. Gently shake, centrifuge at speed 1,500rpm. Then we suck serum for analysis. Serum was stored at –20°C.

Two kinds of pesticides used in the study (Ofatox™ 400EC, Cyperin™ 10EC) were provided by Saigon Pesticides Company. Topsin™ M70WP was provided by Nippon Soda Company, Tokyo, Japan.

All chemicals and reagents used are PAC (purify analysis chemical), that were made by Sigma, Merck, Boehringer–Manheim.

+ Acetic acid, Acetylcholine Chloride, Cholinesterase control, Cholinesterase, was supplied by Sigma Diagnostics and Boehringer–Manheim (Roche Diagnostics)

+ m-Nitrophenol, Sodium chloride, Phosphate buffer, were provided by Merck (Germany) and Sigma (USA).

### 2.2 Methods

The ChE activity was determined by the most commonly used assay described previously by Ellman (1961). The production of thiocholine formed in the hydrolysis of acetylthiocholine is measured by coupling of the reactive thiol with 5, 5′-dithio-bis 2-nitrobenzoate (DTNB) to give a thionitrobenzoate (TNB). The TNB is a yellow anion and its formation can be measured spectrophotometrically. The production of TNB is rapid and the concentration of DTNB used in the assay does not inhibit the enzyme. The rate of change of absorbance at 405nm is directly proportional to cholinesterase activity (Augustinsson, 1978).

## 3.0 Results and Discussion

### 3.1 Effect of Various Parameters

The response of OPH-modified enzyme biosensor was a strong inverse function of the buffer concentration. The magnitude of the response, the lower detection limit, and the response time of the biosensor were better in the weak buffer. Such behaviour can be attributed to the fact that when a concentrated buffer is employed, more of the basic buffer ions permeate through the dialysis membrane and the enzyme layer and neutralize part of enzymatically-generated hydrogen ions. Thus, the hydrogen-ion concentration at the glass-sensing surface is lowered, which produces a smaller response. Because an objective of this work was to develop a rapid and sensitive biosensor for organophosphate pesticides, 1 mM buffer was selected for subsequent investigations. Because it was rather difficult to work with the 1 mM buffer, 100 mM sodium chloride was added to it. Addition of this neutral salt made the buffer easier to work with without affecting the enzyme electrode response characteristic. The response of the enzyme biosensor was a strong function of the starting pH. This profile mirrored the pH profile for the free enzyme. The lowering of the response at high and low pH can be attributed to the reduced activity of the enzyme under these conditions. A starting pH of 8.0, which gave the maximum sensitivity, lowest response time, and largest dynamic range was used subsequently. The operating temperature of the enzyme biosensor affected its response to OP (Amaya, 1996).

In a low temperature range, *i.e.* 20°C–30°C activity of enzyme increased if the temperature increased. In contrary, in a higher temperature range, *i.e.* above 45°C, the activity of the enzyme decreased and even became inactive if the temperature increased further. This may be due to the denaturing of the enzyme with high temperatures. The optimum temperature for activity of AChE is about 30°C. This result is in agreement with the characteristics of acetylcholinesterase derived in human and some animals.

### 3.2 Effect of Ofatox™ on Enzyme Activity

From the experimental results, the acetylcholinesterase activity was 48 per cent of acetylcholinesterase activity of origin fluid when concentration of Ofatox™ was 0.001mg/l. and when the concentration of Ofatox™ was increased by seven times; acetylcholinesterase activity was 0.9 per cent. This meant that a concentration of 0.007mg/l, Ofatox™ can inhibit 99.1 per cent acetylcholinesterase of origin fluid. Thus the acetylcholinesterase activity decreases when concentration of insecticide increases.

### 3.3 Effect of Cyperin™ on Enzyme Activity

From the experimental results, the acetylcholinesterase activity was 30.4 per cent of acetylcholinesterase activity of origin fluid when concentration of Cyperin™ was 0.001mg/l and when the concentration of Cyperin™ was increased seven times; acetylcholinesterase activity was 13.626 U/l. indicating that a mean at concentration of 0.007mg/l Cyperin™ can inhibit 99.2 per cent of acetylcholinesterase of origin fluid. When the concentration of Cyperin™ was increased to eight times, acetylcholinesterase activity was 0 U/l. indicating that a concentration 0.008mg/l Cyperin™ can inhibit 100 per cent of acetylcholinesterase of origin fluid.

### 3.4 Effect of Topsin™ on Enzyme Activity

As Ofatox™ and Ciperin™, Topsin™ also showed the ability to inhibit acetylcholinesterase activity. The acetylcholinesterase activity was 44.2 per cent of acetylcholinesterase activity of origin fluid when concentration of Topsin™ was 0.001mg/l. The acetylcholinesterase activity was 16.813 U/l (=2 per cent acetylcholinesterase activity of origin fluid) when the concentration of Topsin™ was increased to 0.007mg/l.

These results show that acetylcholinesterase activity decreased when the concentration of the insecticide increased (Figure 42.1).

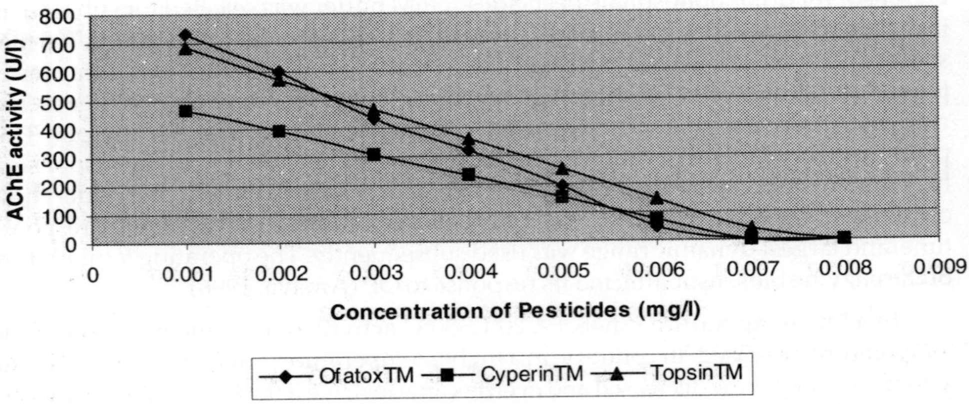


**Figure 42.1**

From the results above, as a first step a test kit to determine OP concentration based on colour intensity is being developed.

| **Color level** | | | | | | | | |
|---|---|---|---|---|---|---|---|---|
| **mg/l of OP** | 0 | 0.001 | 0.002 | 0.003 | 0.004 | 0.005 | 0.006 | 0.008 |

## 4.0 Conclusion

The optimum temperature for testing the activity of AChE in perching duck serum is about 30ºC and the optimum pH is around 8.0. A potentiometric enzyme biosensor for the direct measurement of organophosphate pesticides is being developed. The organophosphate enzyme biosensor has a response time of less than 10 min.

In addition, the ChE-sponges could be used in chemical-biological sensors and incorporated into electronic hand-held telemedicine devices, for instance as electrochemical OP probes. The immobilized enzyme sensors have the unique ability, unlike the current OP ticket, to detect OPs in any environmental condition, such as vegetables, food, etc. Also, the immobilized sensors could be developed into a differential OP detector to identify the type of OP contamination, which would aid in treatment. With the constant threat of chemical warfare, terrorist acts, or spill of pesticides, the development of alternative means of protecting and decontaminating individuals from exposure to OP nerve agents is critical.

## References

Abernathy, M. H., Fitzgerald, H. P., and Ahern, K. M.,1988. An enzymatic method for erythrocyte acetylcholinesterase. Clinical chemistry (34); pp 1055-1057.

Amaya, A., Keifer, M., and McConnell, R., 1996. Comment on EQM Tesmate OP cholinesterase kit. Occupat. Environ. Medicine (53); N0358.

Augustinsson, K. B., Eriksson, H., and Faijerson, Y., 1978. A new approach to determining cholinesterase activities in sample of whole blood. Clin. Chim. Acta, N089; pp 239-252.

Ballantyne, B., and Marrs, T.C., 1992. Clinical and experimental Toxicology of Organophosphates and Carbamates. Butterworth-Heinemann Ltd, Oxford.

Brimijoin, S., 1992. Enzymology and biology of cholinesterase. In "Proceedings of the U.S. EPA Workshop on cholinesterase methodologies", U.S. Environmental protection agency, Washington, DC; pp. 30

Sultatos, L. G., 1994. Mammalian toxicology of Organophosphorus pesticides. J. Toxicol. Eviron. Health (43); pp 271-289.

## Chapter 43

# A Contribution to Medico-Ethnobotany of Kalahandi District, Orissa, on Ear and Mouth Disease

*Nalini Sadangi*[1], *Rabindra N. Padhy*[2] *and Rajani K. Sahu*[3]*

[1]*Kesinga Mahavidyalaya, Kesinga, Kalahandi, Orissa, India*

[2]*Govt. Autonomous College, Bhawanipatna, Kalahandi, Orissa, India*

[3]*B.J.B. Autonomous College, Bhubaneswar, Orissa, India*

**E-mail: sahurajani@yahoo.co.in*

## ABSTRACT

Different herbal methods for treating ear and mouth diseases in ethnomedicinal practice of the tribal people of Kalahandi district are described based on a survey among scheduled caste and scheduled tribe population. Ten species are found to be used as external applications. All most all the species are found to be new from Orissa on a scrutiny of literature.

***Keywords:*** *Ethnobotany, Medicinal plants, Kalahandi, Orissa, Ear and mouth disease.*

## 1.0 Introduction

The district Kalahandi lies between 19° 10′–20°30′ N latitude and 82° 30′–83° 50′ E longitude. The district contains undulating plains to the northeast and extension of Eastern Ghats. The region from east to southeast is covered with high plateau of 300-500 m above M.S.L. Many flat hill tops locally called mali lie between 1200-1200m above M.S.L. Forest of Kalahandi is tropical dry mixed deciduous type with great diversity of flora and fauna. The rivers Tel and the Indravati are the tributaries of large rivers, like Mahanadi and Godavari, respective The district enjoys tropical monsoon climate with average rain fall of 800 to 1200 mm and temperature ranges between 28° and 50°C. Earache, ear sore, and mouth trouble like tongue sore is common problems that are easily cured by the herbal healers. They hardly depend upon doctors for the treatment of these diseases. Scrutiny of literature has revealed that a few data are available regarding the ethnomedicinal treatments for ear disease Ethnomedicinal information of 10 species used in ear and mouth diseases are reported in this paper.

## 2.0 Materials and Methods

An extensive ethnomedical survey was conducted during fieldtrips from 1999 to 2002. The traditional healers and knowledgeable age-old persons were interviewed and the information was collected. The information collected from one village was crosschecked with that obtained from another.

Voucher specimens were collected and are preserved in the Government Autonomous College, Bhawanipatna. The information obtained is enumerated in alphabetical order with family, local name, method of application etc. Abbreviations used–Fam–Family, L–Local name, P–Parts used, Pl.–Place of collection. The details of plant species are enumerated as follows.

## 3.0 Results

*Bambusa vulgaries* Sch ex-wendl earache–Fam Poaceae L. Baunsh P-Culm. Pl-Thuamul Rampur and adjacent villages

Culm is spitted and granules of salt like structure are collected. There are dropped ear in for cure of ear sore.

*Chlorophytum arundinaceum* Baker Fam Liliaceae. L. Kanjer saga, P-Leaf, Pl-Mardiguda.

Leaves placed in hot ash to warm and cleaned with a wet cloth. The warm leaf is squeezed and the lukewarm juice is dropped in ear for the treatment of ear sore and earache.

*Cleome viscosa* Linn: Fam–Capparidaceae, L.Hulhullia, P-Leaf, Pl-Tolbahammi.

Fresh leaf juice is collected and warmed. At a Luke warm temperature, it is dropped in ear for pus in the ear.

*Dendropthe falcata* (L) Etting–L. Fam-Loranthaceae, L. Mahul madang P-leaf Pl-Chianpadar.

Leaf juice is warmed and dropped in ear for the treatment of ear infection.

*Gossipium herbaceum* (Linn): Fam–Malvaceae, L.Kapa P–Fruit Pl-Maskaguda.

Fruit is warmed in fire and is squeezed. The juice in a Luke warm temperature is dropped in ear for treatment of ear infection.

*Leucas aspera Spreng*: Fam Lamiaceae. L-Gubi P-leaf Pl-Kandel, Kesinga

Leaves rolled in the palm and squeezing collects juice. The juice is dropped in ear for treatment of oozing pus from ear.

*Spondias pinnata* (L.F.) Kurz-Fam-Anacardiaceae L. Amda, P-Leaf Pl-Musanal and Kandama

Luke warm leaf juice is dropped in ear for treatment of earache. Fruits rubbed with Fitikiri and bark of *Acacia catechu* (L.F.) Wild are mixed with cow ghee and the mixture is applied on tongue for tongue infection and mouth sore. It is a special method of treatment in case of infants. (Fruit pulp collected by rubbing on stone surface is applied on tongue to cure tongue infection).

*Stachyterpheta indica* (L) Vahl-Fam Verbenaceae L.Gorujhagda, P. Leaf, Pl-Bijepur

Leaves pounded with black pepper and the paste is applied on the ulcerated tongue surface for cure of sore tongue and/or for mouth sore.

*Tricosanthes bracteata*(Lam) Vagt. Fam-Cucurbitaceae, L.Mahakal, P-Leaf and fruit, Pl-Kandama, Musanal

Mustard oil is applied on the surface of leaves and is warmed over a flame. Luke warm leaf juice is collected by squeezing and dropped in ear to cure pus in ear. Fruit is fried with mustard oil till it turns black. This oil is dropped in ear in Luke warm condition to cure all types of ear diseases.

*Vanda tesellata*(Roxb) Don-Fam Orchidaceae L. Rasna (Kaugudi), P-Leaf Pl-Kamarda.

Leaf is warmed under hot ash, cleaned with a wet cloth. It is squeezed to collect the juice. That is dropped in ear for treatment of ear infection.

## 4.0 Discussion

The enumeration shows that ethnomedicine for treatment of ear diseases is based on application of Luke warm juice of plant parts like leaf and fruit. Generally placing the leaf in hot ash and squeezing after cleaning collects the juice.

A scrutiny of literature Das *et al.* (2003) shows that most of the plants are newly reported for ear and mouth disease from the state for the first time. Also scrutiny with Jain (1991), Hussain *et al.* (1992), Kirtikar and Basu (1935), reveals that *Bambusa vulgaris, Gossypium herbaceum* and *Dendropthe falcata* have been reported for use in ear disease but the methods of preparation are different. The species like *Stachyterpheta indica* and *Spondias pinnata* are newly reported for cure of mouth disease. Species like *Tricosanthes bracteata* is used in ear disease all over Western Orissa as a popular remedy.

## 5.0 Conclusion

This is a brief report of the medico-ethno botanical survey of Kalahandi district and more exhaustive studies with reference to ear disease in the state are necessary in order to collect and document the rich and vast knowledge available with the traditional healers. Some of the useful remedies can be screened and investigated for cheap and effective healthcare.

## Acknowledgement

Authors are thankful to Dr. Ramesh Mishra, for his help in botanical identification of the plant species. Thanks are also due to the traditional healers who have shared their valuable experience during the survey.

## References

Das, Sarita, Dash S.K., Padhy, S.N., 2003. Ethnomedicinal information from Orissa, state India, A Review. J. Hum Eco; pp. 165-227.

Hussain, V.O.P., Popli, S.P., Mishra, L.N., Gupta, M.M., Srivastava, G.N., Abraham, Z., Singh, A.K., 1992. Dictionary of India medicinal plants, Central Institute of Medicinal and Aromatic Plant Division, Lucknow.

Jain, S.K., 1991. Dictionary of Indian Folk Medicine and ethnobotany, A reference manual of man plant relationship, Ethnic groups and Ethnobotanist in India (with 433 Illustration) N.B.R.I. Lucknow; pp. 311.

Kritikar, K.R., Basu, B.D., 1935. Indian medicinal plants volume 1-4, Bishen Singh and Mahendra Pal Singh, Dehradun, India.

Chapter 44

# Traditional Veterinary Herbal Practices of Kalahandi District, Orissa, India

**N. Sadangi[1], R.N. Padhy[2] and R.K. Sahu[2]***

[1]*Department of Botany, Kesinga Mahavidyalaya, Kesinga, Kalhandi, Orissa, India*

[2]*Department of Botany, B.J.B Autonomous College, Bhubaneswar, Orissa, India*

**E-mail: sahurajani@yahoo.co.in*

## ABSTRACT

Ethnobotanical data of plant parts of 41 Angiosperms have been documented from the tribal district Kalahandi, Orissa, India, as herbal medicines for animals. Diseases cured by plant species *viz, Achyranthus aspera Annona squamosa, Azadirachta indica, Bidens biternata, Biophytum sensitivum, Cassia fistula, Cleistanthus collinus, Ficus glomerata, Holarrhena antidysenterica. Madhuca indica, Milletia extensa, Leucas cephalotes, Ricinus comunis,* are found. These reports are unique from the district.

***Keywords:*** *Ethnobotany, Veterinary, Kalahandi, Orissa, Medicinal plants.*

## 1.0 Introduction

Adumbrated with a dense forest and valleys, the present Kalahandi District, Orissa, occupies the southwestern portion of Orissa, It is situated with in 19°, 10′ and 20°, 30′ North latitude and 82°, 30′ and 83° 50′ Eastern longitude. The district has variegated plants occupying both exotic and native flora of substantial recuperative utility. Topographically the district is undulating, characterized by hillocks and tributaries. Its eastern to southeastern zone is hilly and locally called as Dongerla Area, which is a part of Eastern Ghats. The other half is almost with few isolated hill-locks and cluster of hills. This tract is locally called as "Pahilpar" Area.

A large rural population inhabits the district. Several scheduled tribes like *Bhunjia, Bhottada, Gond, Kandh, Banjara, Sabar* and scheduled castes like *Chamar, Dhoba, Dom, Ganda and Ghasi.* As a land of nomadic tribes, it has a vast treasure of ethno-veterinary practices. Therefore this study was undertaken to collect information on different plants used as veterinary medicines by the scheduled caste and tribes. The available information on traditional-veterinary medicine in India includes contributions of few workers (Brahmam Dhal and Saxena, 1996; Jain, 1999; Mishra *et al.*, 1996; Pal, 1980,1992; Raja Reddy, Sudarshanam, 1987; Rajan and Sethuraman, 1997; Reddy *et al.*, 1997). The data in this report are based on the information gathered in the field during 1999-2002.

## 2.0 Materials and Methods

The data are based on information gathered from traditional veterinary medical practitioners and through personal observations of authors in the treatment of cattle and buffaloes. Dairy farmers and veterinary practitioners were interviewed for traditional uses of herbal plants, about the plants they collect and use, their local names, plant parts used, preparation of remedies, diseases treated, dose and regimen of the drug. The specimens are collected and preserved in Department of Botany, Govt. Autonomous College, Bhawanipatna, Kalahandi, and Orissa, India.

The plants are arranged in alphabetical order with their family in parenthesis, local name, plants part used and traditional use. (Local name is abbreviated as Ln.)

## 3.0 List of Medicinal Plants

1. ***Abutilon indicum* (L). Sweet (Malvaceae), Ln: Jharbhendi.**

   *Parts used*: Root.

   *Uses*: Roots are fed each day to lactating cows as a galactogogue.

2. ***Achyranthes aspera* L. (Amarantheceae), Ln: Kukurdanti**

   *Parts used*: Leaf.

   *Uses*: Leaves pounded into paste that is applied on genital part and allowed to inhale the same for an easy delivery and retained placenta.

3. ***Aegle marmelos* L. (Rutuceae), Ln: Bel**

   *Parts used*: Leaf.

   *Uses*: Leaves of plant pounded with leaves of lemon grass, *Cymbopogon flexuosus* and rhizome of *Curcuma domestica* into a paste which is fed to cattle twice daily in dyspepsia till cured.

4. ***Allium sativum* L. (Liliaceae), Ln: Lesun.**

   *Parts used*: Bulb.

   *Uses*: One hundred g bulb fried with 100 ml of mustard oil. After cooling it is messaged on neck of cattle for treatment of cold and cough, swollen throat and haemorrhagic septicaemiasis. Decoction prepared by boiling 20g bulbs with 20g of fruits of *Piper longum* and 2g leaves of *Ocimum sanctum,* with 2 litre water until it becomes half a litre. After cooling it is given twice a day for 3 days for cure of haemorrhagic septicaemiasis, cough, cold and swollen throat.

5. ***Anona squamosa* L. (Annonaceae), Ln: Sitafal.**

*Parts used*: Leaf.

*Uses*: Leaf paste is topically applied on wounds for healing.

6. ***Andrographics paniculata* (Burm. f.) Wall. (Acanthaceae), Ln: Bhuinlimba.**

*Parts used*: leaf.

*Uses*: One hundred g of leaves, 100g fruits of *Coriandrum sativum* and 10g of *Piper nigrum* together pounded with water, and the filtrate is given orally to cattle thrice a day as a cure for Babesiosis.

7. ***Anthocephalus cadamba* (Roxb.) Miq. (Rubiaceae), Ln: Kadam**

*Parts used*: Leaf.

*Uses*: Half–a–litre of leaf juice extracted mixed with powder of 21 fruits of *Piper longum* and 20g of rock salt. It is given orally twice a day for abdominal pain.

8. ***Azadirachta indica* A. Juss. (Meliaceae) Ln: Lim.**

*Parts used*: Leaf, Bark.

*Uses*: One hundred g leaf, leaf of *Andrographis paniculata* and *Curcuma longa* are made into a paste and given orally to cattle for worm infection. A concentrated decoction of bark with leaves is used to wash the wounds in foot of cattle, bark powder is also used to sprinkle on wound. Fruit oil is used to drop in ears to cure mouth diseases.

9. ***Bambusa vulgaris* Schrad. Ex wendl. (Poaceae), Ln: Banush.**

*Parts used*: Leaf, Young sprouting,

*Uses*: Two hundred g fresh leaf pounded with 20g of Hendua (a product obtained by drying small cut pieces of tender culms of this plant) and 200 ml of three years old jaggery into a paste. It is fed to cattle and buffaloes for control of diarrhoea.

10. ***Bidens biternata* (Lour.) Merr and Sherff. (Asteraceae) Ln: Bankakhamali.**

*Parts used*: whole plant.

*Uses*: Fresh Whole plant is fed to lactating cows as a galactogogue.

11. ***Biophytum sensitivum* (L) DC. (Oxalidaceae), Ln: Badilajkuri.**

*Parts used*: Whole plant.

*Uses*: Fresh plants are fed to lactating cows as a galactogogue..

12. ***Bombax ceiba* L. (Bombacaceae) Ln: Semel.**

*Parts used*: Seed.

*Uses*: 50g of seed powder are given for 3 days twice daily to cure measles.

**13. *Kalanchoe pinnata* (Lam.) Pers. (Crassulaceae), Ln: Patragaja.**

*Parts used*: Leaf.

*Uses*: One hundred g leaves with 21 black peppers made into a fine paste is given orally (to cattle) twice a day to treat dyspepsia.

**14. *Careya arborea* Roxb. (Barringtoniaceae), Ln: Kum.**

*Parts used*: Root.

*Uses*: Root bark is made into paste and is applied on the body of cattle to kill skin flea and lice.

**15. *Cassia fistula* L. (Caesalpiniaceae) Ln: Sunari.**

*Parts used*: Fruit.

*Uses*: Ghee obtained from cow milk is applied on fruit and warmed up in flame and there after it is applied frequently on cold affected swollen throat of cattle for cure.

**16. *Chloroxylon swietenia* DC. Flindersiaceae, Ln: Bheru.**

*Parts used*: Leaf.

*Uses*: Leaves are fed to goat as galactogogue.

**17. *Cleistanthus collinus* (Roxb.) Benth. and Hk. f. (Euphorbiaceae) Ln: Karla**

*Parts used*: Leaf.

*Uses*: Leaves are crushed and spread on floor of cattle shed to cure foot diseases locally called Chapka.

**18. *Diospyros melanoxylon Roxb.* (Ebenaceae), Ln: Kendu**

*Parts used*–Fruit

*Uses*: The fresh fruit is made into paste and given orally to cattle to cure dysentery. Ten pulp of the fruit mixed with little water to make a lotion and applied on eyes to cure infection.

**19. *Erythrina suberosa* Roxb. (Fabaceae), Ln: Baldia**

*Parts used*: Leaf

*Uses*: Leaves are made into paste that applied externally on neck to cure yoke sore.

**20. *Ficus racemosa* L. (Moraceae), Ln: Dumer.**

*Parts used*: Latex.

Fresh latex is applied on wounds of cattle as a cure.

**21. *Gardenia gummifera* L.f. (Rubiaceae), Ln: Kurudu.**

*Parts used*: Resin.

*Uses*: Resin is made into powder and sprinkled on sores of cattle to keep flies and maggots away.

**22.** ***Geniosporum elongatum*** **Benth, (Lamiaceae), Ln: Ghudatulsi**

*Parts used*: Twigs.

*Uses*: Twigs are tied on tail of cow to expel retained placenta.

**23.** ***Gossypium herbaceum*** **L. (Malvaceae), Ln: Kapa.**

*Parts used*: Leaf.

*Uses*: The leaf juice is given orally as a cure for suppuration of waist after delivery.

**24.** ***Hibiscus cannabinus*** **L. (Malvaeae), Ln: Kanria.**

*Parts used*: Seed.

*Uses*: Seeds are fed to lactating cows to enhance lactation.

**25.** ***Holarrhena antidysenterica*** **(Roxb.ex Fleming) Wall (Apocynaceae), Ln: Kure.**

*Parts used*: Root

*Uses*: Twenty g root bark, 20g fruit pulp of *Punica granatum* and pinch of rock salt are made into a paste and given orally to cattle to arrest diarrhoea.

**26.** ***Justicia adhatoda.*** **L. (Acanthaceae), Ln: Basang**

*Parts used*: Leaf.

*Uses*: Two hundred fifty of leaf paste mixed with 250 curd, 100g of resin powder obtained from *Shorea robusta is* given to cows for easy delivery. Half litre juice obtained from pounded leaves boiled with 20g of *Piper nigrum* and 1 litre of water. This decoction after cooling is given orally to cattle twice a day for bronchial problems. Half a litre of leaf juice mixed with 20g of fruit powder of *Piper longum* is prescribed twice a day for severe cough.

**27.** ***Lawsonia inermis*** **L. (Lythraceae), Ln: Menjati.**

*Parts used*: Bark.

*Uses*: Decoction prepared by boiling 250g bark with 2 litre water is prescribed for constipation in lukewarm condition with a pinch of rock salt in 50ml dose twice daily.

**28.** ***Leucas cephalotes*** **(Koen. ex Roth) Spreng, Ln: Gubi.**

*Parts used*: Whole plant.

*Uses*: Whole plant and 21 fruits of *Piper nigrum* are made into a paste and given orally to cattle as a cure for snakebite.

**29.** ***Madhuca indica*** **J.F. Gmel. (Sapotaceae), Ln: Mahul.**

*Parts used*: Seed.

*Uses*: Cake obtained after oil extraction is applied on chronic wounds to expel worms.

**30.** ***Millettia extensa*** **(Benth.) Baker (Fabacace.), Ln: Mankadmal**

*Parts used*: Leaf.

*Uses*: Crushed leaves spread on cattle shed to cure foot diseases.

**31. *Mimusops elengi* L. (Sapotaceae) Ln: Baulo.**

*Parts used*: Leaf.

*Uses*: The hundred of leaves pounded and squeezed juice is given orally twice a day to cows to cure suppuration of waist after delivery. One hundred of fruits pounded to a fine paste, mixed with 1/2 litre water and given orally twice a day as a cure for urinary problems.

**32. *Nyctanthes arbor-tristis* L. (Oleaceae.), Ln: Kukuda had.**

*Parts used*: Leaf, Bark

*Uses*: Half a litre of extracted leaf juice boiled with 20g fruit of *Piper nigrum* and 1 litre water until it becomes 1/2 litre. After cooling it is given orally for 3 days to cure fever.

Leaf juice is extracted and boiled with 20g *Elettaria cardamomum*, and 1 litre water until it becomes 1/2 litre. This decoction is given orally to cattle as a cure for rheumatism. 1/2 litre of leaf juice mixed with 20 gm of *Piper nigrum* fruit powder is given twice a day for 2 days for cure of cough. The stem bark pounded with 2 fruits of *Terminalia chebula* to a fine paste is applied on bone fracture site as a bone setting.

**33. *Pueraria tuberosa*. (Willd) DC. (Fabaceae), Ln: Bhuin Kumda.**

*Parts used*: Root tuber.

*Uses*: Root tuber pounded with water and given orally to cow as a galactogogue.

**34. *Psidium guajava* L. (Myrtaceae), Ln: Maya (Jam)**

*Parts used*: Leaf

*Uses*: Twenty tender leaves of the plant, *Syzigium cumini* and *Mangifera indica* are pounded together, and the Juice is given orally to cattle for the treatment of dysentery.

**35. *Ricinus communis* L. (Euphorbiaceae) Ln: Jada**

*Parts used*: Seed

*Uses*: Ten ml seed oil is mixed with 10g leaves and rhizome paste of *Curcuma longa*. And applied on burn wounds. Oil obtained from seed is given orally in a 10 ml dose once a day for treatment of constipation of cattle.

**36. *Sachleichera oleosa* (Lour.) Oken (Sapindaceae), Ln: Kusum.**

*Parts used*: Seed

*Uses*: Oil obtained from the seeds is messaged on skin to kill fleas.

**37. *Strychnus potatorum* L.f. (Loganiaceae), Ln: Kaya**

*Parts used*: Fruit

*Uses*: The fruit pulp is made into a paste and applied on wounds for healing.

**38. *Terminalia arjuna* (Roxb. ex DC.) Wight and Arn. (Combretaceae), Ln: Kha**

*Parts used*: Leaf

*Uses*: Two hundred Fifty ml leaf juice is given orally to cows twice a day to cure suppuration of waist after delivery. Leaves fed to cattle to strengthen bones.

**39. *Terminalia chebula* Retz. (Combreataceae), Ln: Harda**

*Parts used*: Fruits

*Uses*: Equal quantities of the dried leaves of *Terminalia chebula, Achyranthes aspera, Leucas cephalotes* and *Ocimum sanctum* are made into a powder with a pinch of hing (asafoctida) is mixed with water to make a lotion and applied on teeth of cattle to cure tooth diseases. Fruit powder of *Terminalia chebula, Terminalia belerica* and *Phyllanthus embelica* in equal amounts and mixed with salt is given orally to cattle for abdominal pain. Epicarp of fruits of *Terminalia chebula, Terminalia belerica* and *Phyllanthus embelica* are made into a paste and applied on skin of cattle to kill lice. Fruit of *Terminalia chebula* is rubbed on stone surface to get pulp, which is mixed with water and applied, on tongue for tongue sore.

**40. *Vitex negundo* L. (Verbenaceae) Ln: Nirgundi.**

*Parts used*: Leaves

*Uses*: Twenty ml leaf juice, 20g *Elettaria cardamomum* are boiled with 1 litre water and it becomes half and after cooling is given orally twice a day to cure rheumatism.

**41. *Cayratia auriculata* (Roxb.) Gamble, (Vitaceae) Ln: Masnia**

*Parts used*: Root

*Uses*: The root is made into a paste that is applied on wounds for a cure.

## 4.0 Discussion and Conclusion

Analysis of the data shows that 41 species of medicinal plants are being used for the management of different conditions and diseases of cattle. Many of the information reported in this communication particularly for the species namely *Abutilon indicum, Aegle marmelos, Andrographis paniculata, Allium sativum, Anthocephalus cadamba Bambusa vulgaris, Kalanchoe pinnata, Bombax ceiba, Careya arborea, Chloroxylon swietenia, Diospyros melanoxylon, Erythrina suberosa, Geniosporum elongatum, Gossypium herbaceum, Hibiscus cannabinus, Justicia adhatoda, Lawsonia inermis, Mimusops elengi, Schleichera oleosa, Strychnus potatorum, Terminalia chebula Vitex negundo* are found to be less known to the literature of Indian medicinal plants used in veterinary diseases (Sharma,1996).

Likewise diseases cured by plant species *viz, Achyranthus aspera Annona squamosa, Azadirachta indica, Bidens biternata, Biophytum sensitivum, Cassia fistula, Cleistanthus collinus, Ficus glomerata, Holarrhena antidysenterica. Madhuca indica, Milletia extensa, Leucas cephalotes, Ricinus comunis,* are found to be similar to the uses by other ethnic groups in other parts of India (Sharma, 1996) indicating their authenticity of usefulness in the treatment diseases but methods of using differed from place to place.

The simultaneous uses of a particular plant for the treatment of number of diseases as observed in present investigation for the species like *Allium sativum, Azadirachta indica, Diospyros melanoxylon, Justicia adhatoda, Mimusops elengi, Nyctanthes arbor-tristis Ricinus communis, Terminalia chebula* may also be considered encouraging with regards to their specific uses reported herein, which are unreported in previous literature.

The plants mentioned here are still very popular in this area and enjoy a good reputation in traditional medicine for treatment of veterinary diseases. Inspite of an extensive modern programme implemented by the governmental organizations and hospitals to uplift the rural health care of domestic animals, the traditional treatments have retained popularity in the district. Most of the drugs are utilized in fresh state or as cooled decoction, infusion etc.

Further activities for conservation of plant biodiversity *in situ* or *ex situ* are needed to protect the extinction of plants having ethno-veterinary importance. Steps could be taken by the Government and Non-Governmental Organizations to enunciate a clear policy of conservation and sustainable use of medicinal plants at this stage where a rapid deforestation is uncontrollable.

The therapeutically significant plants need to be cultivated in a systematic manner to meet Indian system of traditional medicine based drug industry and to validate pharmacologically the efficacy of all ethno-veterinary claims.

## Acknowledgements

The authors are thankful to University Grant Commission, (U.G.C) New Delhi, for providing financial assistance to R.K. Sahu. Our sincerest gratitude is due to those tribals who have cooperated by sharing their valuable knowledge with us.

## References

Brahmam, M., Dhal, N.K. and Saxena, H.O., 1996. In: Jain SK. (Ed.). Ethnobiology in Human Welfare, Deep Publication: New Delhi, pp. 393-396.

Jain, S.K., 1999. Dictionary of Ethno-veterinary Plants, Deep Publication: New Delhi, pp. 199.

Mishra, S., Vidyanath, J. and Shaktinath, J., 1996. In: Jain SK. (Ed.). Ethnobiology in Human welfare. Deep Publication: New Delhi, pp. 189-193.

Pal, D.C., 1980. Bull. Bot. Surv. India (22), pp. 96-99.

Pal, D.C., 1992. J. Econ. Tax Bot. Addl. Ser. (10), pp. 137-141.

Raja Reddy K. and Sudarshanam G., 1987. Int. J. Crude Drug Res. (25), pp. 145-152.

Rajan, S. and Sethuraman, M., 1997. Indigenous Knowledge and Development Monitor (5), pp. 7-9.

Reddy, R.V., Lakkshmi, N.V.N. and Venkata Raju R.R., 1997. Ethnobotany (9), pp. 94-96.

Sharma, S.C., 1996. J. Econ. Tax. Bot. Addl. Ser. (12), pp. 123-127.

# *Part IV*

# Country Reports

*Chapter 45*

# Country Status Report on Traditional Medicine Research and Development in Nigeria

***Emmanuel Orgah***
*Nigeria Natural Medicine Development Agency, Lagos, Nigeria*
*E-mail: emmaorgah@yahoo.com*

## BACKGROUND

Nigeria is a country in the west coast of Africa with a population of about 145 millions. There are more than 250 ethnic cultural groups in Nigeria with distinct Traditional Medical practices in the management and care of various diseases. The current global re-emphasis on Traditional Medicine (TM) in the light of current heavy disease burden and socio-economic crises coupled with the changing role of people in the cultural communities, points to only one health alternative: sourcing public health from TM and a concerted effort towards the sustainable utilisation of natural resources in developing countries.

## 1.0 The Nigeria Natural Development Agency (NNMDA)

The Nigeria Natural Medicine Development Agency (NNMDA) is an Agency of the federal ministry of science and technology established to enable the Nigerian government to actualize its critical strategy in the research, development, documentation, preservation and promotion of Nigeria's TM and facilitate its integration into the National Healthcare Delivery System. The aim is to develop and promote safe and efficacious TM therapies, to redress health inequities and improve the economic wellbeing of Nigerians. (Profile on the Nigeria Natural Medicine Development Agency–Federal Ministry of Science and Technology)

The establishment of the Agency arose from the full appreciation by our government of the vast potentials of the country's Traditional Medicine knowledge

(TMK) and the enormous biodiversity. The Nigerian people and government have made several attempts in the post-colonial era (since the 1960s) for the standardization, quality control, promotion of local production and commercialization of TM (NNMDA, 2007). The establishment of the Agency in 1997 streamlined these efforts and focused TM research. The Agency facilitates national and international cooperative and collaborative research, development and promotion efforts in the TM sector.

## 2.0 Dependence on TM in Nigeria and the Role of TMPS in Building a Positive Health Agenda

Traditional Medicine is the mainstay of primary healthcare in Nigeria, as in other parts of Africa. One may be right to say too that it is the mainstay of the economy since the role-played by people in improving their own health and the availability of supportive knowledge creates both good health and socio-economic growth. Over 85 per cent of our people depend on Traditional Medicine practices and products not only for their healthcare delivery but also for social, economic and community issues. For most of our people, it is the only source of healthcare delivery known, accessible, acceptable and affordable.

The struggle for good health in Nigeria and indeed in most developing countries embodies a struggle for the recognition of Traditional Medicine Practitioners (TMPs), as actual agents of change and health information dissemination. We believe that stakeholders with the most critical role in building a positive health agenda must include TMPs.

We are convinced that the role and services of the Nations Traditional Healers, if appropriately harnessed can strengthen the capacity of the nation's healthcare delivery systems. For example, it is believed that TMPs bear the brunt of the HIV/AIDS pandemic as People Living with HIV/AIDS (PLWHAS) most often return to their communities for care, support and sometimes eventual death. At the same time, some practices of TMPs such as circumcision, facial scarification, bloodletting etc and their bogus claims are believed to encourage the spread of HIV/AIDS, cause complications and constitute risks to the health of the population.

From the numbers that patronize TMPs, it is evident that the people trust them. We have observed that TMPs could become not only the pillars of community-based care and support for people living with HIV/AIDS but also other communicable diseases. Since TMPs can reach over 85 per cent of the people, a population much more than radio and television can reach, they are strategic and vital information disseminators for healthcare improvement.

In line with the foregoing, the Agency sets out to research, document, promote and disseminate researches that would advocate TM for promotion of good health and publicize its wealth and job creation potentials. Our research strategy stems from the acknowledgement of the challenges that TM faces in terms of perception, fiscal policy and industry standards. In spite of the numerous potentials of TM, the following challenges are contended with: disrespect and Denial of the roles of TMPs, mysticism in the practices of TM, inadequate evidence bases for safety and efficacy, attitude of practitioners bordering on secretiveness, complications arising from their activities and bogus and deceptive claims and non availability of Intellectual Property Rights regime etc (Etatuvie, S. O., 2007).

The Agency, mindful of these challenges, and recognizing the role that TM could play in achieving the targets of the Millennium Development Goals (MDGS) (Eradication of extreme poverty and hunger, combating HIV/AIDS, Malaria and other diseases, ensure environmental sustainability and develop a global partnership for development etc) designs its research programs/projects towards maximizing the potentials of the Nation's Natural Medicines for improved healthcare delivery, job and wealth creation, improvement of the quality of life, national economic growth and development.

## 2.1 Specifically

The Agency has ongoing projects for the identification and documentation of Medicinal, Aromatic and Pesticidals (MAPs) Plants, animal/animal parts and mineral used in traditional medicine. These projects documents Medicinal Plants (MPs) of Nigeria in line with the procedures of the World Health Organization (WHO).

The documentation criteria include; the scientific names, names in local languages, medicinal usage by local communities, conditions for cultivation and phytochemical and pharmacological properties.

The primary survey and Photo documentation of medicinal plants in the six geopolitical Zones of Nigeria has been completed. Two books have been published under the titles 'Medicinal Plants of Nigeria', South West and North central Zone Vols.1 respectively. The ones for the other zones are in press. Pictorial canvass display of the surveys has also been developed to provide educational materials for students, researchers and as a raw material resource identifier to practitioners.

## 2.2 A Brief Summary of the Book on the SW Zone Shows

- 117 plant species belonging to 58 families
- 72 species for the treatment of Malaria and other forms of fever
- 52 for skin diseases
- 50 for childbirth and other female reproduction issues
- 30 for worm expelling
- 25 for Rheumatism

*Source*: Okujagu *et al.*, 2004.

## 2.3 A Brief Summary of the Book on NC Zone Shows

- 100 plant species belonging to 45 families
- 12 species for the treatment of Malaria and other forms of fever
- 24 for skin diseases
- 29 for childbirth and other reproductive health issues
- 22 species for diarrhoea and dysentery

- 15 species for ulcer cases
- 20 for worm expelling
- 15 for Rheumatism
- 11 species for eye problems

*Source*: Okujagu *et al.*, 2005.

Ongoing projects to bring to fore and utilize the Nation's indigenous non–medication sciences and technologies–Bone–Setting, Massage therapy, manual technologies and exercises applied singularly or in combination to maintain well–being, as well as to treat, diagnose or prevent illness.

The ultimate objective of these documentation initiatives is to develop a Comprehensive National Inventory of Nigeria's MAPs, animals and animals parts, minerals and non–medication sciences and technologies used for human and veterinary/livestock healthcare management, maintenance, care and support. (Etatuvie, S.O., 2007).

When fully developed, this inventory would: Aid teaching, learning and research. Serve as a key useful resource material for conservation and cultivation, promote entrepreneurs development, wealth and job creation and promote documentation and preservation of indigenous Intellectual Property Rights. (Etatuvie, S.O., 2007).

The Agency has designed and constructed a Pilot Production Plant projected to inter-phase research to industry. This will enhance scale-up studies on simple traditional medicine products, maintain crude drug repository and develop appropriate low cost process technology and formulation of standardized herbal medicines for commercial production. This is critical to the conversion of Nigeria's TMK into a wealth/employment generation resource for poverty reduction.

At the moment, three products have been formulated and are being studied for their full industrial and market potentials.

These products include:

## 2.4 Herbal Mosquito Repellent

These products (mosquito repellent candle, cream, ointment) are based on scientific reports of some Nigeria MPs used traditionally to repel insects. They are targeted at reducing the mosquito–man contact thereby interrupting the transmission of the malaria parasite. Published research reports indicate that the base plants/herbs are environmentally friendly (used in this way) and are of little or no adverse effects on humans.

## 2.5 Herbal Cough Syrup

Our herbal cough syrup combines the soothing and anti–bacteria properties of some Nigerian MPs in a vehicle of pure honey.

## 2.6 Herbal Soap

Most of our traditional communities utilise herbs in the maintenance of skin tones and general dermatological health. They also produce soaps that exploit natural sources of generating lye which they believe is less harsh on the skin while at the same time being economically feasible. The Agency has thus formulated an improved version of herbal medicated soap from the natural resources used by Nigerian people.

These products are undergoing further development and standardization for listing by the Nigeria National Agency for Food, Drug Administration and Control (NAFDAC) and commercialization through Public–Private Partnership arrangements.

## 2.7 Laboratory Support Services

The Agency also provides laboratory support services and product screening of herbal medicine products to small-scale entrepreneurs in the TM sector, who lack the resources and expertise to develop and analyse their products. This is to assist practitioners in the production of safe and efficacious therapies, in other to enhance the development, growth and improvement of healthcare delivery.

The Agency have therefore developed a modern laboratory at the Agency's head office in Lagos Nigeria and moderately equipped it for research and development of screening protocols.

## 2.8 Development of a Digital/Virtual Library

The Agency has developed a full digital/virtual library. The library is a focal Reference Centre for Nigerian Traditional Medicine. The library, among others:

- Assist and stimulate value addition to the abundant raw material resources accruing from the vast biodiversity of Nigeria.
- Stimulate the promotion of e-commerce and create markets for MAPs and other herbal drugs/products of Nigerian origin.
- Assist, preserve and protect our indigenous knowledge, culture and heritage.
- Protect the Nation's Intellectual Property Rights on Natural Medicine knowledge products and practices.

The combined outcome of these initiatives would assist research, preserve and develop the indigenous knowledge, culture and heritage, and protect the Nation's Intellectual property Rights on TMK, products and practices.

## 2.9 Traditional Medicine Manpower Development

Due to globalization, the health sector is undergoing a transformation in terms of focus, access, human resource deployment and distribution, essential care, and technological advances. Capacity building is more challenging than ever and learning must now take place in different forms, under varied circumstances, and for a wide variety of purposes and so must research and development.

In recognition of the forgoing, the Agency developed training modules in collaboration with researchers in Nigerian Universities. The training modules were drawn in line with World Health Organisation's specification for continuing education program for TMPs. Using this modules the Agency have Conducted 26 trainings and interactive sessions involving over nine thousand (9000) TMPs using the village-square model.

The training and interactive programs are designed to enhance the skills of the TMPs, build their confidence, reduce secrecy and improve their practices and products development techniques. It is also to equip them to serve as agents of appropriate medical information dissemination, education, and communication and positive health behavioural change.

The Agency, through her Education, Training and value re-orientation Programs attempts to identify opportunities for cooperation, collaboration and partnership that will strengthen the knowledge base of TMPs and for the provision of good, affordable and accessible healthcare and related information.

The ultimate objective of this initiative is the generation of critical mass of knowledgeable TMPs across the country that would be vehicles of information dissemination and education to combat the spread and control of communicable diseases in the communities where they reside and practice, for improved wellness and health coverage.

This exercise also facilitates collaborations and partnership in the Agency's documentation initiatives hence encouraging TMPs to freely give information bearing on their Traditional Medical Knowledge to enhance research and development (Etatuvie, S. O., 2007).

## 2.10 Collation/Documentation of Published Research Works on Nigerian Traditional Medical Knowledge, Practices, Products and MAPs

Nigerian Scientists have conducted several researches on the use of Nigerian herbs/indigenous sciences and technology for care, management, treatment and cure of various ailments. These are scattered in different journals and publications in Universities and research institutes.

These constitute a vital component of our cultural heritage and national intellectual property that the nation needs to use as base information for value addition. It is a resource for entrepreneurship development, wealth and job creation.

The collation of research works is aimed at: facilitating centralization of all research findings, and ease of referencing, reduction of research duplication, promotion of research gap identification, stimulation of further research, stimulation of commercialization efforts and facilitation of demand driven research by Natural Products scientists.

The 1st Volume of this vital collation, [containing 1050 abstracts on every aspect of Traditional Medicine–(1970–2004)], has been published and distributed to libraries of all higher institutions in Nigeria. This is a part of the materials in our digital library (Okujagu *et al.*, 2006).

## 2.11 Developing Pilot/Experimental Medicinal, Aromatic and Pesticidals (MAPs) Plant Farm/Nurseries in Each of the Six Geopolitical Zones

The Agency is developing pilot medicinal plants farms/botanical gardens in various zones of the country in collaboration with universities and practitioners.

The aim is to: cultivate plants in the areas that they grow best, preserve local knowledge and plants for local use, preserve plants that are about to become extinct, facilitate the study and documentation of the abiotic factors (climatic, soil, altitude, water) and general agricultural conditions needed for medicinal plants to be grown, domesticated and cultivated (Etatuvie, S. O., 2007).

These would promote enhanced species identification, cultivation technique and Good Agricultural and Collection Practices (GACP) for sustainable access, availability and rational use of raw materials for Traditional Medicine products development and commercialization, job and wealth creation.

### 2.12 Facilitating the Development of a Legal Frameworks and Policy for an Intellectual Property Rights (IPR) Regime for Traditional Knowledge, Practice and Products

The Agency is facilitating the development of policies for the institutional, legal and regulatory framework for the practice of traditional medicine in our formal health systems and ensures that intellectual property rights are given priority for the protection and promotion of the indigenous TMK and promote awareness about issues of intellectual property rights with regards to biodiversity and bio-resources.

This is essential to the development and promotion of the Nation's vast biodiversity, bioresources and knowledge not only for health care delivery but also for wealth, job creation and to stem bio-piracy.

### 2.13 Promoting Public Private Partnerships

Through this project, the Agency assist practitioners with technical and scientific support, in addition to training, local and international exposures for the improvement of their products and practices also to assist them meet our regulatory stipulated standards as defined by NAFDAC.

### 2.14 Observational Studies

There have been various claims for cure and management of HIV and other diseases by TMPs. These require scientific and evidence based verification. The Agency in ongoing studies is facilitating observational studies on such therapies in collaboration with research teams in some Nigerian Universities.

## 3.0 Conclusion

Nigeria have a long tradition of mainstream use of traditional medicine and continue to do so mainly for the reason that traditional therapies for various conditions generally cost less than the equivalent pharmaceutical product. Herbal medicines are acceptable, available and accessible to the majority Nigerians.

Traditional medicine in Nigeria approaches healthcare through a variety of techniques and methods that are broadly based on the use of herbs and health foods. Traditional therapies are based on the philosophy that herbal medicines affect the system via a synergistic combination of effects of the natural products in the herbs, animal parts and minerals.

The Nigeria Natural Medicine Development Agency carries out systematic and concerted research in the sector. It is the dedicated national institution for the coordination of research in the herbal medicine sector. Through her many research and infrastructural development, the Agency has crystallized the process for the promotion, Research and Development of TM in Nigeria.

Local production of herbal medicines is a necessary intervention with an immense potential of contributing not only to improved healthcare but to poverty reduction and impact positively on national economic growth and development.

At the moment, Nigeria lacks local technology for efficient processing techniques for herbal medicinal materials leading to high yields; adequate technology for preserving herbal medicines for extended shelf life; low energy losses during processing; methodology for verification of herbalist's claims and local fabrication of equipments. The Agency desires to collaborate with institutions, researchers, industry experts and donors to fully develop and utilise the nation's capacity in these areas. For us, Traditional Medicine is our life, our culture and heritage and our hope for a healthier wealthier tomorrow.

## References

Etatuvie, S. O., 2007. Personal communications.

NNMDA, 2007. Poster: Some Historical Facts on Traditional Medicine Development and Promotion. Nigeria Natural Medicine Development Agency (Federal Ministry of Science and Technology).

Okujagu, T.F. *et al.*, 2004. Medicinal Plants of Nigeria', South West Nigeria Volume 1 Nigeria Natural Medicine Development Agency (Federal Ministry of Science and Technology).

Okujagu, T.F. *et al.*, 2005. Book of Abstracts of Published Research Works and Findings on Nigerian Medicinal Plants and Traditional Medicine Practices. Volume 1. Nigeria Natural Medicine Development Agency (Federal Ministry of Science and Technology).

Okujagu, T.F. *et al.*, 2006. Medicinal Plants of Nigeria', North Central Zone Volume 1 Nigeria Natural Medicine Development Agency (Federal Ministry of Science and Technology).

Profile on the Nigeria Natural Medicine Development Agency (Federal Ministry of Science and Technology).

## Chapter 46

# Most Widely Traded Plant Drugs of Turkey

**K. Hüsnü Can BASER**

*Anadolu University, Faculty of Pharmacy, Department of Pharmacognosy, 26470 Eskisehir, Turkey*

*E-mail: khcbaser@anadolu.edu.tr*

## ABSTRACT

Flora of Turkey which is rich and diverse is well documented in 11 volumes which includes *ca.* 12.000 taxa of vascular plants with over 30 per cent endemism. This natural diversity blended with cultural richness throughout centuries is a rich source of useful plants with use in medicine, food, cosmetics, perfumery, etc. The scope of this paper will cover the most widely traded wild or cultivated medicinal and aromatic plants of Turkey. They include oregano, sage, laurel leaf, aniseeds, cumin, licorice, linden flower, soapwort, storax, sahlep, opium poppy, etc. Information on their traded species, uses and latest export figures will be provided.

*Keywords: Flora, Turkey, Medicinal plants.*

## 1.0 Introduction

Turkey which is situated in between 42°N and 36°N latitudes enjoys three different climates: Mediterranean, Continental, Oceanic, and has an elevation between sea level and > 5500 m. It has land in Anatolia (ASIA) + Thrace (EUROPE). It is considered a passageway between the two continents. Turkey is at the junction of three important phytogeographic regions: Mediterranean, Iran-Turan and Euro-Siberian (Akman and Ketenoglu, 1986).

Therefore, the Flora of Turkey is rich and diverse. 11.700 flowering plant taxa belonging to > 9.000 species have been recorded to grow in Turkey which is *ca.* 2000 less than the number of species growing in Europe. 1/3 of the flora of Turkey comprises aromatic plants. 1000 plant taxa used in folk medicine. *ca.* 30 per cent of the flora consists of endemic species (Baser, 2002.1).

The flora of Turkey is well documented. The flora of Turkey and the East Aegean Islands had been edited in nine volumes and one supplement (Vols. 1-10) between 1965 and 1988 by the Edinburgh University Press in Edinburgh. The 11th volume (2nd supplement) edited by Prof. Dr. Tuna Ekim, Prof. Dr. Adil Güner, Prof. Dr. Neriman Özhatay and Prof. Dr. K.Hüsnü Can Baser was published in 2000 as continuation of the series (Davis, 1965-1985; Davis *et al.*, 1988, Güner *et al.*, 2000)

Turkey annually exports *ca.* $ 100 million worth of medicinal and aromatic plants. Between 2000 and 2003 annual exports of oregano, laurel and sage amounted to $24-26 million with average unit value of 1.7-2.0 dollar per kilogram. In the years 2004 and 2005 annual exports of the same products reached $ 33-34 million ($/kg 1.9-2.0).

## 1.1 Opium Poppy

Turkey is the biggest producer of morphine in the world. Morphine is extracted from poppy straw at the modern Opium Alkaloids Factory in Bolvadin, Afyon.

Annually, 60 tons of morphine is produced from 20.000 tons of poppy straw. Half of the Morphine produced is converted to its salts, and codeine, dionine (diethyl morphine) in the derivatives plant.

Since 1974, the production of Opium by lancing unripe poppy fruits has been prohibited in Turkey to stop illegal trade. Poppies are left to ripen in the field until dry. They are then harvested, crushed to get the seeds. Poppy straw is the seedless crushed fully ripened fruits of Opium poppy. Farmers are required to sell poppy straw to the Turkish Grain Board (Toprak Mahsulleri Ofisi) (TMO). The Morphine Production Plant is run by TMO. The Factory produces also Powdered Opium and Opium Tincture, upon request (Mansfield, 2001).

## 1.2 Rose

Rose oil is produced in Turkey and Bulgaria by water distillation of the fresh flowers of *Rosa damascena* Miller. This species is a natural hybrid of *Rosa gallica* L. and *Rosa phoenicia* Boiss. both of which are found in Turkey. The variety cultivated is "*trigintipetala*" (30 petalled) (Baytop, 1990).

Turkey is one of the two major producers of rose oil together with Bulgaria. Rose oil by water distillation and rose concrete by solvent extraction are produced from fresh flowers of *Rosa damascena* (Rosaceae).

Annually, 7000 tons of roses are worked up to produce 1600 kg of rose oil and 2400 kg of rose concrete. Rose absolute is also produced by some companies in limited amounts. The price of Turkish rose oil varies in the range of $ 3500-5000 per kg. Rose concrete usually sells for $ 475-500 per kg. Bulgarian rose oil sells for slightly less than the Turkish rose oil (Baser, 1992; Baser *et al.*, 2003).

Rose is an entirely cultivated crop and 3500–4000 tons of fresh roses are required to produce 1 kg of rose oil, while 400 kg of fresh roses are sufficient to produce 1 kg of rose concrete. Rose distillation season is between mid-May and mid-June and 100 tons of rose water is also produced annually (Baser, 1992; Baser *et al.*, 2003).

Rose products found in the market include: rose oil, rose water, rose concrete, rose absolute, rose jam, rose soap and dried rose flowers.

### 1.3 Oregano

In Turkey, oregano (kekik) is considered a panacea. Oregano is a collective term referring to members of several genera with the common feature being that they all contain carvacrol as main constituent in their essential oils. Such genera include *Origanum, Thymbra, Satureja, Thymus* and *Coridothymus* of the family Lamiaceae (or Labiatae) and *Lippia graveolens* among others. Plants smelling like Oregano or Thyme are called as "kekik" in Turkish. *Origanum* species constitute the largest portion of Oregano traded around the world (Baser *et al.*, 1993).

Kekik is the most important wild crop of Turkey and Turkey is the world's biggest supplier of oregano. In 2005, dried oregano exports reached an all time high of $17.9 million for 10.4 million kilograms, with a unit value of $1.7 per kg. In 1999, it was $2.2. 1.000 tons is estimated to be consumed domestically (Table 46.1). The rest is either exported or used in essential oil production. At present, Turkey exports an estimated >20 tons of oregano oil. (Baser, 2002).

**Table 46.1: Kekik (Oregano) Exports of Turkey (Anon., 2006)**

| Kekik | 2003 | 2004 | 2005 |
|---|---|---|---|
| Kg | 9.323.572 | 9.776.999 | 10.424.510 |
| US dollar | 14.067.924 | 16.733.271 | 17.882.555 |
| Unit export value ($/kg) | 1.51 | 1.71 | 1.72 |

In 2004, agricultural fields where oregano was cultivated in Turkey reached 5250 hectares and 7000 tons of oregano herb was produced (Anon., 2006).

Majority of kekik exports from Turkey comprises the following five *Origanum* sp. *(in order of significance)* (Baser *et al.*, 1993):

- *O. onites* (Turkish oregano, Bilyali kekik),
- *O. vulgare* subsp. *hirtum (= O.heracleoticum)* (Greek oregano, Istanbul kekigi),
- *O. minutiflorum* (Yayla kekigi, Sütcüler kekigi)[endemic],
- *O. majorana (= O dubium)* (Beyaz kekik, white oregano),
- *O. syriacum* var. *bevanii* (Tarsus kekigi, Israeli oregano)

Other oregano plants include:

- *Thymbra spicata, T. sintenisii* (Sivri kekik, kara kekik, karabas kekik)
- *Coridothymus capitatus* (Timari, Spanish oregano)
- *Satureja cuneifolia, S. hortensis, S. montana* (Zahter, Savory)
- *Satureja spicigera* (Trabzon kekigi) is consumed as kekik in North Eastern Turkey.

- *Thymus* sp. except for *T. kotschyanus* (Bitlis kekigi) are not exported but used in Turkey where ever they grow as herbal tea.
- *Origanum sp.* are successfully cultivated in Aegean Turkey. Cultivation areas exceed 5000 hectares.
- Organic farming of *Origanum onites* also exists in Turkey

A monograph exists in the European Pharmacopoeia on Oregano (*Origani herba*) which allows both *Origanum onites* and *O. vulgare* subsp. *hirtum* in the preparation of this drug (European Pharmacopoeia, 2007).

Pharmacological activities of oregano can be summarized as follows: Oregano (kekik) is mainly used for gastrointestinal system disorders in Turkish folk medicine. We have proven the following activities of oregano oil, oregano water and carvacrol in our biological activity experiments: Oregano inhibits gastrointestinal contractions, choleretic, hypotensive (essential oil); hypertensive (Aromatic water), antimicrobial, antitumor, wound healing activity, antigenotoxic, antimutagenic, antioxidant, free-radical scavenging activity, analgesic and antiinflammatory activity, hepatoprotective/antihepatotoxic activity, antiparasitic against *Leishmannia, Trypanosoma, Plasmodium*, insecticidal, effective in honey bee diseases, food preservative, feed additive (Baser, 2002).

Oregano Water (Kekik suyu) is a herbal drink favoured in Western and Southern Turkey. The distillate of oregano plants left out of the removal of essential oil. It is a hydrosol or aromatic water. It contains 0.12 per cent oil with carvacrol (*ca.*70 per cent) and rare p-menthen-diols (*ca.*10 per cent) as main components. Oregano water is produced using very simple make-shift distillation stills of ingenious design in house kitchens. The oil which floats on top is scooped with a spoon and kept in a separate bottle for rubbing on skin as a remedy for rheumatism. Some distillation companies market oregano water in 1 L or 5 L plastic bottles after diluting it 1:1 with water in urban centres in Turkey. Its uses includes as follows:

Folk medicine: Antiulcer, digestive, antidiabetic, GIS regulation, general prophylaxy.

Pharmacological studies: Bileflow, barbiturate sleeping time, isolated ileum and aorta experiments, inhibition of gastrointestinal contractions, antihypertensive activity, etc (Aydin *et al.*, 1997).

## 1.4 Sage (*Adacayi*)

Dried leaves of *Salvia fruticosa* (Syn. *S. triloba*) (Lamiaceae) are used as herbal tea and for the production of essential oil. In 2004, Turkey exported >1650 tons of dried sage leaves for a return of over 4 million dollars. 300-500 kg of sage oil is produced annually in Turkey. Dried leaves of *S. tomentosa* (syn. *S. grandiflora*) and *S.aramiensis* are also used as herbal tea and marketed locally. *Salvia officinalis* is not a native plant of Turkey but is cultivated in western provinces (Anon., 2006; Baser, 2002.1).

## 1.5 Sideritis (*Dag cayi*)

Dried inflorescenses of several *Sideritis* sp. (Lamiaceae) are used as herbal tea in Turkey. Some species (*S. congesta, S. spicata, S. caesarea*, etc. both endemic) are marketed in Turkey and exported. Flowering spikes have a distinct, mild and pleasant aroma which is extracted by infusing one spike in hot water for about 1 min. (Baser, 1995).

46 *Sideritis* sp. have been recorded in Turkey which is considered to be one of the two main gene centres of this genus together with Spain. In Iberic peninsula and its vicinity, only the Section Sideritis occurs with 69 species and altogether 100 taxa. In Turkey, the Sections Empedoclia and Hesiodia encompass 46 species and altogether 55 taxa. In the geography in between these two peninsulas only a few number of species are recorded (Baser, 2002.1). Pharmacological activity studies by our group revealed its antistress activity.

## 1.6 Mint (*Nane*)

*Mentha spicata* (Bahce nanesi, spearmint) is the most widely cultivated and utilized mint species in Turkey. *Mentha x piperita* (Ingiliz nanesi, tibbi nane, kara nane, peppermint) is not a native plant of Turkey but cultivated in a smaller way. *Mentha arvensis* var. *piperascens* (*M. canadensis*) (Japon nanesi) is not cultivated in Turkey but dementholized mint oil obtained from this species is used widely as Chinese Oil. *Mentha pulegium* (Pennyroyal, Filiskin, Yarpuz) grows wild in Turkey and is worked up for the production of essential oil on a highly limited scale. In 1994, when Turkey suddenly exported 3 tons of pennyroyal oil, an inquiry made by us disclosed the fact that the plant material used did not belong to *M. pulegium*, but to *Micromeria fruticosa* subsp. *brachycalyx* and subsp. *barbata* (Lamiaceae). Both of these species yield pulegone-rich oils like pennyroyal (Baser, 2002.1).

## 1.7 Laurel (*Defne*)

Berries and leaves of *Laurus nobilis* (Lauraceae) are used to produce oil in Turkey (Tanriverdi *et al.*, 1992).

### Berries

Crushed berries are boiled in water and the aromatic fixed oil which floats is scooped out and used mainly in soap making. Laurel soap is used as medicinal soap against dandruff and to invigorate hair.

### Leaves

Dried leaves are used as condiment. They are also distilled to produce essential oil which is used in perfumery and food flavouring.

Turkey exported in 2004, 12.633 tons of dried leaves for a return of over $ 12.6 million. *Ca.* 150 tons of laurel berry oil (Gar yagi, tehnel yagi) is exported annually. Annual production of laurel leaf oil is around 1 ton (Anon., 2006).

## 1.8 Liquorice (*Meyan, biyan*)

Liquorice root is obtained from wild growing *Glycyrrhiza glabra* (Leguminosae). It is, at present, exported as crude drug for use mainly in tobacco, confectionary, soft drinks and pharmaceutical industries. Two processing plants to produce liquorice extract used to exist in Turkey are now shut down due to various reasons. Siirt Factory has been moved to Gaziantep.

Liquorice root and its extract are used as a remedy for gastric ulcers and for cough. A decoction of liquorice roots is consumed in Eastern Mediterranean provinces of Turkey as a refreshment.

In 1997, Turkey exported 2125 tons of liquorice roots for a return of over $ 1.5 million. In 2002, the figures dropped to $372.000 for 654 tons. In 2004, it was 522 tons for a return of $488.000. In 2005, 381 tons for $415.000 (Anon., 2006)

### 1.9 Gypsophila (*Cöven*)

Gypsophila roots (White soapwort) are harvested from wild growing *Gypsophila* sp. (Caryophyllaceae) in Turkey. Aqueous extract of the roots is used in Turkey as the main ingredient of the Turkish delicacy, Helva. Therefore, the drug is mainly consumed in Turkey. Still, annually, around 90 tons of gypsophila roots are exported from Turkey. In 2005, 92 tons were exported for $ 66.000. Abroad, it is utilized to produce crude saponin for use in fire extinguishers, pharmaceuticals and cosmetics (Anon, 2006).

### 1.10 Levant Storax

Crude storax balsam is produced in the south–western corner of Turkey from naturally growing *Liquidambar orientalis* (Hamamelidaceae). The tree trunks are bruised to stimulate the exudation of a sweet smelling balsam.

Balsam smeared bark and wood chips are scraped from the trunks with special scrapers and boiled in water. Floating wood chips and bark are, this way, separated from the balsam which sinks to the bottom.

Crude balsam is used in perfumery after purification and for the production of cinnamic acid and its esters. The crude balsam is locally used for wound healing. Spent bark is used as incense.

Export of levant storax from Turkey shows variation (Anon., 2006):

*In 1994*, 19.6 tons were exported for $ 0.5 million.

*In 1999*, only 266 kg were exported for $3.817.

### 1.11 Anis (Anason)

150 *Pimpinella* L. (Umbelliferae) species grow in the Northern Hemisphere. In Turkey, the genus *Pimpinella* is represented by 23 species and altogether 27 taxa, of which 5 are endemic. *Pimpinella anisum* L. (Anis) fruits (Aniseeds) are used as expectorant, antispasmodic, carminative, diuretic, as broncho-dilator in chronic bronchitis (Baser *et al.*, 2007).

Aniseed is an important agricultural crop of Turkey. Turkey produces *ca.* 10.000 tons of aniseeds of which *ca.* 7.000 tons are used in the manufacturing of RAKI (famous Turkish alcoholic beverage) and the rest is exported (Baser, 1997). In 2005, Turkey exported 2.260 tons of aniseeds for a return of $4.6 million. In 2004, it was 3800 tons for $5.8 million (Anon., 2006). This is due to the fact that state monopoly over alcoholic beverages exists no more since a few years and there are several private brands of Raki increasing local consumption of aniseeds.

## 1.12 Sahlep (Salep)

Salep is obtained from the tubers of terrestrial orchids of the family Orchidaceae. The fat tubers of the species of *Orchis, Ophrys, Platanthera, Serapias*, etc. are collected. After washing, the tubers are either lined up on a string like beads or loaded on a skimmer, and dipped in boiling water for some time in order to kill the enzymes.

The tubers are dried in the sun until they become rock hard. When finely ground and boiled with milk salep makes a pleasant hot drink taken especially in winter months. In summer, salep is a key ingredient of Maras Ice cream, which is hung and cut by knife in hot summer days. Salep plants grow in forests or meadows, and are considered endangered species. In most countries, their collection is prohibited (Kreutz, 1988).

Although its export is banned in Turkey, it is somehow exported. Domestic consumption requires a sizeable quantity of salep tubers to be wild crafted. Its propagation poses problems, as germination of its seeds requires the occurrence of a certain fungus in the soil. Total dependence to the nature for its supply gives shivers to conservationists. However, it can be harvested in a sustainable way. The plant yields two tubers one fat and hard and one weak and soft. After uprooting to collect the fat tuber, if the plant is replanted immediately with its weak tuber, it survives and supplies another fat tuber next year. This example also clearly shows even simple education of the collectors can prevent unnecessary destruction or spoilage.

## 1.13 Other Important Herbs

Export figures of other important medicinal and aromatic plants of Turkey used as culinary herbs are shown in the following Table 46.2 (Anon., 2006).

**Table 46.2: Export Figures of Other Important Medicinal and Aromatic Plants in Turkey**

| | *2004* | | *2005* | |
|---|---|---|---|---|
| *Crop* | *Amount (kg)* | *Value ($)* | *Amount (kg)* | *Value ($)* |
| Cumin | 6.570.066 | 8.461.800 | 7.201.872 | 10.717.522 |
| Fennel/Juniper | 1.738.224 | 1.962.303 | 1.366.678 | 1.576.000 |
| Mahlep | 121.870 | 1.545.388 | 112.696 | 1.406.607 |
| Linden | 175.981 | 781.669 | 253.310 | 1.221.140 |
| Rosemary | 453.207 | 855.916 | 505.424 | 972.079 |
| Sumac | 971.258 | 856.645 | 989.708 | 946.464 |
| Nigella | 68.471 | 113.962 | 45.145 | 88.827 |
| Coriander | 13.338 | 18.548 | 18.151 | 27.968 |
| Caraway | 5.100 | 7.408 | 8.500 | 13.102 |
| Spice mixtures | 139.024 | 642.355 | 107.351 | 547.831 |
| Other spices | 170.118 | 537.288 | 125.781 | 473.689 |
| Other med. plants | 879.944 | 1.788.983 | 1.264.766 | 3.054.789 |

**Table 46.3: Anatolian Vegetable Drugs used in the Hittite Empire (Baytop, 1994)**

| *Latin Name* | *Drug* | *Turkish Name* | *English Name* |
|---|---|---|---|
| *Abies cilicica* | Abietis resina | Köknar | Cilician fir |
| *Agropyron repens* | Graminis rhizoma | Ayrik | Couch grass |
| *Allium cepa* | Allii cepae bulbus | Sogan | Onion |
| *Allium sativum* | Allii sativi bulbus | Sarimsak | Garlic |
| *Amygdalus communis* | Amygdali semen | Badem | Almond |
| *Anethum graveolens* | Anethi fructus | Dereotu | Dill |
| *Armeniaca vulgaris* | Armeniacae semen | Zerdali | Wild apricot |
| *Buxus sempervirens* | Buxi folia | Simsir | Box |
| *Cannabis sativa* | Cannabis herba and fructus | Kenevir | Hemp |
| *Carum carvi* | Carvi fructus | Keraviye | Caraway |
| *Cedrus libani* | Cedri pix | Sedir | Cedar |
| *Coriandrum sativum* | Coriandri fructus | Kisnis | Coriander |
| *Cornus mas* | Corni fructus | Kizilcik | Cornelian cherry |
| *Crocus sativus* | Croci stigmata | Safran | Saffron |
| *Cuminum cyminum* | Cumini fructus | Kimyon | Cumin |
| *Cupressus sempervirens* | Cupressi fructus | Selvi | Cypress |
| *Echinophora tenuifolia* | Echinophorae herba | Cörtük | Echinophora |
| *Foeniculum vulgare* | Foeniculi fructus | Rezene | Fennel |
| *Glycyrrhiza glabra* | Liquiritiae radix | Meyan | Liquorice |
| *Gypsophila* sp. | Gypsophilae radix | Cöven | Soapwort |
| *Hyoscyamus niger* | Hyoscyami folia | Banotu | Henbane |
| *Juniperus oxycedrus* | Juniperi fructus | Ardic | Juniper |
| *Laurus nobilis* | Lauri fructus | Defne | |
| *Lupinus albus* | Lupini semen | Tirmis | |
| *Mandragora autumnalis* | Mandragorae radix | Adamotu | Mandrake |
| *Mentha* sp. | Menthae folium | Nane | |
| *Myrtus communis* | Myrti fructus and folia | Mersin | |
| *Olea europea* | Olivae oleum | Zeytin | |
| *Papaver somniferum* | Papaveris semen and Opium | Hashas | Opium poppy |
| *Peganum harmala* | Pegani semen | Üzerlik | |
| *Plantago* sp. | Plantaginis folia | Sinirli ot | Plantago |
| *Punica granatum* | Granati fructus | Nar | |
| *Quercus infectoria* | Quercinae gallae | Mese mazisi | Oak gall |
| *Q.ithaburensis* | Querci semen | Mese palamutu | Valonea |
| *Rhamnus catharticus* | Rhamni cathartici fructus | Akdiken | Yellow berry |
| *Ruta graveolens* | Rutae herba | Sedefotu | Rue |

*Contd...*

**Table 46.3–Contd...**

| Latin Name | Drug | Turkish Name | English Name |
|---|---|---|---|
| *Salix* sp. | Salicis cortex | Sögüt | |
| *Sesamum indicum* | Sesami oleum | Susam | |
| *Solanum nigrum* | Solani nigri herba | Ýt üzümü | Hound's berry |
| *Tamarix* sp. | Tamaricis folia | Ilgin | |
| *Thymus* sp. | Thymi herba | Kekik | |
| *Veratrum album* | Veratri albi rhizoma | Aksirik out | White hellebore |
| *Zizyphus jujuba* | Jujubae fructus | Hünnap | Jujube |

**Table 46.4: Native Plants Used as Ingredients of Proprietary Medicines in Turkey**

| | |
|---|---|
| Aniseed* (fruit, essential oil) | *Pimpinella anisum* |
| Bay laurel (essential oil) | *Laurus nobilis* |
| Belladonna (leaf, tincture, extract, syrup, alkaloids, atropine) | *Atropa belladonna* |
| Bitter almond* (fixed oil, essential oil) | *Prunus amygdalus* |
| Bitter orange* (flower) | *Citrus aurantium* |
| Black cummin* (seed) | *Nigella sativa* |
| Blackberry (fluidextract) | *Rubus fruticosus* |
| Blueberry (fruit) | *Vaccinium myrtillus* |
| Calendula (flower) | *Calendula officinalis* |
| Calluna (flower) | *Calluna vulgaris* |
| Capsicum* (oleoresin, tincture) | *Capsicum frutescens* |
| Castor oil* | *Ricinus communis* |
| Chamomile (flower, extract, essential oil) | *Matricaria chamomilla* |
| Citrus* (peel, hesperidin) | *Citrus* fruits |
| Colchicum (colchicine) | *Colchicum speciosum* |
| Coltsfoot (leaf) | *Tussilago farfara* |
| Coriander* (fruit) | *Coriandrum sativum* |
| Cummin* (fruit) | *Cuminum cyminum* |
| Datura (Hyoscine) | *Datura stramonium, D. metel* |
| Digitalis lanata (digoxin) | *Digitalis lanata* |
| Everlasting flower (flower) | *Helichrysum plicatum* |
| Fennel* (fruit, extract) | *Foeniculum vulgare* |
| Filipendula (flower) | *Spiraea ulmaria (= Filipendula ulmaria)* |
| Garlic* (allicin, extract) | *Allium sativum* |
| Greek oregano (herba) | *Origanum vulgare* subsp.*hirtum* |
| Hawthorn (leaf, flower, fruit) | *Crataegus monogyna, C. oxyacantha* |

*Contd...*

**Table 46.4–Contd...**

| | |
|---|---|
| Hops* (strobils) | *Humulus lupulus* |
| Horsechestnut (escin) | *Aesculus hippocastanum* |
| Juniper (fruit) | *Juniperus communis* |
| Juniper (tar) | *Juniperus oxycedrus* |
| Lavandin* (flower, essential oil) | *Lavandula angustifolia x latifolia* |
| Lavender* (flower, essential oil) | *Lavandula angustifolia* |
| Lemon* (essential oil) | *Citrus limon* |
| Liquorice (root extract) | *Glycyrrhiza glabra* |
| Mallow (leaf) | *Malva sylvestris* |
| Marshmallow (leaf, extract) | *Althaea officinalis* |
| Mistletoe (leaf, extract) | *Viscum album* |
| Olive* (fixed oil) | *Olea europea* |
| Opium poppy* (morphine, papaverine, codeine) | *Papaver somniferum* |
| Orange* (peel tincture ve essential oil) | *Citrus sinensis* |
| Origanum* (herb, essential oil) | *Origanum onites, O.majorana, O. minutiflorum, O.syriacum var. bevanii* |
| Paprika* (oleoresin) | *Capsicum annuum* |
| Pennyroyal (herb) | *Mentha pulegium* |
| Peppermint*(leaf, extract, essential oil) | *Mentha piperita* |
| Pine* (turpentine, essential oil) | *Pinus brutia, P. sylvestris* |
| Poppy (flower) | *Papaver rhoeas* |
| Psyllium (seed, husk) | *Plantago psyllium* |
| Rose* (distillate, essential oil) | *Rosa damascena* |
| Sage (leaf, extract, essential oil) | *Salvia fruticosa* |
| Scolymus (fluidextract) | *Scolymus hispanicus* |
| Soybean* (fixed oil) | *Soja hispida* |
| Spearmint* (leaf) | *Mentha spicata* |
| Sweet balm (leaf, tincture, essential oil) | *Melissa officinalis* |
| Tea* (theobromine, caffeine) | *Thea sinensis* |
| Tobacco* (nicotine) | *Nicotiana tabacum* |
| Verbascum (flower, extract) | *Verbascum thapsiforme* |
| Wheat* (extract) | *Triticum sativum* |
| Yew (taxol) | *Taxus baccata* |

*: Cultivated.

## References

Akman, Y. and Ketenoglu, O., 1986. The Climate and Vegetation of Turkey, In: Proceedings of the Royal Society of Edinburgh, Ed.: I.C. Hedge, University Press, Edinburgh; pp. 123.

Anon., 2006. State Statistics Office, Ankara, Turkey.

Aydin, S., Baser, K.H.C., Öztürk, Y., 1997. The Chemistry and Pharmacology of Origanum (Kekik) Water, In Essential Oils: Basic and Applied Research, Eds. Ch.Franz, A. Mathe and G. Buchbauer, Proceeding of the 27th International Symposium on Essential Oils, 8-11 September 1996, Vienna, Austria, Allured (USA); pp. 52-60 (1997).

Baser, K.H.C., 1992. Turkish rose oil, Perfumer and Flavorist (17); pp. 45-52.

Baser, K.H.C., 1995. Essential Oils from Aromatic Plants which are Used as Herbal Tea in Turkey, In Flavours, Fragrances and Essential Oils, Ed.: K.H.C. Baser, Proceedings of the 13th International Congress of Flavours, Fragrances and Essential Oils, Istanbul, Turkey, 15-19 October 1995, AREP Publ., Istanbul, Turkey (2); pp. 67-79.

Baser, K.H.C., 1997. The Use of Medicinal and Aromatic Plants in Pharmaceutical and Alcoholic Beverage Industries, Istanbul Chamber of Commerce Publication No 1997-39, Istanbul.

Baser, K.H.C., 2002.1. Aromatic biodiversity among the flowering plant taxa of Turkey, Pure Appl. Chem. 74(4); pp. 527-545.

Baser, K.H.C., 2002.2. The Turkish Origanum Species, In: Oregano, The Genera Origanum and Lippia, Ed.: S.E. Kintzios, Taylor and Francis, UK; pp. 109-126.

Baser, K.H.C., Kürkcüoglu, M., Özek, T., 2003. Turkish rose oil research: Recent results, Perfumer and Flavorist (28); pp. 34-42.

Baser, K.H.C., Özek, T., Tümen, G., Sezik, E.,1993. Composition of the essential oils of Turkish *Origanum* species with commercial importance, J. Essent. Oil Res., 5 (6); pp. 619-623.

Baser, K.H.C., Tabanca, N., Kirimer, N., Bedir, E, Khan, I.A., Wedge, D.E., 2007. Recent advances in the chemistry and biological activities of the *Pimpinella* species of Turkey, Pure Appl. Chem. 79(4); pp. 539-556.

Baytop, T., 1990. Rose oil and oil rose cultivation in Anatolia during the Ottoman era, TAB Bulletin (4); pp. 8-10.

Baytop, T., 1994. A historical overview of the use of medicinal and aromatic plants in Turkey, TAB Bulletin (10); pp. 24-27.

Davis, P.H., 1965-1985. Flora of Turkey and the East Aegean Islands, Vols. 1–9, University Press, Edinburgh

Davis, P.H., Mill, R.R. and Tan, K., 1988. Flora of Turkey and the East Aegean Islands(Supplement),Vol. 10, University Press, Edinburgh

European Pharmacopoeia,2007. 6th Edition, EDQM, Strasbourg.

Güner, A., Özhatay, N., Ekim, T. and Baser, K.H.C., 2000. Flora of Turkey and the East Aegean Islands (Supplement 2), Vol. 11, University Press, Edinburgh.

Kreutz, C.A.J., 1988. Die Orchideen der Türkei, Kreutz Publishers, Landgraaf, Netherlands.

Mansfield, D., 2001. An Analysis of Licit Opium Poppy Cultivation: India and Turkey, FCO, UK

Tanriverdi, H., Özek, T., Beis, S.H., Baser, K.H.C.,1992. Composition of Essential Oils of Turkish Laurel Leaves and Berries, Essays for Science: Felicitation Volume on the 50th Birthday of Prof. Atta-ur-Rahman, 67-74, Hamdard Foundation-Pakistan, MAS Printers, Karachi, Pakistan.

## Chapter 47

# Socio-economic Development and Traditional Medicinal Knowledge Protection in Relwa, Dediapada and Nani Singloti Villages

**Lancelot D'Cruz**
*Department of Biology, St. Xavier's College,*
*Ahmedabad – 380 009, Gujarat, India*
*E-mail: lancy_dcruz@hotmail.com*

## ABSTRACT

This creative venture is the first phase of a project that seeks the agro-productive development of medicinal plants in *Nani Singloti*, *Relwa* and *Dediapada* areas of South Gujarat where the beneficiaries are the *Vasava* tribals. For this purpose, the native plants from Dediapada and their traditional uses as also the demand in the Indian market are being studied. This will enable the groups participating in the project to have enough information to select the plants they want to cultivate. To facilitate round the year cultivation an irrigation system has to be put in place depending on the specific geographical features of the area for which a study of the best system is being undertaken. A bio-prospecting study is also being conducted in the forests of Dediapada to assess the current situation of the native medicinal plants. The project is a collaborative venture involving the coming together of the educational, research, pharmaceutical, and the NGO sectors, the overall objective being the promotion of the socio-economic development and protection of the traditional knowledge of medicinal plants of the Vasava tribes in the Dediapada forests while spreading its uses among the local population. These would be achieved through various capacity building workshops on entrepreneurship, administrative functioning, participatory decision-making, gender equality, health promotion, etc. The genesis of the current project lies in the successful completion of a 3-year project carried out for the Gujarat Ecology Commission entitled *"People-forest-laboratory linkages for conservation of ethno-medicinal biodiversity"*. This involved the setting up of an interactive network of medicine men (traditional healer), the preparation in CD-format of the 100 most significant *Vasavi* medicinal plants, the setting up of five medicinal plant forests in the vicinity of five tribal schools and the use of these for environmental education there, the use of plant tissue culture for conservation of threatened ethno medicinal plant species and ex situ conservation at the College Campus in Ahmedabad.

***Keywords:*** *Ethnomedicine, Biodiversity conservation, Entrepreneurship.*

## 1.0 Introduction

The *Bhil Vasava* tribals inhabiting the *Shoolpaneshwar* sanctuary area in the *Dediapada* region of *South Gujarat* have a rich tradition of indigenous medicine. The Vasavas form a prominent part of the 14.92 per cent tribal population of Gujarat State. They comprise the principal inhabitants of a belt of prime forest cover, the Dediapada forests in South Gujarat, where an estimated one-hectare of forest area is reported to house 1,200 forest species. The significance of this belt of 59,312 hectares of sprawling forest covers stems from the fact that they are the last remnants of a dwindling bio-heritage. The area has assumed greater significance in recent times as it forms the major portion of the *Sardar Sarovar* submergence area.

Dediapada Taluka (subdivision) is situated in the South Eastern tribal belt of the State of Gujarat in India. It is about 70 kms. East of the nearest city and railway station–Ankleshwar–on the Western Railway main line connecting Mumbai with Ahmedabad. The Taluka covers 1027 sq. kms. and has 97,431 inhabitants.

Significantly, Dediapada is a backward tribal taluka–economically, educationally, socially, and politically. According to the 1981 census the total population of Scheduled Tribes amounts to 95 per cent. The low literacy rates among the tribals–14.12 per cent (Gujarat 35.79 per cent) in 1971, 21.14 per cent (Gujarat 43.70 per cent) in 1981, and 36.45 per cent (Gujarat 61.29 per cent) in 1991 is another significant factor which necessitates the documenting of their ethno-medicinal wisdom, since it essentially resides with the elderly practitioners who pass it on by means of oral tradition.

St Xavier's College, through its research arm–Xavier Research Foundation has a long relationship of working together with the *adivasis* of the Dediapada forests through the *Adivasi Samajik Kendra*, Dediapada. They are currently working with three self-help groups created two years ago as an outcome of the project *"People-forest-laboratory linkages for conservation of ethno-medicinal biodiversity"* financed by the Gujarat Ecology Commission and implemented by Xavier Research Foundation. The objective of that project was to strengthen the link between local tribes and forest resources (mostly medicinal plants) while using some of the best methods available in modern science. The project involved the setting up of an interactive network of medicine men, the preparation in CD-format of the 100 most significant Vasavi medicinal plants, the setting up of five medicinal plant forests in the vicinity of five tribal schools for environmental education and ethno-medicinal sensitization; and the use of plant tissue culture for conservation of three threatened ethno-medicinal plant species.

Subsequent to that project, 35 men were invited to participate in workshops aimed at promoting entrepreneurship and leadership. Women were specifically invited for these workshops conducted by an NGO (*MANTHAN*), which continues to collaborate with the group in the current project.

The group members belonging to the Vasava tribe of the Dediapada forest villages are illiterate and suffer abuses and discrimination. Besides cultivating rice and *'tuvar'* (Pulse) mainly for self-consumption, they also collect small quantities of medicinal plants from the forest for their own use. Some of these are sold to middlemen, as they do not have direct access to the larger companies. The groups meet once a month in Dediapada to talk about their problems, to put together the plants they have collected, pulverize the dried plants with mortars and plan their sale strategies.

As a result of several workshops conducted with these self-help groups, several specific problems have been identified. These include vulnerability because of illiteracy, ignorance of the functioning of the market, dependence on rain-fed irrigation, inability to market materials and exploitation by middlemen. Added to this is the psychological factor that they have low self-esteem and are afraid to take leadership.

The situation of the Dediapada forest has to be kept in mind: the rich biodiversity is suffering due to deforestation, and the extinction of native medicinal plants is fast taking place. This extinction means the loss of potential cures for various diseases, which will pose problems at the local and wider level.

## 2.0 Methods

A survey of the ethno-medicinal flora of the Dediapada forests was carried out using a novel methodology which involved the setting up of a unique, interactive, collaborative network of active tribal medicine men (drawn from almost twenty villages spanning the expanse of the Dediapada forests) wherein exchange of ethno-medicinal wisdom could be facilitated in an atmosphere of trust. Thirty-five interactive meetings and three workshops involving eminent botanists and an allopathic doctor of tribal origin helped to confirm, crosscheck, verify, and systematically document the ethno-medicinal flora of the Dediapada forests. The ethno-medicinal usage of significant plants selected on basis of their conservation status, the local name(s), the disease for which used, and the method of usage along with photographic evidence of each plant was presented.

Preliminary phytochemical screening of some ninety-nine ethno-medicinally significant plant species selected on the basis of their medicinal value and conservation status was carried out (D'Cruz, 2002).

Three plant species, significant for their medicinal value to the Vasava tribal but facing a serious threat on account of their restricted presence within the Dediapada forests *Argyreia boseana, Curculigo orchioides* and *Corallocarpus conocarpus,* were selected for clonal multiplication with the twin purpose of developing *in vitro* techniques for ensuring large quantities of plant material throughout the year, as also for restoring these valuable medicinal plants to their original habitat.

Five 'forests' or medicinal plant enclaves were set up around five schools (ranging from a pre-primary *Ashram Shala* at *Nani Singlotti* to a higher secondary school at *Zankhvav*). The group of medicinal men was actively involved in setting up and maintaining these 'forests' which were used for environmental education and ethno-medicinal sensitisation of tribal students through interactive workshops.

Subsequent to the Gujarat Ecology Commission project, thirty-five men were invited to participate in workshops aimed at promoting entrepreneurship and leadership. Women were specifically invited to be part of the group and they attended workshops conducted by MANTHAN (MPS, headed by Mr. Abhay Kothari) in collaboration with the Xavier Research Foundation. MEPS is a non-profit nongovernmental institution which conceives, develops, implements, and disseminates training programmes that focus on the development of entrepreneurial attitude. A panel of experts conducted sessions on Entrepreneurship, Risk-taking, Achievement motivation, Teamwork, and Leadership.

Enhancement of local capacities and promotion of self-management skills will be done through workshops on entrepreneurship and organization as also on gender equality. These will be conducted by the MEPS in collaboration with experts. Modules and work materials are being suitably modified so as to address the group members whose literacy levels are on the lower side.

Entrepreneurship modules will seek to enhance skills like generation of ideas for micro enterprise, assessing and finalizing business ideas, preparing of business plans, sourcing finance, promoting/publishing, costing/pricing the product, understanding cash flow, developing entrepreneurial competencies and client relationships, understanding and adopting possible technologies, planning for expansion and growth, enhancing achievement motivation, risk taking, and communication.

The workshops held to enhance gender equality will deal with the theory of gender, gender attributes, gender and technology, integrating gender concerns into development plans, appropriate technologies, programme implementation, monitoring issues and impact analysis.

The group is being trained by Jeevan Tirth (an NGO with expertise in water harvesting, headed by Raju-Dipti) to understand the basics of water harvesting and to apply these principles to enhance the output of their own lands. They will also participate in a study of the best irrigation systems possible, so as to ensure cultivation of the selected medicinal plants. The members will be involved in the construction of some of these systems as also in the laying down of rules for their maintenance and utilization.

The study carried out under the Ecology Commission project currently forms the basis for an in-depth Market Research Study and Business Feasibility Survey for the commercialization of herbal products from the environs of the Dediapada forests. This study is being carried out in two phases by Sky Quest Labs Private Limited (headed by Mr. Akash Bhavsar and dealing with collaborative research, business research, regenerative medicine and technology transfer) [Appendix 2].

The objectives of the first phase are:

1. To closely survey the 250 plants and reconfirm their availability and usages.
2. To evaluate the initial pre-production potential for these plants while determining the capacity constraint.
3. To identify 25 plants out of 250 based on the literature survey and secondary research keeping in mind availability, commercial and/or medicinal importance and novelty.
4. To understand the life cycle of the selected plants as also the cultural impact of this project on the local market.

This exploratory survey and descriptive market research is to be completed in 160 days [Appendix 3].

The second phase involving product sampling activity, a business feasibility study and the conclusive research, which is to be completed from days 160 to 190, has the following objectives:

1. To identify ten plants out of the twenty-five selected in Phase 1.
2. To evaluate the business and market potential of the ten identified plants and to shortlist five of these for mass cultivation; also to highlight five plants believed to have unexplored potential from a strategic intellectual property creation perspective.
3. To study the supply chain for the herbal selling.
4. To identify the level of value-addition required ensuring the sale of herbs.
5. To narrow down on the best cultivation practices required for industrial level supply of herbs.
6. To define the volume of business likely to be handled in two years and beyond.
7. To identify the regulatory and legal bottlenecks, if any.
8. To develop marketable products and identify price points.
9. To identify the applications areas of the plants to be marketed.
10. To define operational blueprint and evolve strategies for marketing.

Dr. M. R. Almeida of the Blatter Herbarium, St. Xavier's College, Mumbai, is carrying out the botanical study with a view to update the list of ethno-medicinally valuable plants of the Dediapada forests. The study will also help identify the biodiversity-rich forest enclaves and suggest means for conservation of the ethno-medicinal wealth of the Vasavas. The experts will facilitate collection of seeds and planting materials and train the groups to check the quality of herbs collected. They will review the findings of the market survey and be party to the selection of five plants for cultivation.

The groups have been involved in organizing workshops for school students and other local groups and in the setting up of the medicinal plant forests in the three schools at Dediapada, Relwa and Nani Singloti.

The local knowledge to prevent illness will be strengthened by organizing workshops on disease prevention and health promotion addressed to the groups participating in the project.

## 3.0 Results and Discussion

Detailed studies of the ethno-medicinal wisdom of the Vasava tribals has led to the documentation of over 250 plant species of ethno-medicinal significance belonging to over 75 families (D'Cruz, 2002). Over 50 of these are not recorded in the Eco-Environmental Studies of Sardar Sarovar Environs, 1992 [Appendix 1A]. A number of these species are actually facing threats of different magnitudes [Appendix 1B]. Over 30 plant species presently growing in Dediapada forests actually figure in the Threatened List of Biodiversity of Gujarat, 2001 [Appendix 1C]. A number of these are of ethno-medicinal significance to the Vasava tribals (D'Cruz, 2002).

From a botanical perspective, additions were made to the current knowledge of the flora of Gujarat by the addition of nine species of plants to the Flora of Gujarat State by G.L.Shah [Appendix 1D]. Also seven species of Angiosperms as also three species of Pteridophytes were additions to the comprehensive list of Plants of Gujarat (Biological Diversity of Gujarat, GEC, 1996) [Appendix 1E].

More than ten species of plants described in the doctoral thesis were included in the "Medicinal Plants of Gujarat" published by the GEER (Pandey, 2005).

Preliminary phytochemical screening of the 99 selected ethno-medicinally significant plant species was carried out. The presence or absence of secondary metabolites and the distribution of these active principles in the 46 selected plant families/sub-families covered in the study was illustrated (D'Cruz, 2002).

Encouraging results were obtained from experiments to tissue culture of the three selected plant species, significant for their medicinal value and their conservation status. Multiple axillary shooting and root formation was obtained in Argyreia boseana (Vaidya, 2005) and plantlet regeneration was achieved in Corallocarpus conocarpus (D'Cruz, 2002). Entire plantlets could be regenerated directly from the leaf explants of Curculigo orchioides (Vaidya, 2005; Vaidya, 2004). The hardening procedures are being standardized at the Xavier Research Foundation (D'Souza, 2006).

The five 'forests' set up with the active involvement of the medicine men and the tribal children in the local schools were used for conducting a number of interactive workshops for environmental education and ethno-medicinal sensitisation involving the medicine men and the young tribal students. Groups from Zankhvav, Tanakhala, and Narukot and from Nandurbar (in the neighbouring State of Maharashtra) also visited these enclaves and participated in interactive training workshops.

As a result of the training workshops on entrepreneurship held subsequent to the GEC project, women who were specifically invited for the workshops decided to join the group. Three self-help groups (SHGs) were created and registered through the initiative of the group members. One of the groups is composed entirely of women. The three groups keep their own monthly savings. They have currently begun a process of internal borrowing and lending which has enhanced their credibility. The groups decided on a name *"Aaadi Aushadi"* (meaning 'Original Medicine') and a product logo. They have begun to devise small strategies for the local sale of medicinal products. The groups evaluate these strategies from time to time.

Enhancement of local capacities is aimed at promoting self-management skills, along with participatory functioning and an ability to analyse the situation. This will be achieved through the workshops on entrepreneurship and organization, as also on gender equality.

The people from the villages will have the possibility of having more than one crop per year. This will be achieved through the study of the best option of irrigation systems, followed by the construction of some of these systems. The people will be involved in the designing, construction and maintenance of these systems.

The botanical study, the market study, the feasibility of cultivation study and the selection of plants for cultivation through a participatory methodology will empower the groups by providing them with the knowledge of which native plants are commercially and environmentally feasible for initiating their cultivation in the coming monsoon.

Interactive workshops involving tribal medical practitioners and St. Xavier's College students were held at the Xavier Research Foundation, St. Xavier's College in January 2001 and in January 2003. This was appreciated by the NAAC as a "healthy practice" in the Best practice series–3 (NAAC, 2006). Workshops have been held in five tribal schools under the earlier project. These have helped sensitize students to the value of their traditional ethno medicinal wisdom and resulted in increased student participation in the maintenance of these forests. The community linkages in the area and the traditional medicine systems will be strengthened through organizing of workshops for school students and other local groups and through the setting up of the medicinal plant forests in the three schools at Dediapada, Relwa and Nani Singloti.

The groups will benefit by strengthening their local knowledge to prevent illness through the workshops on disease prevention and health promotion that they will attend.

## 4.0 Conclusions

The project is a collaborative venture involving the coming together of the educational (the Staff of the undergraduate St. Xavier's College), research (the Xavier Research Foundation, the Blatter Herbarium), pharmaceutical (Sky Quest Labs Private Limited) and the NGO sectors (Jeevan Tirth and MEPS). The overall objective is the promotion of the socio-economic development and protection of the traditional knowledge of medicinal plants of the Vasava tribes in the Dediapada forests, while spreading its uses among the local population. The venture has been appreciated for its educational and social outreach dimensions (NAAC, 2006).

The direct beneficiaries will be the members of the three self-help groups. Each group has ten registered members, with family size ranging from four to nine. The direct beneficiaries would thus be about 156 people. The indirect beneficiaries will be the entire population of those villages, since the positive effects of the market study and forest study, and the health and traditional uses promotion will be spread around the area, as more people participate in the activity. It is intended that this project serves as a pilot project which could be replicated across tribal south Gujarat, linking together the already existing micro networks of 'Mahila Mandals' (Women's Groups) and other self-help groups to create a macro network which seeks to enhance income generation through usage of their traditional wisdom and bio resources.

The overall project of medicinal plants cultivation is feasible because India consumes and exports large quantities of medicinal plants, which are used by the pharmaceutical sector (western medicine and ayurvedic medicine), by the cosmetic and nutraceuticals sector, as well as in the local markets.

The project (in this the first phase) includes a market and feasibility study, a forest biodiversity study, deciding on the choice of medicinal plants to be cultivated and training for cultivation, training in administration and organization functioning, gender equity, health promotion, etc. The group should be able to decide the kind of organization they wish to set up (cooperative, etc.). In order to provide value addition and protection of their knowledge, the selected plant's properties and active principles will be investigated and patented in the name of the adivasi community (in the next phase).

The entire endeavour will contribute to the preservation of the biodiversity of the Dediapada forest, providing the people an income generating activity (as opposed to the collection of medicinal plants from the wild), while stressing the awareness of the environment protection among the school students and other local adivasi groups.

## Acknowledgements

The author is grateful to Dr. Vincent Braganza and the Xavier Research Foundation, the Gujarat Ecology Commission, ALBOAN, IDOKI and to the collaborating partners in the current project: Mr. Abhay Kothari of MANTHAN (MEPS), Raju-Dipti of JEEVAN TIRTH, Mr. Akash Bhavsar and team of Sky Quest Labs Private Limited and to Dr. M R Almeida and team. A special thanks to the Principal and Staff of St. Xavier's College, Ahmedabad, especially to Fr. Vincent Saldanha, Mr. Saby Vadaken and Ms. Amita Nair for help in preparing this paper. I am deeply indebted to the Adivasi Samajik Kendra, Dediapada and the Adivasi collaborators at Dediapada without whom this venture would not have been possible.

## References

Census of India, 1981. Govt. of India, Directorate of Census Operations, Govt. of India.

Census of India, 1991. Govt. of India, Directorate of Census Operations, Govt. of India.

D' Cruz, L. 2002. Phytochemical and Biochemical studies of some Ethno-medicinal plants of Dediapada forests. Thesis submitted to Gujarat University, Ahmedabad.

D'souza, K., Christian, G., D'cruz, L. and Braganza, V., 2006. In vitro conservation of some ethno medicinal plant species of the Dediapada Forests of South Gujarat.

Manuscript accepted by the Journal of Medicinal and Aromatic Plants. Publication awaited.

Pandey, C.N., Raval, B.R., Mali, Seema, and Salvi, H., 2005. Medicinal Plants of Gujarat. GEER Foundation, Gandhinagar.

Shah, G. L. 1978. Flora of Gujarat State (Part I and II). Sardar Patel University Publication, Vallabh Vidyanagar.

Sabnis and Amin, 1992. Eco-Environmental Studies of Sardar Sarovar Environs. Report of Eco-Environment and Wildlife Management Studies Project, M.S. University of Baroda Press.

Threatened Biodiversity of Gujarat: Baseline Information, 2001. Gujarat Ecological Society, Maharaja Sayajirao University of Baroda, Gujarat Institute of Desert Ecology.

"Using infrastructure and learning resources for social transformation", in Community Engagement: Case presentation. Best practice series–3, NAAC, Bangalore: 2006: pp 30-31.

Vaidya, G., K., D'Cruz, L., Saxena, O., P., Braganza, VJ., 2004. Effect of various sucrose concentrations on plantlet regeneration of Curculigo orchioides Gaertn. Biotechnology for a Better future. Eds. D'souza, L., Anuradha, M., Shashikiran, N., Hegde, S and Rajendra K., SAC Publications, Mangalore: pp.133-137.

Vaidya, G.K., D'Cruz, L., Saxena, O.P., Braganza, VJ., 2005. Initial work for conservation of Argyreia boseana Santapau and Patel by Micro propagation. In: Journal of Current Bioscience (2(2)): 426-430.

Vaidya, G.K., D'Cruz, L., Saxena, O.P., Braganza, V.J., 2005. Effect of Various factors on plantlet regeneration of Curculigo orchioides Gaertn. Plant Cell Biotechnology and Molecular Biology (6 (1 and 2)): pp. 29-34.

## Appendix 1A
## Additions to the List of Plants Recorded in the "Eco-Environmental Studies of Sardar Sarovar Environs" (Sabnis and Amin, 1992)

| Sl.No. | Scientific Name | Vasavi Name | Family/Sub-Family |
|---|---|---|---|
| 1. | *Acampe praemorsa* (Roxb.) Blatt. and McC. | *Vando* | Orchidaceae |
| 2. | *Adansonia digitata* L. | *Vihar amblo* | Bombaceae |
| 3. | *Amorphophallus commutatus* (Roxb.) Bl. ex Decne | *Pebdo, Hevdo* | Araceae |
| 4. | *Aristolochia indica* L. | *Iihavar* | Aristolochiaceae |
| 5. | *Argyreia boseana* Santapau and Patel | *Kumbrao, Amarua* | Convolvulaceae |
| 6. | *Barleria prattensis* L. | *Nanu tundru, Rat muliyu* | Acanthaceae |
| 7. | *Benkara pundulacakai* (Gmelin) Almeida | *Gungari* | Rubiaceae |
| 8. | *Casearia esculenta* Roxb. | *Mano manjo* | Flacourtiaceae |
| 9. | *Ceropegia bulbosa* Roxb. | *Sap okoni* | Asclepiadaceae |
| 10. | *Ceropegia fantastica* Sedgev. | *Mor/Chir okoni* | Asclepiadaceae |
| 11. | *Clematis naravelioides* O. Kuntz. | *Kokarvel* | Ranunculaceae |
| 12. | *Commelina paleata* Hassk. | *Keniyo* | Commelinaceae |
| 13. | *Corallocarpus conocarpus* (Dalz.and Gibs) Hook. | *Mirchi kuvo* | Cucurbitaceae |
| 14. | *Corchorus capsularis* L. | *Kadvi jhiri* | Tiliaceae |
| 15. | *Cordia dichotoma* Forst. | *Gundo* | Ehretiaceae |
| 16. | *Crinum latifolium* L. | *Ukkad kando* | Amaryllidaceae |
| 17. | *Cucumis callosus* (Rottl.) Cogn. | *Sap kachari* | Cucurbitaceae |
| 18. | *Curcuma amada* Roxb. | *Devadu* | Zingiberaceae |
| 19. | *Cyperus eleusinoides* Kunth. | *Gundalu* | Cyperaceae |
| 20. | *Dalbergia lanceolaria* L. | *Tobdikand* | Papilionaceae |
| 21. | *Dioscorea wallichii* Hk. | *Chayru* | Dioscoreaceae |
| 22. | *Ehretia laevis* Roxb. | *Madh movado* | Ehretiaceae |
| 23. | *Embelia basaal* (R. and S.) DC. | *Amtu* | Myrsinaceae |
| 24. | *Eriolaena stocksii* Hook and Thoms. | *Pendvo* | Sterculiaceae |
| 25. | *Erythrina stricta* Roxb. | *Sapilo* | Papilionaceae |
| 26. | *Erythrina suberosa* Roxb. | *Pangaru* | Papilionaceae |
| 27. | *Eulophia herbacea* Lindl. | *Waghmodhu, Madmodhu* | Orchidaceae |
| 28. | *Heracleum grandis* (Cl.) Mukh | *Bokhalo* | Umbelliferae |
| 29. | *Hibiscus hirtus* L. | *Majaniyu* | Malvaceae |
| 30. | *Holostemma rheedei* Wall | *Nani chiri* | Asclepiadaceae |
| 31. | *Lobelia* sp. | *Honuro* | Lobeliaceae |

*Contd...*

**Appendix 1A–Contd...**

| *Sl.No.* | *Scientific Name* | *Vasavi Name* | *Family/Sub-Family* |
|---|---|---|---|
| 32. | *Lygodium microphyllum* (Cav.) R.Br. | *Mor pangiyo* | Schizaceae |
| 33. | *Manisuris clarkei* (Hack.) Bor | *Suthado* | Poaceae |
| 34. | *Marsdenia tenacissima* (Roxb.) Moon. | *Mani Shiri* | Asclepiadaceae |
| 35. | *Nelsonia campestris* (Lam.) Nees. | *Safed chatro* | Acanthaceae |
| 36. | *Nervilia discolor* (Bl.) Schltr. | *Kan khovchiyu* | Orchidaceae |
| 37. | *Pancratium* sp. | *Panjidu* | Amaryllidaceae |
| 38. | *Remusatia vivipara* (Roxb.) Scholt | *Aahuliyo* | Araceae |
| 39. | *Sida orientalis* Cav. | *Movdo bokhiyu* | Malvaceae |
| 40. | *Solena amplexicaulis* (Lamk.) Gandhi | *Togoni, Gumbaliyo* | Cucurbitaceae |
| 41. | *Spigelia anthelmia* L. | – | Loganiaceae |
| 42. | *Spondias acuminata* Roxb. | *Khat aabni* | Anacardiaceae |
| 43. | *Sterculia colorata* Roxb. | – | Sterculiaceae |
| 44. | *Sterculia villosus* Roxb. | *Khodalo* | Sterculiaceae |
| 45. | *Tamilnadia uliginosa* (Retz.) Tirunveng. and Sastre | *Gogadu* | Rubiaceae |
| 46. | *Terminalia paniculata* Roth. | *Hejdo* | Combretaceae |
| 47. | *Trewia nudiflora* L. | *Variya* | Euphorbiaceae |
| 48. | *Trichodesma zeylanicum* Roxb. | *Chachiro* | Boraginaceae |
| 49. | *Trichosanthes tricuspidata* Lour. | *Galundu* | Cucurbitaceae |
| 50. | *Tylophora fasciculata* Ham. ex Wight | *Zher dudhi* | Asclepiadaceae |
| 51. | *Tylophora rotundifolia* Ham. ex Wight | *Paudi phatiyu* | Asclepiadaceae |
| 52. | *Vigna calcaratus* (Roxb.) Kurz | *Gando himdo* | Papilionaceae |
| 53. | *Vigna capensis* Walp. | *Mitho himdo* | Papilionaceae |

## Appendix 1 B

**Plants not reported in the Eco-Environmental Studies of Sardar Sarovar Environs (Sabnis and Amin, 1992) but found present in the Study area and also listed as threatened plants in the list of Threatened Biodiversity of Gujarat: Baseline Information (GEC, 2001).**

| *Sl.No.* | *Scientific Name* | *Vasavi Name* | *Family/Sub-Family* |
|---|---|---|---|
| 1. | *Casearia esculenta Roxb.* | Mano manjo | *Flacourtiaceae* |
| 2. | *Corallocarpus conocarpus* (Dalz. and Gibs) Hook. | Mirchi kuvo | *Cucurbitaceae* |
| 3. | *Dioscorea wallichii* Hk. | *Chayru* | Dioscoreaceae |
| 4. | *Eulophia herbacea* Lindl. | *Waghmodhu, Madmodhu* | Orchidaceae |
| 5. | *Heracleum grandis* (Cl.) Mukh. | *Bokhalo* | Umbelliferae |
| 6. | *Nelsonnia campestris* (Lam.)Nees. | *Safed chatro* | Acanthaceae |
| 7. | *Nervilia discolor* (Bl.) Schltr. | *Kan khovchiyu* | Orchidaceae |
| 8. | *Sterculia villosus* Roxb. | *Khodalo* | Sterculiaceae |
| 9. | *Tylophora fasciculata* Ham. ex Wight | *Zher dudhi* | Asclepiadaceae |

## Appendix 1 C

### List of plants presently found in the Dediapada Forests, which actually figure in the Threatened Biodiversity of Gujarat: Baseline Information (GEC, 2001).

| Sl.No. | Scientific Name | Vasavi Name | Family/Sub-Family |
|---|---|---|---|
| 1. | *Antidesma ghaesembilla* Gaertn. | *Jhad madro, Moto madro* | Euphorbiaceae |
| 2. | *Bauhinia vahlii* Graham | *Aaval Vel* | Caesalpineaceae |
| 3. | *Careya arborea* Roxb. | *Gul Mahudo, Kumbhiyo* | Lecythidacae |
| 4. | Casearia esculenta Roxb. | *Mano manjo* | Flacourtiaceae |
| 5. | Chlorophytum borivilianum Sant. and Fernand. | *Dholi musli, Kuvli* | Liliaceae |
| 6. | *Chlorophytum tuberosum* (Roxb.) Baker. | *Kuvlo* | Liliaceae |
| 7. | *Corallocarpus conocarpus* (Dalz. and Gibs) Hook | *Mirchi Kuvo* | Cucurbitaceae |
| 8. | *Costus speciosus* (Koenig ex Retz.) Sm. | *Pevu* | Zingiberaceae |
| 9. | *Dalbergia volubilis* Roxb. | *Jhino kovado, Goval vitiyo* | Papilionaceae |
| 10. | *Derris scandens* (Roxb.) Benth. | *Kelvo* | Papilionaceae |
| 11. | *Dillenia pentagyna* Roxb. | *Kovlo* | Dillenaceae |
| 12. | *Desmodium heterocarpon* (L.) DC. | *Vandha chipiyo* | Papilionaceae |
| 13. | *Dioscorea wallichii* Hk. | *Chayru* | Dioscoreaceae |
| 14. | *Ensete superbum* (Roxb.) Cheesman | *Jangli Kel* | Musaceae |
| 15. | *Eulophia herbacea* Lindl. | *Waghmodhu, Madmodhu* | Orchidaceae |
| 16. | *Flemingia strobilifera* (L.) R. Br. | *Manitur, Madaro, Femtal madru* | Papilionaceae |
| 17. | *Gloriosa superba* L. | *Nargaiyo* | Liliaceae |
| 18. | *Heterophragma quadrilocularis* (Roxb.) K. Schum. | *Motu jhad* | Bignoniaceae |
| 19. | *Loranthus longiflorus* Desr. | *Vando* | Loranthaceae |
| 20. | *Melia composita* Willd. | *Limbaro* | Meliaceae |
| 21. | *Nelsonia campestris* (Lam.) Nees. | *Safed chatro* | Acanthaceae |
| 22. | *Nervilia discolor* (Bl.) Schltr. | *Kan khovchiyu* | Orchidaceae |
| 23. | *Peristylus plantagineus* Lindl. | | Orchidaceae |
| 24. | *Peucedanum grande* Cl. | *Bokhalo* | Umbelliferae |
| 25. | *Radermachera xylocarpa* (Roxb.) K. Schum | *Ardashishi, Goval vitiyo* | Bignoniaceae |
| 26. | *Spatholobus parviflorus* (Roxb.) O. Ktze. | *Palovein* | Papilionaceae |
| 27. | *Sterculia urens* Roxb. | *Kadayo, Kanav* | Sterculiaceae |
| 28. | *Tecomella undullata* (Sw.) Seem | *Ragat rohido* | Bignoniaceae |
| 29. | *Terminalia chebula* Retz. | *Mani Manji* | Combretaceae |
| 30. | *Tylophora fasciculata* Ham. ex Wight | *Zher dudhi* | Asclepiadaceae |
| 31. | *Uraria rufescens* (DC.) Schindl. | *Vandar chipiyo* | Papilionaceae |
| 32. | *Vanda tessellata* (Roxb.) Hk. f. ex G. Don | *Vando* | Orchidaceae |

## Appendix 1 D
## Additions made by the present study to the Flora of Gujarat State (Part I and Part II) by G.L. Shah (1978)

| *Sl.No.* | *Scientific Name* | *Vasavi Name* | *Family/Sub-Family* |
|---|---|---|---|
| 1. | *Argyreia boseana* Santapau and Patel | *Kumbrao, Amarua* | Convolvulaceae |
| 2. | *Acampe praemorsa* (Roxb.) Blatt. and McC. | *Vando* | Orchidaceae |
| 3. | *Commelina paleata* Hassk. | *Keniyo* | Commelinaceae |
| 4. | *Corallocarpus conocarpus* (Dalz. and Gibs) Hook. | *Mirchi kuvo* | Cucurbitaceae |
| 5. | *Erythrina stricta* Roxb. | *Sapilo* | Papilionaceae |
| 6. | *Eulophia herbacea* Lindl. | *Waghmodhu, Madmodhu* | Orchidaceae |
| 7. | *Spondias acuminata* Roxb. | *Khat aabni* | Anacardiaceae |
| 8. | *Sterculia colorata* Roxb. | - | Sterculiaceae |
| 9. | *Terminalia paniculata Roth.* | Hejdo | Combretaceae |

## Appendix 1 E
## Additions made by the present study to the "Biological Diversity of Gujarat: Current knowledge" prepared by the Gujarat Ecology Commission, 1996

| *Sl.No.* | *Scientific Name* | *Vasavi Name* | *Family/Sub-Family* |
|---|---|---|---|
| 1. | *Argyreia boseana* Santapau and Patel | *Kumbrao, Amarua* | Convolvulaceae |
| 2. | *Erythrina stricta* Roxb. | *Sapilo* | Papilionaceae |
| 3. | *Nervilia disolor (Bl.) Schltr.* | *Kan khovchiyu* | Orchidaceae |
| 4. | *Spigelia anthelmia* L. | - | Loganiaceae |
| 5. | *Spondias acuminata* Roxb. | *Khat aabni* | Anacardiaceae |
| 6. | *Sterculia colorata* Roxb. | - | Sterculiaceae |
| 7. | *Terminalia paniculata* Roth. | *Hejdo* | Combretaceae |

## Appendix 2
## APPROACH

**The ABIRAW (Advanced Bio-business Intelligence, Research and Analysis Wing) team of Sky Quest Labs Private Limited will collect, collate, co-relate and analyze the data collected by means of primary exploratory and descriptive research and coordinated sampling activity, backed by the robust secondary desk research**

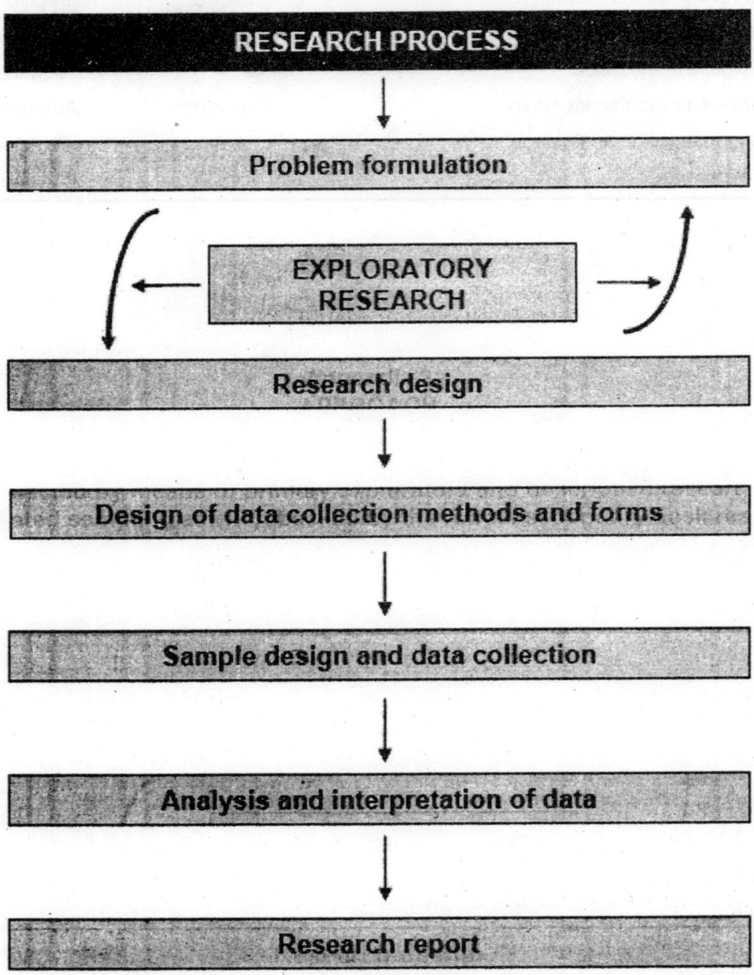

# Appendix 3
## RESEARCH DESIGN

i) Days: 0 to 160:–Phase I (exploratory survey and descriptive market research).

ii) Days: 160 to 190:–Phase II (product sampling activity, business feasibility survey and conclusive research).

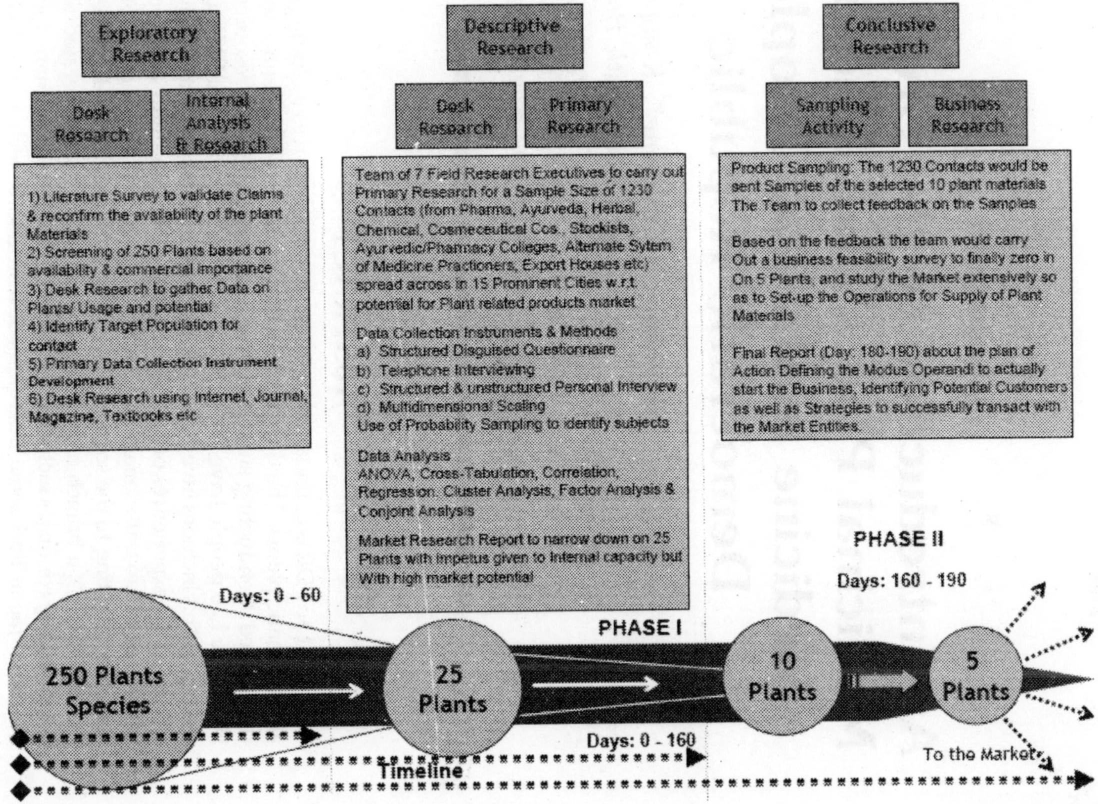

*Chapter 48*

# An Introduction to the Studies of Medicinal Plants and Traditional Medicine in the Lao People's Democratic Republic

***Bounhong Southavong*, Kongmany Sydara and Somsanith Bouamanivong***

*Traditional Medicine Research Centre, Ministry of Health, Vientiane, Lao People's Democratic Republic*

**E-mail: bsouthavong@hotmail.com*

## ABSTRACT

The Lao PDR is abundant with forest product resources including medicinal and aromatic plants. The development and utilization of potential resources is still limited. Conducting studies on the sustainable use of the resources is a key issue. The Lao people have a long history of practicing and studying traditional medicine. This includes investigating the palm leaf manuscripts kept in the temples, as well as the experiences of ancestors in different communities. Data pertaining to the uses of Lao traditional medicine has been studied for selecting, publishing, and disseminating to the society. Since 1998, the Traditional Medicine Research Centre (TMRC), a branch of the Ministry of Health, has cooperated with many neighbouring countries including the Socialist Republic of Vietnam, the Republic of China, Japan and some international institutions such as the International Cooperative Biodiversity Group (ICBG) to study medicinal plants for treating many diseases, including viral diseases, HIV/AIDS, malaria, tuberculosis, and cancer. Some new active compounds from candidate plants have been isolated and biological tests have been carried out. *Asparagus cochinchinensis* (Lour.) Merr., Asparagaceae shows anti-HIV and anti-cancer effects, 18 plants show anti-malarial effects, including *Rourea minor* (Gaertn.) Aubl., Connoraceae; *Gongronema nepalensis* (Wall.) Decnee Asclepiadaceae; *Nauclea orientalis* (L.), Rubiaceae; and *Diospyros quaesita* Thwaites, Ebenaceae.

***Keywords:*** *Lao PDR, Traditional medicine, Medicinal and aromatic plants, Traditional Medicine Research Centre (TMRC), Forest product resources.*

## 1.0 Introduction

The Lao People's Democratic Republic is located in the Indochina peninsula with a land area of 236,800 sq km; mountains and forest areas cover 65 per cent and forest covers 47 per cent of the total territory. Laos has 48 ethnic groups with beautiful cultures, traditions and experiences in healing diseases by their own indigenous medicine. Laos is endowed with abundant forest product resources due to its different types of forests, such as dry dipterocarp, highland mixed deciduous, highland dry semi-evergreen, lowland dry semi-evergreen, lowland mixed deciduous, gallery, coniferous and mixed coniferous broadleaf. The development and utilization of potential resources is still limited; though, the investment for commercialization in the field of medicinal plants is still very low. The Lao government encourages scientific studies and sustainable uses of natural resources, especially medicinal plants for the development of pharmaceutical products.

According to qualitative surveys from 1976 up to present, involving interviewing healers from different ethnic groups about traditional knowledge, Lao people know how to use about 4,000 medicinal plant species; Lao Pharmacopoeia cited about 3,000 species; well-known healers collect about 1,000 species, and about 500 species are being used for treating common maladies in Laos. The Traditional Medicine Research Centre (TMRC), a branch of the Ministry of Health, has collected traditional remedies from old books and manuscripts in Buddhist temples and communities, often written in ancient scripts. Selected remedies have been translated into contemporary Lao language and published for the benefit of our society.

With regards to scientific research on medicinal plants, the TMRC has been collaborating with many institutions in neighbouring countries since 1976. We have cooperated with the Institute of Materia Medica of the Socialist Republic of Vietnam in surveying medicinal plants in various parts of the country. We have also studied the active compounds of the false Culumba, *Coscinium spp*. the moon seed tuber, *Stephania spp*. grown in the country, cooperated with the Vietnamese Academy of Science and Technology (VAST), in the establishment of a pilot for the extraction of artemisinin, an anti-malarial agent from *Artemisia annua* L.. Very recently we joined the International Cooperative Biodiversity Group (ICBG), under the Lao-Vietnam based ICBG Project to study medicinal plants in the country. The main objectives of this project are to produce a documented inventory of tropical forest plant diversity in Laos that includes botanical inventory, ethnobotanical surveys among tribal communities, as well as to discover novel active molecules from plants as possible candidates for drug development in the treatment of various diseases, including HIV/AIDS, tuberculosis, and malaria. In addition, studies on medicinal plants for the treatment of cancer and central nervous system related diseases, including Alzheimer's disease, are being carried out.

## 2.0 Activities

- Interviewing healers to find out their capability in healing diseases (to identify the symptoms related to diseases concerned, for selecting candidates).
- Collection of samples and herbarium specimen for identifying the exact scientific names of the studied species (through references and analysis).
- Extraction of samples.
- Bioassay directed chromatic fractionation for the isolation of biologically active constituents with anti-HIV or anti-malaria activities.
- Elucidation of active compounds through state-of-the-art physical and spectroscopic methods: NMR and LC/MS/MS.

## 3.0 Results

**Table 48.1: Medicinal Plants with Biological Effects**

| *Number* | *Scientific Name* | *Part Studied* | *Effects* |
|---|---|---|---|
| 1 | *Asparagus cochinchinensis* (Lour.) Merr., Asparagaceae | Root | Anti-HIV, anti-cancer* |
| 2 | *Rourea minor* (Gaertn.) Aubl., Connoraceae | Stem | Anti-malaria ** |
| 3 | *Gongronema nepalensis* (Wall.) Decnee, Asclepiadaceae | Stem | Anti-malaria *** |
| 4 | *Nauclea orientalis* (L.) L. Rubiaceae | Stem | Anti-malaria **** |
| 5 | *Diospyros quaesita* Thwaites Ebenaceae | Stem and dried leaves | Anti-malaria |

(*) J. Nat. Prod. 2004, 67, 194-200; (**) Phytochemistry 67 (2006) 1378-1384; (***) Ongoing edited article; (****) Chemistry and Biodiversity, Vol. 2 (2005).

**Table 48.2: The Active Compounds of Studied Species**

| *Species* | *Active Compounds* | *Notes* |
|---|---|---|
| *Asparagus cochinchinensis* (Lour.) Merr. | 1. *asparacoside (spirostanol saponin)*<br>2. *asparacosin A (C-27 spirosteroids)*<br>3. *asparacosin B*<br>4. *3'-3"-methoxyasparenydiol (acetylenic derivative)*<br>5. *asparenydiol (known compound)*<br>6. *3'-hydroxy-4'-methoxy-4'-dehydroxynyasol (a new polyphenol)*<br>7. *nyasol*<br>8. *methylnyasol*<br>9. *1,3-bis-di-p-hydroxyphenyl-4-penten-1-one*<br>10. *Trans-conyferyl alcohol* | Compounds 1, 6 and 8 demonstrated moderate cytotoxicities. Ellipticine was used as a positive control. |

*Contd...*

**Table 48.2–Contd...**

| *Species* | *Active Compounds* | *Notes* |
|---|---|---|
| *Rourea minor* (Gaertn.) Aubl., | 1. *rourinoside*<br>2. *rouremin*<br>3. *1-(26-hydroxy-hexacosanoyl)-glycerol* | All of the 3 compounds showed weak *in vitro* activity against *Plasmodium falciparum.* |
| *Gongronema nepalense* (Wall.) Decnee | *Gongroneside A (Steroidal glycoside)* | This compound showed anti-malarial activity *in vitro* with an IC50 value of 1.54μM *P. falciparum* D6 clone. |
| *Nauclea orientalis* (L.) L. | 1. *naucleaorine [=(16α, 17β)-3 14:15,20-tetrahydro16-ethenyl-17–(β-D-glucopyranosyl-oxy) 19α-methoxyoxayohimban-21-one]*<br>2. *epimethoxynaucleaorine*<br>3. *3α, 19α, 23-dihydroxyurs-12-en-28-oic acid*<br>4. *oleanolic acid* | Shows moderate *in vitro* activities against *P. falciparum.* |
| *Diospyros quaesita* Thwaites., Ebenaceae | 1. *Betulenic acid 3β-caffeate*<br>2. *(-)-pinoresinol*<br>3. *3α-hydroxymethyl-2α, 4β-bis-(3-methoxy-4-hydroxy phenyl) pyran*<br>4. *2,10-dimethoxy-8-propenal-6a-11a-α-pterocarpan*<br>5. *2-ami no-3-phenyl-propyl benzoate*<br>*6.* 6-methoxy-7-hydroxyl coumarine<br>7. *poriferast-5-en-3β,7α–diol* | Substances (1) and (2) showed *in vitro* activities against *P. falciparum.* Substances (3) (4) and (5) were determined to be new natural products. Substances (6) and (7) are known compounds. |

As a matter of fact, realizing the Policy and Guidelines of the Government on health, the integration of Modern medicine with Traditional Medicine in the prevention, treatment and the promotion of people health, the Lao Traditional Medicine Knowledge (LTMK) has been thoroughly searched from the beginning of the foundation of the former Research Institute of Medicinal Plants (RIMP), the now-a days Traditional Medicine Research Centre. Recently, parallel to the implementation of the ICBG Project, Lao traditional medicine has been systematically studied. Lao traditional remedies, the treasure of Lao LTMK have been collected by searching in antique books kept in the temples or pagoda and in tribal communities and by interviewing healers. Aiming at the conservation and the promotion of the use of Lao Traditional Medicine Knowledge (LTMK), the Traditional Medicine Mapping Project (TMMP) has been initiated and is currently underway. During the search for LTMK, many precious remedies for healing acute and chronic diseases have been discovered. Some hundreds of remedies have been translated from Tharm script to modern Lao, published into 3 volumes and widely distributed to society, especially for use in primary health care.

**Table 48.3: Some Examples of Lao Traditional Medicine Remedies**

| | | |
|---|---|---|
| **Remedy for Kidney Stones:** | | |
| 1. | *Aganonerion polymorphum* Pierre in Spire and A. Spire, Apocynaceae | 20 g |
| 2. | *Cassytha filiformis* L., Lauraceae | 20 g |
| 3. | *Achyranthes aspera* L., Amaranthaceae | 20-30 g |
| 4. | *Begonia siamensis* Gagn., Begoniaceae | |
| | Or *Passiflora hispida* D.C., Passifloraceae root | 20 g |
| 5. | Water | 1 liter |
| Decoct for 1 hour, divide into 3 equal parts, and drink 3 times/day. | | |
| **Remedy for Healing Dry Cough:** | | |
| 1. | Root of *Achyranthes aspera* L. | 15g |
| 2. | Root of *Blumea balsamifera* D. C. | 20g |
| 3. | Stem of *Ocimum sanctum* L. | 3 ten-centimeter-long pieces |
| 4. | Root of *Mimosa pudica* L. | 20g |
| 5. | Water | 3 liters |
| Boil for 1 hour; drink as a substitution for drinking water. | | |
| **Remedy for Healing Intestinal Ulcer:** | | |
| 1. | Young fruit of *Aegle marmelos* | |
| 2. | *Tinospora crispa* Miers. | |
| 3. | *Curcuma longa* L. | |
| All ingredients are taken with an equal amount, 15 g decocted with 1 liter of water, dividing into 3 parts, drink in a day | | |
| **Aphrodisiac Recipe:** | | |
| 1. | Ripe banana (*Musa sapientum* L./*M. paradisiaca* L.) | 2 parts |
| 2. | Ripe fruit of *Aegle marmelos Correa* | 1 part |
| 3. | Honey of May | q. s. |
| Make into 0.5 g pills. Take one pill three times a day. | | |

## 4.0 Conclusion

Studies of medicinal plants of Laos are being carried out and some significant results have been found. This includes the discovery of some molecules that have been determined to have biological effects against the related diseases. However, new medicines from these plants have not yet been developed. Parallel to studies of medicinal plants, Lao traditional medicine knowledge is also being sought. Many precious traditional remedies have been found, selected, published and widely disseminated to society for wide uses, especially in Primary Health Care System of the country.

*Chapter 49*

# Herbal Prophylactics in Mauritius: Status of Traditional Use and Research

**Theeshan Bahorun**

*Department of Biosciences, Faculty of Science, University of Mauritius, Réduit, Republic of Mauritius*

*E-mail: tbahorun@uom.ac.mu, hemrazb@yahoo.com*

## ABSTRACT

Over the past few years there has been a resurgence of interest in integrating traditional herbal medicine with primary health care. In that vein, the World Health Organisation has initiated global efforts on traditional medicine to increase research on the untapped plant resources that would hopefully be the source of putative bioactive compounds/extracts with therapeutic relevance. The Republic of Mauritius, a small island state of 1,865 km$^2$ located some 800 km to the south east of Madagascar, harbours a unique flora (700 native flowering plants) with high levels of endemism (45 per cent). Medicinal plants are important elements of indigenous medical systems with at least 460 medicinal plants having been described. Several endemic plant species are also known in the traditional pharmacopoeia and many of their uses are deeply rooted in the Mauritian culture. These endemic and/or medicinal plants represent a reservoir of invaluable resources with therapeutic potentials but remain poorly studied. It is well established that that the therapeutic potential of medicinal plant largely lies in the presence of secondary metabolites including alkaloids, terpenoids and polyphenols. In that regard plant polyphenols, in particular, have been greatly recognized for their pluripharmacological beneficial effects, including antioxidant properties. This country paper gives an insight on the status of traditional/herbal medicine in Mauritius and focuses on research outcomes related to phytophenolic screening, antioxidant characterisation and molecular work initiated to understand the basis of the actions of a number of endemic species with cancer chemo preventive properties.

***Keywords:*** *Mauritius, Traditional medicine, Endemic plants, Polyphenolics, Antioxidants, and Chemonrevention.*

## 1.0 Introduction

Traditional medicine has always had an important place in the therapeutic armoury of mankind. Folklore medicines have regained use in occidental societies whilst they continue to be the cornerstone of therapy in several underdeveloped and developing regions. Plants have formed the basis of sophisticated traditional medicine systems among which are Ayurvedic, Unani, Chinese, and the lesser-known African and Australian systems. In addition to their use as phytomedicines, the science of ethnobotany and ethnopharmacology is very often used as a guide to lead to the discovery of novel sources and classes of therapeutics. Natural products continue to fulfil an important role in the development of therapeutic agents. For more than half of the twentieth century, natural products formed a central pillar of the modern pharmaceutical industry. For instance, 49 per cent of the new chemical entities introduced into clinical use between 1981 and 2002 were of natural product origin or natural product analogs (Newman *et al.*, 2003). Natural products continue to make the most dramatic impact in the area of cancer. Of 155 anticancer drugs developed since the 1940s only 27 per cent could not be traced to natural products, with 47 per cent being either a natural product or a direct derivation thereof (Newman and Cragg, 2007).

The use of traditional medicine in Mauritius has long been described in the pharmacopoeias (Daruty de Grandpré, 1911) and has an important cultural significance besides being readily accessible and affordable. The Republic of Mauritius which is composed of the islands of Mauritius, Rodrigues, Agalega, St. Brandon and a number of outlying smaller islands, all located in the south of the Indian Ocean between latitudes 10° S and 20° S and longitude 55° E and 65° E has evolved a unique flora and fauna with high levels of endemism. Nevertheless the flora originated from several sources and it is believed that 70 per cent of the phanerogams are derived from Madagascar and the African continent, 8 per cent from Asia, 12 per cent are of pan-indo pacific origin and 8 per cent are endemic (Guého, 1988). The island harbours a diversity of important indigenous forest trees but the decline in native forest area has significantly reduced the population level of these species. However, the remnant areas of native vegetation still hold a great diversity of plant species that are of great conservation value. The island of Mauritius is endowed with 681 native species of which 47 per cent are endemic to Mauritius (Bahorun *et al.*, 2007). It is also estimated that more than 1675 species have been introduced in the island (Heeroo, 2000). The level of endemicity far exceeds estimates from the Mascarene neighbouring islands of Réunion and Rodrigues islands both with 35 per cent and other African countries mainly Namibia (17 per cent), Zambia (4.4 per cent), Zimbabwe (2.1 per cent) and Bostwana (0.8 per cent) (Guého, 1988; Maggs *et al.*, 1998). However many of the endemics have become highly endangered, with about 50 taxa being reduced to less than 10 individuals (Atkinson and Sevathian, 2005).

Some 460 medicinal plants from 118 families have been described till date (Gurib-Fakim and Guého, 1995). A number of species of the Mauritian endemic flora is also strongly anchored in the traditional pharmacopoeias contributing to the culture and traditions of the Mauritian people. Mauritian endemic plants have gained significant recognition during the past decades for their reported prophylactic potential. A number of these plants are used for the treatment of bronchitis, rheumatic pain, dysentery, renal stones, hypertension, and migraine and as purgative (Gurib-Fakim and Guého, 1995, 1996). Although the majority of the endemics have not been described for their traditional uses, they represent interesting sources of complementary and alternative medicine. These plants could potentially play an important role in bioprospecting of new pharmaceutical agents, as they are an untapped reservoir of bioactive compounds. They may represent important sources of therapeutics thereby spawning interest in their study. To date, data on their biological, biochemical and phytochemical properties as well as on their molecular mechanisms of action are still limited therefore warranting more in depth studies to delineate their therapeutic potential.

This country paper reviews the status of traditional medicine in Mauritius focusing on research endeavours on medicinal/endemic prophylactic plants with special emphasis on some of the investigations conducted at molecular level with a view to understand the basis of their actions.

## 2.0 Status of Traditional Medicine Use in Mauritius

Current estimates from the World Health Organization suggest that in many developing countries, a large proportion of populations rely heavily on traditional practices. This is the case in Africa, where 80 per cent of the population depends on traditional medicine for their primary health care due to the severe shortage of qualified personal in modern medicine and the high cost of imported pharmaceuticals (Scott, 1993). The demand on traditional medicine is very likely to escalate with the emergence of new diseases and because imported medicine is unsustainable in several African countries including Mauritius under the current economic realities.

In Mauritius, a wide number of plant species from the Apiaceae, Apocynaceae, Asclepiadaceae, Asteraceae, Bombacaceae, Bromeliaceae, Caesalpinaceae, Celastraceae, Convolvulaceae, Erythroxylaceae, Euphorbiaceae, Ebenaceae, Flacourtiaceae, Liliaceae, Myrtaceae, Meliaceae, Orchidaceae, Oxalidaceae, Rubiaceae, Sapotaceae, Verbenaceae are known to contribute to the management of diseases among the population (Table 49.1).

A survey conducted as part of a regional project under the aegis of the Indian Ocean Commission has led to the publication of two volumes on medicinal plants of Mauritius (Gurib-Fakim *et al.*, 1995, 1996). Over and above the database including ethnobotanical, botanical and to a limited extent, phytochemical and pharmacological data, anti-fungal and anti-microbial screens of some endemic medicinal and aromatic plants have also been reported (Jelager *et al.*, 1999). Other species provide active ingredients for drugs and pesticides. For example, extracts of the leaves of *Aphloia theiformis* was found to be active within 24 hours against *Biomphalaria glabrata* snails, the intermediate hosts of *Schistosoma mansoni* (Gopalsamy *et al.*, 1988). Similarly *Polycias dichroostachya* was shown to have strong molluscidal activity. There also exists a score of aromatic plants that are being exploited for commercial purposes and they include the Ylang ylang (*Cananga odorata*), the Vanilla (*Vanilla fragrans*), Pink pepper or Brazillian pepper tree (*Schinus terebithifolius*).

**Table 49.1: Introduced and Endemic* Plants in Traditional Medicine in Mauritius**

| Family | Species | Common Name | Medicinal Purpose |
|---|---|---|---|
| Apiaceae | *Foeniculum vulgare* | Gros anis/fenouil | Treatment for constipation |
| Apocynaceae | *Nerium oleander* | Laurier | Against eczemas |
| | *Allamanda cathartica* | Allamanda | Against jaundice |
| Asclepiadaceae | *Tylophora coriacea** | Ipéca du pays | Treat vomiting |
| | *Sarcostemma sp* | Liane calli | Used against diarrhoea |
| Asteraceae | *Ayapana triplinervis* | Ayapana | Against vomiting, diarrhea |
| | *Psidia viscosa** | Baume de l'île plate | Against asthma and fever |
| | *Psidia terebinthina** | Baume de l'île plate | Against asthma and bronchitis |
| | *Senecio lamackianus** | Bois chèvre | Treatment of influenza and cough |
| Bombacaceae | *Adansonia digitata* | Baobab | Used against diarrhea |
| Bromeliaceae | *Ananas bracteatus* | Ananas sauvage | Against vomiting, also as an abortive |
| Burseraceae | *Canarium paniculatum** | Bois colophane | In cases of rheumatism |
| | *Protium obtusifolium** | Bois colophane bâtard | Intestinal problems |
| Caesalpinaceae | *Cassia fistula* | Fleur cavadee | Laxative |
| Celastraceae | *Maytenus pyria** | Bois à poudre | Use against dysentery. Anti-tumoral, anti-inflammatory, anti-leukemic properties |
| | *Cassine orientalis** | Bois d'olive | Use against hypertension |
| Chryso-balanaceae | *Grangeria borbonica** | Bois de buis | Agaisnt stomach pain and asthma |
| Convolvulaceae | *Ipomoea indica* | Liane bleue | For rheumatic pain and head aches |
| Ebanaceae | *Diospyros neraudii**<br>*Diospyros revaughanii**<br>*Diospyros tesselleria**<br>*Diospyros melanida** | Ebène | Antibacterial, antifungal, antiviral, antihelminthic, antiprotozoan, and antimalarial properties |
| Ericaceae | *Agauria salicifolia** | Bois cabris | Skin disorders |
| Erythroxylaceae | *Erythroxylum * laurifolium* | Bois de ronde | Diuretic, used against renal stones |
| Lamiaceae | *Plectranthus madagascariensis* | Baume du Pérou | Anti-coughing property |
| Liliaceae | *Aloe bardadensis* | Mazambron | Against muscular pain |
| Meliaceae | *Azadirachta indica* | Neem | Anti-diabetic effect, Treatment for hemorrhoids |
| Monimiaceae | *Tambourissa quadrifida** | Bois tambour | Purgative |
| Myrtaceae | *Eugenia tinifolia** | Bois de nèfles | Purgative |
| | *Eugenia uniflora* | Roussaille | Against dysentery, hematuria |
| | *Syzygium glomeratum** | Bois de pomme | Use in the treatment of migraine |
| Orchidaceae | *Vanilla planifolia* | Vanillier | Digestive, aphrodisiac property |
| Oxalidaceae | *Averrhoa bilimbi* | Bilimbi long | Use against hypertension and intestinal infections |

A wide range of exotic and native plants used by traditional practitioners is also part of the diet, in particular mentha (*Mentha piperita*), cloves (*Syzygium aromaticum*), onion (*Allium cepa*), basil (*Ocimum gratissimum*), thyme (*Thymus vulgaris*), amongst others (Adjanohoun *et al.*, 1983). Commonly used herbal medicine in Mauritius includes Ayapana (*Ayapana triplinervis*) used against vomiting and diarrhoea, "bilimbi long" (*Averrhoa bilimbi*) for the treatment of hypertension and intestinal infections, "roussaille" (*Eugenia uniflora*) and neem (*Azadirachta indica*) for their anti-diabetic effect, fenouil (*Foeniculum vulgare*) against constipation and "laurier" (*Nerium oleander*) for the treatment of eczemas.

Several of the native plants have also found effective uses against a range of ailments (Table 49.1). For instance, a decoction of the bark of *Erythroxylum sideroxyloides* is used as a diuretic and against renal stones. Similarly, *Crinum mauritianum* has been found to alleviate rheumatic pain while Mauritian people against hypertension traditionally use *Cassine orientalis*. *Maytenus pyria* is beneficial against dysentery and has anti-tumoral, anti-inflammatory, anti-leukemic properties. The *Diospyros* species mainly *D. neraudii, D. tesselaria, D. mellanida, D. revaughanii* have been reported against a wide range of pathologies as they possess antibacterial, antifungal, antiviral, antihelminthic, antiprotozoan, and antimalarial properties. *E. tinifolia* and *S. glomeratum* have been described in the traditional pharmacopoeia respectively as a purgative and for the treatment of migraine. Plants like *Sarcostemma* sp, *Tylophora coriacea* (Ascleipiadaceae), *Psiadia terebinthina, Psidia viscose, Senecio lamarckianus* from Asteraceae family, *Canarium paniculatum, Protium obstusifolium* from the Burseraceae family, *Maytenus pyria* (Celatraceae), *Grangeria bornonica* (Chrysobalanaceae), *Agauria salicifoila* (Ericaceae), *Erythroxylum laurifolium* (Erythroxylaceae), *Phyllantus lanceolatus* (Euphorbiaceae), *Crinum mauritianum* and *Lomatophyllum purpureum* from the Liliaceae family, *Tambourissa quadrifida* (Monimiaceae), *Badula insularis* (Myrsinaceae), *Eugenia tinifolia* and *Syzygium glomeratum* from the Myrtaceae family have also known traditional uses (Table 49.1).

More recently a number of investigations have focused on the effects of *Momordica charantia* aqueous fruit extract on the modulation of fluid, d-glucose and l-tyrosine transport in vitro (Mahomoodally *et al.*, 2005, 2007), the screening of traditional antidiabetic medicinal plants (*Coix lacryma-jobi* (Poaceae), *Aegle marmelos* and *Vangueria madagascariensis* (Rutaceae), *Articarpus heterophyllus* (Moraceae), *Azaridachta indica* (Meliaceae), *Eriobotrya japonica* (Rosaceae) and *Syzigium cumini* (Myrtaceae) for possible $\alpha$-amaylase inhibitory effects in vitro (Kotowaroo *et al.*, 2006) and the screening for anti-infective properties of several medicinal plants (*e.g. Michelia champaca* and *Antidesma madagascariense*) of the Mauritian flora (Rangasamy *et al.*, 2007).

## 3.0 Current Research in Traditional Medicinal/Endemic Mauritian Plants

Medicinal plants contain an amalgam of phytoconstituents that may act individually, additively or in synergy to improve health. Thus compared to modern allopathic medicine, traditional medicine aims to restore balance by using chemically complex plants or by mixing several different plants to maximise the synergistic effect of the various phytochemicals for a better therapeutic effect. Traditional native plants are promising target for the discovery of novel compounds of pharmaceutical value and in this line, careful phytochemical, pharmacological, and toxicological analyses are necessary to assess their effectiveness. Furthermore molecular mechanisms associated with their actions needs to be comprehensively defined and understood.

The plethora of phytochemicals in plant extracts can simultaneously affect multiple pharmacological targets and provide clinical efficacy beyond the reach of single compound based drugs. This is perhaps the most important factor why the mainstream pharmaceutical research is moving away from single molecule or single target approach to combinations and multiple target approaches using plant extracts. The growing surge of interest in natural products and/or herbal extracts and the role played by ethno medicine during the past centuries, support the need for scientific validation of the purported medicinal properties of these extracts.

In the main, alkaloids, terpenoids and polyphenolics are classes of plant secondary metabolites that have gained significant recognition as therapeutic compounds. Nitrogen-containing alkaloids have contributed the largest number of drugs ranging in effects from anticholinergics (atropine) to analgesics (opium alkaloids) and from antiparasitics (quinine) to anticholinesterases (galantamine) to antineoplastics (vinblastine/vincristine) (Raskin *et al.*, 2002). Terpenoids and phenolics have also made important contribution to the modern pharmacopoeia. Terpenoids range from $Na^+/K^+$ pump-inhibiting cardiac glycosides from *Digitalis* spp. (recognized as a treatment for congestive heart failure), to antineoplastic (paclitaxel) to antimalarial artemisinin (a component of *Artemisia annua* extract used for centuries in traditional Chinese medicine) and steroidal saponins used in birth control pills (Calixto *et al.*, 2000; Cragg, 1998; Abdin *et al.*, 2003). Plant phenolics have contributed aspirin and podophyllotoxin to modern medicine and are considered as valuable prophylactic antioxidants, which are currently sold as dietary, supplements and/or herbal remedies (Ferguson 2001; Erlund 2004).

It is therefore clear that plant secondary metabolites have pluripharmacological properties and a number of *in vitro* and *in vivo* studies have highlighted the antimicrobial, antioxidative, anti-inflammatory, anti-mutagenic, cardioprotective and chemopreventive effects of these compounds, thus indicating why these bioactive constituents are greatly warranted as therapeutics. Among these metabolites, polyphenolic compounds are a particularly attractive class commonly cited for their biological and therapeutic activities including antimicrobial, anti-inflammatory, vasodilatory, expectorant, and anti-mutagenic and antioxidant properties (McGregor *et al.*, 1999; Spignoli, 2000; Soobrattee *et al.*, 2005). In addition, the regulatory activity of phenolic antioxidants on cell signal transduction pathways mainly the MAPK, JNK kinases, transcription factors mainly NF-kB, c-Jun, c-myc, c-fos have been highly emphasized as a strategy for reducing the incidence of diseases induced by reactive oxygen and nitrogen species (Owuor and Kong, 2002; Hou *et al.*, 2004). The prophylactic effects of phenolic antioxidants stem mainly from several epidemiological studies and their ability to arrest the onset of chronic degenerative diseases in animal models and cell cultures (Cao *et al.*, 2004; Dijsselbloem *et al.*, 2004; Kris-Etherton *et al.*, 2002). More than 4000 of these compounds generally referred as flavonoids have been identified in both higher and lower plants. They can be subdivided into six classes: flavones, flavanones, isoflavones, flavanols and anthocyanins with the basic ring skeletons of these classes are shown in Figure 49.1.

**Figure 49.1: Chemical Structures of Flavonoids and Some Examples**

| *Classes* | *Structural Formula* | *Examples* |
|---|---|---|
| Flavanones | 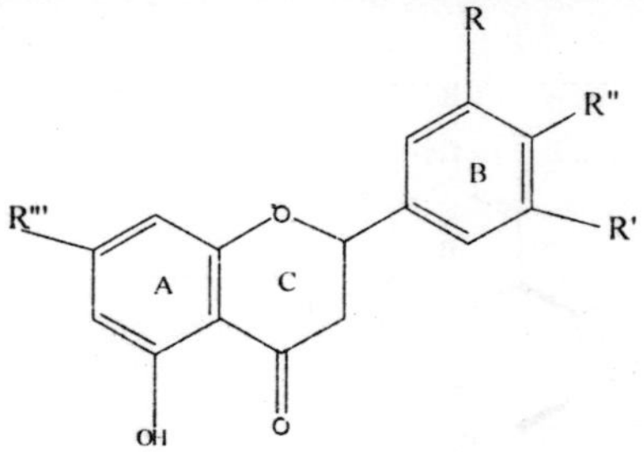  | R=R$^{1}$=H, R$^{11}$=R$^{111}$= OH; Naringenin<br>R= OH, R$^{1}$=H, R$^{11}$=R$^{111}$= OH; Eriodyctiol<br>R=R$^{1}$=OH, R$^{11}$=R$^{111}$= OH; 5$^{1}$-OH–Eriodyctiol |
| Flavones | 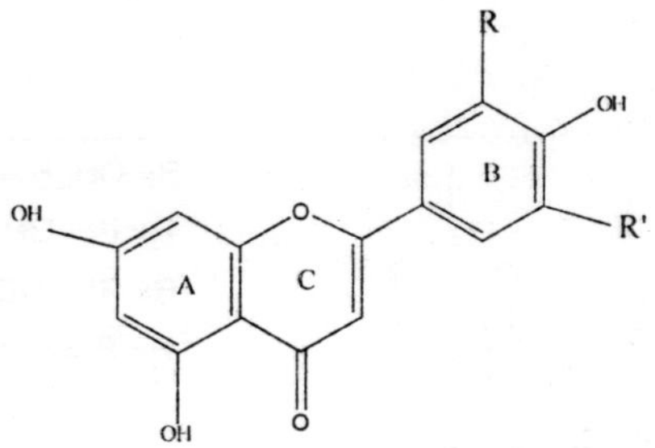  | R=R$^{1}$=H; Apigenin<br>R= OH, R$^{1}$= H; Luteolin<br>R=R$^{1}$=$OCH_3$; Tricetin |
| Isoflavones | 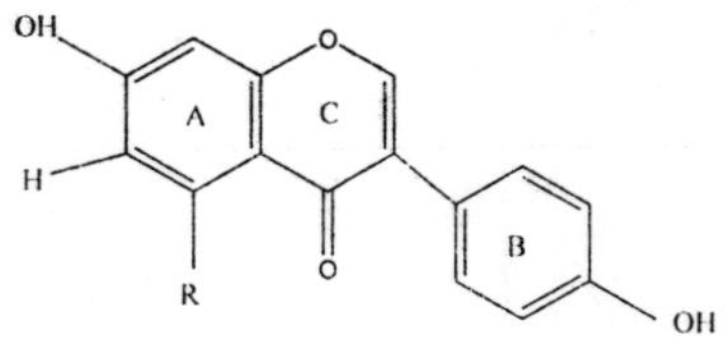  | R = H; Daidzein<br>R = OH; Genistein |
| Flavonols | 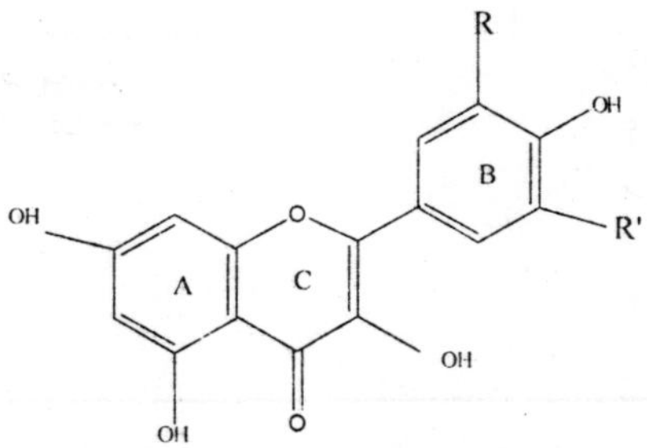  | R=R$^{1}$=H; Kaempferol<br>R= OH, R$^{1}$= H; Quercetin<br>R=R$^{1}$=OH; Myricetin |

*Contd...*

**Figure 49.1–Contd...**

| *Classes* | *Structural Formula* | *Examples* |
|---|---|---|
| Flavanols | 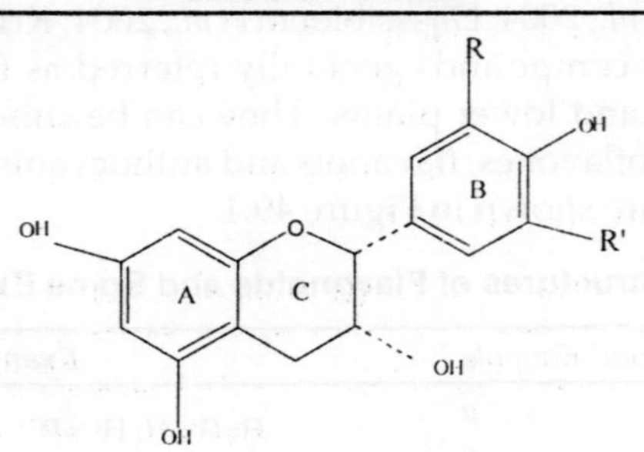 | R= OH, R'= H; (+)-Epicatechin<br>R=R'=OH; (+)-Epigallocatechin<br>R=OH, R'=H; (–)-Catechin<br>R=R'=OH; (–)-Gallocatechin |
| | 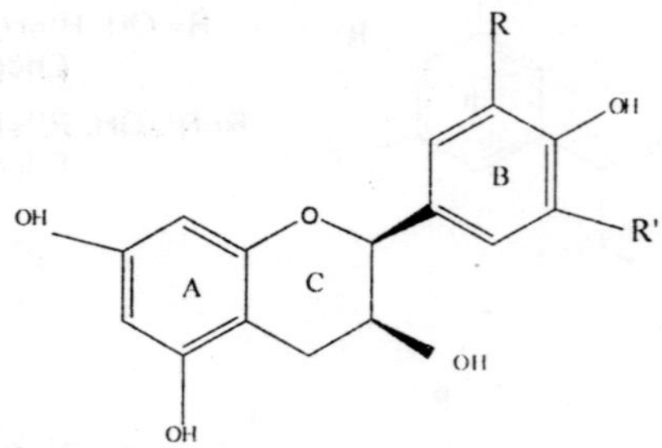 | |
| Anthocyanidins | 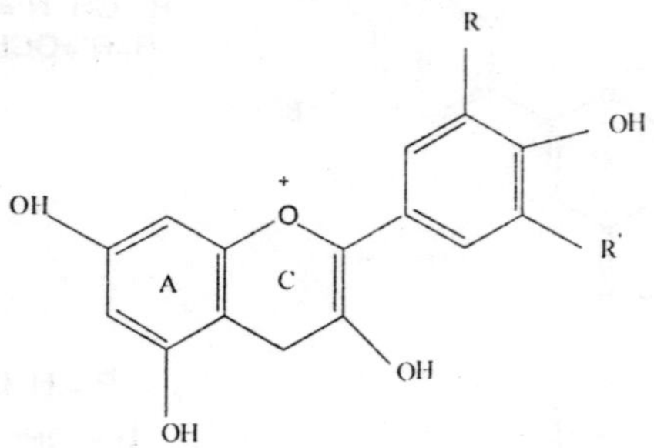 | R= OH, R'= H; Cyanidin<br>R= R'= OH; Delphinidin<br>R= R' = $OCH_3$; Malvidin<br>R= R'= H; Pelargonidin |
| | 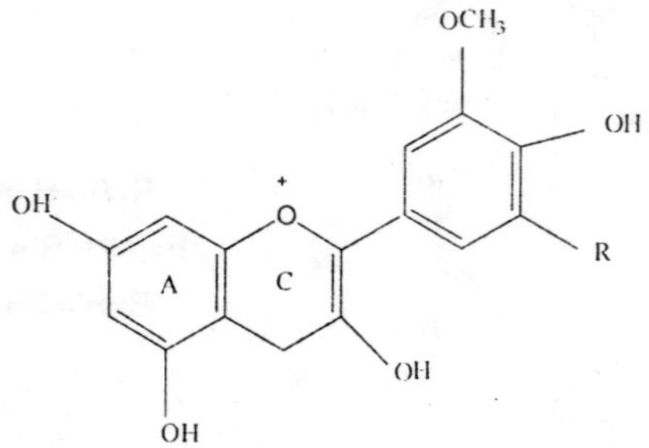 | R= H; Peonidin<br>R= OH; Petunidin |

Literature data abounds in examples where phenolic compounds are the bioactive components responsible for the prophylactic benefits of traditionally used plants sources (Ishige *et al.*, 2001; Ivanova *et al.*, 2005; Spignoli, 2000). For instance, soy estrogens are applied in hormone replacement therapy (Dijsselbloem *et al.*, 2004) and these phytochemicals also have applications in the prevention of atherosclerosis (Cassidy *et al.*, 2003). (-)-EGCG, the major antioxidative component of green tea has been reported for growth inhibitory effects in cancer cells which appear to be mediated by the induction of apoptosis, the arrest of a specific phase of the cell cycle, the inhibition of aberrant arachidonic acid metabolism and the inhibition of proteasome activities (Fujiki *et al.*, 2003; Hou *et al.*, 2004). With the background that high amounts of phenolic compounds in plant extracts is suggestive of putative health benefits, a number of studies have been geared for the past fifteen years, at the University of Mauritius, towards the phytochemical screening and biological activity evaluation of medicinal and/or endemic plants. The outcomes of some of these investigations are reviewed here.

The phytochemical composition of some of the endemic plants of Mauritius mostly with respect to their phenolic compositions have been characterized (Table 49.2)

**Table 49.2: Phytochemical Screening of Traditionally based Botanical Drugs used Mauritius for the Management of Primary Health Care *(Table Adapted from Bahorun et al., 2003)***

| *Plant Names (Families)* | *Phytochemicals Present* | *Traditional uses (Gurib-Fakim et al., 1995-1997)* |
|---|---|---|
| *Psiadia* sp. (Asteraceae) | Phenols, flavonoids, saponins, tannins | Pulmonary infections, asthma, fever, coughs |
| *Canarium paniculatum* (Burseraceae) | Phenols, anthocyanins, tannins, terpenes, coumarins | Rheumatism, skin ulcerations |
| *Senecio ambavilla* (Asteraceae) | Phenols, flavonoids, tannins | Rheumatism, gout, urinary infections, renal infections |
| *Grangeria borbonica* (Chrysobalanaceae) | Phenols, flavonoids, tannins | Stomach pains, asthma |
| *Cnestis glabra* (Connaraceae) | Flavonoids, tannins, pro-anthocyanidins, saponins | Fever |
| *Erythroxylum hypericifolium* | Flavonoids, saponins, tannins | Fever, renal stones, throat infections |
| *E. laurifolium* | Phenols, flavonoids, saponins, tannins | Fever, renal stones, throat infections |
| *E. sideroxyloides* (Erythroxylaceae) | Phenols, flavonoids, saponins, tannins, triterpenes, alkaloids | Fever, renal stones, throat infections |
| *Antidesma madagascariensis* | Phenols, flavonoids, pro-anthocyanidins, saponins, tannins | Fever, astringent, diabetese, dysentery, jaundice |
| *Phyllanthus casticum* | Phenol, flavonoids, pro-anthocyanidins, tanins, saponins. | Fever, diarrhoea, dysentery, urino-genital infections |

*Contd...*

**Table 49.2–Contd...**

| *Plant Names (Families)* | *Phytochemicals Present* | *Traditional uses (Gurib-Fakim et al., 1995-1997)* |
|---|---|---|
| *P. phyllireifolius* (Euphorbiaceae) | Phenols, flavonoids, pro-anthocyanidins, tannins | Colics, diuretic, emmenagogue, cystitis |
| *Aphloia theiformis* (Flacourtiaceae) | Phenols, flavonoids, pro-anthocyanidins, saponins, tannins | Dysentery, fever, rheumatism, gastro-intestinal infections, jaundice |
| *Foetidia mauritiana* (Lecythidaceae) | Alkaloids, proanthocyanidins, saponins, tannins | Laxative, emmenagogue, purgative, diuretic |
| *Leea guinensis* (Leeaceae) | Phenols, flavonoids, pro-anthocyanidins, tanins | Oedemas, antiseptic, colds |
| *Turraea casimiriana* (Meliaceae) | Phenols, flavonoids, tannins, proanthocyanidins, saponins, | Boils, hypotensive, emmenagogue |
| *Tambourissa* sp (Monimiaceae) | Flavonoids, proantho-cyanidins, saponins, tannins | Dermatitis, emmenagogue |
| *Ficus reflexa* (Moraceae) | Phenols, proanthocyanidins | Throat infections |
| *Embelia angustifolia* (Myrsinaceae) | Alkaloids, phenols, flavonoids, saponins | Liver complaints, dysentery, urinary tract infections |
| *Scutia myrtina* (Rhamnaceae) | Phenols, flavonoids, pro-anthocyanidins, saponins, tannins | Diarrhoea, dysentery, astringent, antidote for toxic fish poisoning |
| *Chassalia coriaceae* (Rubiaceae) | Anthocyanin heterosides, saponins, triterpenes, iridoids, flavonoids | Astringent |
| *Dodonaea viscosa* | Flavonoids, saponins, tannins, proanthocyanidins | Rheumatism, gout, throat infections, contusions |
| *Doratoxylon apetalum* | Flavonoids, saponins, tannins, proanthocyanidins | Venereal diseases, skin infections |
| *Molinae alternifolia* (Sapindaceae) | Phenols, flavonoids, flavones, proanthocyanidins, saponins, tannins | Dysentery, throat infections |
| *Mimusops maxima* (Sapotaceae) | Phenols, flavonoids, flavones, proanthocyanidins, tannins | Diarrhoea, dysentery, astringent |
| *Premna corymbosa* (Verbenaceae) | Alkaloids, saponins, flavonoids, phenols | Coughs, influenza |

Fractionations of the extracts of *Canarium* sp (Burseraceae) has led to the isolation and characterization of epicatechin, 3-O-galloylepigallocatechin, epigallocatechin, methyl gallate ester, pentagalloyl glucose, gallic acid, methyl gallate ester, alpha and beta amyrins. The Psiadia species from the Asteraceae family yields kaempferol-3-methyl ether, quercetin-3-methyl ether, kaempferol-3,7-methyl ether amongst others. Quercetin-3-O-glucose rhamnoside has been isolated from the methanol extract of the leaves of *Chassalia coriaceae* (Rubiaceae) (Marie *et al.*, 2000).

Gurib-Fakim *et al.* (2005) showed the potential antimicrobial profile of *Antidesma madagascariensis* (Euphorbiaceae), *Faujasiopsis flexuosa* (Asteraceae), *Toddalia asiatica* and *Vepris lanceolata* (Rutaceae), *Labourdonnaisia* species in particular *L. glauca, L. revolute, L. calophylloides, Sideroxylon* species mainly *S. cinereum, S. puberulum* and *S. grandiflorum, Mimusops species* (*M. maxima, M. erythroxylum,* and *M. petiolaris*), Erythroxylum species (*E. sideroxyloides, E. laurifolium, E. hypericifolium,* and *E. macrocarpum), Canarium paniculatum* and *Protium obtusifolium* (Burseraceae), *Chassalia coriaceae* and *Gaertnera psychotrioides* (Rubiaceae). A similar study conducted by Pedersen *et al.* (1999) had indicated the antibacterial effects of *Gaertnera psychotroides* (Rubiaceae) against the gram-positive *Staphylococcus aureus*, and the gram-negative *Escherichia coli, Pseudomonas aeruginosa,* and *Salmonella typhi*. The same authors showed that *Mussaenda landia, Antirhea borbonica* and *Chassalia coriacea* from the Rubiaceae family were also effective against some bacterial strains (Pedersen *et al.*, 1999). Less recent investigations have also highlighted the screening of traditional plants for cytotoxicity (Chapuis *et al.*, 1988), antiviral (Beuscher *et al.*, 1994) and antineoplastic activities (*Terminalia arjuna*) (Pettit *et al.*, 1996).

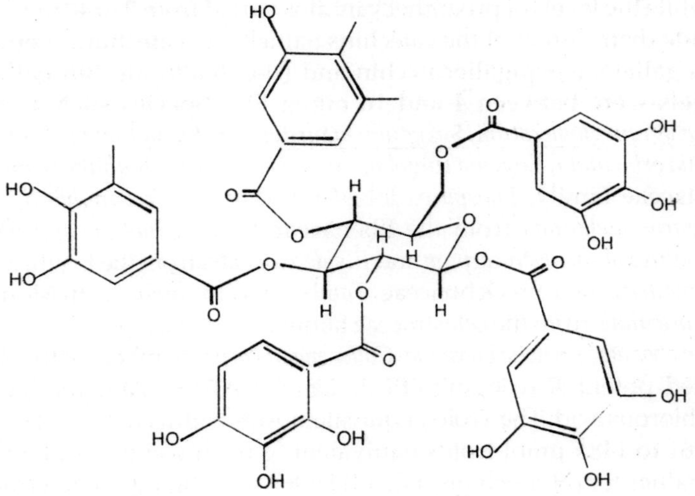


**Pentagalloyl glucose**

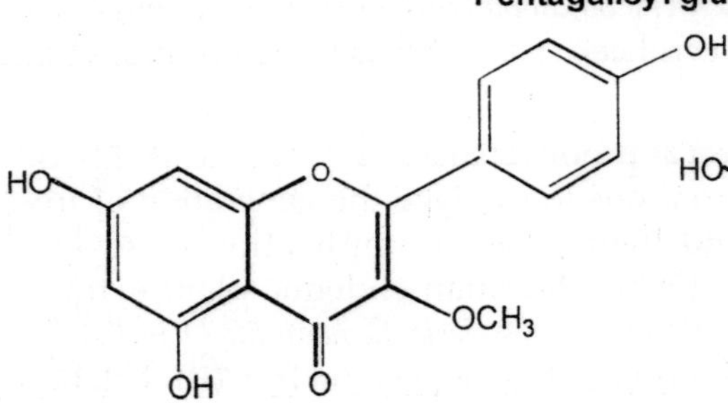


**Kaempferol-3-methyl ether**

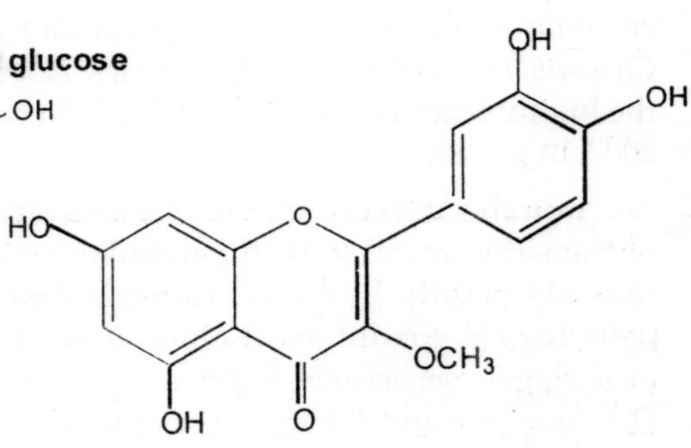


**Quercetin-3-methyl ether**

The implication of oxidative stress in the etiology and development of several acute and chronic pathophysiological disorders has led to the suggestion that antioxidant therapy can be feasible strategy for disease management. The recent explosion in the search for natural antioxidants for food preservation and prophylaxis provided more incentive for the screening of the Mauritian endemic flora. Although there exist several listings of native plants for their medicinal applications, little is known on their active constituents. In an effort to fill that void, our group has initiated since a number of years several research endeavours to comprehensively investigate the prophylactic potential of our endemic flora. In this context we have evaluated the antioxidant propensities and phenolic contents of 36 species from the Myrtaceae, Rubiaceae, Ebenaceae, Celastraceae, Erythroxylaceae, Sterculaceae, Myrsinaceae, Amaryllidaceae, Euphorbiaceae, Erythroxylaceae, Ochnaceae, Asteraceae, Monimiaceae, Asclepadiaceae and Meliaceae families were analyzed for their total phenolics, proanthocyanidins, flavonoids contents, antioxidant and metal chelating potentials (Neergheen *et al.*, 2005, 2007; Soobrattee *et al.*, 2007 in press).

Total phenolics content varied widely and ranged from 1 to 103 mg GA/g fresh weight (FW) while the levels of proanthocyanidins varied from 3 to 40 mg/g FW and there was a wide distribution of the catechins namely (+)-catechin, (-)-epicatechin, (-)-epicatechin gallate, (-)-epigallocatechin and (-)-epigallocatechin gallate. Total Flavonoid levels were between 4 and 16 mg/g FW. Species such as *Syzygium commersonii, Syzygium glomeratum, Syzygium mauritianum, Syzygium venosum, Eugenia pollicina, Eugenia orbiculata, Eugenia tinifolia, Eugenia elliptica, Monimiastrum globosum* from the Myrtaceae family, *Diospyros tessellaria, Diospyros revaughanii, Diospyros neraudii, Diospyros mellanida* from the Ebenaceae family, *Badula multiflora* from *Myrsinaceae, Erythroxylum macrocarpum* and *E. sideroxyloides* from the Erythroxylacaeae family, *Ochna mauritiana* from Ochnaceae, *Tambourissa cordifolia* from Monimiaceae family. *Cassine orientalis* from the celastraceae family, *Gaertnera psychotroides, Myonima nitens, Myonima obovata, Fernelia buxifolia, Coffea macrocarpa* members of the Rubiaceae family indicated potent scavenging effects against $ABTS^{\cdot +}$ And the biologically reactive hypochlorous acid. The Trolox Equivalent Antioxidnt Activity (TEAC) value ranged from 161 to 1485-µmol-trolox equivalent/g fresh weight of plant material while the $IC_{50}$ values for (Hypochlorous acid) HOCl scavenging ranged from 0.15 to 2.27 mg FW/ml. In addition, leaf extracts of *Monimiastrum acutisepalum, Cassine orientalis, Coffea macrocarpa, Eugenia tinifolia, Coffea mauritiana, Chassalia coriacaea, Chassalia lanceolata, Diospyros* species, *Fernelia buxifolia* were effective scavengers of the highly reactive hydroxyl radical (Neergheen *et al.*, 2005, 2007; Soobrattee *et al.*, 2007, in press).

Iron chelators are of potential interest as prophylactics in view of the likelihood of transition metal ions in particular iron ions to catalyze the generation of free radicals mainly hydroxyl radicals and their possible implication in several pathological conditions (Kehrer *et al.*, 1993). Mauritian endemic plant extracts including *S. commersonii, S. glomeratum, E. tinifolia, D.tesseleria, D. neraudii, D. mellanida, D. revaughanii* and *T. boutoniana* showed concentration dependent iron (II) chelation activity with $IC_{50}$s less than 3.2 mg FW/ml. Lipid peroxidation is known to alter the membrane physical properties and to affect a number of cellular processes such as membrane fluidity, membrane fusion, permeability, modulation of membrane-bound enzyme activity and cell adhesion (Kehrer, 1993; Gutteridge, 1995; Teague *et al.*, 2002). The important contribution of lipid peroxidation in a number of disease conditions has led to an increased interest in the role of natural antioxidant inhibitors in protecting membrane lipids. Interestingly, the endemic plant extracts in the main *E. pollicina, D. revaughanii, B. multifkora, E. orbiculata, S. venosum, S. glomeratum, C. macrocarpa, O. mauritianna, D. tesseleria, D. neraudii, G. psychotroides, C. orientalis, D. mellanida* were potent inhibitors of microsomal lipid peroxidation ($IC_{50:}$ 0.06-0.2 mg FW/ml). These extracts are potent inhibitors of free-radical induced peroxidation in membrane mimetic systems and can find applications in the management of clinical disorders as well as in the food industry to protect against lipid oxidation. Further experimental work will define the potential uses of the extracts. It is noteworthy that the antioxidative property of the extracts was observed to be mostly ascribed to the synergistic effect of the various classes of polyphenolics identified (Tables 49.3 and 49.4).

**Table 49.3: Distribution of Flavan–3–ol Derivatives in Some Selected Mauritian Endemic Species**

| *Plant Species* | *Catechins* | | | | | *Procyanidin Dimers* | |
|---|---|---|---|---|---|---|---|
| | *(+)–C* | *(–)–EC* | *(–)–ECG* | *(–)–EGCG* | *(–)–EGC* | *B1* | *B2* |
| *Cassine orientalis* | (+) | (++) | – | – | (+) | (+) | (+) |
| *Chassalia grandifolia* | (+) | – | – | – | Tr | – | – |
| *Coffea macrocarpa* | (+) | (++) | (++) | (+) | (+) | (+) | (+) |
| *Coffea mauritiana* | (+) | (+) | – | (++) | (+) | Tr | (+) |
| *Diospyros melanida* | (+++) | – | (+) | (++) | (+++) | – | (+) |
| *Diospyros neraudii* | Tr | (+) | (+) | (+) | – | – | – |
| *Diospyros revaughanii* | (+) | (+) | (++) | (+) | – | – | (+) |
| *Diospyros tesselleria* | (+++) | – | – | (++) | (++) | (+++) | (++) |
| *Erythroxylum sideroxyloides* | (+) | – | – | – | Tr | – | – |
| *Eugenia elliptica* | (+) | (+) | – | (+) | (+) | (+) | – |
| *Eugenia orbiculata* | (+++) | (+++) | – | (++) | (+++) | (+++) | (+++) |
| *Eugenia pollicina* | (++) | (+++) | (++) | (+++) | – | (+++) | (++) |
| *Eugenia tinifolia* | (+++) | (+++) | – | (+++) | (++) | (+++) | (+) |
| *Fernelia buxifolia* | (+) | – | – | – | (+) | – | – |
| *Monimiastrum acutisepalum* | (+) | (+) | (+) | – | (+) | (+) | – |
| *Myonima obovata* | (+) | – | (+) | – | (+) | (+) | (+) |
| *Syzygium commersonii* | (+++) | – | – | (+++) | (+++) | (+++) | – |
| *Syzygium glomeratum* | (+) | (+++) | (+++) | (++) | (+) | (+) | (+) |
| *Syzygium mauritianum* | (+++) | (+++) | – | (+++) | (+++) | – | (++) |
| *Syzygium venosum* | (+++) | – | (+++) | – | (+) | (+++) | (++) |
| *Trochetia boutoniana* | (+) | – | – | – | – | – | (+++) |

(+++) = very prominent; (++) = prominent; (+) = present; tr = trace; (–) = not detected.
Estimated from the peak area of HPLC profiles.

**Table 49.4: Distribution of Flavonol Aglycones: Kaempferol, Myricetin and Quercetin in the Hydrolysed Plant Extracts**

| *Plant species* | *Kaempferol* | *Myricetin* | *Quercetin* |
|---|---|---|---|
| *Cassine orientalis* | (+++) | (++) | (+++) |
| *Chassalia grandifolia* | (+) | – | (+) |
| *Coffea macrocarpa* | (+) | – | (+) |
| *Coffea mauritiana* | (+) | (+) | (+++) |
| *Diospyros melanida* | (+++) | – | (+++) |
| *Diospyros neraudii* | (+++) | – | (+++) |
| *Diospyros revaughanii* | (+++) | (+++) | (+++) |
| *Diospyros tesselleria* | (+++) | (+) | (+++) |
| *Erythroxylum sideroxyloides* | (+) | (+) | (+++) |
| *Eugenia elliptica* | (+++) | – | Tr |
| *Eugenia orbiculata* | (++) | – | (+++) |
| *Eugenia pollicina* | (+++) | – | (+++) |
| *Eugenia tinifolia* | (+) | – | (+) |
| *Fernelia buxifolia* | – | – | (+) |
| *Monimiastrum acutisepalum* | (++) | – | (+++) |
| *Myonima obovata* | (++) | – | (+++) |
| *Syzygium commersonii* | (++) | (++) | (+) |
| *Syzygium glomeratum* | Tr | – | (+++) |
| *Syzygium mauritianum* | (+++) | – | – |
| *Syzygium venosum* | Tr | – | (++) |
| *Trochetia boutoniana* | (++) | – | (++) |

(+++) = very prominent; (++) = prominent; (+) = present; tr = trace; (–) = not detected.
Estimated from the peak area of HPLC profiles.

Considerable attention has been focussed on the ability of phenolic rich plant extracts to induce apoptosis in cancer cell lines (Herman-Antosiewicz and Singh, 2004; D'Agostini *et al.*, 2005). Apoptosis has been proposed as a novel target for cancer prevention (Steele and Kelloff, 2005) and the rationale is the elimination of neoplastic cells that fail to respond to the cell regulatory signals. Along this line our group has screened 26 endemic plants extracts against the proliferation of the human breast cancer cell lines: MCF-7 and MDAMB 231 showed that *Eugenia orbiculata, Eugenia pollicina, Monimiastrum acutisepalum, Monimiastrum globosum, Syzygium commersonii, Syzygium mauritianum, Syzygium venosum* from the Myrtaceae family, *Myonima obovata* (Rubiaceae), *Cassine orientalis* (Celastraceae) and *Coffea macrocarpa* (Ebenaceae) potentially reduced the growth rate of these cancer cell lines. *E.pollicina* extract inhibited cell proliferation significantly and induced apoptosis in MCF-7 cells at a concentration of 0.5 mg FW/ml. Several experimental studies have suggested the importance of plant extracts and naturally occurring phytochemicals as inducers of apoptosis and their potential application as chemopreventive agents (Chiang *et al.*, 2005; Jo *et al.*, 2005). For instance the extract of *Ganoderma lucidum*, an oriental fungus, at a concentration of 500 μg/ml significantly inhibited the proliferation of MCF-7 cells and the antiproliferative effect was attributed to cell cycle arrest at G1 phase and also to the induction of apoptosis (Hu *et al.*, 2002). The ethanolic extract of *Solagrum nigrum* ripe fruits has been shown to inhibit the proliferation of human MCF-7 breast cancer cells and to induce cell death by apoptosis (Son *et al., 2003*). The mechanism underlying apoptotic induction by *E. pollicina* may result from the phenolic components which have been reported to induce apoptosis via multiple mechanisms in particular by triggering the CD95-CD95L signalling pathway; activating the caspases, decreasing the expression of Bcl-2 and cyclin D1, up-regulating p21 and proapoptotic protein Bax and by the MAPK activation that results in p53 up-regulation (Clement *et al.*, 1998; Hu *et al.*, 2002; She *et al.*, 2001; She *et al.*, 2002). However, this hypothesis needs to be comprehensively elucidated.

Our group has further substantiated the chemopreventive effect of the endemic extracts of *M. globosum, which* exhibited antigenotoxic effects on BaP-induced DNA migration in HepG2 cells (Mersch-Sundermann *et al.*, 2006). The exposure to relatively low concentrations of *M. globosum* (24.4 μgFW/ml culture medium) significantly inhibited the BaP-induced genotoxicity in HepG2 cells. A previous investigation in our laboratory had showed that the total phenolic, proanthocyanidin flavonoid contents of Mauritian endemic species from Eugenia (*E. elliptica, E. fasciculate, E. orbiculata*), Monimiastrum (*M. acutisepalum, M. globusum*) and Syzygium (*S. coriaceum, S. glomeratum, S. guehoii, S. Mauritianum, S. petrinense, S. venosum*) were proportionately associated with Cu,Zn-SOD promoter activity and inversely correlated with catalyse promoter activity suggesting that the chemopreventive potentials of the extracts might reside in their abilities to modulate the expression of antioxidant enzyme genes (Toyokuni *et al.*, 2003).

In addition substantial body of evidence from experimental studies has identified Gap Junction Intercellular Communication (GJIC) as a key target for chemoprevention (Passani *et al.*, 1998; Trosko *et al.*, 2005) and several naturally-occurring compounds including green tea, resveratrol, caffeic acid phenyl ester, epicatechin, ginsenoside $Rb_2$ have been shown to either upregulate GJIC in stem cells or prevent the down regulation of GJIC by tumour promoters (Kang *et al.*, 2000; Na *et al.*, 2000; Nielsen *et al.*, 2000; Sigler and Ruch, 1993). Mechanistic studies have shown that tumour promoters have the ability to down-regulate GJIC via the activation of protein kinase C, MAPK, hyperphosphorylation of the major gap junction protein called connexin 43, the disappearance of gap-junctional plaques in plasma membrane and also through an increase in intracellular $Ca^{2+}$ levels which can trigger closure or degradation of the gap junctions (Matesic *et al.*, 1994; Warn-Cramer *et al.*, 1998). Our work with endemic plants demonstrated that leaf extracts of *C. orientalis, E. pollicina* and *S. commersonii* significantly restored GJIC at a concentration of 0.5, 0.5 and 0.25 mg FW/ml respectively. The molecular mechanism of the preventive effect of the plant extracts on the inhibition of GJIC by $H_2O_2$ has to be further studied to provide additional details on the chemopreventive nature of the endemic plant extracts.

## 4.0 Conclusion

This review highlights the current status of traditional herbal medicine in Mauritius and the potentiality of the endemic flora as an important source of naturally occurring bioactive compounds, hence providing an impetus to delineate their possible uses as prophylactic agents. One of the major motivations of our investigations remains the deep concern regarding the declining number of endemic plant species (surveys have revealed that less than 1.9 per cent of the land area of the island supports native vegetation) and the subsequent lost of potential sources of phytochemical richness and antioxidant propensities. Considering the uniqueness of the Mauritian flora and its prophylactic propensity, there is an urge to reinforce existing conservation strategies to safeguard the threatened endemics with medicinal and potential therapeutic uses. This paper thus additionally provides for justification to the development of a sustained policy towards conservation.

The safety and efficacy of these products are of paramount importance and future perspective points to scientific research that will identify and/or confirm therapeutic benefits to these medicinal/endemic plants in order to validate efficacy. In addition the potential toxicity resulting from the interaction of plants' phytochemicals with conventional drugs also need to be addressed. Fallacies are often associated with use of traditional medicinal plant and include: (i) traditional plants, being natural are absolutely safe; (ii) traditional plants do not have side effects; (iii) efficacy can be obtained over a wide range of doses. Considering these viewpoints, pharmacological and toxicological studies are vital to establish the true value of the traditional plants. Further investigations on phytochemical discovery and subsequent screening on the endemic flora will surely open new opportunities to exploit their properties as chemopreventive agents and to develop pharmaceuticals based on their constituents. In fact this has been the driving force behind research of our group.

In addition to safety and efficacy, another important issue relating to the protection of knowledge, innovations and practices of traditional and indigenous medicine has been receiving increasing international attention in recent years. The Council of TRIPS of the WTO is revising articles in the respective agreements dealing with patent ability of traditional knowledge. Vast majority of plant resources originate from developing countries and it is to be recognized that traditional knowledge plays a key role in the protection and sustainable use of biodiversity. In the past, several multi-nationals corporations have exploited these resources by converting them into products of commercial value without paying compensation for the knowledge that was transferred with the material. At the Earth Summit in Rio in 1992, member states accepted the principle that bio-resources are the sole-property of sovereign states and that they have the freedom to use them as tradable commodities. However many countries have so far not enacted legislation to implement the resolutions passed at the Convention. While considering the protection of intellectual property rights of traditional medicine, the obligations of TRIPS/WTO must be taken into account. Many developing countries will need to revise their legislation in order to make it TRIPS compliant. Access to plant resources and the associated traditional knowledge can provide substantial benefits to companies and research institutions in both developing and developed countries. There is a growing concern that knowledge of traditional medicines is at times appropriated, adopted and patented by scientists and industry with little or no compensation to its custodians, and without their prior informed consent. The need to protect traditional medicine knowledge and to secure fair and equitable sharing of benefits derived from the use of biodiversity and associated traditional medicine knowledge have been fully recognized. At present, existing conventional patent law protection requirements are not applicable to 'traditional' knowledge and needs to be revisited.

## References


Abdin, M. Z., Israr, M., Rehman, R. U., Jain, S. K., 2003. Artemisinin, a novel antimalarial drug: biochemical and molecular approaches for enhanced production. Planta Med. (69); pp. 289–299.

Adjanohoun, E. J., Assi, L. A., Eymé, J., Gassita, J. N., Goudoté, Guého, J., Ip, F. S. L., Jackaria, D., Kalachand, S. K. K., Keita, A., Koudogbo, B., Landreau, D., Owadally, A. W., Soopramanien, A., 1983 Médecine traditionelle et pharmacopée: Contribution aux études ethnobotaniques et floristiques à Maurice (Iles Maurice et Rodrigue. ACCT; pp. 214.

Atkinson, R., Sevathian, J. C., 2005. A guide to the plants in Mauritius. Mauritius: Mauritius Wildlife Foundation.

Bahorun, T., Neergheen V.S.,. Soobrattee M.A, Luximon-Ramma V. A. And Aruoma O.I., 2007. Prophylactic phenolic antioxidants in functional foods of tropical island states of the Mascarene Archipelago (Indian Ocean). In Angiogenesis, Functional and Medicinal Foods, Ed: Jack Losso, Fareidoon Shahidi and Debasis Bagchi, Marcel Decker, Inc. New York; pp. 149-176.

Bahorun, T., Neergheen, V. S., Aruoma, O. I., 2005. Phenolic constituents of *Cassia fistula*: an overview. African Journal of Biotechnology (4); pp. 1530-1540

Bahorun, T., Gurib-Fakim A., and Aruoma O.I., 2003. Plant bioactive components as prophylactic agents. In Molecular and Therapeutic Aspects of Redox Biochemistry, T. Bahorun and A Gurib-Fakim, Ed; OICA International (UK) Limited; pp 171-189.

Beuscher, N., Bodinet, C., Neumann-Haefelin, D., Marston, A., Hostettmann, K., 1994. Antiviral activity of African medicinal plants. J. Ethnophramacology (42); pp101-109

Calixto, J. B., Beirith, A., Ferreira, J., Santos, A. R. S., Filho, V. C., Yunes, R. A., 2000. Naturallly occurring antinociceptive substances from plants. Phytother Res. (14,); pp. 401-418.

Cao, J., Ren, L. L., Liu, J. W., Li, Y., Qu, H. Y., 2004. Gene expression spectra in human leukemia HL-60 cells treated with EGCG. Mutat Res (556); pp. 193-200.

Cassidy, A., Teresa, S. P., Rimbach, G., 2003. Molecular mechanisms by which dietary isoflavones potentially prevent atherosclerosis. Exp Rev Mol Med (5); pp. 1-15.

Chapuis, J.C., Sordat, B., Hostettmann, K., 1988. Screening for cytotoxicity of plants used in traditional medicine J. Ethnopharmacol (23); pp. 273-284.

Chiang, L. C., Ng, L. T., Lin, I. C., Kuo, P. L., Lin, C. C., 2005. Anti-proliferative effect of apigenin and its apoptotic induction in human Hep G2 cells. Cancer Lett (11); pp 1-8.

Clement, M. V., Hirpara, J. L., Chawdhury, S. H., Pervaiz, S., 1998. Chemopreventive agent resveratrol, a natural product derived from grapes, triggers CD95 signalling dependent apoptosis in tumour cells. Blood (92); pp. 996-1002.

Cragg, G. M., 1998. Paclitaxel (Taxol): a success story with valuable lessons for natural product drug discovery and development. Med. Res. Rev. (18); pp. 315–331.

D'Agostini, F., Izzotti, A., Balansky, R. M., Bennicelli, C., De Flora, S., 2005. Modulation of apoptosis by cancer chemopreventive agents. Mutat Res. (591); pp. 173-186.

Daruty de Granpré, C. 1911. Plantes Médicinales de l'Ile Maurice et des pays intertropicaux. The Mauritius stationery and printing establishment R.de Spéville and Co2

Dijsselbloem, N., Berghe, W. V., Naeyer, A. D., Haegeman, G., 2004. Soy isoflavone phytochemicals in interleukin-6 affections. Multipurpose nutraceuticals at the crossroad of hormone replacement, anti-cancer and anti-inflammatory therapy. Biochem Pharmacol (68); pp. 1171-1185.

Erlund, I., 2004. Review of the flavonoids quercetin, hesperetin, and naringenin. Dietary sources, bioactivities, bioavailability and epidemiology. Nutr Res (24); pp. 851-874.

Ferguson, L. R., 2001. Role of plant polyphenols in genomic stability. Mutat Res (475); pp 89-111.

Fujiki, H., Suganuma, M., Kurusu, M., Okabe, S., Imayoshi, Y., Taniguchi, S., Yoshida, T., 2003. New TNF-$\alpha$ releasing inhibitors as cancer preventive agents from traditional herbal medicine and combination cancer prevention study with EGCG and sulindac or tamoxifen. Mutat Res (523-524); pp. 119-125.

Gopalsamy, N., Vargas, D., Gueho, J., Ricaud, C., Hostetmann, 1988. Saponins from leaves of Aphloia theiformis. Phytochem (27); pp. 3593-3595

Guého, J. 1988. La végétation de l'île Maurice. Edition de l'Ocean Indien, Mauritius.

Gurib-Fakim, A., Guého, J., 1996. Plantes médicinales de Maurice. Edition de l'Ocean Indien, Mauritius (Tome 2) pp. 531

Gurib-Fakim, A., Guého, J., 1995. Plantes médicinales de Maurice. Edition de l'Ocean Indien, Mauritius (Tome 1) pp. 485

Gurib-Fakim, A., Subratty, H., Narod, F., Govinden-Soulange, J., Mahomoodally, F., 2005. Biological activity from indigenous medicinal plants of Mauritius. Pure Appl. Chem. (77); pp. 41–51.

Gutteridge, J. M. C., 1995. Lipid peroxidation and antioxidants as biomarkers of tissue damage. Clin Chem (41); pp. 1819-1828.

Heeroo, R., 2000. Documentation of the weed status of exotic plants in Mauritius based on the records of the Mauritius Herbarium. Bsc Thesis, University of Mauritius.

Herman–Antosiewicz, A., Singh, S. V., 2004. Signal transduction pathways leading to cell cycle arrest and apoptosis induction in cancer cells by Allium vegetable-derived organosulfur compounds: a review. Mutat Res (555); pp 121-131.

Hou, Z., Lambert, J. D., Chin, K. V., Yang, C. S., 2004. Effects of tea polyphenols on signal transduction pathways related to cancer chemoprevention. Mutat Res (555); pp 3-19.

Hu, H., Ahn, N. S., Yang, X., Lee, Y. S., Kang, K. S., 2002. Ganoderma lucidum extract induces cell cycle arrest and apoptosis in MCF-7 human breast cancer cell. Int J Cancer (102); pp 250-253.

Ishige, K., Schubert, D., Sagara, Y., 2001. Flavonoids protect neuronal cells from oxidative stress by three distinct mechanisms. Free Radic Biol Med (30); pp 433-446.

Ivanova, D., Gerova, D., Chervenkov, T., Yankova, T., 2005. Polyphenol and antioxidant capacity of bulgarian medicinal plants. J Ethnopharm (96); pp. 145-150.

Jelager, L., Gurib-Fakim, A., Adsersen, A., 1999. Antibacterial and antifungal activity of some medicinal plants in Mauritius. Pharmaceutical Biol (36); pp 153-161.

Jo, E. H., Kim, S. H., Ra, J. C., Kim, S. R., Cho, S. D., Jung, J. W., Yang, S. R., Park, J. S., Hwang, J. W., Aruoma, O. I., Kim, T. Y., Lee, Y. S., Kang, K. S., 2005. Chemopreventive properties of the ethanol extract of Chinese licorice (Glycyrrhiza uralensis) root: induction of apoptosis and G1 cell cycle arrest in MCF-7 human breast cancer cells. Cancer Lett (230); pp 239-247.

Kang, K. S., Kang, B. C., Lee, B. J., Che, J. H., Li, G. X., Trosko, J. E., Lee, Y. S., 2000. Preventive effect of epicatechin and ginsenoside $Rb_2$ on the inhibition of gap junctinal intercellular communication by TPA and $H_2O_2$. Cancer Lett (152); pp 97-106.

Kehrer, J. P., 1993. Free radicals as mediators of tissue injury and disease. Crit Rev Toxicol (23); pp 21-48.

Kotowaroo, M. I., Mahomoodally, M. F., Gurib-Fakim, A., Subratty, A. H., 2006. Screening of traditional antidiabetic medicinal plants of Mauritius for possible alpha-amylase inhibitory effects in vitro. Phytother Res (20); pp. 228-231.

Kris-Etherton, P. M., Hecker, K. D., Bonanome, A., Coval, S. M., Binkoski, A. E., Hilpert, K. F., Griel, A. E., Etherton, T. D., 2002. Bioactive compounds in foods: their role in the prevention of cardiovascular disease and cancer. Am J Med (113); pp 71S-88S.

Maggs, G. L., Craven, P., Kolberg, H. H., 1998. Plant species richness, endemism, and genetic resources in Namibia. Biodiversity Cons (7); pp. 435–446.

Mahomoodally, M. F., Gurib-Fakim, A., Subratty, A. H., 2005. Antimicrobial activities and phytochemical profiles of endemic medicinal plants of Mauritius. Pharmaceutical Biol (430; pp. 237-242.

Mahomoodally, M. F., Gurib–Fakim, A., Subratty, A. H., 2005. Effects of Erythroxylum macrocarpum (Erythroxylaceae), an endemic medicinal plant of Mauritius, on the transport of monosaccharide, amino acid and fluid across rat everted intestinal sacs in vitro. J Cell Mol Biol (4); pp. 93-98.

Marie, D., 2000. The isolation and characterization of bioactive molecules from endemic medicinal plants of Mauritius. PhD Thesis, University of Mauritius, Mauritius.

Matesic, D. F., Rupp, H. L., Bonney, W. J., Ruch, R. J., Trosko, J. E., 1994. Changes in gap junction permeability, phosphorylation and number mediated by phorbol ester and non-phorbol ester tumor promoters in rat liver epithelial cells. Mol carcinogen (10); pp. 226–236.

McGregor, L., Bellangeon, M., Chignier, E., Lerond, L., Rouselle, C., McGregor, J. L., 1999. Effect of a micronized purified flavonoid fraction on in vivo platelet functions in the rat. Thrombosis Res (94); pp. 235-240.

Mersch-Sundermann, V., Bahorun, T., Stahl. T., Neergheen, V.S., Soobrattee, M.A., Aruoma, O.I., Wohlfarth, R., Sobel, R., Brunn, H.E., Schemeiser, T., 2006. Monimiastrum globusum, an endemic Mauritian plant, exhibited both DNA-damaging potency and chemopreventive effects towards BaP-induced genotoxicity in human derived cells. Toxicology in vitro (20); pp. 1427-1434

Na, H. K., Wilson, M. R., Kang, K. S., Chang, C. C., Grunberger, D., Trosko, J. E., 2000. Restoration of gap junctional intercellular communication by caffeic acid phenylester (CAPE) in a ras-transformed rat liver epithelial cell line. Cancer Lett (157); pp 31-38.

Neergheen, V. S., Bahorun T., Jen L-S, Aruoma O. I. 2007. Inhibition of lipid peroxidation and free radical scavenging potential of Mauritian endemic plants used in ethnomedicine. Pharmaceutical Biology (45); pp. 9-17

Neergheen, V. S., Soobrattee, M. A., Bahorun, T., Aruoma, O. I., 2006. Characterization of the phenolic constituents in Mauritian endemic plants as determinants of their antioxidant activities in vitro. J Plant Physiol. (163); pp 787-799.

Newman, D. J., Cragg, G. M., 2007. Natural products as sources of new drugs over the last 25 Years. J. Nat. Prod. (70); pp 461–477.

Newman, D. J., Cragg, G. M., Snader, K. M., 2003. Natural products as a source of new drugs over the period 1981–2002. J. Nat. Prod. (66); pp.1002–1037.

Nielsen, M., Ruch, R. J., Vang, O., 2000. Resveratrol reverses tumor promoter-induced inhibition of gap-junctional intercellular communication. Biochem Biophys Res Comm (275); pp. 804-809.

Owuor, E. D., Kong, A. T., 2002. Antioxidants and oxidants regulated signal transduction pathways. Biochem Pharmacol (64); pp. 765-770.

Passani, M. B., Luceri, C., Caderni, G., Dolara, P., 1998. Intercellular communication in normal and aberrant crypts of rat colon mucosa. Cancer Lett (123); pp 77-81.

Pedersen, O., Gurib-Fakim, A., Subratty, H., Adsersen, A., 1999. Pharmocological properties of seven medicinal plants of the Rubiaceae from Mauritius. Pharmaceutical Biol. (37); pp. 202-207.

Pettit, G. R., Hoard, M.S., Doubek, D. L., Schmidt, J. M., Pettit, R. K., Tackett, L.P., Chapuis, J.C., 1996. Antineoplastic agents 338. The cancer cell growth inhibitory. Constituents of *Terminalia arjuna* (Combretaceae). J. Ethnopharmacol. (53); pp 57-63.

Raskin, I., Ribnicky, D. M., Komarnytsky, S., Ilic, N., Poulev,A., Borisjuk, N., Brinker, A., Moreno, D. A., Ripoll, C., Yakoby, N., O'Neal, J. M., Cornwell, T., Pastor, I., Fridlender, B., 2002. Plants and human health in the twenty-first century Trends Biotechnol. (20); pp. 522–531.

Rangasamy, O., Raoelisen, G., Rakotoniriana F.E., Cheuk K., Urverg-Ratsimamanga S., Quetin-Leclercq J., Gurib-Fakim A., Subratty A.H. 2007. Screening for anti-infective properties of several medicinal plants of the Mauritian flora. J. Ethnopharmacol (109); pp. 331-337.

Scott, G., 1993. Medicinal and aromatic plants. Healthcare, economics and conservation in South Africa. Veld and Flora (79); pp 84-87.

She, Q. B., Bode, A. M., Ma, W. Y., Chen, N. Y., Dong, Z., 2001. Resveratrol induced activation of p53 and apoptosis is mediated by extracellular-signal-regulated protein kinases and p38 kinase. Cancer Res (61); pp 1604-1610.

She, Q. B., Huang, C., Zhang, Y., Dong, Z., 2002. Involvement of c-Jun NH (2)-terminal kinases in resveratrol-induced activation of p53 and apoptosis. Mol Carcinog (33); pp 244–250.

Sigler, K., Ruch, R. J., 1993. Enhancement of gap junctional intercellular communication in tumor promoter-treated cells by components of green tea. Cancer Lett (69); pp 15-19.

Son, Y. O., Kim, J., Lim, J. C., Chung, Y., Chung, G. H., Lee, J. C., 2003. Ripe fruits of Solanum nigrum L. inhibits cell growth and induces apoptosis in MCF-7 cells. Food Chem Toxicol (41); pp 1421-1428.

Soobrattee, M. A., Neergheen, V. S., Googoolye K., Aruoma O. I., Bahorun T. Phenolics content and antioxidant actions of the Rubiaceae, Ebanaceae, Celastraceae, Erythroxylaceae and Sterculaceae families of Mauritian endemic plants. Toxicology in vitro. Doi: 1001016/j.tiv.2007.07.012

Soobrattee, M. A., Neergheen, V. S., Luximon-Ramma, A., Aruoma, O. I., Bahorun, T., 2005. Phenolics as potential antioxidant therapeutic agents: Mechanism and actions. Mutat Res (579); pp 200-213.

Spignoli, G., 2000. Protective effects of dietary flavonoids on cardiovascular system and circulation. Eur Bull Drug Res (8); pp 1-8.

Steele, V. E., Kelloff, G. J., 2005. Development of cancer chemopreventive drugs based on mechanistic approaches. Mutat Res (591); pp 16-23.

Teague, W. E., Fuller, N. L., Rand, R. P., Gawrisch, K., 2002. Polyunsaturated lipids in membrane fusion events. Cell Mol Biol Lett (7); pp 262-264.

Toyokuni, S., Tanaka, T., Kawaguchi, W., Lai Fang, N. R., Ozeki, M., Akatsuka, S., Hiai, H., Aruoma, O. I., Bahorun, T., 2003. Effects of the phenolic contents of Mauritian endemic plant extracts promoter activities of antioxidant enzymes. Free Radic Res (37); pp 1215-1224.

Trosko, J. E., Chang, C. C., Upham, B. L., Tai, M. H., 2005. The role of human adult stem cells and cell-cell communication in cancer chemoprevention and chemotherapy strategies. Mutat Res (591); pp 187-197.

Warn-Cramer, B. J., Cottrell, G. T., Burt, J. M., Lau, A. F., 1998. Regulation of connexin 43-gap junctional intercellular communication by mitogen activated protein kinase. J Biol. Chem (273); pp 9188-9196.

*Chapter 50*

# Research on Some Indigenous Medicinal Plants of Myanmar

***Soe Soe Win***

*Lecturer, Department of Engineering Chemistry,*
*Mandalay Technological University, Mandalay, Myanmar*
*E-mail: soesoewinmdy@gmail.com*

## ABSTRACT

In Myanmar, the study of traditional indigenous plants and their uses in therapy plays a very important role. Potential medicinal plants for six priority diseases namely Malaria, Tuberculosis, Diabetes, Hypertension, Diarrhoea and Dysentery are studied extensively in Myanmar. Moreover, medicinal plants which are potential for anti-hepatitis, anti-HIV and anticancer are also being conducted. Botanical identification and preparation of extracts are made on respective plants. The effectiveness of herbal medicinal plants for anti-malarial activity as well as toxicity is being screened by using *In vitro* and *In vivo* methods. In addition, antibacterial and antifungal activities of the natural products of plants are being tested. Chromatographic methods are used for isolation of natural organic compounds. Structural identification and elucidation of isolated pure compounds are also done with spectroscopic methods. In the case of malaria, the isolated pure compounds are again tested for anti-malarial activity singly or after combining with other extracts or compounds. Only after having good results in *In vitro* tests, formulated drugs and extracts are tested to *Plasmodium falciparum* infected persons as a clinical trial for their activity as well as side effect with the permission of ethical committee from Myanmar. A pentacyclic triterpene compound, betulinic acid which was found to be reported an anti-HIV agent, anti-melanoma and anti inflammatory has been isolated (yield 1.34 per cent, m.p.286C) from a new plant source, *Tectona hamiltoniana* Wall locally known as Da-hat.

***Keywords:*** *Anti-malarial, Plasmodium falciparum, Tectona hamiltoniana Wall, Anti-HIV, Anti-melanoma, Anti-inflammatory, Spectroscopic methods.*

## 1.0 Introduction

As a vast country with diverse geographical and climatic conditions, Myanmar is home of the various plants. Many of them are traditionally used to cure various diseases. Traditional medicine has stood a long history of self-sufficiency even before the use of modern medicine in Myanmar. Researches are being carried out using traditional medicinal plants to develop reliable documents for herbal medicine.

Even the Head of state showed an immense interest on indigenous medicinal plants and his Excellency himself gave guidance on production of medicines for six major common diseases in Myanmar based on research of Myanmar traditional medicines, herbal plants and roots of medicinal plants. Systematic arrangements are being made for conducting research on potent Myanmar herbal plants, pilot plantation, conducting research on production and finding process in cooperation with ministries concerned (The New Light of Myanmar, 2004).

In Myanmar, the national health plan has been aimed to solve the problem of six priority diseases identified as top priority in accordance with their prevalence and their burden inflicted upon the health sectors (http://www.myanmar.com/newspaper/nlm). The six priority diseases include malaria, tuberculosis, diabetes, hypertension, diarrhoea and dysentery. One of the objectives is to effectively control and treat the diseases utilizing the locally available resources, including traditional drugs and indigenous practices. The main aim is to prevent the loss of valuable traditional remedies with time to under use, misuse and abuse following the lack of research, documentation and quality control.

## 2.0 Role of Herbal Medicine

According to Myanmar traditional medical belief, there are 96 diseases which afflict human kind. Using fresh or dried roots, stems, barks, leaves, buds and flowers of medicinal plants, and the hair, fat, bones and organs of certain insects, reptiles and mammals, Myanmar indigenous medicine is able to heal and cure all 96 maladies. Indigenous medicines are administered as powders, mixtures, decoctions, infusions, percolates, pastes, extracts, preserves, pills or tablets. (http://www.allmyanmar.com)

The utilization of traditional medicine is growing day by day, not only in Myanmar but also in very part of the world including both developing and developed countries. The quality of traditional medicines depends on good manufacturing practice and high quality plant based raw materials (Sein Win and Thein Swe, 2005).

Traditional medicine is a truly inherited profession whose development has interrelations with the natural and climatic conditions, thoughts and convictions and the social system of Myanmar. Throughout history and till now, it has been a potent medical science, helping raise health and fitness and intellectual level of Myanmar people.

Myanmar traditional medicine is a broad, deep and delicate branch of science covering various basic medical knowledge, different treatises, a diverse array of therapies and potent medicines. So, systematic preservation, protection and promotion are required for its perpetuation and flourishing. All will have to make collective efforts to integrate the different branches of traditional medicine into a comprehensive national medical science in essence through advanced standardization processes.

In accord with the vision, the government has been providing protection and assistance for the emergence of private firms manufacturing standard and harmless indigenous medicines. In addition, the Medical Research Departments of the government have been running research projects to accelerate scientific development of the traditional medicine. The programmes which are to discover effective drugs and record their potencies; to produce potent drugs for common diseases; to set up herbal gardens for medicinal plant conservation; to promote potent traditional medicines; to discover effective therapies that can cure diseases incurable by the western drugs; and to find means to treat patients with the combined potency of the western and traditional medicines; are being carried out by the government research centres for scientific development of Myanmar traditional medicine.

Every year traditional medicine practitioners from all over the nation assemble at the conference, exchanging knowledge and holding discussions with unity for perpetuation and propagation of Myanmar traditional medicine, for the standardized progress of the science and for providing more effective and broader health care services through the profession. Truly, the practice of convening the annual conference will bring good results not only to the field of traditional medicine, but also to the nation and the people ((http://www.Myanmar.information.net).

## 3.0 Status of Research on Herbal Medicinal Plants

Throughout the world today, especially in the developing countries, people has been focusing on the value of medicinal plants in treating and preventing common diseases such as AIDS, malaria, hepatitis, diabetic, and so on. Much scientific work has been done to isolate and identify the chemical constituents and the active principles from these plants which ensure the therapeutic effect to a particular disease.

Also in Myanmar, the study of traditional plants and their uses in therapy plays a very important role. Many Research Departments which are placed under various Ministries are doing research work, either directly or indirectly on indigenous medicinal plants.

Ministry of Health, Ministry of Industry (1) and Ministry of Science and Technology are the three main Ministries which are carrying out research work on herbal medicinal plants. In addition, under the Ministry of Education, the Department of Chemistry is the main Department, where extensive research papers are being produced on medicinal plants. Assignments or Thesis Topics are given to MSc and PhD candidates, who work on the specific plants to extract, isolate and identify the chemical constituents and the compounds present in those plants, and to test the bioactivity of the isolated compounds. *In vivo* as well as *in vitro* examinations are being carried out. Tests with various strains of viruses, bacteria and micro organisms are also carried out in the course of their work. The chemical structures of isolated compounds are also elucidated by modern spectroscopic methods such as UV, FT-IR, Mass Spectral analysis, and NMR etc.

Ministry of Forestry and Ministry of Agriculture are two Ministries which support and help the research proceedings through supplying the plant raw materials, in many cases cultivating and planting the needed kinds of plants.

Guidance and instructions as well as strong support have been given by the Government to promote production and distribution of herbal medicines for the above mentioned six major prevailing diseases. The concerning Ministries and the Departments are making much effort to fulfil the Guideline and Instructions of the Government. Some achievements and research progress will be presented in this paper.

## 3.1 Ministry of Science and Technology

In Myanmar, the Ministry of Science and Technology (MOST) takes responsibility for development in the field of science and technology and it is organized with six departments.

Under the Ministry of Science and Technology, there are Departments in which extensive research works have being carried out on medicinal plants for six major diseases namely malaria, tuberculosis, diabetes, hypertension, diarrhoea and dysentery. Moreover, researches of medicinal plants which are potential for anti-hepatitis, anti-HIV and anticancer are also being conducted.

They are Pharmaceutical Research Departments (PRD) in Yangon and Kyaukse, Department of Biotechnology, and Department of Engineering Chemistry in Mandalay Technological University.

Vision of the Departments are to conduct research for a variety of region-wise medicinal plants for various diseases, to produce potential herbal medicine for better health care and to ensure fully effective drug for consumption. Pharmaceutical Research Departments as well as Department of Engineering Chemistry are carrying out research on medicinal plants and collaborative activities are also made with the department of Biotechnology with the aim to promote the role of herbal medicine with approved scientific data especially for malaria.

## 3.2 Development Strategy for Herbal Medicinal Products

Botanical identification and preparation of extracts were made. The effectiveness of herbal medicinal plants for anti-malarial activity as well as toxicity is being screened by using *In vitro* and *In vivo* methods. In addition, antibacterial and antifungal activities of the natural products of plants are being tested. Chromatographic methods are used for isolation of natural organic compound. Structural identification and elucidation of isolated pure compounds were also done with spectroscopic methods.

Myanmar medicinal plants which are potential for anti-malarial were extracted and isolated to obtain pure compounds. The isolated pure compounds are again tested for anti-malarial activity singly or after combining with other extracts or compounds. Only after having good results in *In vitro* tests, formulated drugs and extracts are tested to *Plasmodium falciparum* infected persons as a clinical trial for their activity as well as side effect with the permission of ethical committee from Myanmar. Some examples are: Different medicinal plant extracts and pure compounds from *Plumbago zeylanica* Linn, *Piper aurantiacum* Wall., *Zingiber officinale* Rose., *Momordica dioica* Roxb., *Trewia nudiflora* Linn, *Caesalpinia bonducella* Flem., *Scoparia dulcis* Linn, *Blumea balsamifera* DC. *Swietenia macrophylla* King, *Cassia siamea* Lam, *Andropogon citratus* DC. and *Piper longum* Linn were made and tested for their anti-malarial activity.

Conducted research findings and the results from the research departments are collected and published through various Journals and Media in order to give information to the traditional medicine practitioners as well as to the public. A combined Research report (in Myanmar language) has been published as Vol. 1 and Vol. 2 in 2002 entitled "The effective Myanmar Medicinal Plants" in which research reports for 67 medicinal plants are described in detail. The book "Potential plants for Malaria and Other Diseases" (in Myanmar language) including research reports of 25 plants has also been published. In addition, research articles for some Myanmar medicinal plants are issued in the Journal of Myanmar Academy and Technology (JMAT). Some more publications are still under process. Moreover, there are 124 medicinal plants which have been screened for bioactivity. Myanmar traditional medicine can be considered to have entered new era, becoming more scientific, it has gained wide acceptance and has now been incorporated into curriculum in University of Medicine.

The research on medicinal plants corresponding to the diseases such as diarrhoea, dysentery, diabetes as well as anti-tumour and anticancer are carried out by some M. Sc and Ph.D. candidates from the Technological Universities under the Ministry of Science and Technology for their thesis. At present, determination of the activity of medicinal plants for anti tuberculosis is also being conducted and achieved success to some extent.

In Myanmar, there are many medicinal plants which are not much under investigation. According to Literature survey (San Khin U., 1969; Tha Myat U., 1972; MOST, 2002; MOST, 2003), some useful medicinal plants are described in the Tables 50.1–50.7.

## 4.0 Other Related Ministries

### 4.1 Ministry of Health

The Ministry has seven functioning departments. They are Department of Health Planning, Department of Health, Department of Medical Science, Department of Medical Research (Lower Myanmar), Department of Medical Research (Upper Myanmar), Department of Medical Research (Central Myanmar) and Department of Traditional Medicine. All these departments are further divided according to their functions and responsibilities. Maximum community participation in health activities is encouraged. Collaboration with related departments and social organizations has been promoted by the ministry. Among them Department of Medical Research (Lower Myanmar), Department of Medical Research (Upper Myanmar), Department of Medical Research (Central Myanmar) and Department of Traditional Medicine are carrying out the research on herbal medicinal plants. (http://www.moh.gov.mm/file/Health%20Infrastructure.pdf.)

**Table 50.1: Some Useful Myanmar Medicinal Plants for the Treatment of Malaria**

| Sl.No. | Myanmar Name | Scientific Name | Family Name | Parts Used |
|---|---|---|---|---|
| 1. | Kathawbok | *Cassia occidentalis* L. | Caesalpiniaceae | Root |
| 2. | Kaphi | *Coffee arabica* L. | Rubiaceae | Leaves, Fruit |
| 3. | Kyaung-ban-gyi | *Vitex negundo* L. | Verbenaceae | Leaves |
| 4. | Kyaung-ban | *Vitex trifolia* L. | Verbenaceae | Leaves |
| 5. | Kyet-hin-ga | *Momordica charantia* | Cucurbitaceae | Leaves, Fruit |
| 6. | Ka-det | *Cratavea religiosa* | Capparidaceae | Bark |
| 7. | Kha-ye | *Mimusops elengi* | Sapotaceae | Bark |
| 8. | Khan-dauk | *Thalictrum foliolosum* DC. | Ranunculaceae | Root |
| 9. | Khu-than | *Hymenodictyon excelsum* | Rubiaceae | Bark |
| 10. | Nga-yok-kaung | *Piper nigrum* L. | Piperaceae | Seed |
| 11. | Say-ga-gyi | *Andrographis paniculata* | Acanthaceae | Whole Plant |
| 12. | Sindon-ma-nwe | *Tinospora cordifolia* | Menispermaceae | Bark, Leaves |
| 13. | Sa-nwin | *Curcuma longa* L. | Zingiberaceae | Rhizome |
| 14. | Pazun-sa | *Alternanthera sessilis* R.Br. | Amaranthaceae | Whole Plant |
| 15. | Taung-mayo | *Alstonia scholaris* R.Br. | Apocynaceae | Leaves, Bark |

**Table 50.2: Some Useful Myanmar Medicinal Plants for the Treatment of HIV**

| Sl.No. | Myanmar Name | Scientific Name | Family Name | Parts Used |
|---|---|---|---|---|
| 1. | Kyaung-sha | *Oroxylum indicum* | Bignoniaceae | Bark |
| 2. | Kyet-hin-ga | *Momordica charantia* | Cucurbitaceae | Leaves, Fruit |
| 3. | Danta-thu-kha | *Scoparia dulcis* L. | Scrophulariaceae | Whole Plant |
| 4. | Pon-nyet | *Calophyllum inophyllum* L. | Guttiferae | Bark |
| 5. | Phan-ga | *Terminalia chebula* | Combretaceae | Fruit, Bark |
| 6. | Ye-chin-ya | *Flueggea microcapa* | Euphorbiaceae | Bark |
| 7. | Kon-chin-ya | *Flueggea leucopyrus* Willd. | Euphorbiaceae | Bark |
| 8. | Ye-yo | *Morinda angustifolia* Roxb. | Rubiaceae | Fruit |
| 9. | Thanat-kha | *Limonia crenulata* | Rutaceae | Leaves |
| 10. | Thara-phi | *Calophyllum amoenum* | Guttiferae | Bark |
| 11. | Thetyin-gyi | *Croton oblongifolius* Muell. | Euphorbiaceae | Root |
| 12. | Ada-lut | *Curcuma angustifolia* | Zingiberaceae | Rhizome |
| 13. | Thit-sein | *Terminalia belerica* | Combretaceae | Bark |
| 14. | Da-hat | *Tectona hamiltoniana* Wall. | Verbenaceae | Bark |
| 15. | Taw-banda | *Terminalia catappa* | Combretaceae | Bark |

**Table 50.3: Some Useful Myanmar Medicinal Plants for the Treatment of Hepatitis B**

| *Sl.No.* | *Myanmar Name* | *Scientific Name* | *Family Name* | *Parts Used* |
|---|---|---|---|---|
| 1. | Ka-nyut | *Asparagus officinalis* | Liliaceae | Root |
| 2. | Kyeik-hman | *Eclipta alba* Hask. | Compositae | Whole Plant |
| 3. | Kon-khaya | *Argemone mexicana* L. | Papaveraceae | Latex |
| 4. | Gon-ga-man | *Crocus sativus* L. | Iridaceae | Pollen |
| 5. | Zee-byu | *Emblica officinalis* Gaertn. | Euphorbiaceae | Fruit |
| 6. | Thinbaw Zee-byu | *Phyllanthus distichus* Muell. | Euphorbiaceae | Seed |
| 7. | Dan-gyi | *Lawsonia inermis* L. | Lythraceae | Bark |
| 8. | Payan-nawa | *Boerhaavia diffusa* L. | Nyctaginaceae | Whole Plant |
| 9. | Pan-tama | *Melia azedarach* L. | Meliaceae | Leaves, Bark |
| 10. | Pauk-pan-byu | *Sesbania grandiflora* Pers. | Papilionaceae | Leaves, Bark |
| 11. | Pinzein-net | *Ocimum sanctum* L. | Labiatae | Leaves, Root |
| 12. | Mahogany | *Swietenia microphylla* King. | Meliaceae | Seed |
| 13. | Min-go-ga | *Argyreia bargigera* Chois. | Convolvulaceae | Root |

**Table 50.4: Some Useful Myanmar Medicinal Plants for the Treatment of Cancer**

| *Sl.No.* | *Myanmar Name* | *Scientific Name* | *Family Name* | *Parts Used* |
|---|---|---|---|---|
| 1. | Thin-baw-manyo | *Catharanthus roseus* | Apocynaceae | Whole plant |
| 2. | Kyauk-htin-shu | *Taxus baccata* L. | Taxacaceae | Leaves, Fruit |
| 3. | Ye-yo | *Morinda angustifolia R*oxb. | Rubiaceae | Fruit |
| 4. | Kyat-thon-byu | *Allium sativum* L. | Liliaceae | Rhizome |
| 5. | Sha-saung-laput | *Aloe vera* L. | Aloaceae | Leaves |
| 6. | Mayo | *Calotropics procera* | Asclepiadaceae | Whole plant |
| 7. | Kyet-hin-ga | *Momordica charantia* | Cucurbitaceae | Fruit |
| 8. | Su-lar-na-pha | *Oldenlandia diffusa* Roxb. | Rubiaceae | Whole plant |
| 9. | Piset | *Eupatorium odoratum* L. | Asteraceae | Flowers |
| 10. | Tha-la‘ | *Punica granatum* L. | Punicaceae | Fruit shell |
| 11. | Pan-tama | *Melia dubia* Cav. | Meliaceae | Leaves, Bark |
| 12. | Ngu-shwe-wa | *Cassia fistula* L. | Caesalpiniaceae | Fruit |
| 13. | Tabin-tai-mya-nan | *Vitis repens* | Vitaceae | Rhizome |
| 14. | Da-hat | *Tectona hamiltoniana* Wall. | Verbenaceae | Bark |

**Table 50.5: Some Useful Myanmar Medicinal Plants for the Treatment of Tuberculosis**

| Sl.No. | Myanmar Name | Scientific Name | Family Name | Parts Used |
|---|---|---|---|---|
| 1. | Gamon-kyet-thun-byu | *Fritillaria roylei Hook.* | Liliaceae | Bulbs |
| 2. | Sein-na-ban | *Lantana camara* L. | Verbenaceae | Leaves, Root |
| 3. | Taw-lay-nyin | *Jussiaea suffruiticosa* L. | Onagraceae | Whole Plant |
| 4. | Pan-tama | *Melia azedarach* L. | Meliaceae | Leaves, Bark |
| 5. | Maya-gyi | *Adhatoda vasica Nees.* | Acanthaceae | Leaves |
| 6. | Lauk-thae | *Desmodium triqueterum DC.* | Papilionaceae | Leaves |
| 7. | Shaw-byu | *Sterculia foetida L.* | Sterculiaceae | Leaves, Seed |
| 8. | Thanat | *Cordia dichotoma* Frost. | Boraginaceae | Fruit |

**Table 50.6: Some Useful Myanmar Medicinal Plants for the Treatment of Diabetes**

| Sl.No. | Myanmar Name | Scientific Name | Family Name | Parts Used |
|---|---|---|---|---|
| 1. | Kinbon | *Coccinea indica* W. and A. | Cucurbitaceae | Leaves, |
| 2. | Kabaung-ye-kyi | *Strychnos potatorum* L. | Loganiaceae | |
| 3. | Zawgyi-mok-seik | *Nardostachys jatamansi* | Valerianaceae | Root |
| 4. | Kyet-hin-ga | *Momordica charantia* L. | Cucurbitaceae | Leaves, Fruit |
| 5. | Yar-khan-hwhite | *Gymnema acuminatum* Wall. | Asclepiacaceae | Leaves, Root |
| 6. | Danta-thu-kha | *Scoparia dulcis* L. | Scrophulariaceae | Whole Plant |
| 7. | Peik-thingat | *Cassia auriculata* L. | Caesalpiniaceae | Flower |
| 8. | Pyiban-nyo | *Cassia glauca* Lam. | Caesalpiniaceae | Leaves, Flower |
| 9. | Beda | *Eichhornia crassipes* Solms. | Pontederiaceae | Flower |
| 10. | Tha-kyar-ma-kite | *Orthosiphon aristatus* | Labiatae | Leaves |
| 11. | Thabye | *Syzygiumcumini* L. | Myrtaceae | Seed |
| 12. | Ega-yit | *Millingtonia hortensis* L. | Bignoniaceae | Leaves |
| 13. | Zee-byu | *Emblica officinals* Gaertn. | Euphorbiaceae | Fruit |
| 14. | Thit-kyabo | *Cinamomum tamala* F.Nees. | Lauraceae | Bark |

### 4.1.1 Department of Medical Research (Lower Myanmar)

The Department of Medical Research (DMR) was first established in 1963. It was expanded in 1990 and further reorganized as Department of Medical Research (Lower Myanmar). The missions of the Department are: to conduct biomedical research; to promote, support, organize and coordinate all biomedical research in the country; to provide the infrastructure necessary for effective biomedical research; and to provide training in health research. It consists of six research centres; Socio-Medical Research Centre, Bio-Medical Research Centre, Clinical Research Centre, Diagnostic and Vaccine Research Centre, National Blood Research Centre, National Poison Control

Centre and one Hepatitis B vaccine plant. The Department has carried out research in anaemia, ascariasis, dengue haemorrhagic fever, diabetes, diarrhoea, dysentery, health systems research, hepatitis, HIV/AIDS, human reproductive health, hypertension, leprosy, malaria, nutrition, snake bite, sport medicine, toxicology, traditional medicine, tuberculosis and hepatitis B vaccine production (http://www.moh.gov.mm/file/Health%20Infrastructure.pdf).

**Table 50.7: Some Useful Myanmar Medicinal Plants for the Treatment of Diarrhoea and Dysentery**

| Sl.No. | Myanmar Name | Scientific Name | Family Name | Parts Used |
|---|---|---|---|---|
| 1. | Kok-ko | *Albizzia lebbek* Benth. | Mimosaceae | Leaves, Bark |
| 2. | Kyaung-sha | *Oroxylum indicum* | Bognoniaceae | Fruit, Bark |
| 3. | Kabaung-gyi | *Strychnos nux-vomica* L. | Loganiaceae | Root |
| 4. | Ngu-shwewa | *Cassia fistula* L. | Caesalpiniaceae | Root, Bark |
| 5. | Sein-na-ban | *Lantana camara* L. | Verbenaceae | Root, Bark |
| 6. | Sa-nwin phyu | *Curcuma zedoaria* Rose. | Zingiberaceae | Root |
| 7. | Pinle-ka-bwee | *Casuarina equisetifolia* Forst. | Casuarinaceae | Bark |
| 8. | Peik-thingat | *Cassia auriculata* L. | Caesalpiniaceae | Whole Plant |
| 9. | Pan-nu | *Saussurea lappa* Clarke. | Compositae | Whole Plant |
| 10. | Ponna-yeik | *Ixora coccinea* | Rubiaceae | Root |
| 11. | Thit-sein | *Terminalia bellerica* Roxb. | Combretaceae | Fruit, Bark |

### 4.1.2 Department of Medical Research (Upper Myanmar)

Department of Medical Research (Upper Myanmar) was established in Pyin Oo Lwin in 2001. Aiming to conduct studies on Traditional Medicine and herbal plants, herbal medicinal plants all over the country are collected and nurtured in the herbal garden of DMR (Upper Myanmar). Current Research activities undertaken in DMR (Upper Myanmar) includes study on efficacy of some traditional medicine formularies used for treating common diseases in Myanmar, especially in treatment of diabetes mellitus, hypertension, and malaria (http://www.moh.gov.mm/file/Health%20Infrastructure.pdf).

### 4.1.3 Department of Medical Research (Central Myanmar)

A newly established department is situated in central Myanmar at Pyinmanar and has become operation since 2003. Research activities can be expanded further and more collaborative research activities can be undertaken with health and medical universities situated in central and upper Myanmar. As science graduates could be recruited locally, the department is also creating new jobs and opportunities for the advancement for the local youths. Preliminary studies and surveys on malaria and rubella infections in Pyinmanar Township have been conducted (http://www.moh.gov.mm/file/Health%20Infrastructure.pdf).

#### 4.1.4 Department of Traditional Medicine

The Department of Traditional Medicine is one of the departments under the Ministry of Health. The department has 4 major sections with one university and one institute. There are two 50 bedded traditional medicine hospitals and 12 sixteen bedded hospitals situated each in one state and division throughout the country. There are 237 township traditional medicine clinics over the country providing the basic traditional medical treatment at the primary health care level. Traditional medicine used for health care delivery is produced from two pharmaceutical factories under the Department of Traditional Medicine and distributed free of charge to the public (Sein Win and Thein Swe, 2005).

#### 4.1.5 Production of Traditional Medicine Drugs

There are two pharmaceutical factories under the Department of Traditional Medicine. One is situated in Yangon, which produced drugs for lower Myanmar and another one situated in Mandalay which produced drugs for upper Myanmar. The drugs are formulated according to the officially recognized Myanmar Traditional Medicine Formularies or pharmacopoeia (Sein Win and Thein Swe, 2005).

The total of 232 different kinds of raw materials is used to formulate the traditional drugs. Among them 183 (79 per cent) are from plant origin and other from animal origin, minerals and aquatic origin. Main parts used of medicinal plants are stem and root. Flower, leaf, bark, rhizome, fruits are also used in formulation. Most of the raw materials are available in the country, some bought from the raw material dealers and some obtained from the herbal garden and cultivation (Sein Win and Thein Swe, 2005).

### 4.2 Ministry of Industry (1)

#### 4.2.1 Myanmar Pharmaceutical Industries (MPI)

Myanmar Pharmaceutical Industries (MPI) is one of the six state-owned Myanmar Industries under the Ministry of Industry (1) engaged in the production of variety of specific pharmaceutical and consumer goods.

Under MPI, there are altogether 20 factories at present. Those factories consist of Myanmar Pharmaceutical Factory, Soap Factories, Soap Raw Oil Factory, Plastic Factories and Cosmetic Industry. Apart from these factories there is a Development Centre for Pharmaceutical Technology in Gyogon, Yangon that was established by the financial and technical assistance of Japanese International Cooperation Agency. In addition to, the projects of New Pharmaceutical Factory (Pyin Oo Lwin) and New Pharmaceutical Factory (Inyaung) are under implementation stage, and the Spirulina Microalgae Factory (Myanmar Spirulina Factory) in Yekhar, Sagaing division is recently implemented and now entering into full swing production stage.

Myanmar Pharmaceutical factory is producing the range of commodities for pharmaceutical and related products in the form of powder, liquid, Ointment, tablets and capsules (including provimin tablets), injections (including liquid transfusion in plastic bottles), biological products (including Anti-snake Venoms) (http://www.myanmar.gov.mm).

## 5.0 Private Industries in Myanmar

Production of herbal products is now developing according to the encouragement for systematic development by the Government. Public trust is more concentrated on natural products for their effectiveness, reliability and safety for long term use. The private sector also sees the emergence of modern traditional medicine and herbal products industries.

There are also more than 1000 private traditional medicine manufacturers and they produced various kinds of traditional drugs according to the Traditional Drug Law promulgated in 1996 (Sein Win and Thein Swe, 2005).

Private industries such as FAME pharmaceutical Co Ltd, Kyaw Traditional Medicine, Tun Shwe War Traditional Medicine are well-known industries in Myanmar.

FAME pharmaceutical Co Ltd has been manufacturing a variety of herbal products from *Garnodama lucidum*, *Tinospora cordifolia*, *Panax ginseng*, *Ginkgo biloba*, *Hyperium perforatum*, *Brucea javanica Momordica charantia*, and *Morinda citrifolia*. In addition antimalarial drug including plant extracts from *Dichroa febrifuga*, *Artimisia annua* and *Coptis teeta*; and spirullina products are also produced.

## 6.0 Results and Discussion

Medicinal plants were screened for their anti-malarial activity in the ministry of Science and Technology. The potential medicinal plants for anti-malarial were extracted and isolated to obtain pure compounds.

The drugs are formulated by combined plant extracts as well as pure compounds. With the permission of ethical committee from Myanmar, formulated drugs and extracts are tested on *Plasmodium falciparum* infected persons as a clinical trial for their activity as well as side effect.

Regarding the *in vitro* antimalarial activity of the plant extracts after screening, potential plants including *Valeriana wallichii*, *Trewia nudiflora* Linn and *Piper longum* Linn (Sa Bai, 2002), *Tridax procumbens* Linn, *Clerodendum serratum*, *Caesalpinia crista*, *Alstonia scholaris* R.Br., *Zigiber officinale*, and *Cyperus rotundas* Linn (MOST, 2002) are noted for their activity *in vitro* and some are in the progress for *in vivo* in the Department of Biotechnology.

Clinical trial to *Plasmodium falciparum* infected patients for their effectiveness of some herbal drugs and plant extracts are planned to be conducted by collaboration with other Ministries.

The study for diarrhoea and dysentery reveals that polar extracts (Water extract, 95 per cent EtOH extract and 50 per cent EtOH extract) are effective for *In vitro* test. *Leucania gluca*, *Quisqualis indica*, *Eugenia jambolana*, *Euphorbia splendens* and *Piperbetal* are promising traditional medicinal plants (Nwe Yee Win *et al.*, 2001).

Clinical trials on dysentery patients were conducted at the Clinical Research Unit (Traditional Medicine). It was found that giving 5 kernels of *Brucea javanica* once a day for 5 days possess strong amoebicidal action, and effectively curing the dysentery with little or no adverse effects. *In vivo* study showed that the effect of watery extract of *Orthosiphon aristatus* is found to be potential for diabetes mellitus. (http://www.moh.gov.mm).

A pentacyclic triterpene compound, betulinic acid which was found to be reported an anti-HIV agent, anti-melanoma and anti-inflammatory has been isolated (yield 1.34 per cent, m.p.286C) from a new source of Myanmar indigenous plant, *Tectona hamiltoniana* Wall locally known as Da-hat by solvent extraction, column separation and structural elucidation methods using chromatographic techniques (Soe Soe Win *et al.*, 2006).

Research out comings is being compiled and some papers are now in process for publication. Some plant extracts are planned to pursue further research up to the stage of clinical trials. After obtaining permission from ethical committee for drug control, the process of formulating Drugs and clinical trials will be continued and fruitful results are hoped to be materialised in the near future.

DMR LM has successfully produced hepatitis B vaccine with mass production in the near future. Medical research work has been developing in Myanmar since 1970 and is now flourishing, with several major medical research projects in progress. Currently, herbal research places its emphasis on treatments for malaria, tuberculosis, diabetes, hypertension, dysentery and diarrhoea (http://www.moh.gov.mm).

DMR LM transferred research findings on hypoglycaemic drug and anti-amoebic drug to the Department of Traditional Medicine and Myanmar Pharmaceutical Factory for mass production. DMR LM is also conducting anti-TB activity on five Myanmar medicinal plants on *in-vitro* and *in vivo* toxicity studies. A clinical trial is also being carried out on TB patients and the results have been found to be promising (http://www.moh.gov.mm).

Medicinal plants were screened for their anti-hypertensive activity at the DMR. *Plantago major* Linn was found to be most promising in animal models. The plant was further subjected to short-term and long term studies in humans. Plants for hypertension have now been scientifically documented for clinical use (http://www.moh.gov.mm).

Ministry of Health is concerned with the aspect of disease control, treatment of malaria, drug production procurement and finally to conduct research against malaria. Technical transfer of research findings to the Myanmar Pharmaceutical Industry under the Ministry of Industry (1) was affected for mass production and for economic and safe use by the community.

In connection with the production of anti-malaria drugs, research on vaccines was conducted successfully from the Ministry of Industry-1. The important anti-malarial drugs such as quinine from cinchona bark and artemisinine compounds from *Artemisia annua* can now be produced locally without importation or outside assistance (The New Light of Myanmar September 27, 2004).

Although some medicines have not been produced on a commercial scale, their potency levels have been tested and some pilot productions have been performed.

## 7.0 Conclusion

Overall, it can be concluded that all the above research and developments have been undertaken under the guidance of the Head of State with a strong support from the National Health Committee.

The departments from different ministries are conducting scientific and advanced research on potential traditional drugs and therapies; recording their potency levels; launching research project to manufacture traditional medicines to cure common diseases of the nation and also to try out ways to treat weird diseases that are incurable with the modern medicines; and inventing new treatments through combination of modern medicine, advanced hospital equipments and indigenous medicine.

Systematic arrangements are being made for conducting research on potent Myanmar herbal plants, establishing pilot plantation and conducting research on production processes in cooperation with other related ministries concerned so that the country will have a reliable health care system with the aid of indigenous herbal medicine.

## Acknowledgements

I especially wish to express my most sincere thanks and deepest gratitude to His Excellency, the Honourable Minister U Thaung, Ministry of Science and Technology, for his permission to attend the International Workshop on: "Herbal Medicinal Plants and Traditional Herb Remedies, Hanoi, Vietnam, 20-21 September 2007".

My grateful thanks are also due to Dr. Ko Ko Oo, Director General, Department of Atomic Energy for sending necessary document and information for this workshop.

I also wish to sincere thanks to the Centre for Science and Technology of the Non-Aligned and Other Developing Countries (NAM S&T Centre) as well as Institute of Natural Products Chemistry (INPC), Vietnamese Academy of Science and Technology (VAST), Hanoi, Vietnam.

## References

Bai, S., July, 2002. Screening of Antibacterial and Antimalarial Activities of Some Medicinal Plants" Department of Engineering Chemistry, Yangon Technological University Yangon Myanmar.

http://www.allmyanmar.com, Traditionnal Medicine Myanmar.

http://www.moh.gov.mm.

http://www.myanmar.gov.mm.

http://www.moh.gov.mm/file/Health%20Infrastructure.pdf.

http://www.myanmar.information.net, Myanmar Information Committee, November 26, 2006

MOST (Ministry of Science and Technology), 2002. The Effective Myanmar Medicinal Plants (In Myanmar language), 1 and 2, Win Light Colour, Yangon.

MOST (Ministry of Science and Technology), 2003. The Potential Myanmar Medicinal Plants for Malaria and Other Diseases (In Myanmar Language), Shwe Hin Tha, Yangon.

San Khin U., 1969. Some Medicinal and Useful Plants, both Indigenous and Exotic of Burma (Botanical, English and Burmese Names and Family).

Tha Myat U., 1972. A Dictionary of Medicinal Plants in eleven Languages, Agricultural Corporation, Yangon Myanmar.

The New Light of Myanmar September 27, 2004. Potent medicines can be produced for six major common diseases. Work coordination meeting 1/2004 of committee for production of medicines for six major diseases held. http://www.myanmar.com/newspaper/nlm.

Win, N.Y., Nyein, M.M., Wynn, N., Myint, W., Myint, S.H. and Khine, M., January, 2001. Antibacterial and Activities of selective Myanmar Medicinal Plants. JMAT (Journal of Myanmar Academy of Technology) (1(1); pp.75-88.

Win, S. and Swe, T., 2005. Herbal Gardens and Cultivation of Medicinal Plants in Myanmar. Regional Consultation on Development of Traditional Medicine in the South East Asia Region, Pyongyang, DPR Korea, 22-24 June 2005.

Win, S.S., Aye, M., Khine, M. and Wynn, N., 2006. Isolation and Structural Assingnment of the Anti-HIV Agent (Betulinic Acid) from New Plant Source, the back of *Tectona Hamiltoniana* Wall (Da-hat). JMAT (Journal of Myanmar Academy of Technology) (6(1-2)); pp. 28-36.

## *Chapter 51*

# Status of Medicinal Plants and Prospects of their Cultivation in Dang

***Chiranjivi Regmi***
*Nepal Academy of Science and Technology,*
*Khumaltar, P.O.Box 3323, Kathmandu, Nepal*
*E-mail: cregmi@hotmail.com*

## ABSTRACT

Nepal is rich in biodiversity due to its vertical microclimatic zones ranging from tropical to alpine due to the altitudinal variation of the topography. Nepal's share of world's land is no more than 0.1 per cent but the country is ranked between 25 and 30 positions in global context and 11th position in the continental scale of biodiversity richness. In this relatively small, area, more than 700 species of medicinal plants have been reported, of which 250 species are endemic to the country. Nepal Academy of Science and Technology (NAST) and Nepal Sanskrit University (NSU) jointly conducted a research project entitled "Conservation and Management of Medicinal and Aromatic Plants in Dang" during 2001-2005. The objectives of the project were identification of medicinal plants growing in the ecological conditions of dang, conservation of medicinal plants including endangered species by establishing a herbal garden and development of cultivation technology of some important medicinal and aromatic plants. The study has revealed 255 species of medicinal plants and 154 local traditional healers in Dang. Germplasms of 85 important species have been collected, planted and maintained in the form of an Herbal garden at Beljhundi in Dang covering about 3 ha of land. These include five threatened species; *Pterocarpus marsupium* (critically endangered), *Rauvolfia serpentina* (vunerable), *Oroxylum indicum* (critically endangered), *Asparagus racemosus* (vulnerable) and *Tinospora cordifolia (Vulnerable)* stated at different levels of threat according to IUCN red list categories. Field trials were conducted on domestication of *Rauvolfia serpentina, Piper longum and*

*Withania somnifera*. The results show that these crops grow very well with the average production of 200-400 kg/ha in the ecological conditions of Dang. The technology has been recommended to the community forest user groups of the district for their cultivation.

***Keywords:*** *Medicinal plants, Herbal garden, Local healers, Endangered species, Cultivation of medicinal plants.*

## 1.0 Introduction

Nepal is located in the Himalayan Region. The total area of the country is 147,181 sq. km. Variations in altitude; geology and soils covering the short distances have resulted in forming a region with a wealth of natural ecosystems. This includes more than 2168 species of fauna and more than 8350 species of flora of which 370 species are endemic, 700 species with medicinal properties, 500 species edible and 200 species cultivated in Nepal. Nepal's share of world's land is no more than 0.1 per cent while its share in flowering plant species is over 2 per cent (IUCN 1999). The country is ranked between 25$^{th}$ and 30$^{th}$ position in global context and 11$^{th}$ position in the continental scale of biodiversity richness. Out of 700 species of medicinal and aromatic plants (MAP's) 250 species are endemic to the country (Rawal *et al.*, 2001).

People collect the herbs from the nearby forest that indicates the danger of depletion of germplasm of valuable medicinal plants. Although they collect and sell useful parts of medicinal plants from the nearby forest, they are very eager to cultivate them and develop small processing industries. Conservation of germplasm of such plants is the need of today. *In vitro* and cryopreservation of such plants are very expensive for Nepal. Conservation of germplasm in the field is indisputably the best option because necessary applied research can be also conducted in the field for their cultivation in the marginal land.

Dang, the project area is located between Siwalik and Mahabharat (latitude 27,37'–28.21'N and longitude 82.2'-85. 544' E) with altitude 213 m to 2058 m above sea level of Mid-Western Development Region of Nepal. Climatically, Dang links areas extending from tropical to temperate zones. Total area of the district is 297339 ha out of which forest including community forest covers 197273 ha and agricultural land covers 80784 with huge potential of cultivation of medicinal plants in community forest and marginal agricultural land.

*Rauvolfia serpentina, Asparagus recemosus, Curculigo orchioides Operculina turpethum* and *Piper longum* are some of the important medicinal plants that grow in Dang district in the wild. As these crops are in high demand in the internal as well as external market, roots of first four species are collected from the wild without taking adequate conservation practices so far. These species once abundant in Dang have become almost extinct due to the extensive collection of roots. Few other species are popular cash crops in the area that could contribute to improve economic status of local farmers. Hence, the Government of Nepal has given priority for the development of cultivation packages of these crops.

Nepal is rich in ethnic diversity too. Within the small territory, there are 101 ethnic groups among which several ethnic groups are unique and indigenous to Nepal. Different communities such as Tharu, Abadh, Magars, Khas and other under privileged groups are residing in Dang district. Each ethnic group has traditional knowledge of using medicinal plants to cure common diseases. In Nepal, ayurvedic system is predominantly followed. However, Chinese system of using traditional medicine is also practiced in some quarters making chances of amalgamation of two ancient compendia.

Only 25 per cent of the Nepalese people are using modern allopathic medicine, rest of the people are dependent on natural herbal and ayurvedic medicines in Nepal. Hence, there are quite a large number of practitioners of the traditional medicine actively working throughout the country.

It was therefore, felt necessary that Academic institutions such as Nepal Academy of Science and Technology (NAST) and Nepal Sanskrit University(NSU) take the initiative for the conservation and sustainable utilization of MAP's and traditional knowledge on them by conducting scientific studies and research. This project was carried out jointly by these two organizations NAST and NSU. NSU owns more than 1000 ha of land in Dang. It provided the required area of land to establish an herbal garden to carry on research as envisaged by the project where as the research team was from NAST. The research was carried out during 2001-2005.

The objectives of the project were identification of medicinal plants growing in the ecological conditions of Dang, conservation of medicinal plants including endangered species by establishing an herbal garden and development of cultivation technology of some important medicinal and aromatic plants.

## 2.0 Methodology

Participatory approach was applied for the survey of medicinal plants and local healers. For this purpose, first of all a questionnaire was developed for getting primary (first hand) information from the local traditional healers. Considering the fact that the local healers hesitate or become conservative to disclose their knowledge on traditional medicine to outsiders, it was decided to involve local people. Accordingly two ten-day trainings were organized for the representatives of CFUGs and NGOs of Dang. All the trainees had at least SLC pass recommended by the District Forest Office of Dang. Hence all the trainees were local and capable of filling the questionnaire as per the given instructions.

The germplasms were collected from different nurseries belonging to GOs, NGOs, private nursery men while some of the local germplasms were collected from wild.

Emphasis was not given to the number of individual plants of a particular species. Therefore the number of individual plants of different species was different based on their availability, economic importance and purpose of conservation

Cultivation trials have been conducted on domestication of *Rauvolfia serpentina, Piper longum* and *Withania somnifera* for three years in the premises of NSU in Dang.

## 3.0 Results and Discussion

### 3.1 Medicinal Plants

Survey was carried out in the two municipalities and 32 Village Development committees (VDCs) out of 40 VDCs. The survey revealed that there are 255 species of medicinal plants in Dang traditionally used by local healers. All these medicinal plants have been scientifically identified. *Khanal and Bhandary* (1988) reported 217 species of plants from Dang used by local people for different purposes including traditional medicine, fibre, forages and fodder etc. However, the current study has been focused on recording the plant species specifically used by local healers. Similarly *Acharya* (1996) has reported 65 species of medicinal plants belonging to 40 families from Pawan Nagar VDC. The number of species recorded in this study is higher than those reported earlier. The list also contains some species that are at different level of threatened status under IUCN categories.

All the species (255) belong to 85 families. However the number of species belonging to families varies from only one to maximum 35. We have considered the families that have five and more than five species as major families. Major families with the number of species found are given in Table 51.1.

**Table 51.1: Major Families of Medicinal Plants Found in Dang**

| Sl.No. | Family | No. of Species |
|---|---|---|
| 1. | Leguminosae | 35 |
| 2. | Compositae | 18 |
| 3. | Moraceae | 13 |
| 4. | Graminae | 12 |
| 5. | Euphorbiaceae | 10 |
| 6. | Labitae | 10 |
| 7. | Apocynaceae | 8 |
| 8. | Rutaceae | 7 |
| 9. | Lauraceae | 6 |
| 10. | Rosaceae | 6 |
| 11. | Oleaceae | 5 |
| 12. | Solananceae | 5 |
| 13. | Zingiberaceae | 5 |

The study also has revealed that there are equally important species in terms of their commercial and medicinal value as those found at high altitudes. Although the species recorded by our study outnumbers the earlier reported number, it is still not final one and needs further survey extensively to establish the ultimate figures.

### 3.2 Local Healers

Total population of Dang is 354413. Khas (Brahman, Chhetry and Dalit) are in majority with 233707 population followed by Tharu 105018, Abadh 5378, Magar

1993 and Newar 397(District profile 2006). They do have different cultures but they live in good harmony respecting each other's culture. All of these ethnic groups have their system of traditional medicine developed since time immemorial and continuously enriched since then. In each Community there are traditional healers who are given respected positions in the society as "Guruwa" in Tharu community, "Vaidya" "Khas" and Dhami Jhakri in other communities. They are very rich in traditional knowledge on medicinal plants and healing systems. They are the living sources of such traditional knowledge and in many cases their knowledge has not been yet documented in written form but transferred from one generation to another practically and vocally from parents to their off springs.

The results of the survey on local healers show that there are 154 local traditional healers in Dang. This is the first attempt to record them and many such healers might have not been covered and there is need for a separate survey for this purpose.

The number of local healers by age is very important. Table 51.2 shows the number of local healers by age group. Maximum number of local healers was recorded of age group above 60 followed by 50-59, 40-49 and minimum below 30.

**Table 51.2: Local Healers by Age Group**

| *Ethnic group* | *> 30 years* | *31–39 years* | *40–49 years* | *50–59 years* | *60+ years* |
|---|---|---|---|---|---|
| Tharu | 4 | 10 | 21 | 16 | 21 |
| Khas | 9 | 7 | 9 | 13 | 15 |
| Dalit | – | 4 | 2 | 4 | 4 |
| Kumal | – | 2 | 2 | 1 | 1 |
| Magar | 1 | – | 3 | 1 | 1 |
| Newar | – | – | 1 | – | – |
| Ahir | – | 1 | – | – | – |
| Total | 14 | 24 | 38 | 45 | 42 |

The declining tendency of local healers of younger age might be explained simply by the fact that they are less interested in acquiring the traditional knowledge from their elders. It is the indicator of danger that the traditional knowledge on medical use of medicinal plants will be lost very soon after the demise of the elderly local healers as the average life expectancy of Nepali people is 56 years. There is a risk that such a traditional knowledge might be lost in the near future.

## 3.3 Establishment of a Herbal Garden in Beljhundi, Dang

Selection of species for the conservation was carried out based on the economic importance, IUCN threatened status and National conservation strategy policy for the particular species. Some other locally available species were also selected with an objective to use them for demonstration purpose.

Germplasms of 85 species of medicinal plants have been collected, planted and maintained in the land of NSU covering about 3 ha of land. These include five threatened species; *Pterocarpus marsupium* (critically endangered), *Rauvolfia serpentina* (vulnerable) *Oroxylum indicum* (critically endangered), *Asparagus racemosus* (vulnerable) and *Tinospora cordifolia* (vulnerable) stated at different levels of threat according to IUCN red list categories assessed by CAMP Pokhara, 2001. This might serve as the milestone for the establishment of the Herbal Garden and thereafter for the establishment of Conservation and Research and Development Centre of Medicinal Plants in Beljhundi, Dang.

The number of individual plants established is different for example the number of threatened species such as *Oroxylum indicum* and *Pterocarpus marsupium* and others were limited to few numbers from 4-5 to 10–15 individuals where as number of plant species such as *Cinnamomum glaucesens, Ocimum sanctum* and others were in few hundreds.

## 3.4 Cultivation Trials

### 3.4.1 Assessment of Productivity of Pipla (*Piper longum*) in Dang

*Piper longum* is an important medicinal plant. The fruits, roots and thicker parts of the stem are used in Ayurvedic and allopathic medicine for cough, bronchitis, asthma, insomnia, and epilepsy. There is a high demand of this crop in the internal as well as international market. Pipla grows in wild in mid-hills and plains of Terai and inner Terai of Nepal. Although some farmers grow as hedges all-around., it is mainly collected from the wild. It can very well fit in the agro forestry system of terai and inner terai because it grows very well under shade. The field experiment was laid out under the sisoo plantation in randomized complete block design (RCBD) in Beljhundi, Dang in September 1999. There were two treatments using support and without support with 6 replications. The crop was harvested in October 2002 because Pipla is the perennial plant and starts giving fruits only on third year after plantation. The average yield of dry fruits obtained from the treatment without support was 175 kg/ha and with support was 215 kg/ha. The results show that Pipla grows well under sisoo plantation area in Dang.

### 3.4.2 Assessment of Performance of Aswagandha (*Withania somnifera)* in Dang

*Withania somnifera* is used for treating male sexual impotency. There is a high demand for Ashwagandha in Ayurvedic medicine. Although the agro climatic conditions suitable for Ashgwagandha exist in Terai and Inner Terai regions of Nepal, no information about its cultivation is available so far in the country. It grows well in sandy loam or light soil, with good drainage. Considering the economic importance and appropriate agro climatic conditions in Dang, attempt was made to introduce Ashwagandha and evaluate its performance. The experiment was carried out in 1999 in the premises of Nepal Sanskrit University, Dang. The seeding was carried out in June by broadcasting method in small experimental plots of 10mx20 m. and harvesting was carried out in January-February 2006. No fertilizers were applied to the experimental plots. The average yield was about 200kg/ha. Although this yield is low as compared to average commercial yield (300-500kg/ha), it indicates that with application of good cultivation practices, Ashwagandha can be successfully grown in Dang.

### 3.4.3 Trials on Spacing of Sarpagandha (*Rauvolfia serpentina*)

*Rauvolfia serpentina* is well known for its reserpine content. The roots of Rauvolfia are widely used in Ayurvedic medicine for hypertension in crude form and extracts such as reserpine and other alkoloids in pure form of this plant are also used in allopathic medicine. It is one of the endogenous plants growing in the wild and was abundant in Dang until few years ago. As it has a high demand in the market, plants were collected indiscriminately from wild in the past. It almost was at the state of extinction in Dang district and other parts of the country. The government of Nepal has included it, in the list of plants that cannot be exported without processing. Since this plant is still in high demand, it was felt necessary to develop its cultivation technology. Experiment was carried out to develop agro-technology applicable to cultivate it in the community forests since the farmers are not willing to use their arable land for its cultivation, rather they are interested in growing it in community forests under/along with other forest trees. The field experiment was laid out in randomized complete block design (RCBD) in Beljhundi, Dang in September 1999. There were five treatments with different spacing (0.5mx0.15m, 0.5mx0.3m, 0.5mx0.45m. 0.5mx0.6m and 0.5mx0.75m). The crop was harvested in December 2002 because it takes three years to get maximum economic production of roots with high content of reserpine and along with other important alkaloids. The average yield of dry roots obtained from the treatment ranged from 1300-2800 kg/ha.

The preliminary results show that these crops grow very well with the average production almost equal to other places in Dang. However these trials have to be further tested on a larger scale before making final recommendations.

## Acknowledgements

The author expresses sincere gratitude to Prof. Dr. Hom Nath Bhattarai, Vice Chancellor of NAST for providing all the support to participate and present this paper in this workshop. Sincere thanks to NAST and NSU authorities for their support to carry the research. The author acknowledges the support of research team members I.P. Khanal, V. Singh and B.P. Yadav.

## References

Acharya, S.K., 1996. Folk Uses of some Medicinal Plants of Pawannagar, Dang district. J.Nat. Hist. Mus. (Nepal).

CAMP Workshop Report, 2001. Conservation Assessment and Management Prioritization Workshop held in Pokhara Nepal.

IUCN Report, 1999. Nepal Country Report on Biological Diversity. World Conservation Union (IUCN) with contributions from Bishnu Bhandari and Narayan Belbase Published by IUCN, Nepal.

Joshi, K.K. and Joshi,S.D., 2001. Genetic Heritage of Medicinal and Aromatic Plants of Nepal Himalayas. Budha Academic Publishers and Distributors Pvt. Ltd. Kathmandu Nepal; pp. 239.

Khanal, B. and Bhandary, H.R., 1988. A Study on Natural Environment of Dang Valley. Final report submitted to the NAST; pp. 32-62.

Ministry of Forest and Soil Conservation, 2006. Nepal Biodiversity strategy implementation Plan (2006-2010).

Rawal, R.B., Acharya, B. and Subedi, B.P., 2001. Jaributi marketing and policy issues in Nepal. Paper presented in Seminar on Biodiversity Support Program in Workshop organized by East West Centre Hawaii, USA.

Regmi, C., Khanal, I.P. and Yadav, B.P., 2006. Performance of Ashwagandha (*Withania somnifera*) in Dang. In Proceedings 4th Conf. of Sc. and Tech. NAST; pp. 2207-22014.

Regmi, C. and Khanal, I.P., 2006. Assessment of productivity of pipla (*Piper longum* L.) in Dang. In Proceedings 4th Conf. of Sc. and Tech. NAST; pp. 372-375.

*Chapter 52*

# The Role of Indigenous Knowledge Systems in Bioprospecting and Product Development in South Africa: A Policy, Research, Development and Innovation Perspective

***Hlupheka Chabalala***

*National IKS Office, National Office on Indigenous Knowledge Systems, Brummeria, Republic of South Africa*

*E-mail: hlupheka.chabalala@dst.gov.za, amenrai@gmail.com*

## ABSTRACT

The significance of indigenous knowledge systems [IKS] to the socio-economic development cannot exclude local communities, their knowledge and natural resources. It is for this fact that the South African government is committed to improving the quality of life for all its citizens through the development of African Traditional Medicines [ATM]. The ageless wisdom of indigenous communities declares that ATM has unlimited potential in management both infectious and chronic diseases. This paper therefore seeks to explore the role of IKS in research and development of ATM within the South African National Systems of Innovation [NSI]. This is being done through the implementation of the Bioprospecting and Product Development Platform [BPDP]. The expected outcome and long term impact of this initiative is wealth creation and skills development. It is common knowledge that valuable discoveries are easier with the help of indigenous knowledge. The role of indigenous communities therefore includes knowledge of biodiversity, locally developed technologies and their utilisation, product development, innovation, service delivery, commercialisation, marketing, and equitable benefit sharing. Multinationals and researchers continue to unethically use IK as a precursor to screening for products, with little or no regard for the protection of indigenous intellectual property and benefit sharing. The aim of the BPDP is to coordinate, develop, and promote innovation using indigenous resources and knowledge for improved quality of life using ATM, indigenous food and natural cosmetics. The Department of Science and Technology [DST] identified bioprospecting as a niche for innovation and entrepreneurship. Moreover the NSI in South Africa has evolved significantly over the years and lead to the development of enabling policies and strategies, *e.g.* Research and Development Strategy and Indigenous Knowledge Policy, which recognize the role of ATM in science and technology.

***Keywords:*** *African traditional medicine, Bioprospecting, Indigenous knowledge systems, Product development, National system of innovation.*

## 1.0 Introduction

The establishment of the "Health for All" initiative recognised the role of traditional medicines in addressing health challenges in the world. This was due to the fact that all countries in the world have traditional or indigenous knowledge related to health and healing (WHO, 2000). The advent of allopathic medicine and other foreign practices in Africa, in particular, led to the undermining of this ancient science of healing. However, the rise of indigenous knowledge systems has seen the recognition of natural or herbal products regaining their position in the world (WHO, 1999).

The South African government also recognizes its wealth embedded in its rich biodiversity and indigenous knowledge under the custodianship of its practitioners or holders. It is estimated that there are over 24 000 medicinal plants in South Africa (Light ME, 2005). The use of herbal remedies is on the increase, and as a result there is a concern over the safety, quality and efficacy of these medicines. There is still a challenge in terms of regulating its use, even within the national health system. In order to address these challenges, various initiatives and strategies were developed and implemented (DST [R&D Strategy], 2002, DST [IKS Policy], 2004).

The National Department of Health [NDoH] implemented pieces of legislation on Traditional Medicines; however the act is still being amended (NDoH, [Traditional Health Practitioners Act] 2004). Together with other government agencies like, the Medical Research Council [MRC] and the Council for Scientific and Industrial Research [CSIR], the Department of Health initiated the National Reference Centre for African Traditional Medicines [NRCATM]. The objectives of the NRCATM include investigating the safety, quality and efficacy of ATM, registration and control of marketed traditional medicines, and collection and dissemination of information to promote, regulate and register ATM (DST [R&D Strategy], 2002, NDoH [NRCATM], 2004).

The establishment of the Traditional Medicines Directorate by the Department of Health will ensure that all legislations related to ATM are well implemented. There are initiatives to provide for a statutory council to separately address traditional medicines issues. With over 70 per cent of South Africans primarily using ATM or consulting traditional health practitioners, it was necessary to classify ATM differently from imported complementary or alternative medicines (NDoH [Traditional Health Practitioners Act] 2004; Ham, C., 2006).

The approval of the IKS Policy by Cabinet in 2004 was followed by the establishment of the National IKS Office [NIKSO] in April 2006. The mandate of the Office is to coordinate all IKS-related issues in the country, with a special focus on science, technology and innovation. The Knowledge Development Unit of the NIKSO is responsible for research and development, IKS laboratories, research chairs, innovation and entrepreneurship. These four areas involve extensive work on herbal remedies through the bioprospecting and product development platform (DST [R&D Strategy], 2002; DST [IKS Policy], 2004).

## 2.0 The Significance of Indigenous Knowledge Systems

The importance of indigenous knowledge to indigenous and local communities and its application to modern life cannot be underestimated. Indigenous knowledge also constitutes much of the world's medicinal and agricultural knowledge (DEAT, 2004; WHO, 1999). Indigenous and local communities around the world rely on this knowledge for their survival, daily life, healing and nutrition needs. South Africa is of course no exception to the field of bioprospecting, innovation and product development (Tabi, MM., 2006).

Bioprospecting therefore is viewed as any research on, or development of or application of, indigenous biological resources for commercial or industrial purposes. Its processes include a systematic search, collection or gathering of resources or making extractions from such resources for the purpose of such research, development or application. The utilization for the purpose of such research or development of any information regarding any traditional use of indigenous biological resources by indigenous communities is critical. Research on, or the application, development or modification of any traditional uses for commercial or industrial exploitation is also central in bioprospecting (DEAT, 2004, DST [IKS Policy], 2004).

### 2.1 Role of Indigenous Communities

Bioprospecting requires the knowledge and skills of local communities. It is common knowledge that major drug discoveries were made easier with the help of indigenous communities. The role of indigenous communities therefore includes specific knowledge of biodiversity, primary research on biodiversity and its local use and development of products using natural resources. The custodians of indigenous knowledge in South Africa are considered as main role-players in innovation and service delivery (Tabi, MM., 2006; King, SR., 1996). Their role is well recognised in commercialisation and marketing of their products, hence they must be given the privilege of ownership and benefit sharing. The various initiatives that the DST is implementing included full participation of civil society and non-governmental organisations involved in IKS (DST [IKS Policy], 2004).

## 2.2 Bioprospecting and Product Development: African Traditional Medicine

South African indigenous communities have been practicing bioprospecting and product development for millennia. The establishment of the Convention on Biodiversity [CBD] significantly addresses issues of access and sharing of benefit. While the CBD opens the way for much progress in these areas, certain critical issues remain unresolved (DST [IKS Policy], 2004). These include legalizing and formalizing the bioprospecting process in a way, which ensures that there is full and prior informed consent of fair as well as fair and equitable benefit sharing with the originator/originators of the knowledge. It is for this reason that the DST initiated the BPDP to primarily benefit knowledge holders.

On the other hand, BPDP in South Africa has been the preferred field of research by universities and science councils. These institutions also worked in close collaboration with multinational companies, with little or no recognition of indigenous communities. However these illicit activities will be discouraged by national legislation. Recently, there has been a steady growth of interest in ATM as it is viewed by pharmaceutical industries as a source of lead in the identification of active compounds for use in the production of synthetic modern drugs (DST [IKS Policy], 2004).

Moreover, medicinal herbs and plants are under the threat of extinction as a result of growth-exploitation, environment-unfriendly harvesting techniques, and loss of growth habitats and unmonitored trade. As a result, the promulgated Biodiversity Act and approval of the accompanying regulations will legally control access to South Africa's biodiversity. The act promotes the sustainable use of natural resources, provides for the fair and equitable benefit sharing and calls for the establishment of a National Trust Funds. It also compels bio-prospectors to enter into a benefit-sharing agreement with all providers of resources and knowledge, and also to obtain their prior informed consent before proceeding with research, etc (DEAT, 2004).

South Africa is still concerned that that multinationals and other foreign establishments use its indigenous knowledge as a precursor for product screening, with little or no regard for the protection of indigenous intellectual property. The Research and Development Strategy and the IKS Policy support the further development of resources for socio-economic development and respect of intellectual property.

## 2.3 Aim and Objectives of the BPDP

The main aim of the BPDP is to coordinate, develop, and promote innovation using indigenous resources and knowledge using ATM for improved quality of life. This is being done through establishing sustainable partnerships with other government departments, IK Holders/Practitioners, private sectors, science councils, universities, non-government organisation and community-based organisations. Specific objectives are as follows:

- To facilitate collaboration within the different organisations involved in bioprospecting and product development in South Africa;
- To drive the development of necessary business concepts that will be beneficial to the knowledge holders/practitioners and for general public good;
- To coordinate the development of bioprospecting research programmes that are appropriate and will lead to commercialisation, economic growth, job creation, international competitiveness and wealth creation;
- Create a culture of technical development in the field of pharmaceutics and drug development for technology, skills development and utilisation;
- Develop partnerships with communities and scientists in the industrialisation of IK for retention of intellectual property and technical skills;
- Create a culture of responsive research to current challenges of the nation, *e.g.* HIV/AIDS, Poverty, Skills shortage.

Using existing resources specifically designated to bioprospecting and product development, the platform is in the process of creating flagships for a well-coordinated and regulated bioprospecting industry, enshrined in ethics, fair and equitable benefit sharing. The DST established a BPDP, which has four committees, which in the process of carrying the following mandate.

- Coordinate bioprospecting initiatives related to innovation and technology in traditional medicines, natural cosmetics, indigenous food and jewellery.
- Develop an inventory of IKS bioprospecting activities in various institutions in the country; and further support those with developmental potential.
- Assist to facilitate in drawing up specific contractual arrangements between indigenous communities and professional organisation working in the field, *e.g.* pharmaceutical, cosmetic companies etc;
- Investigate and validate research and developmental initiatives related to serendipitous discoveries, including benefit-sharing models.

## 2.4 South African BPDP Initiatives

The DST has identified BPDP as a niche for innovation and included it in its 10-year plan. The South African National System of Innovation has also evolved significantly over the past years and has lead to the development of enabling environment for the implement its strategies. Following the establishment of the National IKS Office in 2006, the first meeting on BPDP was organised in June 2007. Stakeholders ranged from government departments, science councils, universities, NGO's CBOs and IK Holders/Practitioners. The NIKSO thereafter developed the initial draft of the strategy, thus providing leadership in the area [see Figures below].

For the past five years, the DST through the IKS Unit has been supporting research projects through various organisations in the country. The establishment of the Medical Research Council-IKS Lead programme is one of such instruments the department is using. The MRC established a laboratory that focuses on the development of African traditional medicines. The focus of these IKS Laboratory is on priority health conditions in South Africa, *e.g.* HIV/AIDS, TB, Malaria, Diabetes, Cancer and Hypertension.

Through the South African Research Chairs initiative, the Department awarded the University of KwaZulu-Natal a Chair in Traditional Medicines. The main objectives of this Chair will also include investigation of ATM, thus seeking best methods of interfacing the indigenous knowledge and traditional medicine into the national health systems and other knowledge systems.

The CSIR was also given the responsibility of developing and populating databases with herbal remedies. The Biosciences unit is also fully involved in the development of ATM, in close collaboration with knowledge holders. The role of indigenous knowledge holders is well respected and recognised. It is important to note that though there are different initiatives ongoing in the country, the BPDP is an attempt by the DST to coordinate the research and development; as well and innovation and entrepreneurship strategies.

Figures 52.1–52.3 were developed to provide a simplified framework of the processes used to plan and implement the BPDP platform. The Figures are generic and can be used as models for any process involving product development.

## 3.0 Discussion

Figures 52.1–52.3 show various processes and systems already set in motion by the DST in order to fully implement BPDP. Figure 52.1 illustrates the basic and fundamental stages used in product development. However, what is critical in this model is the access and benefit sharing stage, which is place high in the priority of events to be followed. Also is the monitoring and evaluation phase, which is often ignored.

Figure 52.2 shows the various stages involved in the development of African Traditional Medicines including clinical trials. An important part of this system is that different role players are brought together to share limited resources and expertise. The smooth implementation of this initiative lies in the coordination of roles and responsibilities of individual partners. The DST also recognizes the role that the private sector is already playing in this field, and therefore recommends private sector's full participation.

Figure 52.3 shows a strategic roadmap, agreed upon with various stakeholders. Given all resources made available, the 2007 financial year was dedicated towards planning, organisation and development of the implementation strategy. The strategy includes consultation with senior management for advocacy and leadership purposes. It should also be noted that the DST has in the past, and is stilling supporting various academic institutions in further developing various aspects of this platform, *e.g.* Medical Research Council IKS Laboratories, Centre for Industrial and Scientific Research's Bioscience Unit, The University of KwaZulu-Natal. Large numbers of

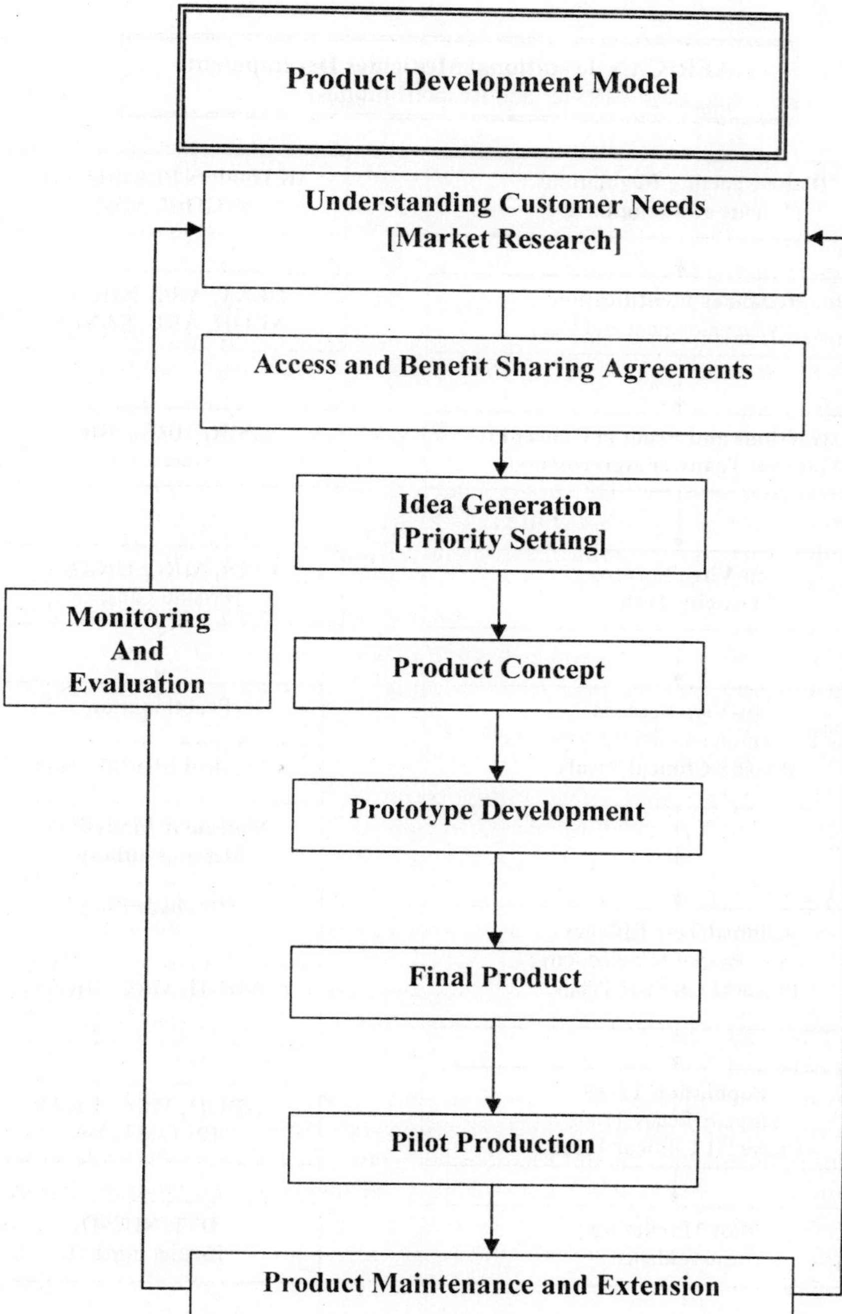


**Figure 52.1: Proposed Generic Product Development Model (Adapted from Hatting, 2006)**

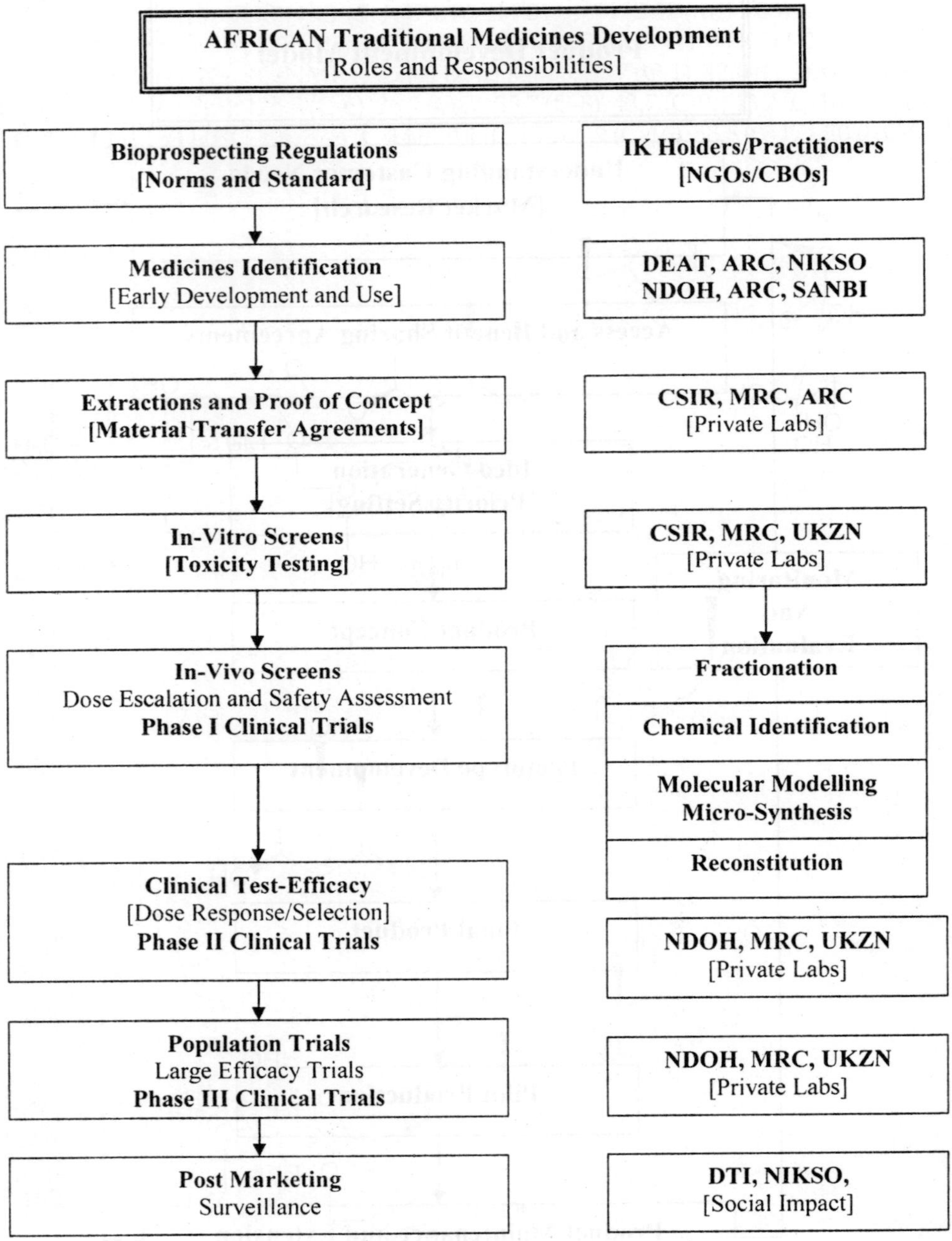


**Figure 52.2: Proposed African Traditional Medicines Development Process**

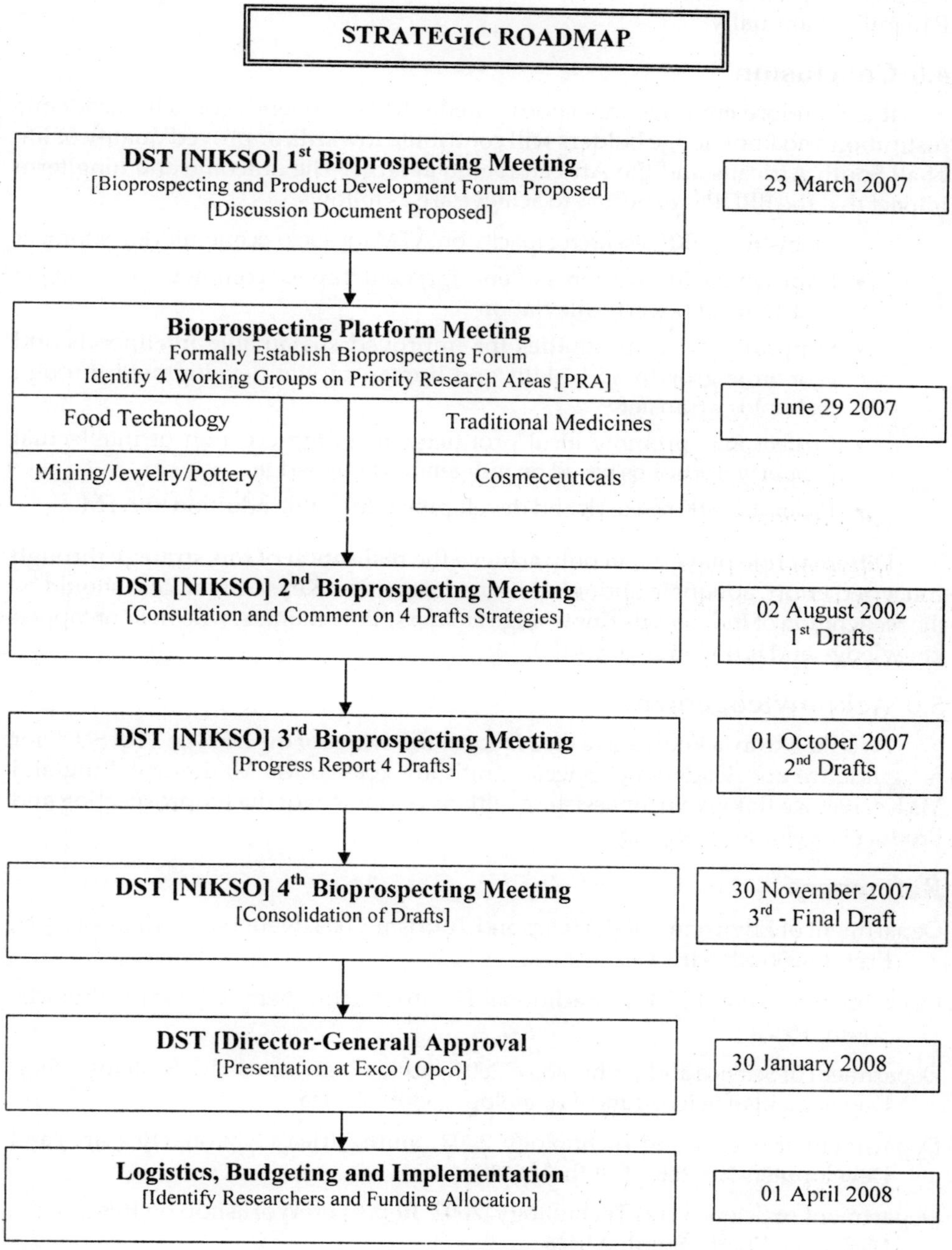


**Figure 52.3: Strategic Roadmap for African Traditional Medicines Development**

research projects are carried out by the National Research Foundation (NRF) using R10 million annually.

## 4.0 Conclusion

It is therefore envisage that coordinated efforts of science councils, academic institution and knowledge holders will contribute towards improved quality of life of all South Africans and the African region at large. The outcome and long term impact that the BPDP is expected to achieve are as follows:

- Mainstream IKS research capacity on ATM for socio-economic development
- Improve the innovation and entrepreneurship for commercialisation job creation and poverty alleviation
- Support local communities for improved sustainable livelihoods and economic growth and, skills and human capital development through technology transfer
- Protect and promote local products, including creation of intellectual property portfolios based on indigenous knowledge
- Promote of IK research and development for value addition to ATM

Different role players can only achieve the realisation of this strategy through concerted effort, adequate budget, skills and expertise. Key to its success should be the recognition of Indigenous Knowledge Holders/Practitioners, who hold untapped knowledge and innovation potential.

## 5.0 Acknowledgements

I would like to acknowledge the National IKS Office of the DST, *i.e.* Prof Seleti for his guidance and leadership. Special gratitude goes to Ms Mammone Tang and Ms Keabetswe Rakgwale for assisting with development of the Bioprospecting and Product Development strategy.

## References

Department of Environmental Affairs and Tourism. 2004. National Biodiversity Act, Pretoria, South Africa

Department of Health, 2004. Traditional Health Practitioners Act. (35) 1, Pretoria, South Africa

Department of Science and Technology, 2004. Indigenous Knowledge Systems Policy. Department of Science and Technology, South Africa

Department of Science and Technology, 2002. South Africa's National Research and Development Strategy. South Africa

Department of Science and Technology, 2002. Report on Workshop on Research in Medicinal Plants. South Africa

Ham, C., 2006. Commercialising medicinal plants: A South African guide. Gardening News

Hatting, A., 2006. Innovation, entrepreneurship and technology diffusion: The role of the University of Technology in the NSI. Proceedings of the 1st All Africa Technology Diffusion Conference, Tshumisano Partnership in Technology, South Africa: pp. 79-100

King, S.R., Carlson, T.J. and Moran, K., 1996. Biological diversity, indigenous knowledge, drug discovery and intellectual property rights: creating reciprocity and maintaining relationships. Journal of Ethnopharmacology (51(1-3)): pp. 45-57

Light, M.E. *et al.*, 2005. Riding the wave: South Africa's contribution to ethnopharmacological research over the last 25 years. Journal of Ethnopharmacology. (100 (1-2)); pp. 127-130.

National Department of Health, 2004. National Centre for African Traditional Medicines: A South African Model. South Africa.

Tabi, M.M., Powell, M. and Hodnicki, D., 2006. Use of traditional healers and modern medicine in Ghana. International Nursing Review (53): pp. 52-58.

World Health Organisation, 2000. Promoting the role of Traditional Medicine in Health Systems: a strategy for the African Region 2001-2010. Harare, World Health Organization

World Health Organisation, 1999. Traditional, Complementary and Alternative Medicines and Therapies, Washington DC, WHO Regional Office for the Americas/Pan American Health Organisation

## Chapter 53

# Indonesia Country Report on Herbal Medicinal Plants and Traditional Herbs Remedies


*Adriana Marthiany Lubis*

*Medicine and Nutrition Division of the Deputy Minister for Program Development, Ministry of Research and Technology, Indonesia*

*E-mail: adri@ristek.go.id*



## ABSTRACT

Indonesia is known as the second mega biodiversity country in the world, with 30,000 species of flowering plants growing in vast tropical rainforest. About 1,000 species possess significant medicinal potential. Indonesians have been using traditional herb remedies for preventive or curative purposes since the ancient time. National Agency of Drug and Food Control reported that 9,737 items of traditional herb remedies are registered. Traditional herb remedies resources in Indonesia vary in terms of its nature. The first scheme is *jamu* or herbal mixture, which has been used empirically as medicine for self-medication. Secondly, it is the standardized natural extract, followed phytopharmaca as the third scheme. The development of traditional herb remedies in Indonesia faces several significant factors: (a) low interest of conventional health providers including that of the medical doctors, (b) the absence of traditional medicines knowledge in medical school curricula, and (c) lack of standard, either raw materials, simplicia, or extract.



*Keywords: Medicinal plants, Mega biodiversity, Traditional herb remedies.*


## 1.0 Introduction

Indonesia is an archipelago comprising some 17,000 islands. Although it covers only 1.3 per cent of the earth's surface, it contains almost 15 per cent of all higher plants, as well as a significant share of the world's animal diversity. Indonesia is one of the world's top two mega-centres of biodiversity (alongside Brazil). Indonesian soils and oceans are very rich in various sources for medicinal materials or simplicia. Indonesia has the largest biologic varieties in the world with ca 30.000 types of plants, and part of those plants is sources of natural medicinal materials. This is a very big opportunity to produce medicinal materials as well as completed products domestically by us.

It is also a country of enormous cultural diversity. Among its 210 million inhabitants, there are no fewer than 336 different cultures, speaking over 250 languages. The fact that the country is an archipelago has serious implications to the country's politics, economy and infrastructure. Indonesian governments and non-governmental organizations (NGOs) foster the use of the rich natural resources that are to be found all over the country in an effort to make it less dependent on imports.

This article focuses on Indonesian flora, specifically those plants which have therapeutic properties. The Indonesian Country Study on Biodiversity (ICSBD, 1993) put the number of species of flowering plants in Indonesia at between 25,000 and 30,000. Some 10 per cent of the total flora of Indonesia is thought to have medicinal value. Some 40 million Indonesians depend directly on biodiversity, and Indonesian communities make use of around 6,000 plant species, 1,000 animal species and 100 microbe species on day-to-day basis (Bappenas, 2003; Government of the Republic of Indonesia, 2003). Many plants, which are useful for medicinal purposes, have been imported, together with details of their use. In some cases this has led to the development of new uses, while formerly unknown species are regularly integrated into traditional Indonesian medical systems.

Today, *jamu* (herbal mixture) plays a decisive role in the national development. *Jamu* is an important component of national health care. It plays a major role in the economy of the rural areas. As a result of the continuous exchange of information between various cultural groups, traditional systems of medicine are not static but dynamic, regularly incorporating new knowledge and uses. While all the various systems are based on more or less the same plant material, users are limited by what is available in their own locality and the existing knowledge with regard to their use. This has resulted in an interesting series of often-complex patterns of use.

## 2.0 The Legacy of Indonesia's Traditional Medicine Industry

Traditional medicine industry in Indonesia shows an interesting trend of growth, particularly in terms of numbers small traditional medicine industries. In a 1992 survey, it was recorded 429 small traditional medicine industries or home industries) producing traditional herbal medicine *(jamu)* for the country's domestic demand. In 1999 the number has skyrocketed to 833, and in 2002 it was estimated as much as 1,000 small traditional medicine industries operating in many parts of the country. On the other side, large traditional medicine industries are also growing from 20 large factories in 1992 to 87 in 1999. Some well-known herbal medicine industries are Mustika Ratu, Sari Ayu, Air Mancur, Nyonya Meneer, and Sido Muncul. The total money involved in the industries reached IDR 10 trillion or about US$ 10.6 billion (at the estimate 1 US$ = IDR 9,400). As comparison, similar transaction in Brazil reaches US$ 20 billion, China US$ 6.6 billion, and Malaysia US$ 1.2 billion.

The impressive figures of herbal medicine transaction in Indonesia was strongly related to rural people's economy as well as their faith to their ancestor's customs in maintaining family health as part of their social obligation to stay socially productive. In terms of labour force, the large sum of money involved also shows that the *jamu* industry is able to absorb considerable number of labour to help rural economy going.

The complex utilization patterns of medicinal plants in Indonesia is related to the purpose of utilization, type of sickness, the availability of raw materials, as well as to local condition in terms of social habit and customs. As a general rule, people use specific plant species to cure specific diseases. In Kampung Gumpang, Aceh (North Sumatra), the Acehnese use *puding hitam* or black pudding *(Graptophyllum* sp.) to cure eye diseases, *besibesi (Justicia gendarussa Burm.f.,syn. Gendarussa vulgaris Nees.)* for stomachache, and *rutih* or *geceh*, devil's tree, ditabark tree *(Alstonia scholaris (L.) R.Br.)* to cure malaria (Anon,1995). However, a particular plant species may also be utilized to cure different diseases within different ethnic communities in different regions of the country. For example, *alang-alang* or *lalang*, known widely as cotton grass *(Imperata cylindrica (L.) Beauv.)*, one of the most widespread grass species in Indonesia, which is found as high as 3,000 m above sea level is often use to cure different diseases or sickness in different ethnic or area in the country. *Alang-alang* grows wild in dry forest, open fields and dry land. The roots of this species are often used to cure high blood pressure, fever, cough, and hepatitis. Another example is *temulawak (Curcuma xanthorrhiza Roxb.)*, which is often used to cure a wide variety of different diseases.

Another possibility is that different ethnic groups in different geographic areas use different plant species for the same disease. For malaria, people in Aceh use *rutih* or *geceh (Alstonia scholaris (L.) R.Br.)*. In Bengkulu, *medang (Beilschmiedia madang Blume)* is used to cure malaria. East Timor, *bidara laut (Strychnos lucida R.Br.)* is used to cure the same disease. This pattern reflects the geographic variability within the same area (Aceh and Bengkulu are both in Sumatra) and on different islands within Indonesia (Sumatra, Timor).

People also make use of plant mixtures. For instance, the Seberida people from the Province of Riau (Sumatra) treat large wounds with a mixture of barks of *loban* or wild pepper *(Vitex trifolia L.)*, *dukuh* or *langsat (Lansium domesticum Correa)* and *rambutan (Nephelium lappaceum L.)*. It is clear that the greater the geographic distance, the more pronounced the differences between the systems of traditional medicines used by the respective communities. However, in some cases different ethnic communities living close to each other maintain distinct traditions and different healing systems. The most obvious example is the case of "modern" Indonesian ethnic groups such as the Sundanese or Javanese living next to "older" ethnic groups such as the Kubus and Talang Mamak tribes of Sumatra, the Penan of Kalimantan, the Asmat of Irian Jaya, and the Baduy of West Java. But even ethnic groups like the Sundanese of West Java and the Javanese of Central Java use different methods of healing and disease prevention. For liver infections, for instance, the Sundanese eat Curcuma domestica (turmeric) as *lalaban* or fresh salad, fresh vegetable, while the Javanese use boiled dried turmeric to treat the same ailment.

The above information shows that many ethnic groups in Indonesia possess and believes strongly in the effectiveness of traditional herbal medicine as their heritage. Their ancestors are believed to develop such herbal medicine due to their local wisdom and knowledge to help maintaining their societal needs. Such knowledge on herbal medicine was gradually improved and developed through centuries of experiences and empirical evidences so it reached particular position in the existing social and medicinal systems of the respective ethnicity. The knowledge has been transmitted through generations, which at the end it has faced empirical and academic test and experiment which lead Indonesia's *jamu* as part of the society's daily life with standardized phytopharmacia. Indonesia's herbal medicine or *jamu* has undergone pre-clinical and clinical tests to obtain its standardized status in the pharmacological world.

## 3.0 The Concern

As Indonesia's herbal medicine grows and faces ever increasing demand, it is then important to consider the utilization of the country's natural resources properly and wisely, particularly in terms of traditional herbal plants which has proven to be able to enhance better health and economic service. Scientists have repeatedly expressed their concern that many medicinal plants are already endangered and others are likely to become so in the near future. There are listed 29 species of medicinal plants, grouping them according to the IUCN criteria. The majority of the species were considered rare, others were classified as "status unknown", vulnerable, or endangered. It is compiled a list of 1,260 species of medicinal plants, which originate in Indonesian forests. On the basis of an analysis of study together with our own observations, a number of conclusions can be drawn. First, the majority of rare medicinal plants are trees. Second, most of the rare plants are rain forest species. Third, the potentially endangered species include *jamu* plants which are still collected from the wild: of the 55 most important species of plants used for jamu, about 25 per cent are still collected from the forests. Fourth, highly regarded species like *purwoceng (Pimpinella pruatjan)*, which is used as an aphrodisiac, have already become extremely rare or even locally extinct due to over-harvesting of wild populations. Given the commercialization of the *jamu* system, the importance of traditional herbal medicine in Indonesia, and its role as an export commodity, ways must be found to maintain the biological diversity of medicinal plants in Indonesia, while ensuring that the peoples of Indonesia will still be able to make use of their traditional medicines.

## 4.0 The Expected Effort of the Government

To maintain and support the production of both medicinal plants and their positive use as herbal medicine, several suggestions are made:

1. The government should provide supporting policy and programs related to education, monitoring and control of traditional medicine. Such programs should be executed and implemented in a professional way, responsible,

independent and transparent. On the other side, herbal medicine producer and industry should assure and bear responsibility of the quality of traditional medicine they produce.

2. The government should also provide a conducive environment to provide, produce, and distribute quality traditional medicine, safe, and proven to have positive effect, scientifically tested and can be used for personal use or with formal health service and advice. The user community of herbal medicine has the right on the information regarding a good and correct traditional medicine that leads them to the right track of medication and better health.

## 5.0 The Needs

Traditional medicine in Indonesia still relies to a large extent on plant materials taken from the wild. Most of these plants are species typical of more or less undisturbed forest ecosystems. It follows then that the harvesting of these natural resources must be carried out on a sustainable basis, in the interest of the long-term maintenance of the health care system of Indonesia. The most urgent needs can be categorized as follows:

1. The government should promote the plantation and conservation of traditional medicine plant resources.
2. The government should guarantee the safety and effectiveness of traditional medicine, the usable quantity, types, packaging forms, dosage, proper indication and composition that do not lead the consumer to the wrong direction.
3. The government should clearly distinguish and standardize both traditional medicine and material.

## 6.0 The Potential

Indonesia's potential in traditional medicine industry relies primarily on both the available medicinal plant resources and large consumer of herbal medicine. As already mentioned in the previous chapter, the country's traditional herbal medicine industry has soared dramatically during the period of 1992 to 2002. The huge transaction on herbal medicine throughout the country is a potential strength in the effort to improve the quality and standardization of Indonesia's herbal medicine industry and distribution. Such facts are also supported by the government's policy on Mid-term Development Plan 2004-2009, which put traditional medicine as part of the government's programs of development. Furthermore, herbal medicine development is also part of the government's Seven Priorities of Knowledge and Technology Implementation Program and as the first priority in Health Knowledge and Medicinal Development Program of the State Ministry for Research and Technology. Indonesian has Indigenous Drug Development and Cultivation Program. The aim of this program is to develop and increase Indonesian indigenous drugs, which have high quality and safety as well as have real efficacy that is strictly tested, and which have been used widely for self-treatment by the society or used in the formal health services (Health Development Plan, 1999).

The target of this program is Indonesian indigenous drugs (OAI) to be developed and utilized widely primarily in the formal health services and for export.

The principle activities included in this program are:

1. Standardization of simplicia including the extracts of OAI;
2. Development of agri-medicine and cross-sectoral cooperation;
3. Leading the use of OAI phytopharmaceuticals in hospitals and puskesmas;
4. Mapping OAI and ethno-pharmacognoxy;
5. Construction of OAI information centre;
6. Increasing export of OAI; and
7. Development of cooperation network between OAI industries and research institution in environment.

## 7.0 Programs of the State Ministry of Research and Technology, Division of Health and Medicine: The Expected Accomplishment of 2009

### 7.1 Research and Development Program on Natural Medicine Material

The 2009 program of the Division of Medicine and Health on Natural Medicine is a program that aims the improvement of herbal medicine in broad terms. This program intends to develop the existing potential and position of herbal medicine material into a better utilization. The primary targets of the program are:

1. Improving the number of standardized herbal medicine to 50 and phytopharmacyst to 15.
2. Improving the number of standardized medicinal plant extract package to 20 plants per year.
3. Developing a manual on stability test on selected biochemistry and phytochemistry features of medicinal plants with focus on anti cancer, immunomodulator, anti dengue and anti avian influenza.

### 7.2 Program of Diffusion and Utilization of Knowledge and Technology on Natural Medicine Material

Program of Diffusion and Utilization of Knowledge and Technology on Natural Medicine Material of the Division of Medicine and Health aims at the proper application of technology package of herbal medicine by various stakeholder and beneficiaries of herbal medicine, industries, and the communities. The expected accomplishments of the program are:

1. Proper application of the technology related to standardized extract of herbal plants by stakeholder industry.

2. The application of technology package of natural resource products by stakeholder industry to the proportion of as much as 50 per cent of total medicine market in Indonesia.
3. The application of technology package of fermented-base medicine material (new generation of antibiotics, cholesterol depressant, vitamins, hormones) by stakeholder industry.
4. The application of production technology of medicine material and herbal supplement with proper quality and safety to the consumer.

## 7.3 Knowledge and Technology Institutional Capacity Improvement Program in the Production of Natural Medicine Material

The program on Knowledge and Research Capacity Improvement in the Production of Natural Medicine Material is aimed particularly to improve the existing facilities in research and knowledge related to herbal medicine in broad terms. The expected accomplishments of 2009 are:

1. The availability and operationalization of research and development laboratories that fulfilled the standard.
2. The augmentation of qualified human resource with suitable training and experience in advanced industry.

## 8.0 The Development Targets of 2025

1. Local industry should be able to produce and market natural herbal medicine obtained through natural exploration in Indonesia.
2. Indonesia's natural microbes should be listed in a nomenclature as indigenous to Indonesia and should be utilized to produce medicine groups of antibiotics, vitamins, hormones, and enzymes for pharmacy industry.
3. All superior medicinal plants should already possess standardized value as determined by the Board of Control of Medicine and Food.
4. The integration of validated natural medicine of herbal and other natural resources through phytochemistry and pharmacology tests into the existing formal health service system and it should also be able to be posed as an alternative and complement to modern medicine.

## References

Anon, 1995. National Conservation Plan for Indonesia (3 A-H) Ministry of forestry, Directorate General of Forest Conservation, Jakarta

Bappenas, 1993. Indonesian Biodiversity Strategy and Action Plan. Indonesia National Development Plan Agency.

Bappenas, 2003. Indonesian Biodiversity Strategy and Action Plan, 2003-2020 IBSAP. Indonesia National Development Plan Agency.

Health Development Plan of republic of Indonesia, 1999. Ministry of Health

Kementerian Negara Lingkungan Hidup. (KLH), 2002. From Crisis to Sustainability. Paving the Way for Sustainable Development in Indonesia. Overview of the implementation of Agenda 21, Jakarta.

National Research Agenda, 2006-2009. National Research Council for State Ministry of Research and Technology of Republic of Indonesia, Jakarta.

White Paper for Research, Development and Application on Science and Technology for Health and Medicine, 2005-2025. State Ministry of Research and Technology of Republic of Indonesia, Jakarta.

*Chapter 54*

# Some Frontline Medicinal Plants of Kashmir Himalaya Used in Unani Medicine: Present Status and Role

***Tariq Ahmad Butt* and M.K. Siddiqui***

*Central Council for Research in Unani Medicine,*
*New Delhi, India*
**E-mail: tariqbutt66@yahoo.co.in*

## ABSTRACT

After a brief rendezvous with modern medicine, people throughout the world are shifting back to traditional medicine. Perhaps because they have apprehensions regarding the safety and toxicity of western medicine. High cost of production of synthetic drugs and the lack of adequate primary health care programme in rural and tribal belts of the third world have also contributed to this resurgence of interest in traditional medicine whatever the reason may be the demand for green medicine is continuously increasing. In India the total trade in ISM and H sectors is claimed to be well over Rs5000 crore per year. Trend has become a compelling reason to evolve a mission mode approach towards medicinal plants. It is a well-known fact that there is an abundance of knowledge regarding the medicinal properties and uses of plants incorporated in native cultures of people throughout the world. Before it vanishes it is important to make salvage of some of the native folklore especially regarding the medicinal use of plants. Such studies have shown promising results and made some new therapeutically effective drugs available to us. In India the territory of J&K State is considered a rich repository of medicinal plants particularly those areas as which fall under the great Himalayan range and constitute what is common known as "Kashmir Himalaya". The floristic diversity is mainly due to presence of wide range of topography and climatic conditions. Because of difficult terrain and severe climatic conditions many areas of Kashmir have no surface communication with outside world for about 3-5 months a year. Therefore, the people have properly relying on plants growing around for the basic necessities of life, be it fond, fodder, fuel or medicine. About 570 plants species are claimed to be of medicinal importance. More than 50 per cent plant based medicine prescribed in British pharmacoepia is to grown in this region. The presentation describes some important medicinal plants, which attributes to Unani system of medicine and their use by local population in primary health care. Most of the plant species are endemic to Kashmir Himalaya and its adjoining areas. Some frontline plant species are *Aconitum heterophyllum*, Sps of *Artemisia, Berberis lycium, Conchicum luteum*, and *Delphinium denudatum*.

***Keywords:*** *Traditional medicine, Status is wild, Propagation and conservation, Bioactivity, Kashmir Himalayas.*

## 1.0 Introduction

Till few decades back the traditional systems of medicine were prevalent only in the rural areas of developing countries because of their limitations to afford the high cost of production of modern synthetic drugs. But the increasing resistance of some disease-producing microorganisms against synthetic drugs has made the policy makers even in developed countries to incorporate traditional herbal medicine in their health care programmes. Besides, because of increasing apprehensions regarding the toxicity and safety of modern drugs people all over the world is shifting back to traditional medicine. This global resurgence of interest in traditional herbal remedies has become a compelling reason to evolve a mission mode approach towards medicinal plants.

There is an abundance of knowledge about the medicinal properties and uses of plants incorporated in the native cultures of people throughout the world. Failure to document this indigenous ethnobotanical knowledge would result in its perpetual loss to humanity. Therefore, Central Council for Research in Unani Medicine (CCRUM) in India has included the ethnobotanical exploration as one of the programmes in its multidirectional research activities. The Survey of Medicinal Plants unit of RRIUM (CCRUM), Sgr has been continuously making efforts to make salvage of some of the native folklore, especially regarding the medicinal use of plants. For this ethnobotanical survey tours are conducted continuously in the far-flung and tribal areas of Jammu and Kashmir State (J&K). The present paper deals with the gamut of information generated from such field studies.

All those areas of J&K, which fall in the mighty mountain ranges of Western Himalaya, constitute what is commonly known as "Kashmir Himalaya". It serves as a unique natural area and is very rich in floristic wealth. A wide range of climatic and topographic diversity has endowed it with a broad spectrum of vegetation pattern ranging from sub-tropical–temperate and sub alpine/alpine to the cold arid conditions of Ladakh. It has been a source of variety of medicinal plants, which have been put to use from the time immemorial. Kashmir valley has enjoyed the reputation of being the home of herbal Medicine. It is said that the veteran Ayurvedic scholar Charka was Kashmiri Brahmin.

Due to difficult terrain and severe climatic conditions many areas in the Kashmir Himalaya have no surface communication with outside world for about 3-5 months a year. Therefore, the people have been largely relying on plants growing around for their basic necessities of life, be it food, fodder, fuel or medicine. The plants growing in this region have high medicinal properties but unfortunately most of the species have become rare and threatened and need special attention for their survival.

## 2.0 Methodology

The ethnobotanical survey tours (both one day and multi day) were conducted across the J&K. The information on each plant was recorded in the field through interviews with the persons having knowledge of medicinal plants or practicing as local medicine–men. The claims collected from one locality were crosschecked with another locality for confirmation. For each plant species information was collected on local name, medicinal use, parts used and mode of application. A review of literature for general information, bioprospection, use in Unani system of Medicine and bioactivity etc for the plants described in the paper was carried out thoroughly. Voucher specimens were deposited in the herbarium of RRIUM, Srinagar. Besides certain analytical characters were measured for each plant species during field studies.

## 3.0 Results and Observations

Although a large number of folk claims have been collected during ethno pharmacological explorations, however, only 15 plant species having attributes to Unani system of medicine, high demand in the local market and seem to have better prospects for commercial production have been discussed in the paper. The folk medicinal use with local name or names and parts used are summarized in Table 54.1. The uses in Unani System of Medicine (USM) Unani name, some main phytochemical constituents and the bioactivity of the plant species are briefly given below:

### *Achillea millefolium* L

**Unani Name**

Biranjasif

**Use in USM**

Laxative, diuretic, anthelmintic, analgesic, abortifacient.

**Phytochemical**

Aerial part yields essential oil, Achillicin, achillin, austrirein, Constituents: millefin and achilifolin, flavone, derivatives like apigenin, luteolin, rutin, etc were recently found (Innocente *et al.*, 2007)

**Bioactivity**

Essential oil shows antioxidant and antimicrobial activity (Ferda, *et al.*, 2003); Hepatoprotective, antispasmodic (Yaeesh, *et al.*, 2006); Anti protozoan activity in essential oil on Trypanosoma cruzi (Giani, *et al.*, 2007)

**Table 54.1**

| *Name of the Plant (Botanical Name)* | *Local Name* | *Parts Used* | *Folk Medicinal Use* |
|---|---|---|---|
| *Achillea millefolium* L. (Asteraceae) | Pehl gass, Panjoli | Flowering spikes and Leaves | Leaves made into paste to cure tooth and head aches. Powdered leaves and flowering spikes used as tonic and antipyretic |
| *Aconitum heterophyllum* wall ex Royle (Ranunculaceae) | Patris, Pivak | Root | Root taken orally to cure abdominal pain and as anthelmitic. Decoction of root is used in fevers |
| *Artemisia absinthium* L (Asteraceae) | Tethwan | Aerial part | Taken with water as vermifuge, leaves are used as insecticides |
| *Asplenium adiantum* nigrrum L. (Polypodiaceae) | Dade | Whole plant | It is used to treat diarrhoea, jaundice and as diuretic. Young leaves taken as vegetable and considered healthy food. |
| *Berberis lycium* Royle (Berberidaceae) | Kawdach | Fruits, Root and Bark | Fruit is eaten raw as tonic and anticoagulant. Decoction of root and bark is used for eye infections and boils. Decoction of root taken as antidiabetic. |
| *Paeonia emodi* wall ex H.K.f | Mid | Root | Powdered roots are used as purgative in dyspepsia. Fleshy roots are used in uterine disease, biliouness, dropsy and nervous affections. In fusion of flowers is given to control diarrhoea. |
| *Colchium luteum* Baker (Liliaceae) | Verikeom | Bulbs | The extract of bulbs is used to cure sciatica, rheumatism, swollen joints and as aphrodiasic. |
| *Cydonia oblonga* Miller (Rosaceae) | Bum Chunt | Fruit | Fruit taken as vegetable and considered as cardiac tonic. Jam of fruits is used in winter to prevent cough and other chest complaints. Dried seeds are used to cure mouth ulcers. |
| *Delphiunm denudatum* Wall. ex HandT (Ranunculaceae) | Nirbisi | Root | Roots are used to cure gastritis and enlargement of liver, root paste externally applied to cure arthritis and as antiseptic. Leaves are used as insecticide. |
| *Picorhiza kurooa* Royle ex Benth (Scrophulariacae) | Kour | Root | Extract of the roots is used in stomach troubles, fevers. Root paste applied externally to cure hyperpigimentation. |
| *Podophylum hexandrum* Royle (Podophulariaceae) | Banwangun, Papra, Drenmokshu | Fruit and Root | Fruit is eaten raw to cure chest congestion. Root extract is used to cure rheumatism, stomach and hepatic troubles. |

*Contd...*

**Table 54.1–Contd...**

| Name of the Plant (Botanical Name) | Local Name | Parts Used | Folk Medicinal Use |
|---|---|---|---|
| *Prunella vulgaris* L. (Lamiaceae) | Kalveoth Ust-e- Kudus | Whole plant | Flowers boiled in water and vapours inhaled to relieve body ache. The decoction of whole plant is taken orally to cure upper respiratory ailments, Jaundice and obesity and as antipyretic. |
| *Salix caprea* L. (Salicaceae) | Breidmushk | Flowers | Decoction of flowers is used to cure chest congestion and as vitalizer and tonic. The leaves are cooked as vegetables and given to the women during pregnancy as general and uterine tonic. |
| *Taraxacum officinale* Webber (Asteraceae) | Hundh | Aerial part | Decoction of leaves is also used against diabetes and as anti-inflammatory |
| *Viola odorata* L. (Violaceae) | Nun Posh Bunafsha | Whole plant | The infusion of flowers or whole plant is taken orally to cure acute bronchitis and as antipyretic. |

## *Aconitum heterophyllum* wall ex Royle

### Unani Name

Atees

### Use in USM

Antiperiodic, aphrodiasic, astringent, tonic, dyspepsia and cough

### Phytochemical Constituents

Hetisine, heterophylline, heterophyllisine, heterophyllidene, atidine, and constituents dihydroatisine.

### Bioactivity

Preparation of Aconitum species showed marked influence on development of inflammation (Pashinskii *et al.*, 2006). Plant extract inhibited spinach Mosaic virus (Zaidi *et al.*, 1986) immunomodulatory activity (Atal *et al.*, 1988). Antihypertensive activity (Raymond *et al*, 1954)

## *Artemisia absinthium* L

### Unani Name

Afsantin

### Use in USM

Used in epilepsy, hemiplegia, and facial palasy and as melancholic, antispasmodic, antiseptic. Also used in fevers, swelling and inflammation of viscera.

**Phytochemical Constituents**

Yields volatile oil called absinthe and contains thujylalcohol, cadinone, constituents etc. bitter glucosides absinthin, anabsinthin, artemetin and Artebsin, absintholide, artenolide. 2 new diastercomeric homoditerpene peroxides from aerial parts (Rucker *et al.*, 1992)

**Bioactivity**

Steroid sparing has shown significant effect in crohn's disease (Omer *et al.*, 2007). Crude extract exhibited hepatoprotective action, thus validates traditional use (Anwar *et al.*, 1995) Antimalarial activity (Rucker *et al.*, 1995). Also shows antimicrobial activity.

## *Asplenium adiantum-nigrum* L

**Use in USM**

Not found in Unani literature but widely used by Unani physicians in Kashmir for the diseases of spleen and ophthalmology.

**Phytochemical Constituents**

Flavonoids like some glucosides and rhamnosides found in aerial parts constituents (Filippo, 1991). Also conatins hydroxycinnamic acid, stearic acid, vitamin K3

**Bioactivity**

Expectorant, laxative, purgative, diuretic, anti jaundice and anti- constipative (Vasudeva, 1999)

## *Berberis lycium* Royle

**Unani Name**

Dharhald

**Use in USM**

Fruit astringent, sedative, anti pyretic. Roots used as resolvent, lithotryptic, diuretic, anti–rheumatic, anti paralytic and in hemicrania.

**Phytochemical Constituents**

Berberine, Tertiary dihydroprotoberberine and Barbamine

**Bioactivity**

Himalayan plant showed pesticide effect (Tewery, 2005). Berberine sulphate shows anti-inflammatory effect. Berberine produced antagonistic effect on ventricular arrhythmia following myocardial ischemia in wistar rats (Zhongguo *et al.*, 1993). Berberine also increases required dose of aconitine and oubain to induce ventricular premature beats, ventricular fibrillation and tachycardia and cardiac arrest. Barbamine shows hypotensive action.

## *Colchicum luteum* Baker

### Unani Name

Suranjan

### Use in USM

To treat gout, rheumatism and diseases of liver and spleen.

### Phytochemical

Seeds and corm contains colchicines, 2–demethylcolchcine, N-formyl- N–deacetycolchcine and β and γ-lumicolchicine. Seeds also contain carnigerine corms, contain non tropane alkaloids lutein and luteidine, collutene, colchamine, 3–dimethylcolchamine, 3–demethyl, β-lumicolchicine and luteunine and also reported form plant.

### Bioactivity

Colchicine analogs–deactyl thiocolchicine (DTC), deactylmethyl colchicine (DMC) and trimethylcolchine acid (TMCA) were effective in the treatment of Gout: DMC and DTC may alicit argranulocytosis.

## *Cydonia oblonga* Miller

### Unani Name

Behi

### Use in USM

Used as cardiac stimulant, tachycardia, antianxiety and in flatulence and liver complaints. Seeds have laxative and cooling effect.

### Phytochemical Constituents

A homo–monoterpenic compound recently isolated by Soura, *et al.* constituents 2007. Caffeoylquinic and dicaffeeoylquinic acids, lucenin, stellarin (Silva *et al.*, 2005); 4 hydroxy–7,8–dihydro–B–ionone in fruits juice; Marmelolactones A and B from fruit (Rastogi and Mehrotra, 1980)

## *Delphinium denudatum* Wall ex H. and.Th.

### Unani Name

Jadwar

### Use in USM

Stimulant, tonic, alterative, anti–epileptic and hemiplegia.

### Phytochemical Constituents

Delphinidine, denudatidine, isotalatizidine, condelphine. New constituents diterpenoid alkaloid and acetyllheterophyllisine isolated (Rahman *et al*, 1997)

**Bioactivity**

Ethanolic extract showed protective effect in a rat model of Parkinsons disease (Ahmad *et al.*, 2006). Root extract showed anti epileptic activity (Raza *et al.*, 2001). Memory enhancing activity (Nizami *et al.*, 2005) and antifungal activity (Rahman, 1997)

## *Paeonia emodi* Wall ex H. F

**Unani Name**

Odd–e–Saleeb

**Use in USM**

Epilepsy, facial palsy, uterine diseases, biliousness, dropsy and hysteria.

**Phytochemical Constituents**

Monoterpene glycosides, triterpene (Muhammad *et al.*, 1999), Gallic constituents acid, methyl gallate, emodinol (Riaz *et al.*, 2003), Paeoninol and Paeonin isolated from the fruit (Riaz *et al.*, 2004)

**Bioactivity**

Lipoxygenase inhibiting and antioxidant activity shown (Riaz *et al*, 2004); Plant has shown sedative, anti–inflammatory activities and also anticonvulsant (Yu *et al.*, 1990) and Anti anxiety activities.

## *Picrorhiza Kurooa* Royle ex Benth

**Unani Name**

Kutki

**Use in USM**

Antieplieptic, swollen piles, cough, leucoderma, ascitis, anti flatulent, tranquilizer, abortificent, anti-inflammatory and antipyretic.

**Phytochemical**

Root extract yields picroliv which contains constituents like picrosides I, II and IV. Kutkoside, minecoside, scroside B (Kumar *et al*, 2004); Extract of seeds yielded a new tritepenoid, 2$\alpha$, 3$\beta$, 19 $\beta$, 23 tetrahydroxyolean–12–en–28–0–D–$\beta$-glucoside along with other known triterpenoids.

**Bioactivity**

Water extract of the plant showed hypolipemic effect in hyperlipemic mouse (lee *et al.*, 2006). The biopolymeric fraction (RLJ–NE205) isolated from rhizomes improves the immune system (Gupta *et al.*, 2006). Apocyanin proved effective in arthritis, colitis and athero–sclerosis (Worm *et al.*, 2001). The methanolic extract exhibited anti-inflammatory, antistress and immunomodulatory and antihepatotoxic actions (Russo *et al.*, 2001; Ansari *et al.*, 1991)

## *Podophylum hexandrum* Royle

**Unani Name**

NA

**Use in USM**

Unani physicians use powdered rhizomes as hepatic stimulant and purgative.

**Phytochemical Constituents**

Podophyllotoxin identified from high altitude sps (Puri *et al.*, 2006) constituents Aryltetralin lignans and podophyllone.

**Bioactivity**

Modulates gamma radiation induced immumosuppresion in balb/mice implications in radioprotection (Goel *et al.*, 2007). Rhizome extract exhibited cytotoxic and radioprotective properties, (Shukla *et al.*, 2006). Podophyllotoxin is important for it's anti cancer activities. It is used as a precursor for the chemical synthesis of anticancer drugs etopside, teniposide and etopophose (Fartya *et al.*, 2004). Lignans from the leaf extract showed antifungal activity.

## *Prunella vulgaris* L

**Unani Name**

Ust–e–Kudus (In Kashmir only)

**Use in USM**

In the upper respiratory tract infections and the diseases caused due to accumulation of phelgum. The decoction of the plant is also used in hepatitis and ascites. Externally applied on painful joints to reduce inflammation.

**Phytochemical Constituents**

Lupeol, stigmasterol, olenolic acid, ursolic acid (Beijing *et al.*, 1985). constituents Prunellin (Tabba *et al.*, 1989). Penta and Hexa cyclic acids from roots (Kojima *et al.*, 1987, 1988)

**Bioactivity**

Aquous extract showed, a high antiviral activity against herpes simplex virus (HSV)–1,2 and acyclovir (resistant) strain (Nolkeuper *et al.*, 2006) and a concentration dependent photo-protection against UVA induced oxidative stress and may be beneficial as a supplement in photo protective dermatological preparations (Psotova *et al.*, 2006). Polysaccharides extracted from the plant exhibited both immune stimulatory and anti-inflammatory effect against microbial invasion (Fang *et al.*, 2005). Prunellin has shown anti HIV activity (Tabba, *et al.*, 1989)

## *Salix caprea* L

**Unani Name**

Beid mushk.

**Use in USM**

Flowers, leaves and stem bark are used as stimulant, refreshing, cardiac and brain tonic sedative, laxative, antipyretic and in Jaundice and the enlargement of spleen

**Phytochemical Constituents**

1,4–dimethoxybenezene (Floral scent compound) Dotterl *et al.*, 2005. constituents Stem wood and knots were found to contain the phenolic compounds like vanillic acid, naringenin, coumaryl alcohol, coniferyl alcohol, sinapylaldehyde, dihydrokaempferol, catechin, gallocatechin and taxifolin (Pohjamo, *et al.*, 2003)

**Bioactivity**

Anti-oxidant and hepatoprotective activity (Alam *et al.*, 2006). Inhibits skin carcinogenesis in murine skin, oxidative stress, ornithine decarboxylaase activity in DNA synthesis (Sultana *et al.*, 2004)

## *Taraxacum officinale* Webber

**Unani Name**

Kasni (In Kashmir only)

**Use in USM**

In ascitis, jaundice, choleocystitis and as, liver and spleen tonic, resolvent deobstruent. Seeds are used in tachycardia and enlargement of spleen. Root is used as blood purifier.

**Phytochemical Constituents**

Lutein epoxide from petals (Martinez *et al.*, 2006). Sesquiterpene constituents lactones, taraxinix acid derivatives, benzyl glucoside, syringin etc were isolated from roots (Kisiel *et al.*, 2000). Taraxalisin isolated from root latex (Ruden Skaya *et al.*, 1998) Hydroxycinamica acids, chicoric acid, monocaffeyltartaric acid and chlorogenic acid through out the plant; coumarins, chichorin and aesculin found in leaf extracts (Williams *et al.*, 1996).

**Bioactivity**

Flower extract possesses antioxidant activity (Hu *et al.*, 2005) hot water extract of the plant shows correlation with anti tumour activity (Baba *et al.*, 1981) with some other plants has shown to decrease glucose and fructose amine levels in non obese diabetic mice (Petlvki *et al.*, 2001). It has shown increase in Nitric oxide production in mouse. Nitric oxide has diverse functions like vasodilation, neural communication, cell growth regulation and host defence.

## *Viola odorata* L

**Unani Name**

Bunafsha

**Use in USM**

Antipyretic, resolvent, laxative and demulcent. Also used in eczema and to cure certain eye disease and bronchitis.

**Phytochemical Constituents**

Linear cyclotide, violacin A (Ireland *et al.*, 2006) two polypeptides–constituents vodo M and vodo N isolated (Svangard *et al.*, 2003.)

**Bioactivity**

Plant extract exhibited 100 per cent repellency effect against *Aedes aegypti*, *Anopheles stephensi* and *Culex quinquefasciatus* (Amer *et al.*, 2006). The chemical and biological stability of cyclotides of V. odorata have potential as pharmacological tools and as leads to anti tumour agents (Lindholm *et al.*, 2002). Significant oral antipyretic activity comparable to asprin shows by hexane extract (Khattak *et al.*, 1985)

## 4.0 Discussion

India is considered one of the 12-mega biodiversity centres of origins in the world (J.I.N Kumar *et al.*, 2005). The J&K state contributing part to this treasure is also rich in ethnic folklore, culture and heritage. The people have their own food habits, some indigenous beverages, cultural practices and the art of herbal healing. The present studies indicates that the man–plant relationships are strong and the concept of traditional medicine is well established and the people have deep faith on the effectiveness of the herbal cure. Although the modern medicine has attracted the attention of the people of J&K, particularly in main towns but still, there is a large population who prefer to use natural herbs in primary health care. These herbs are used by locals in crude form and have successfully cured their ailments for generations. Since the climate of the area is extremely cold during winters the people are usually susceptible to chest congestion, dyspnoea, throat infections and some skin diseases like frostbites and ulcers. However, the people have developed effective therapies to prevent themselves from these diseases.

A perusal of literature indicates that the use of some medicinal plants likes *Artemisia absinthium*, *Achillea millefolium*, *Cydonia oblonga* and *Viola odorata*, etc have already been reported in literature. However, the modes of application in many cases are different as far as the part of the plant used, method of preparation of drugs and modes of administration are concerned. This suggests that folk medicinal therapies developed through personal experience in tribal and other folk communities are mostly endemic in nature. It can be further ratified by the fact that in some cases different names have been given to the same plant sps even within the same state as *e.g. Achillea millefolium* L. is known as pehlgass in the southern and eastern parts of the state and as Panjoli in the northern parts. Similarly podophyllum hexandrum known as Drenmokshu in Kargil area, papra in upper reaches of Naranag and ban–wangun in rest of the state. Prunella vulgaris which is locally known as Kalveout but as Ustekudoos in the local market which is the name given to Lavendulla stoechs in Unani literature. It is quite confusing and strongly suggests a thorough investigation to develop a sort of common code of nomenclature to all species used in the traditional system of medicine. As is evident in the observations/results part the present biological investigation of plants showed promising activities and in some cases that coincides with the traditional uses and thus, proves the authenticity of the traditional medicines. Indeed, the revelation of such proofs has been an impetus towards the modern biological activities and has laid the foundation of reverse pharmacology.

Therefore, all such plants growing here in Kashmir Himalaya have considerable importance, actual and potential–for both traditional and modern system of medicine. There is a need to undertake detailed phytochemical and pharmacological studies of the medicinal plants growing locally in this region as it may lead to the discovery of new compounds of therapeutic value for the treatment of specific ailments for which there is no satisfactory treatment in modern medicine.

The foregoing discussion reveals that there is no dearth of potential in the medicinal plants growing in Kashmir Himalaya. But unfortunately the picture is not so bright as far as the present status of many important medicinal plant species in natural habitats is concerned. They have fallen prey to the unplanned human activities and are faced with the onslaught of ecological crisis that has rendered them at the brink of extinction. During the ethnobotanical exploration certain analytical characters like frequency, dominance, abundance etc were also studied to make the assessment of the germplasm. There are number of factors responsible for the depletion of medicinal plants. Most of the medicinal plants in this region grow at higher altitudes and usually in the habitats that are vulnerable. However, our observations in the field showed that the pressures of over grazing are as much responsible for the depletion of important medicinal plants as is the indiscriminate exploitation for commercial gains. The distribution and status of the plant species included in this paper is given in Table 54.2. Apart from measuring analytical characters the local herbal drug markets were survived in different districts to ascertain the availability of medicinal plants. It was found that Delphinium denudatum was rarely available in the market and for Rs. 3600 kg when the same drug before 4-5 years was selling at Rs. 800 kg and was easily available. Paeonia emodi was not available in the local market at all. The cost of *Aconitum heterophyllum* has gone from Rs. 500 (2 years back) to Rs. 3500 at present. All these details and the findings in Table 54.2 evidently shows that there is an urgent need to plan strategies for the conservation of the rare and threatened medicinal plants. Conservation should be done involving both conventional and biotechnological approaches. Guidelines for *in situ* conservation and *ex situ* cultivation in near to natural conditions are needed to be prepared and implemented. It is imperative to make more use of biotechnological methods, which will not only help in achieving the target quickly, but it will also provide a tool for generating variability. Thus the vanishing germplasm can not only be rescued from extinction but also improved genetically. Domestication of some high altitude medicinal plants like *Aconitum heterophyllum*, Podophyllum hexandrum, Picrorhiza kurooa, Colchium leutum, Paeonia emodi etc is a challenge. In such cases more modern techniques are required for the identification and isolation of novel genes and development of transgenics for designer plants that will be of great help and will prove frugi ferrous.

**Table 54.2: Local Distribution and Present Status of the Plant Species**

| *Name of the Plant Species* | *Local Distribution* | *Present Status* |
|---|---|---|
| *Achillea millefolium* L | Pakistan to Uttar Pradesh. Temperate–subalpine1500–3500m | Common |
| *Aconitum heterophyllum* wall ex Royle. | Pakistan to Central Nepal. Subapline/alpine, 2700–4000 m | Rare |
| *Artemisia absinthium* L | Pakistan to Kashmir, temperate Sub alpine1700–3600m | Threatened |
| *Asplenium adiantum-nigrum* L | Kashmir–Himachal Pradesh Temp. Subalpine, 2000–3000m | Common |
| *Berberis lycium* Royle | Pakistan to Central Nepal Temperate zones 2000–3000m | Threatened |
| *Colchicum luteum* Baker | Pakistan–Himachal Pradesh Temperate zones1500–2600m | Very rare |
| *Cydonia oblonga* Miller | Cultivated in temperate regions | Not common in wild |
| Delphinium denudatum Wall ex H. C.T. | Western Himalaya Temperate Subalpine 2000–3000m | Rare |
| *Paeonia emodi* Wall ex H. F | Afghanistan to west Nepal 2200–3000 subalpine | Threatened |
| Picrorhiza kurooa Royle ex Benth | Pakistan–Uttar Pradesh Alpines 3300 - 4500m | Rare |
| *Podophylum hexandrum* Royle | Afganistan–SW China Subalpine/alpine 2700–4000m | Threatened |
| *Prunella vulgaris* L | Afghanistan to BhutanTemperate Subalpine, 1500 - 3600m | Common |
| *Salix caprea* L | Cultivated in temperate regions | Not common in wild |
| *Taraxacum officinale* Webber | Temperate Himalayas 1500–3000m. Also cultivated | Common |

Our extensive field studies make us to propose following few suggestions for overall improvement:

1. The existing laws should be reviewed to plug the loopholes.
2. The laws should be implemented strictly to prevent indiscriminate collection of rare and threatened sps.
3. The random grazing at higher altitudes should be stopped and pasturelands should be earmarked for the grazing of cattle
4. The availability of medicinal plants should be periodically assessed.
5. Drug Co-operatives be set up to make systematic collection of the plants and to organize training programmes to train the local people on different aspects of medicinal plants, like collection, cultivation, harvesting etc.
6. An inventory of the rare and threatened medicinal plants must be prepared which should include a detailed survey of the size and structure of the natural populations and their distribution.

7. To maintain quality assurances and GMP (as recommended by WHO) for the production of herbal drugs Govt. should intervene to regulate the purchasing of crude drugs by the industry, particularly, in those countries where the markets are still in juvenile stage.

## References

Ahmad, M., Yousuf, S., Khan, M.B., Ahmad, A.S., Saleem, S., Hoda, M.N. and Islam, F. 2006. Protective effect of ethanolic extract of *Delphinium denudatum* in a rat model of *Parkinson's* disease. *Human Experimental Toxicology*. 25(7): 361-368.

Alam, M.S., Kaur, G., Jabbar, Z., Javed, K. and Athar, M. 2006. Evaluation of anti-oxidant activity of *Salix caprea* flowers. *Phytother. Res.* 20(6): 479-483.

Amer, A. and Mehlhorn, H. 2006. Repellency effect of forty one essential oils against Aedes, Anophlese and Culex Mosquitoes. *Parasitol. Res.* 99(4): 478-490.

Ansari, R.A., Tripathi, S.C., Patnaik, G.K. and Dhawan, B.N. 1991. Anti hepatotoxic properties of *Picroliv:* an active fraction from rhizomes of *Picrorhiza kurroa. Journal of Ethnopharmocology*. 34(1): 61-68.

Anwar, H.G. and Khalid, H.J. 1995. Preventive and curative effects of *Artemisia absinthium* on acetaminophen and $CCL_4$ induced hepatotoxicity. *General Pharm,.acology*. 26 (2): 309-315.

Atal, C.K., Sharma, M.L., Kau1, A. and Khajuria, A. 1986. Immuno modulating agents of plant origin. Preliminary screening. *Journal of Ethnopharmacology*. 18(2): 133–41.

Atta-u-Rehman., Ashraf, M., Choudhary, M.I., Habib-ur-Rehman. and Kazmi, M.H. 1995. Antifungal aryltetrallin lignans from leaves of *Podophyllum hexandrum. Phytochemistry. 40(2):* 427-431.

Beijing Y.D. and Xuebao 1985. Isolation of ~ amyrin, Daucosterol, Oleanolic acid and Ursolic acid. *Chemical abstract*. 17: 297.

Chandler, R.F., Hooper, S.N. and Harvey, M.L 1982. Ethnobotany and phytochemistry of yarrow, *Achillea millefolium*. Compositae. *Economic Botany*. 36: 203-223.

Chawla, R., Arora, R., Puri, S.C., Shawl, A.S., Sultan, P., Krishan, T. and Qazi, G.N. 2006. r–*Podophyllum hexandrum* offers radioprotection by Modulating Free Radical Flux: Role of Aryltetralin Lignans. *Evidence-based Complementary and Alternative Medicine (eCAM)*. 10(1-9): 1093.

David, E., Jackson. and Dewick, P.M. 1984. Aryltetralin lignans from *Podophyllum hexandrum* and *P. peltatum. Phytochemistry*. 23(5): 1147-1152.

Dotterl, S., Fussel, U., Jurgens, A. and Aas. G. 2005. 1, 4-Dimethoxybenzene, a floral scent compound in willows that attracts an oligolectic bee. *Jour. Chem. Ecol.* 31(12): 2993-2998.

Farkya, S., Bisaria, V.S. and Srivastava, A.K. 2004. Biotechnological aspect of the production of the anti cancer drug: podophyllotoxin. *Appl. Microbiol. Biotechnol.* 65(5): 504-5 19.

Fattouch, S., Caboni, P., Coroneo, V., Tuberoso, C.L., Angioni, A., Dessi, S., Marzouki, N. and Cabras, P. 2007. Antimicrobial activity of Tunisian quince *(Cydonia oblonga* Miller.) pulp and peel polyphenolic extracts. *Jour. Agric. Food Chem.* 55(3): 963-969.

Ferda, C., Mehmet, U., Bekta, *T.*, Dimitra, D., Moschos, P., Atalay, S. and AskIn, A.H. 2003. Antioxidant and anti-microbial activity of the essential oil and methanol extract of *Achillea millefolium* subsp. *millefolium* Afan *(Astaraceae). Journal of Ethnopharmacology. 87(2-3):* 215-220.

Fillipo, I. 1991. Xanthone 2, 4–di–c–glycosides from *Asplenium-adiantum–nigrum. Phytochemistry.* 30(1 I): 3839-3840.

Fillipo, I. 1980. A Xanthone–*a*–glycoside from *Asplenium-adiantum–nigrum* L. *Phytochemistry.* 19(9): 2030-2031.

Goel., H.C., Prakash, H., Ali, A. and Bala, M. 2007. *Podophyllum hexandrum* modulates gamma radiation-induced immunosuppression in the *Balblc* mice: Implications in radioprotection. *Molecular Cell Biochem.* 295(1-2): 93-103.

Gulam, A.M. 1973. Tertiary di-hydroprotoberberine alkaloids of *Berberis lycium. Phytochemistry.l2(7): 1822-1823.*

Gupta, A., Khajuria, A., Singh, J., Bedi, K.L., Satti, N.K., Dutt, P., Suri, K., Suri, A.P. and Qazi, G.N. 2006. Immunomodulatory activity of biopolymeric fraction RLJ-NE–205 from *Picrorhiza kurroa. International immunopharmacology.* 6(10): 1543-1549.

Hamauzu, Y., Yasui, H., Inno, T., Kume, C. and Omanyuda, M. 2005. Phenolic profile, anti-oxidant property and anti-influenza viral activity of Chinese quince *(Pseudo cydonia sinensis* Schneid.), quince *(Cydonia oblonga* Mill.) and apple *(Malus domestica* Mill.) fruits. *Jour. of Agri. and Food Chem..* 53(4): 928-934.

Hu, C. and Kitts, D.O. 2005. Dandelion *(Taraxacum officinale)* flower extract suppresses both reactive species and nitric oxide and prevents lipid oxidation in vitro. *Phytomedicine. 12(8):* 588-597.

Ikram, M., Shafi, N., Mir, 1., DO, M.N., Naguyon, P. and Le Quesne, P.W. 1987. 24–zetaEthylcholesta–7; 22–dien–3 beta–01; a possible anti-pyretic constituent of *Artemisia absinthium. Planta Medica.* 53: 389.

Innocente, *G.*, Vegeto, E., Dall, S., Acqua, P., Ciana, M., Giorgetti, E., Agradi, A., Fico, S. and Tome, F. G. 2007. Invitro estrogenic activity of *Achillea millefolium* L. *Phytomedicine. 14:* 147-152.

Ireland, D.C., Colgrave, M.L., Nguyencong, P., Daly, N.L. and Craik, OJ. 2006. Discovery and Characterization of a Linear Cyclotide from *Viola odorata:* Implications for the Processing of Circular Proteins. *Journal of Molecular Biology.* 357(5): 1522-1535.

Kasimov, S.Z., Abdusamatov, A. and Malikov, V.M. 1987. Sesquiterpene lactones of two species of *Artemisia. Khim Prir Soedin.* 4: 607-608.

Khan, 1., Qayum, A. and Qureshi, Z. 1969. Study of hypotensive action of barbamine, an alkaloid isolated from *Berberis lycium. Life Sciences.* 8(17): 993-1001.

Khattak, S.G., Gilani, S.N. and Ikram, M. 1985. Antipyretic studies on some indigenous Pakistani medicinal plants. Journal ofEthnopharmacology. 14(1): 45-51.

Kim, H.M., Oh, e.H. and Chung, C.K. 1999. Activation of inducible nitric oxide sythase by *Taraxacum officinale* in mouse peritoneal macrophages. *General Pharmacology.* 32(6): 683688.

Kisiel, W. and Barszcz, B. 2000. Further sesquiterpenoids and phenolics from *Taraxacum officinale. Fitoterapia.* 71(3): 269-273.

Kojima, H., Tominaga, H., Sato, S. and Ogura, H. 1987. Pentacyclic triterpenoids from *Prunella vulgaris. Phytochemistry.* 26(4): 1107-1111.

Kojima, H., Tominaga, H., Sato, S., Takayanagi, H. and Ogura, H. 1988. Two novel hexacyclic triterpenoids from *Prunella vulgaris. Phytochemistry.* 27(9): 2921-2925.

Kumar, V., Mehrotra, N., Lal, J. and Gupta, R.e. 2004. Pattern profiling of the herbal preparation picroliv using liquid chromatography-tandem mass spectrometry. *Journal of Chromatography A.* 10456(1-2): 145-152.

Lindholm, P., Goransson, D., Johansson, S., Claeson, P., Gullbo, J., Larsson, R., Bohlin, L. and Backlund, A. 2002. Cyclotides: a novel type of cytotoxic agents. *Mol. Cancer Ther. 1(6):* 365-369.

Lee, H.S., Yoo, E.B. and Ku, S.K. 2006. Hypolipemic effect of water extracts of *Picrorhiza kurroa* in high fat diet treated mouse. *Fitoterapia.* 77(7-8): 579-584.

Nizami, Q. and Jafri, M.A. 2005. Convulsant, anti-anxiety and memory enhancing activities of *Delphinium denudatum. European Neuro-Psycho-Pharmacology.* 15(3): S 683.

Nolkemper, S., Reichling, 1., Stintzing, F.e., Carle, R. and Schnitzler, P. 2006. Antiviral effect of aqueous extract of the Lamiaceae family against *Herpes simplex virus* type 1 and type 2 in vitro. *Planta Medica.* 72(15): 1378-1382.

Ochir, G., Budesinsky, M. and Motl, O. 1991. 3–oxa-guaianolides from *Achillea millefolium. Phytochemistry.* 30: 4163-4165.

Omer, B., Krebs, S., Omer, H. and Noor, T.D. 2007. Steroid sparing effect of wormwood *(Artemisia absinthium)* in crohn's disease. *Phytomedicine.* 14: 87-95.

Ovezduriev, A., Abdular, N.D. Ucunov, M.l. and Kasimov, S.Z. 1987. Artenolids–a new disesquiterpene from *Artemisia absinthium. Khim Prir Soedin.* 5: 667-671.

Pashinskii, V.G., Gaidamovich, N.N., Poveteva, T.N., Vetoshkina, T.V., Nesterova, Iu.V. and Pushkarskii, S.V. 2006. Influence of *Aconitum* preparations on the development of chronic inflammation. *Eksp Klin Farmakol.* 69(2): 55-57.

Pelletier, S.W., Aneja, R. and Gopinath, K.W. 1968. The alkaloids of *Aconitum heterophyllum* wall.: Isolation and characterization. *Phytochemistry.* 7: 625-635.

Petlevski, R., Hadzila, M., Slijepcevic, M. and Juretic, D. 2001. Effect of 'anti-diabetis' herb preparation on serum glucose and fructosamine in NOD mice. *Journal of Ethnopharmacology.* 75(2-3): 181-184.

Pohjamo, S.P., Hemming, J.E. Willfor, S.M., Reunanen, M.RT. and Holmbom. B.R. 2003. Phenolic extractives in *Salix caprea* wood and knots. *Phytochemistry._63(2): 165-169.*

Puri, S.C., Handa, G., Bhat, B.A, Dhar, K.L., Spiteller, M. and Qazi, G.N. 2006. Characterization of two epimers, 4alpha and 4beta, of a novel podophyllotoxin-4-0-(D)-6-acetylglucopyranoside from *Podophyllum hexandrum* by LC-ESI-MS-MS. *Jour. of Chromatogr. Sci.* 84(3): 167174.

Rastogi, R.P. and Mehrotra, B.N. 1980-1984. *Compendium of Indian Medicinal Plants.* 3: 78. PID New Delhi.

Rastogi, R.P. and Mehrotra, B.N. 1990-1994. *Compendium of Indian Medicinal Plants.* 5: 11. PID New Delhi.

Rahman, A., Nasreen, A., Akhter, F., Shekhani, M.S., Clardy, J., Parvez, M. and Choudhary, M.l. 1997. Antifungal diterpenoid alkaloids from *Delphinium denudatum. Journal of Natural Products.* 60(5): 472-474.

Raymond, H. 1954. Anti hypertensive action of *Aconitum heterophyllum.* C *R Seances Soc. Bio!' Fif.* 108(13-14): 1221-1224.

Raza, M., Shaheen, F., Choudhary, M.l., Suria, A., Rahman, AU., Sombati, S. and DeLorenzo, R.J. 2001. Anticonvulsant activities of the FS-l sub fraction isolated from roots of *Delphinium denudatum. Phytother. Res.* 15(5): 426-430.

Roder, L.A., Schneider, M. and Winter, RP. 2002. Isolation oflonone glycosides, 9–0–beta–D-glucopyranoside of (6R)–3–oxo–4–hydroxyl–7, 8–dihydro–alpha–ionol; 3–oxo5, 6–epoxy beta–ionol from the leaves of *Cydonia oblonga. Natural Product Letters.* 16(2):119-122.

Tewery, D.K., Bhardwaj, A. and Shanker, A. 2005. Pesticidal activity in five medicinal plants collected from mid-hills of western Himalayas. 22(3): 241-247.

Tucker, A.O., Maciarello, M.J. and Sturtz, G. 1993. The essentials of *Artemisia,* Powis Castle and its putative parents *A. absinthium* and *A. arborescens. Journal of Essential Oil Research.* 5: 239242.

Vasudeva, S.M. 1999. Economic importance of Pteridophytes. *Indian Fern Journal.* 16(1-2): 130-152. Williams, C.A., Goldstone, F. and Greenham, J. 1996. Flavonoids, cinnamic acids and coumarins from the different tissues and medicinal preparations of *Taraxacum officinale. Phytochemistry.* 42(1): 121-127.

Worm, E.V., Beukelman, C.J., Berg, AJJ.V., Kroes, B.H., Labadie, R.P. and Dijk, H.V. 2001. Effects of methoxy1ation of apocyanin and analogs on the inhibition of reacted oxygen species production by stimulated human neutrophills. *European Journal of Pharmacology. 433(2-3):* 225-230

Yaeesh, S., Jamal, Q., Khan, A.U. and Gilani, A.H. 2006. Studies on hepatoprotective, anti-spasmodic and calcium antagonist activities of the aqueous-methanol extract of *Achillea millefolium. Phytother. Res.* 20 (7): 546-51.

Zafar, S., Aftab, A.M. and Siddiqui, *T.A.* 2002. Effect of root aqueous extract of *Delphinium denudatum* on morphine-induced tolerance in mice. *Fitoterapia.* 73(7-8): 553-556.

Zaidi, Z.B., Gupta, V.P., Samad, A. and Naqui, A.Q. 1988. Inhibition of spinach mosaic virus by extracts of some medicinal plants. *Current Science.* 57: 151-152.

Zhongguo, Y., Du1ixue, Yu. and Zazhi. 1993. Antagonistic effect of berberine on ventricular arrhythmia following myocardial ischemia. *Chem. Abstr.7: 119.*

Zhongguo, Y. and Zazhi. 1990. Effect of berberine on ventricular arrhythmia similar to that of quinidine. *Chem. Abstr.* 25: 113.

*Chapter 55*

# Perceptions, Attitudes, Knowledge and Practice of Traditional Medicines Among Bruneians: A Pilot Study

***Nurolaini Pg Haji Muhd Kifli[1]*, Zaw Wint[1] and Linda Lim[2]***

*[1] Institute of Medicine, University Brunei Darussalam, Jalan Tungku Link, Gadong, Brunei Darussalam*

*[2] Outpatient Pharmacy, Raja Isteri Pengiran Anak Saleha (RIPAS) Hospital, Gadong, Brunei Darussalam*

**E-mail: ineh799@yahoo.com, nurol@im.ubd.edu.bn*

## ABSTRACT

The usage of traditional medicine (TM) has become very popular in Brunei but no available data are presently available. This study was undertaken to investigate the extent of TM use in Brunei; to study Bruneian's perception, attitude and practices on the use of TM; to quantify the usage of TM against prescriptive medicines; to address the cost implication; and to support future studies. Questionnaire survey was designed by the researchers and pre-tested before distribution. The sampling was done by randomly using the snow balling method. 250 survey forms were administered to patients at the tertiary referral Hospital (Raja Isteri Pengiran Anak Saleha Hospital), University staff, friends and families. Analysis was done by SPSS package version 15. Overall, the response rate was good (60 per cent, *n=150*). 68.5 per cent of Bruneians had used some form of TM in their life (88.2 per cent of Chinese used TCM; 40 per cent of Malay used Local herbs and 38.8 per cent used TCM). Of the total, 82 per cent respondents who had used TM are within 31-45 years ($p<0.05$). The significant race of the users was Chinese (85 per cent, $p<0.05$). Interestingly, the genders of the users were equal. 70 per cent indicated TM is readily available. Among those using prescribed medicines (common cold remedies, antipyretics and antibiotics), 14 per cent were using TM. Interestingly, more than 70 per cent of respondents mentioned that they would not inform the doctors if they used TM or not. 77 per cent claimed that there are no adverse effects and the rest had reported that TM is associated with minor side effects (such as weight loss, weight gain, abdominal pain, nausea and vomiting and others). The total value of TM used around USD$140 millions/annum. TM usage is widely practiced among Bruneians due to the availability and believes. More than 50 per cent of TM users do not know their effectiveness and safety and perceived them as safe as these have been used for generations and from natural sources.

*Keywords: Traditional medicine, Usage, Bruneians, TCM, Perceptions.*

## 1.0 Introduction

The usage of traditional medicine includes local and Indonesian herbal remedies (Jamu), traditional Chinese medicines, Indian Traditional Medicines (Ayurveda), and many more has become very popular especially in the Asian regions (Williamson, 2006; Mukherjee, 2006; Lim, 2006). Traditional Medicine (TM) is a comprehensive term used to refer both to Traditional Medicine systems such as Traditional Chinese Medicine, Indian Ayurveda and Arabic Unani medicine, and to various forms of indigenous medicine. World Health Organisation (WHO) (WHO, 2002–2005) defines traditional medicine as including diverse health practices, approaches, knowledge and beliefs incorporating plant, animal, and/or mineral based medicines, spiritual therapies, manual techniques and exercises applied singularly or in combination to maintain well-being, as well as to treat, diagnose or prevent illness. The data and figures for Brunei Darussalam are unavailable but its use is likely to be of the same order. Currently traditional medicine is not regulated as medicines and can be freely purchased from outlets ranging from health and local food stores to Internet sites. This has led to concerns about their safety and quality. There is also the potential for interactions with conventional drugs (Shaw *et al.*, 1997; Izzo, 2001).

This pilot study investigated the extent, perception, attitude and practices on the use of traditional medicine in Brunei Darussalam, which involved questionnaire survey. There are several aims in this study: (*i*) to investigate the extent of traditional medicine usage in Brunei; (*ii*) to study Bruneian's perception, attitude and practices on the use of traditional medicine; (*iii*) to quantify the usage of traditional medicine against prescriptive medicines; (*iv*) to address the cost implication with the use of traditional medicine; and (*v*) to support future study in this area.

## 2.0 Methods

Questionnaire survey was designed by the researchers and was pre-tested to public before distribution. Modification were made on the 28-item structured questions which consists of demographic data (gender, age, races, identity card (i/c) number, occupation), history of usage of traditional medicine, sources and expenditure of traditional medicine per month, use of prescribed medicines and side effects. This pilot study was conducted over a period of 3 months, *i.e.* from December 2006 until February 2007. Random sampling by snow balling method did the sampling. 250

survey forms were distributed to patients at a tertiary referral hospital (RIPAS Hospital) located in Gadong, University's staff member and students, friends and families. Participants self-administered the questionnaire with information sheet about the aim of study. The survey form mostly required the participant to answer a yes, no or not sure response and it was translated bilingually (Malay and English).

Definition of Traditional Medicine is also included in the survey form. [Traditional Medicine in ASEAN definition is any medicinal product for human use consisting of active ingredients derived from natural sources (plants, animals and/or minerals) used in the system of traditional practice. This may include botanical and herbal medicines used traditional for therapeutic purposes over an undefined period of time]. Traditional Medicine were defined as any remedies prepared using traditional recipes or purchased as commercialised products from dispensaries, supermarkets or others. Specific enquiries were made into the types of the traditional medicines they used, duration, frequency, period and reasons of administering it. Opinion about traditional medicine was also asked from the respondents. Minor adverse effects of traditional medicine were also enquired such as weight loss, weight gain, abdominal pain, nausea and vomit and others. In order to quantify the usage of traditional medicine against prescriptive medicines, participants were also asked on any prescribed medications taken together with the traditional medicine. The subjects will state the name of the medications that they are using.

The data were coded and analysed using the SPSS (Version 15.0 software). The univariate analysis and bivariate analysis were carried out to analyse the relationships between variables. The significant level was taken when $p$ value was less than 0.05.

## 3.0 Results

Overall, the response rate is good (60 per cent, $n= 150$). It was reported from this study that 68.5 per cent of Bruneians had used some form of traditional medicine in their life (Chinese race had used 88.2 per cent of TCM; Malay race had used 40 per cent Local herbs and 38.8 per cent TCM). Bruneians were defined as local respondents who possess a yellow i/c colour (98 per cent) and permanent residents with a red i/c colour (2 per cent). The used of traditional medicines was highest among the 31-45 years age group (82 per cent, $p < 0.05$), refer to Figure 55.1. Quite an insignificant number of ethnic backgrounds from Dusun, Iban, Murut and kedayan participated in this study. Interestingly, the gender's of the users were in equal ratio (~ 1:1 male: female) and nearly 90 per cent of the users occupation either working with the government or students.

Majority of the respondents has stated that they have used multiple types of traditional medicine. Most respondents agreed that they used traditional medicines as recommended by friends and families (for both Chinese communities and Malay ethnic group), refer Figure 55.2. Other reasons to using traditional medicines such as for minor conditions, chronic conditions, infectious diseases, and any abnormality were not reported significantly.

Among those using prescribed medicines, 14 per cent were using traditional medicines. The types of prescribed medicines that the respondents were using are

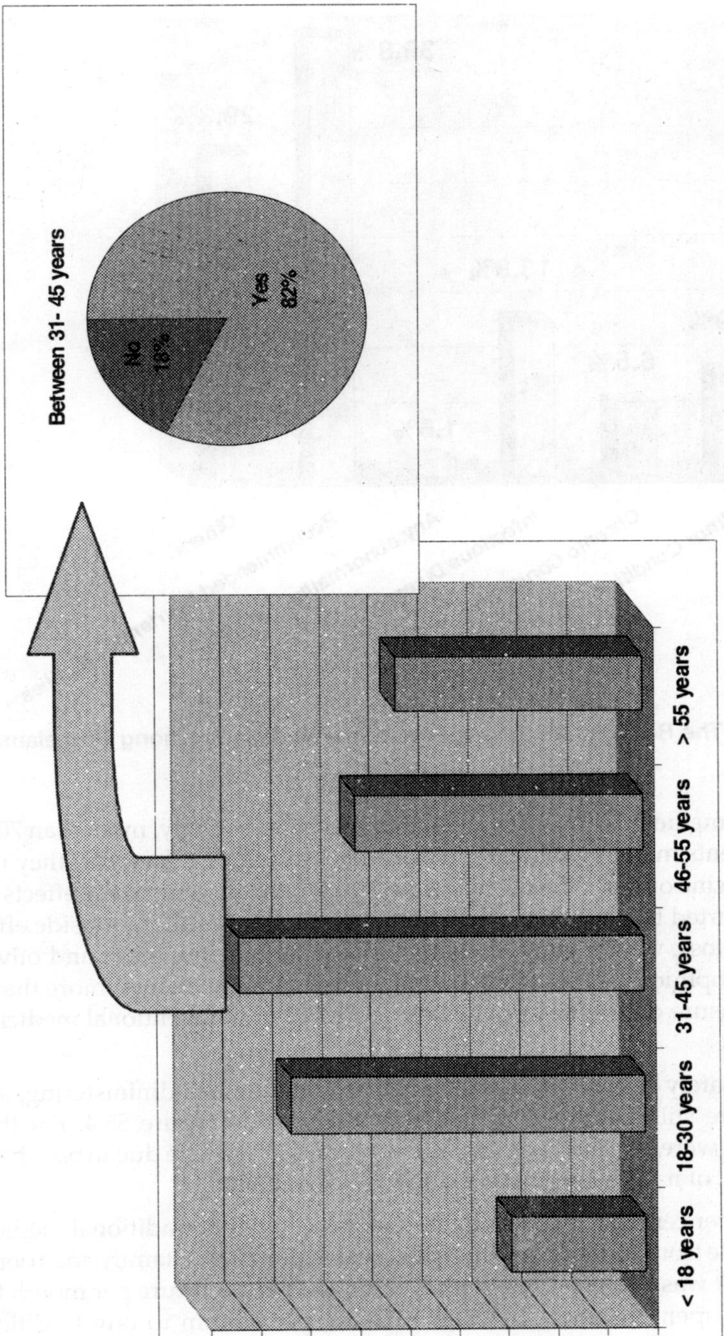


Figure 55.1: The Age Range of Bruneians who have used TM in their Lives

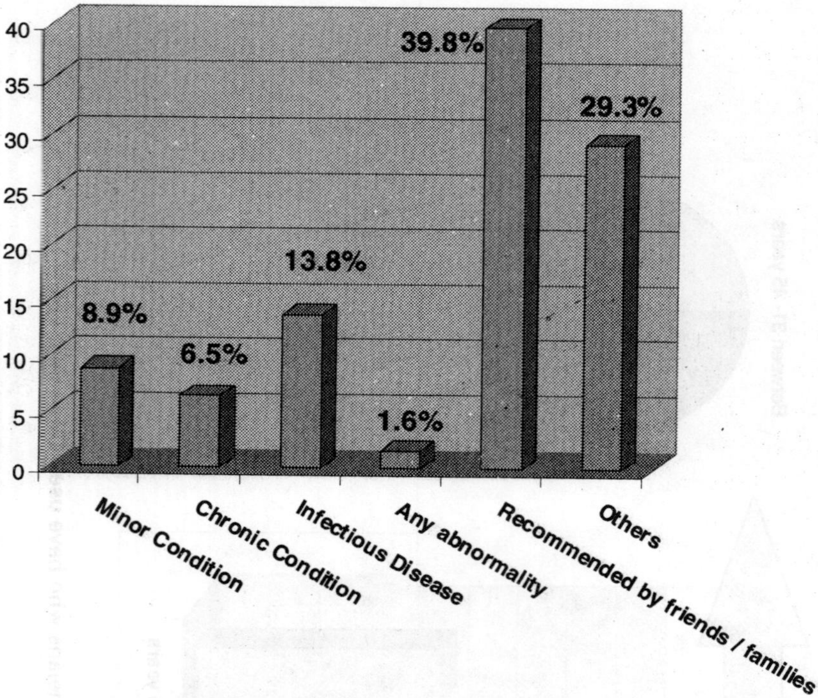


**Figure 55.2: The Reasons for Taking Traditional Medicines among Bruneians**

common cold remedies, antipyretics and antibiotics. Interestingly, more than 70 per cent of respondents mentioned that they would not inform the doctors if they used traditional medicine or not. 77 per cent claimed that there are no adverse effects and the rest had reported that traditional medicine is associated with minor side effects (such as weight loss, weight gain, abdominal pain, nausea and vomit and others). Regarding their opinion on the effectiveness of traditional medicines, more than 60 per cent were unsure of its efficacy when compared to the conventional medicines, refer Figure 55.3.

In terms of safety of the traditional medicines that they are administering, most respondents were still unsure of its safety as indicated in Figure 55.4. For those respondents that were certain those traditional medicines are safe due to no adverse effects were seen, of natural origins and due to cultural belief.

Overall, 70 per cent of the respondents had indicated that traditional medicine is readily available from Chinese dispensaries, local supermarket, family and friends. From the study, it was projected based on an estimated expenditure per month that Bruneian would spent around USD $140 millions per annum to buy traditional medicine either commercialised or natural sources of traditional medicine (either from the roots, bark, leave, flower or others).

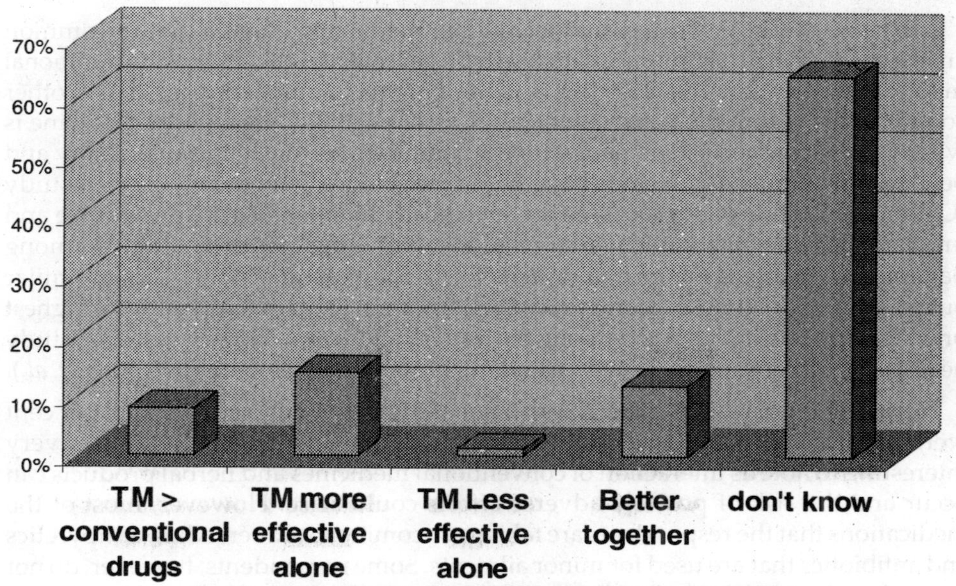


**Figure 55.3: Opinion Regarding the Effectiveness of Traditional Medicine versus Conventional Medicines**

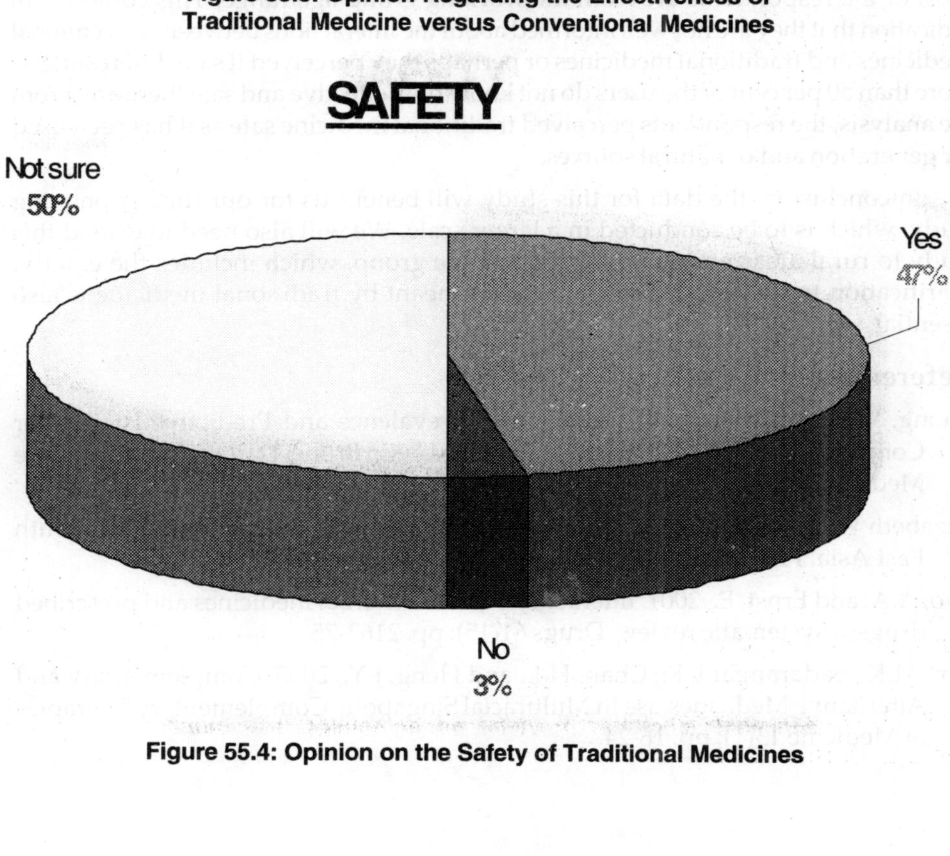


**Figure 55.4: Opinion on the Safety of Traditional Medicines**

## 4.0 Discussion and Conclusions

This pilot study showed that traditional medicines usage is not uncommon among the Bruneian community with nearly 70 per cent reported ever using traditional medicine within their life. This figure is comparable to other studies done in other communities within the Asian countries (Lim *et al.*, 2005). Traditional Medicine is widely practice among Bruneians Chinese communities due to the availability and believes that family and friends have used them before. In another reported study (Chong *et. al.*) done in our local setting specifically looking into the prevalence and predictive factors for complementary and alternative medicines (CAM) use among patients and relatives whom had visited RIPAS hospital (*n*=568) has shown similar outcomes; where Chinese communities are the highest users of CAM with the highest prevalence of CAM user were among the 30 to 39 age group. However, in that study health supplement such as vitamins and minerals was also included (Chong *et. al.*).

Among those respondents whom have used traditional medicines, 14 per cent were reported to have used conventional medicines concurrently. This is very interesting to note as interaction of conventional medicines and herbal products can occur and the risk of possible adverse effects could arise. However, most of the medications that the respondents are taking are common cold remedies, antipyretics and antibiotics that are used for minor ailments. Some respondents, however, do not remember the name of the medicines that they are taking. This is quite alarming as most of the respondents are from the working group age range. This could be an indication that they are not well informed about the interactions between conventional medicines and traditional medicines or perhaps they perceived it safe. Interestingly, more than 50 per cent of the users do not know how effective and safe there are. From the analysis, the respondents perceived traditional medicine safe as it has been used for generation and of natural sources.

In conclusion, the data for this study will benefit us for our further ongoing study, which is to be conducted in a larger scale. We will also need to extend this study to rural areas and various range of age group, which includes the elderly. Clarification to the respondents of what is meant by traditional medicine is also essential.

## References

Chong, V.H., Rajendran, M. and Wint, Z. Prevalence and Predictive Factors for Complementary and Alternative Medicine Use in Brunei Darussalam, Singapore Medical Journal, in press.

Elizabeth Williamson, 2006. System of traditional medicine from South and South East Asia. Pharmaceutical Journal (276): pp. 539-540.

Izzo, A.A. and Ernst, E., 2001. Interactions between herbal medicines and prescribed drugs: a systematic review. Drugs 61(15): pp. 2163-75.

Lim, M.K., Sadarangani, P., Chan, H.L. and Heng, J.Y., 2005. Complementary and Alternative Medicines use in Multiracial Singapore. Complementary Therapies in Medicine 13(1): pp. 16-24.

Mukherjee, P.K. and Wahile, A., 2006. Integrated approach towards drug development from ayurveda and other Indian systems of medicine. Journal of Ethnopharmacology (103): pp. 25-35.

Shaw, D., Leon, C., Kolev, S. and Murray, V., 1997. Traditional remedies and food supplements: a five-year toxicological study (1991-1995). Drug Safety (17): pp. 342-56.

World Health Organisation Traditional Medicine Strategy 2002-2005 (www.who.int/).

## Chapter 56

# Herbal Remedies and Utilization of Medicinal Resources in Bhutan

**Phurpa Wangchuk**
*Institute of Traditional Medicine Services, Department of Medical Services, Ministry of Health, Thimphu, Bhutan*
*E-mail: phurpaw@yahoo.com*

## ABSTRACT

Plenty of medicinal plants were found growing in the crags and valleys of Bhutan and for this reason, Bhutan was also known as "sMan-jong", the land of medicinal plants in olden days. Like any other countries, Bhutan host two forms of Indigenous medicines, the Local Healing Practices and the Formalized Traditional Medical System, which is locally known as *gSo-ba-rig-pa*. Its history goes back to the 8th century when Bhutan embraced Mahayana Buddhism and thusly, Buddhist philosophy remained as the mainstream of *gSo-ba Rig-pa* despite infectious influences by the principles of Greco-Roman, Ayurvedic, Chinese and Tibetan Medicine. Mainly owing to its historical significance and rich documentation supported by long clinical use and their effectiveness, *gSo-ba-rig-pa* medical system has been officially recognized and included in the mainstream of the national health care system in 1967. Today, there are 25 traditional medicine units attached to modern District Hospitals and the Basic Health Units (BHUs) and functions efficiently under the guardianship of the Institute of Traditional Medicine Services (ITMS), providing high quality traditional medical care free of cost. The ITMS based in Thimphu, comprises of three sections, each mandated with different responsibilities. About 98 essential traditional herbal medicines are manufactured at the Pharmaceutical and Research Unit (PRU) using 300 different medicinal ingredients. Both the raw materials and the finished products are subjected to strict quality control processes. The future priorities of the PRU and the Medicinal and Aromatic Plant Section (MAPS) under Ministry of Agriculture are inventory development, domestication trials, cultivation involving farmers, establishment of herb gardens, human capacity development, building research infrastructures, building collaborative partners, improving quality of traditional medicines through research and development and protecting the intellectual property rights of the uniquely propounded Bhutanese traditional medicine.

***Keywords:*** *Bhutan, Traditional medicine, Herbal remedy and Medicinal plants.*

## 1.0 Introduction

Like any other countries in the world, Bhutan host two forms of Indigenous medicines, the Local Healing Practices and the Formalised Traditional Medical System, which is locally known as *gSo-ba-rig-pa*. While the former Local Healing Practice is being transmitted orally from father to son or master to apprentice lacking in proper documentation, the *gSo-ba-rig-pa* medical practice is the classical and codified medical system which was officially recognized and included in the national health care system of the country in 1967 (Wangchuk *et. al*, 2007). Today, it is functional under the umbrella of the Institute of Traditional Medicine Services (ITMS) and has three sections: National Traditional Medicine Hospital (NTMH), National Institute of Traditional Medicine (NITM) and Pharmaceutical and Research Unit (PRU).

The NTMH is responsible for the development and provision of quality traditional medical care that range from behavioural modification, prescription of herbal medicines, herbal therapies including accupressure and herbo-aqua therapy, minor surgey and spiritual healing. Currently, there are 25 Traditional Medicine Units attached to the district hospitals and BHUs in Bhutan. It is fully integrated with modern health care delivery system and is provided free of cost for the patients (Wangchuk *et. al*, 2007). There is a plan to establish Traditional Medicine Units in all the Basic Health Units in the country.

The NITM is responsible for the development of human resources required for the provision of the traditional medical services in the country. The Institute offers five years degree course (B.Sc. Traditional Medicine), 3 years diploma and planned refreshers courses.

The PRU is responsible for manufacturing and production of herbal/traditional medicines, conducting quality control for both raw materials and finished products, carrying out research and product development activities, and ultimately marketing of the herbal products.

This paper presents the history of Bhutanese herbal remedies (gSo-ba Rig-pa) at a glance, treatment regimens, collection, utilization and sustainability of medicinal resources, research and development, constraints and future directions.

## 2.0 Origin and Development of gSo-ba Rig-pa in Bhutan

The term *gSo-ba Rig-pa* consists of two words, *gSo-ba* which means to heal, feed, nourish, correct, and *Rig-pa* which means science, knowledge, perception or erudition (Semichov, 1981). Thus, *gSo-ba Rig-pa*, means 'Science of Nourishment' and most often referred to as the 'Art of Healing Sciences'. This medical system has been an inextricable part of the Bhutanese health care tradition for generations.

Historically, it is reported that Lord Buddha taught medicine simultaneously with the teachings of the Buddhism mostly using disease and healing as metaphors to illustrate his philosophy of the human condition. Though Buddhism spread to many Asian countries, *gSo-ba Rig-pa* became prominent Tibet, Bhutan and Mongolia. While some sources noted that *gSo-ba Rig-pa* in Bhutan took shape with the advent of Mahayana Buddhism from Tibet in the 8th century (Dompnier, 1998), there are other sources stating that *gSo-ba Rig-pa* developed subsequently in Tibet and Bhutan. However, the information is sketchy and the historical data have not been verified but definitely, Greeco-roman, Ayurvedic and Chinese medicines, and the country's own Bon-Shamanistic cultures and traditions greatly influenced the way *gSo-ba-Rig-pa* evolved in Bhutan. Thus, Bhutanese traditional medicine is a synthesis of all the above elements including that of Tibetan medicine.

Bhutan saw the peak development of *gSo-ba Rig-pa* only in the 17th century, during the reign of Shabdrung Ngawang Namgyal. A later record shows that *gSo-ba Rig-pa* was greatly supported especially after 1885 when the secular (*Poenlops* and *Dzongpoens*) and the religious leaders (*Debs* and *Desis*) patronized the profession (Dharmananda, 2002). It is said that their courts privately employed or kept at least one or two esteemed physicians. The successive rulers including first King of Bhutan had many personal physicians. Thus, in olden days, this herbal remedy (*gSo-ba Rig-pa*) was accessible only to few elites.

In 1967, with the objectives of preserving the rich medical tradition and to broaden the health care choices for patients, the third King Jigme Dorji Wangchuk included the Traditional medical system in the National Health System of Bhutan. In 1968, a dispensary was opened in Thimphu (capital of Bhutan) and in 1971; formal training for Drungtshos (Traditional Doctors) and sMenpas (Traditional Compounders) was initiated, providing a solid professional base for gSo-ba Rig-pa. Today, ITMS has the following mandates:

- To preserve, promote and propagate the unique traditional medical system.
- To provide the quality traditional medical health care in the country.
- To develop human resources required for the provision of the traditional medical health care in the country.
- To conduct research and quality control of raw materials and finished products.
- To manufacture high quality traditional herbal drugs

This traditional medicine treats about 20-30 per cent of the total daily OPD patients of the district hospitals in the country as an integral part of the modern health care system (Wangchuk *et al.*, 2007).

## 3.0 Treatment Regimes

The treatment regimen in *gSo-ba Rig-pa* includes five kinds of healing methods like behavioural modification, physiotherapy, herbal medicines, minor surgery and spiritual healing. The behavioural and lifestyle changes include diet modification such as recommending right food, advising to abstain from bad habits like smoking and alcoholism, recommending to sleep for optimal time and advising to do physical exercise.

Physiotherapy includes acupressure and herbal therapy. Acupressure comprises of golden and silver needle therapy. Herbal therapy comprises of herbal bath, herbal steaming, nasal irrigation, and medicinal water bath. Medicinal water bath includes taking bath in the hot springs (Tsha-chus) and other waters that have medicinal properties (sMen-chus). Hot springs are very popular in Bhutan and are mainly used as a therapy for treating diseases instead of using them for a recreational and relaxation purposes. Mindful of the health benefits that the tshachus deliver to the Bhutanese people, the ITMS carried out a series of research on these popular hot springs. It is reported that most of the tshachus present in Bhutan are effective in treating patients with skin diseases, arthritis, old age syndromes, paralysis, venereal diseases and urinary tract infections (Wangchuk and Yeshi, 2007).

Unlike western medicine, prescription of herbal medicines and surgery are the last resorts of treatment. The herbal medicines are multi-ingredient compounds and can be used for various purposes. Some herbal compounds contain certain toxic ingredients like Aconitum species and may be dangerous if the intake dose is exceeded than what is being prescribed. So, physicians prefer to use them judiciously. Presently, minor surgery is almost never practiced in Bhutan, simply because the western surgical methods are more efficient.

Spiritual healing includes meditation and other faith related practices and it is currently applied in mental health care in Bhutan.

The side effect of Bhutanese traditional medicine is unknown till date and many believe that it has none. However, to comply with the international norms, a Pharmacovigilance Centre was established at the ITMS under the direct jurisdiction of the Drug Regulatory Authority of Bhutan. It monitors the side effect and adverse drug reaction of the traditional medicines manufactured and provided by PRU.

## 4.0 Collection and Utilization of Medicinal Resources

Meyer (1995) and Bagozzi (2002) reported that the Bhutanese traditional medical texts contains the formularies for as many as 2200 traditional multi-ingredient drugs and uses about 2990 medicinal plants. However, only 98 formularies are selected for the current national essential drugs list based on the prevalent disease patterns and trends in the country. These 98 formularies use 300 different types of ingredients, which according to *gSo-ba-rig-pa* medical texts, are classified into seven categories:

- Three are of vegetable origin, which is further classified, as *Sngo-sman* (high altitude medicinal plants), *Khrog-sman* (low altitude medicinal plants) and *Rtsi-sman* (resins and extracts).
- Three are of mineral origin comprising of *Rin-po-che-sman* (precious stones/ gems), *Rdo-sman* (base minerals/stone) and *Sa-sman* (medicinal soils).
- One of animal origin called *Srog-chags-sman*.

Due to the strategic topographical and climatic condition, Bhutan is blessed with mysterious zoological and botanical creations because of which almost 70 per cent of all categories of raw materials classified above are available within the country (Bagozzi, 2002). In fact, owing to plentiful availability of the medicinal plants, Bhutan was also known as *'sMan-jong'*, the land of medicinal plants in olden days (Yeshi, 2005). Most rare herbs grow in the alpine zone that supports tundra vegetation.

While the procurement of the raw materials that are imported from India is done through open bidding, the farmers through the involvement of the PRU Staff collect those raw materials available within the country. This is to make farmers realize the importance of medicinal resources and encourage them to sustainably utilize the resources.

The collection season is June to September for the high altitude (2500 to 5000 meters) medicinal plants and November to February for the low altitude (95 to 2500 meter) medicinal plants (Wangchuk, 2006). About 99 per cent of the high altitude medicinal plants used in the Bhutanese traditional medicine grow wild and are collected for their root, bulb, stem, flower, leaf and whole plant (Wangchuk, 2004). After harvesting, the farmers bring the medicinal plants to the drying units (Lingzhi for high altitude medicine plants and Langthel for the low altitude medicinal plants) and there, all the processes such as sorting, cleaning, seizing and drying are carried out. While drying the plant materials, three types of drying methods are followed; sunshine drying, shade drying and the hot air-drying. Shade drying is suitable for those medicinal plants that are sensitive to light. After drying properly, medicinal plants from the drying centres are transported to PRU either in horses or by vehicles. In 2006, PRU have procured about 13 metric tons of raw materials mainly medicinal plants (Wangchuk, 2006).

The raw materials, upon reaching PRU, are then subjected to quality control processes. Those medicinal plants that pass QC examinations are then stored in the raw material stores. From there, all the raw materials are issued for formulations of products. Using those 300 raw materials, Traditional Medicines are formulated into different dosage forms like pill (40 per cent), tablet (30 per cent), ointment (4 per cent), syrup (2 per cent), capsule (13 per cent), powder (4 per cent), crude extract (1 per cent) and un-established dosage forms (6 per cent) (Wangchuk, 2004). In 2006, the production section of PRU has manufactured about 14 metric tons of products, out of which 8 tons were core traditional medicines (Wangchuk 2006).

## 5.0 Sustainability of Medicinal Plants

Despite sound policy on environmental conservation and protection, there are issues and challenges related to the sustainability of medicinal plants and traditional medicines in Bhutan. Many medicinal plants such as *Aquilaria agallocha, Rawolfia serpentine, Ephedra gerardina, Taxus bacccata, Rheum nobile, Rheum accuminata, Picorrhiza* species, *Nardostachys jatamansi, Aconitum* species, *Artemisia* species, Panax pseudo-ginseng sub species himalaicus and *Cordyceps sinensis* are in high demand for pharmaceuticals and have potential international market value. As a result, there are highly executed operational network of illegal traders across the borders and thus the pressures on these medicinal plants have increased. Pressures on some of the medicinal plants also stems up from the following:

- Since Bhutan is an agricultural country, removal of forest for farming had adverse impact on the environment and the loss of the species.
- The cattle, yak and sheep rearing is country's another significant economic activity. Overgrazing of the forest by such animals has detrimental effect on the survival of the grazed plant species. As a result many species is becoming rare. For example, it is believed that intense browsing by yaks checks the growth of seedlings of the Himalayan yew-*Taxus baccata*.
- Some plants that contain pyrrolizidine alkaloids serve as natural feeding deterrents. Severe losses of yaks were reported in eastern part of Bhutan due to intake of *Senecio* species and the *Ligularia* species. These plants contained exceptionally high concentration of pyrrolizidine alkaloids (0.5 per cent/dry matter) and have become the object of menace to the cattle and sheep. So the herders vehemently uproot them. Such acts significantly contribute to the extinction of many alkaloids containing plant species.
- The logging activities, though minimal in Bhutan, have also impacted the growth of medicinal plants.
- Other forest based industries poses significant threat to the medicinal plants of Bhutan.

All these activities and the phenomena raise the issue of concern about the sustainability of some of the rare and threatened medicinal plants in Bhutan. This ultimately raises the doubt on the sustainability of some of the traditional medicine formularies, which uses those rare plants. With this concern and to preserve, promote and perpetuate the sustainability of the traditional medicine through the sustainable supply of useful medicinal plant species, ITMS in collaboration with the Medicinal and Aromatic Plant Section (MAPS) under Ministry of Agriculture initiated the domestication and cultivation trials on 16 prioritized medicinal plant species. The PRU and MAPS have also jointly established medicinal plant gardens in some selected districts like Thimphu, Haa and Bumthang for the high altitude medicinal plants; and Mongar, Tsirang and Trongsa for low altitude medicinal plants. Through such initiative, it is expected to enhance the production of herbal medicine, preserve threatened species and encourage bio prospecting of the medicinal plants in near future.

## 6.0 Research and Development Activities

At PRU, although the research and development is still in embryonic stage, research are being carried out in the following areas:

- Standardization of raw materials and finished products including botanical nomenclature, formulations and extracts.
- Scientific validation of traditional medicine including pharmacological analysis, which consists of clinical trials, claim validation and the fixation of expiry dates for the raw materials and the finished products.
- Pharmacognostical and phytochemical analysis including morphological, cellular, extraction, isolation and identification of bioactive phytochemicals.

These sections together produced first volume of monograph on twenty high altitude medicinal plants and are ready with the second volume of Monograph.

- Product development activities under six product categories such as pharmaceutics, over the counter products, fragrance and essence, cosmetics and toiletries, health promoting and nutraceuticals. Many products are under development.
- Building quality control test parameters and standards and monitoring the quality of the finished products and raw materials
- Operational research including the survey and documentation of medicinal plants, local healing practices and hot springs in Bhutan.

Recently, a research carried out by the author at the University of Wollongong on two Bhutanese medicinal plants *Aconitum orochryseum* and *Corydalis gerdae* was a great success. Former plant which was used in treating fever, snake bite and infections; furnished three new hetisine-type diterpenoid alkaloids and were named as Orochrine, 2-*O*-acetylorochrine and Lingshinaline (Wangchuk *et.al*, 2007). The later plant, from which known protoberberine alkaloids were isolated, was used in treating malaria and infections. These alkaloids and the extracts of both the plants gave significant antimalarial activities against *Plasmodium falciparum*. The antimalarial activity of the two plant isolates was in line with what they have been indicated and used for in Bhutanese traditional medicine. This has proved for the first time at the molecular level that Bhutanese traditional medicine had been founded on the empirical based sciences rather than hypothetical and theoretical assumptions. Such study and revelation was just the tip of an iceberg in an ocean full of ethnomedical informations. Subjection of Bhutanese medicinal plants, including the component of mixtures, to scientific objectivity and interpretational study would further enhance and validate the Bhutanese traditional medicine. The study would also result in obtaining many novel compounds and unknown new mechanisms of drug action. Thus, our traditional medicine has lot to offer both in terms of primary health care needs as well as in natural product-based drugs discoveries.

## 7.0 Constraints, Challenges and Future Directions

Having reported so much about achievements and opportunities, it doesn't mean that there is no constraints or challenges. In fact, there are lots of constraints and challenges. The most important of all is the constraints in research and development, challenges in ensuring sustainability of raw materials especially green resources and ultimately challenges in protecting our intellectual property rights. If there is strong research and development (R&D), all the later challenges can be taken care off. To make R&D well equipped and fully resourceful, it means huge investments in expensive equipments and developing specialized technical competency of the R&D staffs. But PRU cannot have that choice of investing heavily on R&D as the priorities of the ministry of health is on providing basic and free health care services through building Hospitals and BHUs to the communities in a view to reaching the un-reached. Therefore, PRU's future priorities are to:

- Achieving sustainability of medicinal resources
- Developing human capacity and research infrastructures
- Building collaborative partners for research and contract manufacturing
- Protecting the intellectual property rights of the uniquely propounded Bhutanese traditional herbal medicine.

## Acknowledgements

The author is indebted to the Royal Government of Bhutan for funding my participation in the Hanoi Workshop. The author also acknowledges the Head of PRU, Director of ITMS and the Authorities of Ministry of Health for their support in attending this important workshop.

## References

Anonymous, 2005. An introduction to traditional medicine services in Bhutan. Institute of Traditional Medicine Services, Ministry of Health, Royal Government of Bhutan, Thimphu, 2nd edition.

Bagozzi, D., 2002. Traditional and alternative medicine. Fact Sheet No. 297: WHO. Available from: http://www.who.int.

Dharmananda, S., 2002. Traditional medicine of Bhutan. Institute for Traditional Medicine, Portland, Oregon, available from http://www.itmonline.org/arts/bhutan.htm.

Dompnier, R., 1998. The art of healing. Tashi Delek, Druk air's in-flight magazine.

Meyer, F., 1995. The World of Tibetan Medicine. Oriental medicine-An Illustrated Guide to Asian Arts of Healing, Serindia Publications, London: pp. 107-143.

Semichov, B.V., 1981. Foreword. Tibetan Medicine, Library of Tibetan Works and Archives. Dharamsala (4): pp.1-11.

Wangchuk, P., 2004. Bioactive alkaloids from medicinal plants of Bhutan. Department of Chemistry, University of Wollongong, Australia.

Wangchuk, P., 2006. Processing and utilization of non wood forest product by Menjong Sorig Pharmaceuticals. Proceedings of the National Workshop on Development of Non-Wood Forest Products in Bhutan, Forest Resources Development Division, Department of Forest, Ministry of Agriculture, RGoB, Thimphu, Bhutan: pp. 92-97.

Wangchuk, P. and Dorji, Y., 2007. Historical Roots, Spiritual Significance and the Health Benefits of mKhempa-Jong gNyes Tshachu (hot spring) in Lhuntse. Journal of Bhutan Studies, Summer (16): pp. 112-127.

Wangchuk, P., Wangchuk, D. and Agaard-Hansen, J., 2007. Bhutanese Traditional Medicine (gSo-ba-rig-pa): An Integrated Part of the Formal Health Care Services. SEAJTMPH (38 (1)): pp.161-167.

Wangchuk, P., Samten, Ugyen, Thinley, J. and Afaq, S.H., 2007. High altitude medicinal plants of Bhutan. Indian Journal of Ethnobotany.

Wangchuk, P., Bremner, J.B., and Samosorn, S., 2007. New Hetisine-type Diterpenoid Alkaloids from the Bhutanese Medicinal Plant *Aconitum orochryseum* Stapf. J.Nat.Prod (70): pp. 1808-1811.

Yeshi, D., 2005. Sman-ljong zer-wai khungs. Proceedings of the 5th Colloquium on Tangible and Intangible Culture of Bhutan, National Museum of Bhutan, Paro, Bhutan: pp.55-64.

# *Chapter 57*

# A Preliminary Study on the Lowering of Cholesterol Levels by a Combination of Black Seed and Garlic

*M.H.A. Tissera[1]*, K.M.M. Kadudunkorala[1] and K. Withanarachchi[2]*

*[1]Gampaha Wicramarachchi Ayurveda Institute,*
*University of Kelaniya, Yakkala, Sri Lanka*
*[2]Ayurveda Hospital, Galle, Sri Lanka*
**E-mail: mhati@isplanka.lk*

## ABSTRACT

In Sri Lanka, *Nigella sativa* is called *"kaluduru"* which is included in most of the *Ayurveda* preparations used in cerebro-vascular diseases. The *Allium sativum* is a herb known as *suduloonu.* Sanskrit documents reveal a record that garlic had been in use approximately for the last 5000 years as a medicinal ingredient. Clinical research has revealed that oil of *Nigella sativa* has hypocholesterolemic effect on patients with hyperlipidemia. It is also, reported that when it reduces the LDL, there is a tendency to reduce HDL also which is not expected in the treatment. Garlic has shown significant hyperlipidemic effect with the increasing effect of HDL. Therefore the combination of these two drugs may show the more favourable effect on patients with hypercholesterolemia. The aim of this experiment was to study the effect of the combination of both these drugs on the patients with hyperlipidemia. 43 patients were given capsule with 250mg fresh oil of *Nigella sativa* and 250 mg of *Allium sativam*. Each patient was treated with one capsule two times a day, for a period of 30 days. It was found that the treatment of one month with the drug effectively reduced the serum cholesterol level in most of the patients except in 10 patients out of 43. The data analysis shows a decrease of total cholesterol and low-density lipoproteins when the serum HDL level was increased.

***Keywords:** Nigella sativa, Allium sativum, Hyperlipidemia, Hypocholesterolemic effect, Black seed.*

## 1.0 Introduction

Coronary artery diseases (CAD) have been a global problem since long. It prevails in the high-class society as well as in the lower class society and effect all ages specially the middle age group (Park, 2004). The major cause of CAD is atherosclerosis (Satyavati). With reference to major and minor etiological and pathological factors associated with atherosclerosis, hyperlipidemic states especially hypercholesterolemia have been under consideration on a large scale (Jain, 1976). High level of serum LDL with positive and HDL with negative correlation pertaining to atherosclerosis have been found by many workers (Dubey *et al.*, 1986). Diets containing monounsaturated fatty acids (MUFA) have been reported to decrease serum LDL and may raise the HDL cholesterol as well (Ahmed *et al.*, 1992).

In Sri Lanka, Nigella Sativa is called "*Kaluduru*" which is used in most of the Ayurveda preparations used in cerebro-vascular diseases. The useful part of *kaluduru* is the seed, which contains essential oils, fatty acids, nutrients and moisture. Total oil contains saturated fatty acid 18 per cent MUFA 23.8 per cent and PUFA 58.1 per cent (Le, 2004). The major fatty acids are Myristic (0.5 per cent), Palmitic (13.7 per cent), Palmitoleic (0.1 per cent), Stearic (2.6 per cent), Oleic (23.7 per cent), Linoleic (57.9 per cent), Linolenic (0.2 per cent) and Arachidic (1.3 per cent) acids. The *Allium sativum* is a herb known as *Suduloonu/Garlic*. The useful part is the bulb. Sanskrit documents record that use of garlic remedies approximately 5000 years ago. Garlic is used for hypertension, atherosclerosis and hyperlipidemia (Rotzch *et al.*, 1992; Phelp, 1993; Legnani *et al.*, 1993).

Clinical research has revealed that oil of *Nigella sativa* has hypo-cholesterolemic effect on patients with hyperlipidemia (Tissera *et al.*, 2002). It is also reported that when it reduces the LDL, there is a tendency to reduce HDL also, which is not expected in the treatment (Tissera *et al.*, 2000). Garlic has shown significant hypolipidemic effect with the increasing effect of HDL (Arora *et al.*, 1981; Augusti, 1977). Therefore the combination of these two drugs may show the more favourable effect on patients with hypercholesterolemia.

## 2.0 Materials and Methods

Patients were selected from Ayurveda teaching hospital in Boralla and Ayurveda general hospital in Galle. Their serum cholesterol levels were checked consequently twice in two weeks. The patients whose serum cholesterol levels have been high and stagnant were selected for the trials. Some of them were using allopathic medicine, but they were selected only if they were using those drugs for a period more than one year and still the serum cholesterol levels have not reduced.

The experiment has been done over a 10-month period from February 2005 to January 2006. Before starting the experiment their Serum Lipid levels were checked {Total Cholesterol (TC), Tri Glycerides (TG), Low Density Lipoproteins (LDL) and High Density Lipoproteins (HDL)}. They were strictly advised not to increase or decrease the doses of other medicines, which are been taken by them. They were given the Garlichol Capsules, which contain fresh oil of *Nigella sativa* and fresh juice of *Allium sativum* in therapeutic doses. Each patient was treated with one capsule two times a day after meals with some water, for a period of 30 days.

Proforma was filled for each patient twice a month to see whether there are any side effects or unwanted effects. The serum lipid levels were checked at the end of treatment for one month.

## 3.0 Results and Discussion

Nearly hundred of patients were directed to the clinic and 62 patients were selected for the trial. Only 43 patients remained at the end of the trial and there were 11 males and 32 females. All the patients were between the ages of 40 and 80 years.

**Table 57.1: Number of Patient having Different Cholesterol Levels**

| *Sl.No.* | *Total Cholesterol Level Range (mg/dl)* | *Before Treatment* | *After Treatment* |
|---|---|---|---|
| 1 | 120–160 | 00 | 04 |
| 2 | 160–200 | 00 | 21 |
| 3 | 200–240 | 17 | 04 |
| 4 | 240–280 | 19 | 13 |
| 5 | 280–320 | 07 | 01 |
| | Total | 43 | 43 |

It was found that the treatment of one month with Garlichol reduced the serum cholesterol level in most of the patients except in 10 patients out of 43 although 18 of them had levels above 200. The data analysis shows a decrease of total cholesterol and Low-density lipoproteins. The serum HDL cholesterol level also increased.

**Table 57.2: Mean Values of Lipids, Before and After Treatment**

| *Parameters* | *Before Treatment* | *After Treatment* |
|---|---|---|
| TC (Mg/dl) | 244.16 ± 35.53 | 217.39 ± 41.15 * |
| TG (Mg/dl) | 160.24 ± 54.04 | 156.68 ± 45.56 |
| HDL (Mg/dl) | 49.86 ± 11.88 | 52.70 ± 15.44 |
| LDL (Mg/dl) | 171.2 ± 33.70 | 152.93 ± 39.28 ** |

* *$p<0.001$* as compared to the treatment value.

** $p<0.05$ as compared to the treatment value.

These results suggest that Garlichol has some effect on atherosclerosis due to its hypolipidemic action. Lowering of the Total cholesterol and LDL cholesterol will also reduce their ratio with HDL cholesterol, thus reducing the risk for coronary artery diseases. This could be promising in the prevention and management of hypercholesterolemia. At the end of one month of treatment, Garlichol reduced the triglycerides level in most of the patients but the final mean values did not show a significant difference.

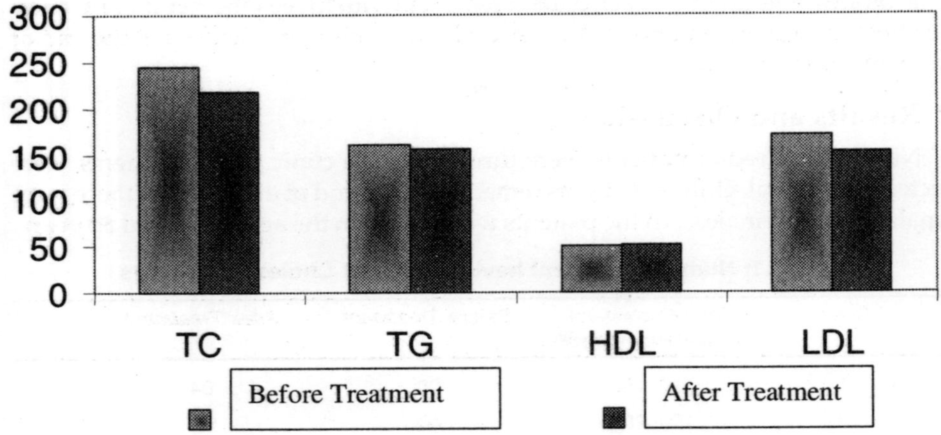


**Figure 57.1: Mean Value of Lipids (mg/dl)**

## 4.0 Conclusion

On the basis of these findings it is concluded that combination of the oil of *Nigella sativa* and garlic shows a hypolipidemic effect in one third of patients who had increased levels of cholesterol. Further investigations are needed to identify the exact effect of the combination of Black Seed and Garlic.

## References

Ahmed, M.M., Jeyalingam, K., Hassan, A.M. and Marinah, T., 1992. Dietary fats and hypercholesterolemia in an experimental model of Macaca Fascilaris. Pak Pathol (3); pp. 5-10.

Arora, R.C., Arora, S. and Gupta, R.K., 1981. The long-term use of garlic in ischemic heart disease–an appraisal. Atherosclerosis (40); pp. 175-179.

Augusti, K.T., 1977. Hypocholesterolaemic effect of garlic Allium sativum lin. Ind J Exp Biol (15); pp. 489-490.

Dubey *et al.*, 1986. Prevention and Management of Coronary Heart Disease by an Indigenous Compound Abana. Alternative Medicine (Zurich, Switzerland) (3); pp. 241.

Jain, R.C., 1976. Onion and garlic in experimental cholesterol induced atherosclerosis. Ind J Med Res (64); pp.1509–1515.

Lata, S., Saxena, K.K., Bhasin, V., Saxena, R.S., Kumar, A. and Srivastava, V.K., 1991. Beneficial effects of *Allium sativum*, *Allium cepa* and *Commiphora mukul* on experimental hyperlipidemia and atheroscierosis–a comparative evaluation. J Postgrad Med (37); pp. 132-5.

Le, P.M., Benhaddou-Andaloussi, A., Settaf, A., Cherrah, Y. and Haddad, P.S., 2004. The petroleum ether extract of *Nigella sativa* exerts lipid-powering action in rats. J Ethanopharmacol (94(2-3)); pp. 251-9.

Legnani *et al.*, 1993. Effects of dried garlic preparation on fibrinolysis and platelet aggregation in healthy subjects. Arzneim Forsch (43); pp.119-21.

Park, K., 2004. Parks textbook of preventive and social medicine. Jabalpur India: Banarasi Das Bhanot (24); pp.272–73.

Phelp, S and Harris, W.S., 1993. Garlic supplementation and lipoprotein oxidation susceptibility. Lipids (28); pp. 475-7.

Rotzch *et al.*, 1992. Postprandial lipaemia under treatment with *Allium sativum,* Controlled double blind study in healthy volunteers with reduced HDL–cholesterol levels. Arzneim Forsch (42); pp.1223-7.

Satyavati, G.V.. Effect of an indigenous drug on disorders of lipid metabolism with special reference to atherosclerosis and obesity (medoroga). Thesis submitted for the degree of Doctor of Ayurvedic Medicine. Banaras Hindu University.

Tissera, Serasinghe, P., Karunanayake, K.S., 2000. "Study on the effect of Baraka oil on the level of serum cholesterol in human blood". Abstract of International seminar on Ayurveda G.A.U. Jamnagar, India. January; pp. 23.

Tissera. *et al.*, 2002. Study the Biological Activity of the oil of *Nigella sativa*. Abstract book, 3rd International seminar on Ayurveda, February, G.A.U. Jamnagar, India; pp. 23.

*Chapter 58*

# The Brief History and Development of Traditional Medical Science in Mongolia

**A. Altantsetseg* and Ch. Chimedragchaa**
*Traditional Medical Science,*
*Technology and Production Corporation of Mongolia, Mongolia*
**E-mail: tradmedcorp@unet.mn, altai03mn@yahoo.com*

## ABSTARCT

This paper gives a brief account of the history and development of traditional medicine in Mongolia. It points out that the first modern scientific research on medicinal plants and traditional medicine began in 1959. This included the first Pharmacological Investigative Facility in Mongolia. From there onwards, it traces the evolution of the Traditional Medical Science, Technology and Production Corporation of Mongolia (TMSTPCM) as the leading national research centre and a base for future development of traditional medicine with activities including scientific research, treatment of patients, and production of medicine. It finally highlights the achievements of traditional medicine and describes the efforts being carried for education, training and research to work in unison with the modern medicine in Mongolia.

***Keywords:*** *Traditional medicine, Folk medicine, Education and training, Research and development, Modern medicine, Mongolia.*

## 1.0 Introduction

Mongolia is situated in the heart of Central Asian Plateau, between 88-120 degrees east longitude and 42-50 degrees north latitude with an area of 1,564,116 sq km. It is the 19[th] largest and least densely populated independent country in the world with a population of around 2.9 million people. Approximately 30 per cent of the country's population is nomadic or semi-nomadic.

Mongolian Traditional medicine is one of the most valuable cultural heritages of the Mongolian people and reflects their nomadic lifestyle. It dates back to more than 2500 years. However, the history of traditional Mongolian medicine arts and its achievements were known only among the Asians and were forgotten for many decades during the 20th century. Folk medicine was the main tool of health care for nomadic Mongolians and was widely practiced for thousands of years under the name of "Black Heal" (Mendsaikhan Z, 2007). Until 10-12$^{th}$ century, the folk medicine was based on mysterious perception of health and illness. It used spring water, mud, diet treatment, bloodletting as well as "Baria zasal–point massage" extensively for various ailments. During the reign of Changez Khan (1154–1226), application of hot metal on wounds was also used. Due to climate, cold diseases were very common in Mongolia and to treat these Moxa (moxibustion) therapy was practiced widely.

Although, the Mongolian people adopted and developed their traditional medicine based on the fundamentals of Ayurvedic and Tibetan medicines, it has also preserved its own distinct art of medicine. Accordingly, the Mongolian and the Tibetan medicines have almost the same theory, diagnostic methods and treatments. The basic theory of Mongolian traditional medicine is the theory of five elements, three essences (khii–wind; shar-bile; badgan-plegm), the theory of five zang organs (heart, liver, kidney, lungs, and spleen) and six fu organs (gallbladder, urinary bladder, large intestine, small intestine, stomach and pericardia) and the theory of white and black vessels. It is believed that all kinds of physical, mental and psychological disorders and ailments can be cured through the use of herbs, mineral water, plants and animal parts (Khaidav, Ts., 1977; B., Bold, 1999; Tumurbaatar, N., 2006).

However, with the political and economic changes in the Twentieth Century, the Mongolian traditional practitioners were prohibited and thus traditional medicine was almost extinguished. Government policies snubbed the traditional medicine practice and during some periods even prohibited its practice and training outright. The Communist government destroyed almost all the Buddhist culture including the records and literature of traditional medicine. From the 1930's until the restoration of democracy in 1990, practitioners barely maintained traditional medical arts and the doctors were forced to go underground.

## 2.0 Development Stages

Mongolian traditional medicine can be divided into the following stages (Lkagvasuren, T.S., *et al.*, 2006; Tumurbaatar, N., *et al.*, 2007):

- Folk medicine (BC IV-AD XIII)
- The Creation of Mongolian Traditional Medicine (AD XIII-AD XVI)
- Flourishing stage of Mongolian Traditional Medicine (AD XVI-1937)
- Stagnant period of Mongolian Traditional Medicine (1937-1989)
- Renaissance of Mongolian Traditional Medicine (since 1989 to present)

In the second half of the sixteenth century, Buddhism affected the whole social life of Mongolia. During the mid 16th century and thereafter when Buddhism flourished throughout the country, Mongolian medicine was replaced by Indo-Tibetan traditional medicine. With it, many medical books were imported from India and Tibet. During the 16th-20th centuries, after the advent of Buddhist culture, traditional systems of Indo-Tibetan medicine became deeply rooted in Mongolia. Medical educational centres called 'Manba Datsan' were established, not only in Mongolia, but also in Inner Mongolia and propagated health education from one generation to another (Boldsaihan, B., 2004; Bold, Sh., 1999; and Ligaa, U., 2005). Yet, over time, scholars and doctors developed a unique style of traditional medicine peculiar for Mongolia's natural bounty, flora and fauna, unique climate, and specific culture and lifestyle of the nomadic people. Thus the Mongolian traditional medicine has two major features: One, it is based on empirical experience of the population to fight against the diseases for hundreds of years; and Second, it is also based on theoretical fundamentals, experiences and methods of the ancient Eastern traditional medicine.

Further, the Mongolian traditional medicine was also based on the creative absorption of the theory and practice of medicine as one of the five pillars of Buddhism. The medicines were prepared according to one's metabolism, the weather and the season. Discovery of medicinal materials in ancient times was closely related to the life, activity, and the natural living conditions of the people and observation of their flora and fauna during the changing season. Legends and folklore had a strong impact on preserving information for the treatment of diseases. In order to ease from sufferings of the diseases, the ancient Mongolians instinctively used sharp-edged stones and heat, used readily accessible resources available in their natural surroundings to relieve the aching parts of the body. The life style of that period was martial and people in the process of household work, taking care of animals, hunting and battle, usually received different types of injuries and wounds, and while treating these by themselves, discovered minor surgery and fracture treatment methods. Along with the use of drugs from plant remedies, special treatment methods were also used to treat war wounds, to stop bleeding, and split fractures. Mongolians have been importing medicinal plants from the neighbouring countries from the ancient times. Many historical documents also confirm about Mongol's vast experience of identifying natural resources of grass and plant species for livestock, and for making potential use of these products in medicine. In this way, Mongolians have used different kinds of herbs to cure and prevent human and animal ailments. Treating concussion of brain, bloodletting therapy, moxibustion application are the few examples of Mongol's independent distinct art of medicine.

After the 12th century when Buddhism spread over the country, many classical works of India and Tibet were introduced, and the theory of five elements and three essences (Hii, Shar, Badgan) was accepted. Some raw materials began to be imported from China, Tibet and India. In the process a large number of lama doctors skilled in traditional medicine, as well as healers educated in the five medical arts (bloodletting, moxibustion, hydrotherapy, massage and acupuncture) were trained. In the beginning of the 20th century, there were more than 700 monasteries where thousands of lamas and monks were engaged in study of all branches of knowledge including medicine.

About 100 medical schools were established. During the period many medical schools of traditional medicine were built near the monasteries and the traditional medical art was taught and practiced over a long period of time. Well-known physicians and scholars, who were born during this period, profoundly studied Indo-Tibetan medicine and developed traditional medicine enriching it with own unique medical practice. Many medical treatises were translated from Tibetan and published into Mongolian. Many schools were constructed and conducted training courses for Maramba-traditional doctors all over the country.

After the victory of people's revolution in 1921, the western medicine started replacing traditional medicine. However, the doctors trained in Western Medicine were also allowed to work side by side with traditional doctors. From the 1930s, while encouraging and supporting Western style medicine in each possible way, the Mongolian government, by radically rejecting and suppressing traditional medicine, caused this precious wealth of tradition to be forgotten for over 30 years. Later, it was only in 1950s that systematic study of traditionally used plants, animal and mineral medicinal substances began and included areas such as stockpiling and dissemination of medicinal plants, the comparison of Mongolian, Tibetan, and Latin names, the botanical traits and specific nature of traditional compounds, their chemical composition, structure, and medical applications and effects (Khaidav, T.S., 1962, 1978, 1985).

Mongolians have thus been using traditional herbs remedies for preventive and curative purpose since the ancient times. Each region is a source of unique natural product and herbal remedies used in the traditional medicine. According to the survey conducted by researchers of Institute of Botany, and Complex Biological Expedition of Mongolia, there are around 800 species of medicinal plants that have a great significance today in both scientific and traditional medicine (Ligaa, U., 1996, 2005; Boldsaihan, B., 2004). These natural resources are basic conditions for experiments in healing, eventually leading to a core of empirical knowledge. Our ancestors were able to discover treatments for illness, which grew out of their lifestyle, and introduced it to the world at that time. Traditional medicine was first established without any kind of scientific background. In ancient Mongolia people were simply developing treatments through trial and error.

## 3.0 Traditional Medicine and Scientific Research

The first modern scientific research on medicinal plants and traditional medicine began in 1959 under the initiative of Academician Ts. Khaidav, founder of the first Pharmacological Investigative Facility in Mongolia. He has been a leading scholar and researcher in the field of traditional medicine. The founding of the first scientific laboratory of traditional medicine was the most important step for research and education in this field. Commencing in 1959, the government revived the research and investigation of astrology and traditional Mongolian medicine. Systematic scientific studies began, especially the preparation of plant catalogues used in folk medicine. Since traditional medicine began to flourish again, medicines produced from indigenous raw plant materials were discovered, and the first works of investigations and pharmaceutical production were published. One important work was Khaidav's monograph "Some Historical Features of Oriental and Medicinal plants used in Mongolian Folk Medicine" (1965). The historical survey discussed selected medicinal plants and their traditional uses. It clearly resulted in the revised interest in developing traditional medical studies and became an important field of research. (Munkh-Amgalan, Yu., *et al.*, 2002).

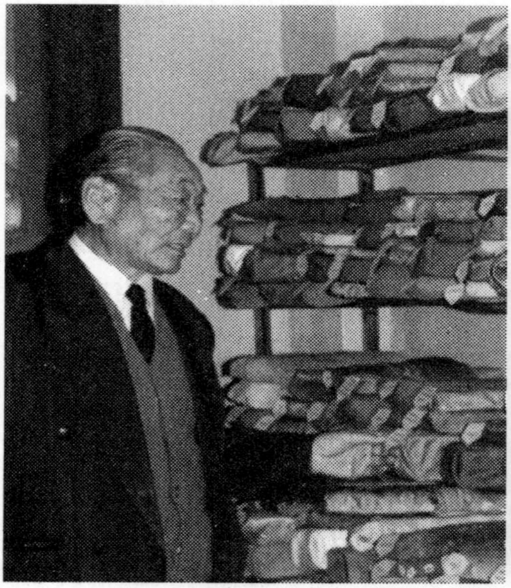

**Academician Ts. Khaidav**

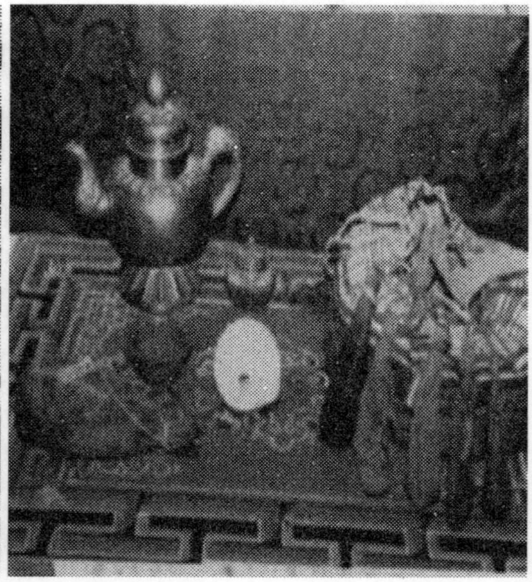

**Doctor's Instruments and Sack for Medicine**

Khaidav's work became the foundation for the present research centre of Mongolian Traditional medicine. Khaidav aimed that the facility would study the history and heritage of Eastern medicine; and safeguard and maintain original documentary evidence, rare books and other papers and artworks; and compile notes and interviews from old and experienced physicians and scholars to be passed on to the future generations. The mission of this Centre was to study the history, heritage and original documentation of Eastern medicine, collect rare books and documentations along with meetings with old experienced physicians and scholars to learn from them. Over the years, the research facility has gone through several changes in the name. In 1973 under the supervision of the Academy of Sciences, it was reorganized as the Institute of Natural Compounds. A decade later in 1981 the Institute was restructured and named as the Institute of Traditional Medicine under the Ministry of Health. The main responsibility of the Institute of Traditional Medicine was to provide pharmacological and clinical studies, to create new medications, to train young researchers and establish new research laboratories, which became the base of the new development of Traditional Medical science in Mongolia. Finally this organization expanded and evolved into the Traditional Medical Science, Technology and Production Corporation of Mongolia (TMSTPCM) as the leading national research center and a base for future development of traditional medicine with activities including scientific research, treatment of patients, and production of medicine (TMSTPCM introduction book, 2005).

### 3.1 TMSTPCM Mission

The main tasks of TMSTPCM are:

- Study ancient traditional system of medicine in all aspects on scientific basis..
- Investigate the effectiveness of combining diagnosis, treatment, and prevention principles of traditional medicine with the modern methods of treatment thereby upgrading the quality of medical services and treatment,
- Improve standardization and technology of the traditional drugs and produce effective drugs and remedies from natural sources and put into medical practice.
- Carry out the tasks assigned by the government through scientific projects, involving current traditional medicine issues and,
- Supply consultative services for medical students and doctors by organizing training courses and consultations on traditional medicine.
- Put into medical practice the results of the research in the form of new medicine, methodology, standardization, technology, brochures and instructions.
- Develop directives on traditional medicine at the government policy level.
- Control and act as the professional representative for practitioners of traditional medicine and guide the State and the private medical institutions, producing traditional drugs, for proper techniques for patient treatment,
- Provide expertise across a range of issues, including export, import of medicinal raw materials and other related matters on behalf of the government.
- Carry out field expeditions to determine the resource of medicinal herbs, define the specificity of reproduction and utilization of the natural medicinal plants.
- Work out the technology for some rare plants for cultivation.

The structure and organization of the TMSTPCM is as under:

- The Research Center
- Traditional medical education and training
- Traditional Medical Polyclinic Department
- Traditional Medical Drug Factory

### 3.2 The Research Centre

The Research Center conducts research on Mongolian medicinal plants to identify the ingredients of centuries-old remedies and help to develop new health products.

TMSTPCM has promoted some important investigations which had not been previously possible. Consequently, it has revealed more than 60 new natural substances; introduced more than 30 preparations based on plant, animal, and mineral products; isolated about 50 methods and methodologies on diagnosis and treatment, and standardized 130 products; and provided more than 160 technical conditions, technological instructions and 28 patents. Moreover, TMSTPCM members have published 30 books on traditional medicine and related subjects. In the past 40 years, have published 600 scientific articles and presented about 700 papers and reports to various seminars and symposia at national and international level. The TMSTPCM journal "Tejeehui uhaan" is published yearly with full review of the works executed on science subjects.

Various Departments under the Research Centre are:

**Theory Department**

This division deals with theoretical issues in traditional medicine. Its mission is to gather information from old literature and study fundamental principles of traditional medicine and research into the effectiveness of combining diagnosis, treatment and prevention principles of traditional medicine with the modern treatment methods.

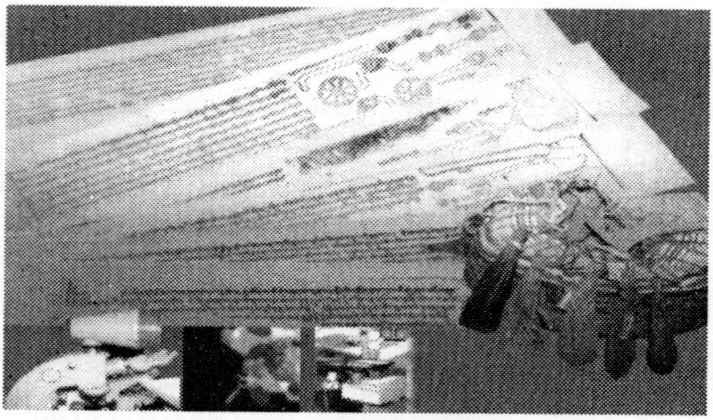

**Ancient Books**

**Pharmacology Department**

This division studies the pharmacological mechanisms of the drugs and undertakes pharmacological researches on plant, animal and mineral origin by biomedical methods to produce new preparations and introduce them into medical practice.

**Department of Phyto-chemistry**

The activities include:

- Carry out phyto-chemical tests of the compounds, extract biologically active substances, determine the structure and work out standardization and technology,
- Work out standardization principle of multi and few component recipe drugs of traditional medicine.

## Achievements

The researchers of this organization, on the theory and methodology of traditional and modern medicine, have suggested two new scientific hypotheses: One, that of relation of khii shar, badkhan-membrane structure of organisms; and Second, the theoretical principle of traditional composition method of mono and multi component drugs (Ambaga, M, 1999, 2006; Dagvatseren, B. 1996, 2006). The Centre has invented many new technologies, produced new medicaments, updated methods of medical practice and made a comparative analysis between traditional medicine and conventional medicine.

The TMSTPCM has been actively engaged in several important scientific projects:

- "Mongolian medicine", "Othoch", "Khuder" or Musk–deer (1991-1993),
- "Mongolian Traditional medicine–1 (1994-1996)
- "Mongolian-Tibetan Traditional medicine database', a project sponsored by Canadian International Research Development Center (1995-1998)
- "Traditional Drug–Medicine–3", "Mongolian Astragal", "Musk–deer and musk",
- Study on Mongolian drug used against aging" (1997-1999)
- Innovative methods of treatment, prophylactic and diagnosis of traditional medicine and new medicine (2000-2002)
- Theoretical and practical problems of traditional medicine (2003-2005)

We have put into medical practice more than 200 scientific achievements on the basis of scientific projects.

### 3.2.1 Exploration and Cultivation of Medicinal Plants

One of the vital elements in the development of traditional Mongolian medicine, initiated by our colleagues is the domestication of animals and cultivation of very rare plants used in traditional medicine. Consequently, in order to cultivate rare medicinal plants and accelerate research and development activities, the TMSTPCM established a Plantation facility in Bulgan aimag in 1991.This Plantation has been undertaking cultivation, collection and utilization of rare medicinal plants that would accelerate traditional medicine and development of research activities.

Most of the important medicinal plants are continuously being threatened under the danger from anthropogenic actions and many of the species that are used as raw materials for drug production are limited in resource. Further, the rare species are vanishing due to desertification, frequent drought, fires and hay mowing, timber cutting, logging, harvesting for medicinal and food use, and grazing of animals. In view of this it has become necessary to take steps and find ways for domestication and cultivation of some kinds of medicinal plants in order to provide raw materials for already existing factories. Therefore, the problem of restoration of medicinal plants in the nature and in artificial ways has become crucial not only for Mongolia but also worldwide. According to the appendix of Law on Natural Plants (1995), there are 88 registered very rare species of medicinal plants, which is 66.2 per cent of the common and very rare plant species in Mongolia.

The scientific investigations on the study of ecological and biological characteristics of regeneration of wild growing medicinal plants and study of the habitat of their natural conditions show that, these can be cultivated in artificial man-made conditions and successfully regenerated without loosing their medicinal value.

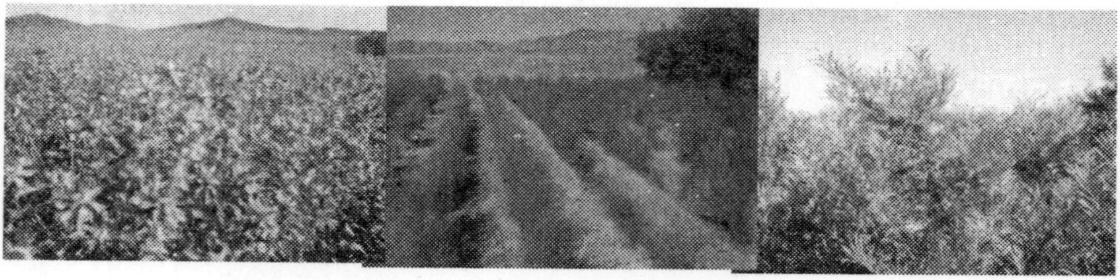

**Medicinal Plants Cultivated in Plantation Centre**

Here more than 20 species of rare and imported medicinal plants such as Inula *Helenium* L, *Asparagus officinalis, Silybum marianum* L., *Fritellera palladiflora* L.,*Glicine max* L.,*Syringa wolfii* Schneid., *Coriandrum sativum* L.,*Cassia tora* L., *Carthamus tinctorios.*, Lycium *chinence* L, etc. and acclimatized and cultivated rare and medicinal plants such as *Mentha longifolia* L., *Eleaegnus angustifolia* Bunge.,*Calendula officinalis* L., *Glycyrrhiza uraensis* Fisch., *Hyppophae rhamnoides* L.,*Sophora alopecuroides* L., *Artemisia sphaerocephala* Krasch. and *Polygonatum odoratum* L have been planted. Our scientists are working to study and implement agricultural technology for acclimatizing plants to different soil, water and climatic conditions, for extracting and preserving their active biochemical components, and for planting and raising them as well.

### 3.2.2 Musk Deer Breeding Sector

This division studies the biological aspects of the Musk deer and determines the research and experimentation of musk, which was widely used in traditional medicine. Accordingly, methods for breeding, raising and domesticating rare animals, such as musk deer in captivity, and removing musk from them without causing any

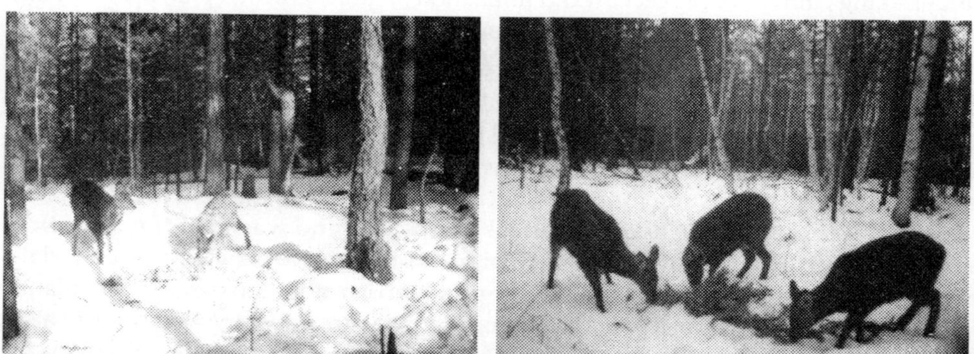

**Musk Deer**

harm to the deer, are being improved. Male musk deer produces musk, which is about 25 g per year by weight. The main component of musk is muscone and its chemical structure is L-3 methylcyclophentadecanon.

The Musk-deer breeding operation is located at Gachuurth, just outside Ulaanbaatar city.

### 3.3 Drug Factory

The Traditional Medicine Drug Factory conducts research and production of new medicaments from traditional recipes.

In Mongolia the method of preparing prescriptions of herbal drugs is carried in old traditional way, but the researchers are also conducting studies in scientific ways for producing medicaments based upon the knowledge and methods of traditional medicine. To date, the facility has screened and produced more than fifty kinds of traditional medicaments of plant, animal or mineral origin for the domestic medical practice. Further, it manufactures more than 160 types of traditional drugs in pill, syrup, and powder forms and provides throughout Mongolia. Some medicines are also exported to Poland and Russia. The TMSTPCM pharmaceutical production is also assessing the possibilities to market its herbal products to the West.

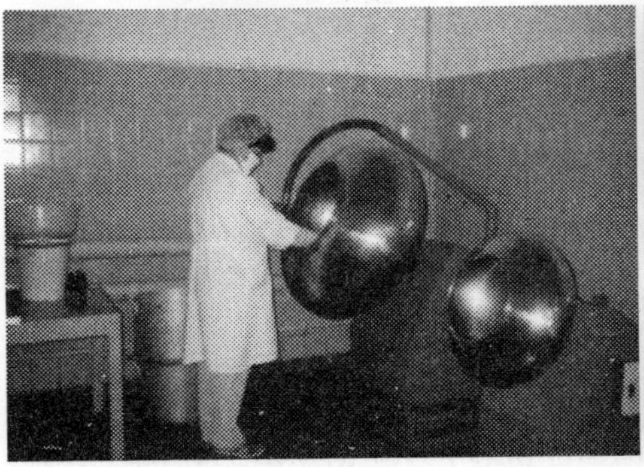

**In the Drug Factory**

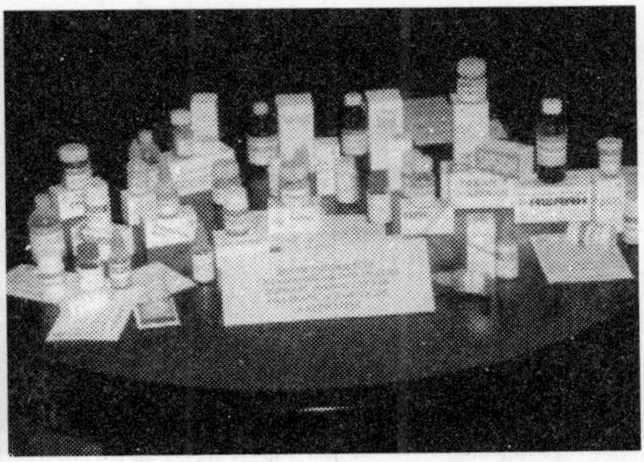

**New Medicines Developed in the Pharmacological Laboratory**

### 3.4 The Traditional Medical Hospital

The Hospital boosts an 85-90 per cent healing rate, administers 50,000 outpatients and 4,500 in-patients in the Polyclinic. It offers cardio-vascular, gynecological, and neurological therapies, physical therapy, spring water and balneotherapy, X-ray screening and ultra-sonography service. Additionally, our modern facilities are equipped with clinical and biochemical laboratories.

Mongolian traditional medicine has its own unique integrated theoretical system considering the body as a whole entity containing within itself eternal contradiction and, at the same time, unity. The main diagnostic methods used by doctors rely upon the three fundamentals, which are observation, interviewing the patient and pulse feeling. In addition, checking of urine, examining eyes and tongue, as well as palpation, auscultation and olfaction is also carried. They also use modern medical laboratory and diagnostic methods. After observing a patient, the doctor will formulate a synthetic analysis based on information gained from these examinations, determine the disease and make an ultimate diagnosis. The doctor then develops a principle for treatment and prescribes appropriate medication. These treatments are supported by different oriental medical methods and therapies such as herbal drugs, decoctions, acupuncture (general electro-acupuncture, fluid needling, hot needling, gold and silver needling), moxibustion, traditional massage techniques Baria Zasal (soft massage, hot oil, broth, milk, spring water massage, massage of the different parts of body), mud therapy (balneotherapy), spring water therapies, bloodletting-venesection, cupping, bone setting and medicated bathing etc.

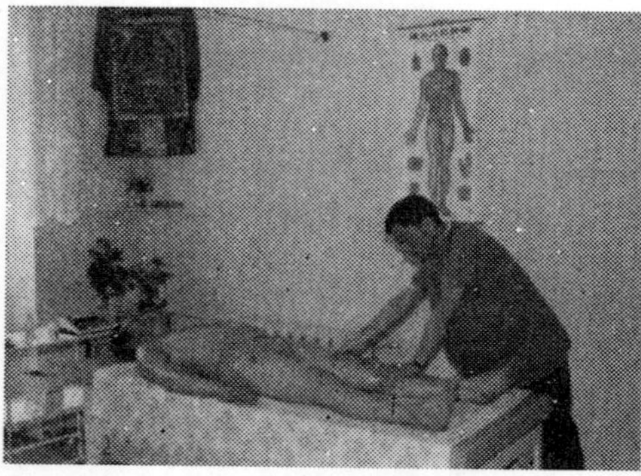

**Massage**

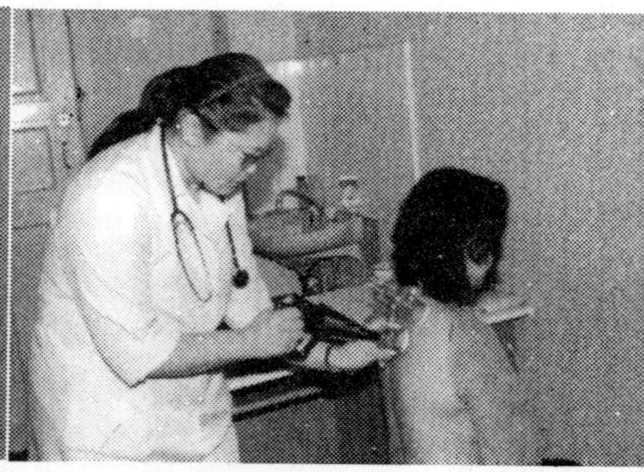

**Cupping**

**Traditional Methods of Treatment**

Moxibustion is considered a traditionally Mongolian method of treatment. It is well suited to our cold conditions, changing weather and to nomadic living. Due to this "cold disease" is widespread in Mongolia and moxa therapy is used very commonly. Mongolians also call it "heat therapy". Moxibustion method means the burning of an herb above the surface of the skin to warm the active points. It is often used in conjunction with acupuncture or other treatments. Mongolian traditional skills like brain re-adjustment used to treat cerebral concussion, the bone-adjustment for fractures and dislocation, and medicated bathing for curing certain skin and rheumatic conditions, are also very effective.

Mongolian art of bone setting, called "Bone art" in Mongolia, is a fascinating subject. It developed mainly during the Qin dynasty. Bonesetters used many interesting methods such as applying cupping glasses to treat broken bones, or an herbal compress, and if necessary, used surgery with the aid of ice as a local anesthetic. Bone art is a completely independent branch of the Mongolian medicine. Bone-manipulators would simply hold the fractured or dislocated limb in their hands and give it the twist. The bones would heal quite soon afterwards. Such healers usually came from a family of traditional bonesetters.

Cupping is the practice of putting a cup on the surface of a patient's skin, thus drawing their flesh up into the cup. This practice is used to treat anything from backaches to kidney problems. Both conventional and traditional medicine practitioners practice it in order to increase blood circulation. Along with massage it is the most common treatment of Mongolia.

## 3.5 Education and Training

A department of traditional medicine was the first to be set up at the National Medical University of Mongolia in 1990. For the graduates, the curriculum is of five years, which includes two years of modern medicine and biological sciences, and three years of traditional medicine. There is no restriction today for modern doctors to practice traditional medicine. Since 1990, training courses on traditional medicine of 3 to 6 months are offered for modern doctors by the Institute of Traditional medicine in cooperation with the Union of Mongolian Traditional Medicine and the Medical University (Tumurbaatar, N., *et al.*, 2006). Till now, about 400 doctors have obtained qualification. Training courses on acupuncture was started in 1970. Intensive studies on diagnosis and treatment principles of folk medicine were made in a short period (Khaidav Ts., 1988, 1998; Boldsaikhan, B., *et al.*, 1990; Ambaga, M., *et al.*, 1999; Dagvatseren, B., 1996, 2006; Bold, Sh., 1999, 2002). There were no clinical facilities engaged in traditional medicine until 1989. Thereafter, the government opened a department of traditional medicine in each of the provinces and at present, all hospitals of 21 aimags (administrative units), territories and secondary hospitals of UB and its districts have traditional medicine departments. Around 160 private traditional medicine clinics are operating in Mongolia (Bold, Sh., 1999). Today, 3 government and 3 private pharmacology factories are manufacturing more than 5 tonnes of 270 kinds of traditional medicine drugs under the quality control of State Inspection department. Each herbal medicine has 2-30 compounds in it and they use 200 kinds of plants, which are grown in Mongolia and 100 kinds of plants are imported from other countries (Mendsaikhan, Z, 2007).

Mongolian researchers have published the biological, geo-botanical, pharmacological effects of more than 800 plants, which grow in Mongolia and the proper way to use them in the oriental treatment (Khaidav, Ts., 1962, 1978, 1985; Ligaa, U., 1996, 2005; Boldsaihkhan, B., *et al.*, 1990, 2004). Lately, modern doctors also use traditional medicine for diagnosis and medical treatment very widely.

Nowadays, Mongolian government is paying much attention on tradition, culture and scientific heritage of the country. In the early Twenty-first century, TMSTPCM has ensured that traditional medicine is a well-developed aspect of Mongolian culture, and that Mongolia will maintain this knowledge legacy despite the fact that the communist regime had prohibited the practice of the traditional medical arts for several decades in the prior century.

At present, traditional medicine is fully appreciated in the society, and supplied along with developed modern medical service. In 1999, Mongolia's Parliament took positive steps to create a legal environment for the future development of traditional medicine and issued its national policy on Traditional Medicine in the "State policy for Development of Mongolian Traditional medicine". The basic strategy is to focus on staff training, standardization of the training curriculum, improving research and applying it to medical practice, translating ancient medical literature from old Mongolian and Tibetan scripts, and expanding the manufacturing base of herbal remedies. The national expert committee was established in 1991, called as the Professional Committee for Traditional Medicine. Regulations on herbal medicines were issued in 1998 and 2001. The laws are the same for herbal medicines as for the conventional pharmaceuticals. Thus herbal medicines in Mongolia belong to the over-the-counter medicines and can be sold without restriction (Health Minister's order No 169 of 2001). By law, herbal medicines may be sold with medical health and nutrient claims. National herbal monographs are found in the Manual of Traditional Medicine Raw materials and Prescriptions Control (2003). The regulatory requirements for herbal medicine manufacture are the same GMP rules that apply to conventional pharmaceuticals. Implementation of the requirements is ensured by the State Professional Inspection Agency, which inspects manufacturing processes. There are 22 registered herbal medicines in Mongolia; however none is included on the essential drug list.

### 3.6 International Cooperation

Traditional Mongolian medicine has attracted the attention of doctors and researchers at home and abroad. Confidence in traditional treatments is increasing every year and traditional medical hospitals are becoming more and more popular worldwide. In consequence, at the international level, the World Health Organization's National Center of Traditional Medicine for Asia recognized TMSTPCM as a contributor to the discipline. TMSTPCM has been a member of the International Association of Asian traditional medicine since 1994. Business cooperation has been established with similar research organizations in Russia, China, Japan, Poland, Germany, Greece, Vietnam, India and Korea. The Corporation had organized an international symposium on: The Second International Symposium on Chemistry of Herbal Medicine and Mongolian drug in 2006 in Ulaanbaatar.

## References

Ambaga, M., Sarantsetseg, B., Bold Sh, 1999. The membrane mechanism and some theoretical problems of traditional medicine. Ulaanbaatar; pp. 76.

Ambaga, M., 2006. The scientific-methodological basis for creating an integrated system of oriental traditional and modern medicine, basing on a new definition about cells, The Second International Symposium on Chemistry of Herbal Medicine and Mongolian drug, Ulaanbaatar; pp.56-57.

Ayur Vijnana a periodical on Indo-Tibetan an allied medical cultures, 2002. Vol.8, India. http://www.ittm.org/publications/Ayurvijnana

Bold, Sh., 1999. Traditional medicine in Mongolia. Workshop on development of national policy of TRM. Beijing, China; pp. 34-40.

Bold, Sh., Ambaga M., 2002. The history and fundamentals of Mongolian Traditional Medicine, UB; pp. 1-120.

Boldsaihan, B., Baavgai, Ch., 1990. Mongolian Traditional medicine. UB.; pp. 384.

Boldsaihan, B., 2004. Encyclopedia of Mongolian medicinal plants. UB; pp. 1-160.

Dagvatseren, B., 1996. Practical and methodological foundation of Mongolian and Tibetan medicine. UB; pp. 170.

Dagvatseren, B., 2006. Theory and methodology of integrative medicine and traditional drugs. Abstracts. The second international symposium on chemistry of herbal medicine and Mongolian drug. Ulaanbaatar; pp. 15-16.

Khaidav, Ts., 1962. Medicinal Plants of Mongolia. UB; pp.89.

Khaidav, Ts., 1977. Animal originated medicine in Mongolian Traditional Medicine. UB; pp.156.

Khaidav, Ts., Menshikova, A., 1978. Medicianal plants in Mongolian traditional medicine UB; pp. 189.

Khaidav, Ts, Altanchimeg, B., Varlamova., T.S, 1985. Medicinal plants in Mongolian medicine, UB; pp.390.

Khaidav, Ts., 1988. The tradition of Folk medicine and its scientific basis. Ulaanbaatar; pp. 1-75.

Khaidav, Ts., 1998. The origin of Mongolian medicine and main stages of its development. Ulaanbaatar; pp. 1-48.

Legal Status of Traditional Medicine and Complementary medicine, a worldwide review, WHO., 2001 Geneva.

Ligaa, U., 1996. Medicinal plants of Mongolia used in Mongolian traditional medicine; pp. 416.

Ligaa, U., Davaasuren, B., Ninjil, N, 2005. Mongolian medicinal plant's uses in Eastern and Western medicine. UB; pp. 654.

Lkhagvasuren, Ts., Tumurbaatar, N., Oldokh S., 2006. History and national policy of Mongolian traditional medicine. The second International Conference on Traditional Medicine: Current situation and future status. Abstract book. Ulaanbaatar; pp. 12-14.

Mendsaikhan. Z., 2007. Current situation of traditional medicine in Mongolia. Book of abstracts. International workshop on Herbal Medicinal Plants and Traditional Herb Remedies. Hanoi, Vietnam; pp. 32-34.

Munkh-Amgalan, Yu., Tsend-Auysh, G., Ts., Khaidav, 2002. Innovator of traditional Mongolian Medicine. AyurVijnana (8).

http://www.ittm.org/publications/Ayurvijnana

Tumurbaatar, N., 2006. The basic understanding of Traditional Medicine. Ulaanbaatar; pp. 1-348.

Tumurbaatar, N., Tsend-Ayush, D, Tserendagva, D, Enkhjargal, N., 2006. Education and training of Mongolian traditional medicine. The 2nd International Conference on "Traditional Medicine: Current situation and future status. UB.; pp. 15.

Tumurbaatar, N., Ganbayar, Ya, 2007. The historical review of mongolian traditional medicine. 8th international conference on prophylactic and rehabilitation medicine. Èðêóòñê, Russia; pp.160-162.

Traditional Medical Science Technology and Production Corporation of Mongolia, Introduction book, 2005. Ulaanbaatar; pp. 1-10.